JEWS, MEDICINE,
AND MEDIEVAL SOCIETY

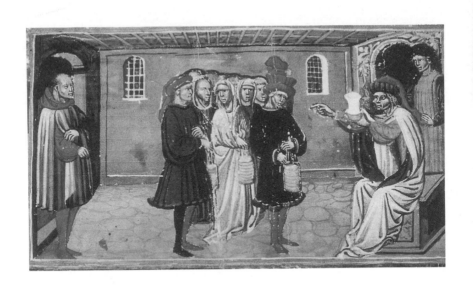

JEWS, MEDICINE, AND MEDIEVAL SOCIETY

Joseph Shatzmiller

UNIVERSITY OF CALIFORNIA PRESS
Berkeley   Los Angeles   London

University of California Press
Berkeley and Los Angeles, California

University of California Press
London, England

Copyright © 1994 by
The Regents of the University of California

Library of Congress Cataloging-in-Publication Data

Shatzmiller, Joseph.
  Jews, medicine, and medieval society/Joseph Shatzmiller.
    p.   cm.
  Includes bibliographical references and index.
  ISBN 0-520-08059-9 (acid-free paper)
    1. Physicians, Jewish.   2. Medicine, Medieval.   I. Title.
  R694.S52   1994
  610.69'52'08992404—dc20
                                                        93-2810
                                                          CIP

Printed in the United States of America

2 3 4 5 6 7 8 9

Contents

Preface vii

Introduction ix

1 **Jews and the Medicalization of Society in the Middle Ages** 1

The Medicalization of Society, 1250–1450:
   The Growing Need for Doctors 2
Church Opposition to the Clerical Practice of
   Medicine 8
The Opening: The Entry of Jews into the
   Profession 10

2 **The Making of the Jewish Doctor** 14

Supervision of the Medical Profession and
   Licensing Procedures 14
Private Medical Education: The Masters and the
   Students 22
Jewish Students in the Faculties of Medicine 27

3 **The Hebrew Medical Library** 36

Required Bibliography: Examinations 36
Hebrew: The Language of Medical
   Instruction 38
The Economics of Translation 42
Building the Hebrew Medical Library:
   Strategy and Timing 48

4   Reputation: Brilliant Medical Careers   56

Doctors in Princely Courts   57
A Successful Medical Dynasty:
    The Abenardut   60
Luminaries: Jewish Doctors of International
    Repute   64
Royal Favors Bestowed on Doctors   70

**5   Rejection: Apprehensions about Jewish
Doctors   78**

Failures, Accidents, Incompetence   78
Suspicions   85
Ecclesiastical and Secular Legislation against
    Jewish Doctors   90
The Ineffectiveness of Legislation   93

**6   Jewish Doctors in the Medieval City:
Numbers and Status   100**

Doctors as Part of the Social Scenery: Literary
    Evidence   100
The Number of Jewish and Non-Jewish
    Doctors   104
Women in the Medical Profession   108
Doctors Hired by Municipalities   112

**7   Private Practice: Doctors and Patients in
Daily Encounters   119**

Was There a "Mystique" about Jewish
    Doctors?   120
Jewish Patients and Christian Doctors   121
Patients, Doctors, and the Rule of the Law   124
Master Bonafos: Surgeon in Manosque before
    1348   131
Other Economic Activities   135

Conclusion   140

Notes   143
Select Bibliography   211
Index   235

Preface

Maimonides: Whenever I have talked about my wish to write about Jewish doctors in the Middle Ages the name of this most illustrious man has immediately arisen. Little wonder, since Moshe ben Maimon (1135–1204) is one of the best-known personalities in the history of the Jews. He was a rabbinic scholar; he was a powerful philosopher; he was a community leader. He was also a doctor, a successful practitioner, and a prolific medical writer. Could one write about Jewish doctors without making him the center of the story? Let me therefore state immediately that this is not a book about Maimonides. The great man lived in the Moslem world—Cordoba, Fez, and Cairo were the cities where he spent most of his days—while for the most part my documents come from Christian Europe: Spain, Italy, and the south of France. The story this book will tell gains momentum around the year 1250; Maimonides died almost fifty years beforehand. And while most of our knowledge about him as a doctor comes from his medical writings, I am interested in the history of the medical *profession* and medical services, not in the development of medical sciences or the art of healing.

But I am afraid I run too fast. This is not the point where I intended to be in this short preface. Let me, therefore, come back to square one and express my thanks first to the Hannah Institute for the History of Medicine, whose headquarters are in Toronto, for helping me to pursue my interest in the subject. I have expressed my gratitude to the directors

of this institution on previous occasions and I do so here again gladly. The two anonymous readers for the University of California Press made useful suggestions and offered penetrating criticism. The reader will find their fingerprints throughout the book, and I thank them both for their efforts. I should also like to warmly thank Gérard Jobin, my collaborator at the Université Jean Moulin in Lyon, for helping with the bibliography; my daughter, Ira, who suggested the title of this book; Susan Mersky, Edward Shorter, Dr. Malcolm Marshall, and Beth McAuley for looking over my English; and Beth for her word processing of this complicated manuscript. Many colleagues offered me materials and ideas. I hope that I did not forget any of them in the appropriate notes.

Introduction

Sooner or later doctors and their patients come to the attention of medievalists involved in archival research. Scholars most likely to come into contact with medieval doctors are those carrying out research into the history of Mediterranean Europe. Interested researchers have almost insurmountable quantities of written records to examine in order to discover these medical practitioners, but they may be sure that the documents exist and that once they have found them the effort will be amply compensated. They will encounter real, live doctors whose names, dates, and locations are known and flesh and blood patients who disclose the illnesses that afflicted them. At times the doctors' methods of cure are specified, and in many instances the question of remuneration is openly discussed.

In principle there should be no difficulty in identifying medieval physicians or in distinguishing those who were Christians from those who were Jews. The Latin title *medicus* was then the equivalent of today's "doctor" and follows the name of the practitioner in our documents. People were well able to distinguish between the superior *medicus physicus*, well-rounded in his education, and the more inferior surgeon, or *medicus cirurgicus*, of limited medical capacity who was expected to deal with wounds and to perform a variety of surgical operations. Jews appear both as "physicians" and "surgeons" in these documents, and they are easily recognizable by the label *judeus* attached to their name. Thus, there is

no doubt at all as to the religious and professional identity of a "magister Leo phisicus judeus" or a "magister Bonafos chirurgicus judeus," both of whom lived in Manosque in Haute Provence during the first half of the fourteenth century.

Since I began my work in the Provençal archives, I have found a myriad of documents about doctors and their activities in the notarial registers and in the court registers of Marseilles and Manosque. Manosque, a small city in northern Provence, especially caught my attention because of its dozens of court records that start as early as the 1240s, records that are accompanied by numerous notarial cartularies. Over the years I have published some of the most interesting of these documents, but such publications did not allow me to deal with more encompassing questions. Limiting this particular enquiry to the world of Jewish doctors, I have endeavored to discover how many were practicing during this period and what proportion of the profession they represented. Were they really overrepresented in the medical profession? Did they represent, say, half of the practitioners of the medieval city? In which regions? When? Where did these Jewish doctors obtain their medical education, considering that the universities of the time were clerical institutions. In particular, I wanted to understand the social and economic conditions that gave birth to such professional opportunity for Jews in a world that tended to exclude them from almost all other professions. Here we see Jews engaged in a lucrative profession that awarded its practitioners power and prestige. We have no difficulty understanding why so many young Jews were attracted to medicine, but the complexity of Christian attitudes toward Jewish practitioners is a particularly difficult subject of inquiry. After all, medieval society was marked by blatant bigotry, fostered by superstitions as well as fears, almost all of which were sanctioned in one way or another by the church. How was it then that Christians accepted the Jewish doctor and allowed him (or her) to inspect their bodies, to prescribe for them, and in that way to determine their survival? Moreover, since most of our evidence comes from contemporary legal documents, questions have to be answered about the status of these doctors in law and about the degree to which the prevailing legal system

was intended not only to supervise their activities but also to protect them. Were they a legitimate part of the profession? Did the law come to their aid when misunderstandings occurred between them and their Christian patients?

Provençal archives are famous for the insights they provide into the social and economic realities of the Middle Ages. To rely only on these repositories for this study, however, would have been a mistake. Other archives in southern Europe offer no less exciting possibilities. Spanish scholars working in Catalonia, Murcia, and elsewhere as well as Italian investigators in Umbria and Sicily have uncovered fascinating documents pertinent to the questions just posed. These documents often surpass those of Provence in both numbers and content. One can only wonder how much richer this study might have been had I access to all the relevant studies, which are often published in remote provincial journals. Yet although the geographical scope of this study is limited and evidence is only rarely brought from Germany, England, or northern France, I hope that a better understanding of the dynamics of the medical profession in these southern regions may help us to ask the right questions about developments in other parts of medieval Europe. Moreover, the insights gained from this inquiry will no doubt prove valuable not only for the history of the medical profession but also for the understanding of the entry of Jews and other minority groups into the professions in general both in the past and in the present. Is it merely coincidence that medicine is so predominant in Jewish life today as well? How are we to explain this lasting attraction? Is there something in Judaism which drives its adherents into the medical field? Or, as I tend to believe, is this concentration simply a coincidence, the result of a felicitous conjuncture, the product of an unprecedented growth of the European economy (the "boom" of the twelfth century) and its urban civilization? Since so much of the following discussion will depend on the answer to this last question, I address it without further delay.

1

Jews and the Medicalization of Society in the Middle Ages

In the countries of Mediterranean Europe during the High or Late Middle Ages (1250 onward), one can hardly find a Jewish community that did not count at least one medical doctor among its members. Next to moneylending, medicine seems to have been the most preponderant profession among Jews. To give just one example—more will be found in chapter 5—the city of Avignon, in the Comtat Venaissin, listed at least thirty-four Jewish doctors in the fourteenth century, while Rome had fifteen medical practitioners residing in the city between 1454 and 1482.[1] Similar numbers occur in many other cities and villages.[2] They attest to the extensive participation of Jews in the medical profession, a participation out of proportion with contemporary demographics and the place of Jews in society. Why is it then that a minority group accounting for less than 1 percent of the overall population and representing at most 5 percent or 8 percent of the population in great cities[3] occupied such a significant place in this profession, at times accounting for 50 percent or more of the practitioners? To answer these and similar questions we must examine the development of medical services during the Mid-

dle Ages in order to shed light on the changes in the collective mentality of the people which brought about the "medicalization" of the medieval West.

The Medicalization of Society, 1250–1450: The Growing Need for Doctors

What I call the "medicalization" of medieval society or "the growing interest in and appreciation of scientific medicine"[4] seems to have gained tremendous momentum between 1200 and 1250. This process implied first and foremost that the services of learned professional practitioners were no longer limited to members of the princely class of feudal lords and prelates of the church but proliferated and penetrated all layers of society. Regimens for health (*regimina sanitatis*), for example, which up to this time were written for the benefit of kings and princes, now found their way into the houses "of merchants, members of the liberal professions, or clerics."[5] People of modest income became dependent on medical services and were ready to put aside part of their earnings in order to benefit from the expertise of a doctor. A prime example of this new concern for health is a contract made in Manosque in the year 1310 between a Jewish doctor named Isaac and an unassuming citizen named Raimundus Saunerii.[6] Nothing seems to have been wrong with Raimundus or with any member of his family. What he wished to establish with this contract was a relationship, which today we would call insurance, with a doctor in which during the next four years Raimundus, his wife, and his children would benefit from the services of the practitioner. As for the doctor's remuneration, Raimundus was prepared to commit himself to a yearly payment of four sestarii of wheat, about 320 kilograms in modern weight. Other contracts found in the Manosque archives[7] and elsewhere give the names of peasants and artisans who also considered expenditures on medicine and healing entirely normal. Indeed, after the medical catastrophe of 1348 ("The Black Death"), pressure was exerted on members of municipal councils to hire doctors at public expense in order to provide some help to the

poor who could not handle such expenditures on their own. (Chapter 5 discusses these issues in more detail.)

These developments in the social history of medicine, which were, let us remind ourselves, just one aspect of the overall and momentous changes then taking place in society and its organization, were also expressed in the attitudes and collective sensitivities of Europeans at this time. Medical argument and medical certification now made their appearance in society and in the justice system, with the aim of justifying an individual practitioner's behavior or misbehavior. From about the year 1300, civil courts in Provence, Italy, and Spain ceased to give verdicts in cases of bloodshed or death without having first heard and officially acknowledged the expert opinion of one or, better still, several doctors.[8] Ecclesiastical courts in Marseilles or in Paris would not rule on the dissolution of a marriage on the grounds of impotence without first allowing doctors to deliberate the case.[9] By this time interested parties knew well when to insist on a medical expert's opinion and how to ask for an official document.

While I shall dwell more on medical experts in chapter 7, here I will describe briefly some of the notarized medical certificates. The first one, which comes from Spain, was presented by Don Juan de Leon, a professor at the university of Salamanca, in the year 1472. He wished to justify on health grounds his absence from classes for several months.[10] In 1325, in similar circumstances, a Provençal soldier named Salvatus Ricardi who lived in Trets was unable to fulfill his obligation after enlisting in a military expedition. He also used sickness to explain his absence.[11] On the island of Sicily three medical certificates were issued between February 12 and February 25, 1299, in which sailors, with the help of local doctors, registered their inability to embark as scheduled with the royal navy.[12] In Manosque more than forty years later two prominent city businessmen confined to quarters because of a financial conflict with the representatives of the king of France cited health reasons in order to be released. One of them, the very respectable Andreas Davit, claimed to be "old and disabled," while the other, Bertrandus Rebaunti, was found by court messengers confined to his bed and so sick that he was "unable

to consume meat and the likes."[13] Similarly, in Marseilles a medical consideration brought about the release of a detainee from the local royal prison in 1309.[14] The man, a Jew named Jussonus de Posqueriis, citizen of Marseilles, had not repaid a debt he owed to a certain Amiguetus Vincentii. Before obtaining his freedom he had to find a relative to vouch for him and promise to pay the money, "otherwise to return to before-mentioned jail." Yet Jussonus was freed at least "for several days" because "it so pleased" the judge, mostly by reason of his "poor health." The judge registered his decree in the court register and probably even made it public. Finally, we notice that the medical argument also became an element in the slave trade of the time. In Catalonia, for instance, transactions were annulled if the doctor was not ready to issue a medical clearance certifying the state of health of the human merchandise.[15]

The value society attached to medical certification is also clearly revealed in documents concerning leprosy, the most frightening sickness of the period. Municipalities, representing the interest of the public, were usually eager to officially declare a sick person a leper in order to isolate him. They spent as much as eleven florins at times to hire a doctor to carry out the examination. Suspected individuals, quite naturally, wanted to avoid the stigma at all costs. Both sides were prepared to go a long way in order to obtain the right document. For example, on October 19, 1441, a Manosque citizen named Pierre Filhole sought notarial certification of an examination in Aix-en-Provence by the doctor Pierre Contier.[16] "I have seen, I have touched, and I have diligently examined," stated the doctor, clearing the man of the disease. In the case of a man named Petrus Barbavayre, however, the municipal authorities of Istres, the small city where he lived, sought such a document from a notary. The findings of the doctors did not leave much doubt as to the man's condition: his skin, his eyes, and his nose, which was partially wasted, all witnessed against him.[17]

At times these "leprosy" documents reveal real legal battles between the parties concerned. Around 1446 when a certain Pons Vendran was declared a leper by the master Vitalis Cohen of Marseilles, he did not accept the diagnosis but asked

for another examination. To his great relief a new committee, composed of masters Pierre Contier and Boniac Cohen of Aix-en-Provence in addition to the above-mentioned Vitalis Cohen, was appointed and reversed the first verdict.[18] In the trial of Vendran's contemporary Louis Bermond, a three-act scenario took place. Bermond was first declared healthy by the doctor Pierre Contier of Aix, but this decision was challenged by the authorities of Ginasservis, his village of origin. When a second jury found Bermond to be indeed a leper, Pierre Contier took his colleagues to court. Not only was Bermond cleared a second time but the members of the jury received considerable fines for having arrived at a false decision. The description of this medical embroglio appears in a recently discovered notarial document dated April 9, 1435.[19]

But the medicalization of society meant much more than new attitudes toward the legalities of medicine; it also implied the introduction of structural changes in the practice of the profession itself. Medical services had to depart from the realm of Christian charity and become part of the marketplace, where not only goods but also services were sold.[20] Instead of clerics, old men, experienced women, or other well-meaning volunteers, we now see the emergence of professional, secular practitioners, mostly male, who wished to be remunerated for the expertise they possessed and for the effort they exhibited and who were expected to take responsibility for misdeeds and failures. These practitioners soon became subject to public regulation. They were expected to possess a certain degree of medical knowledge and demonstrate it during an official examination in order to obtain a license to practice. The professionals, now called *magister* and *medicus*, claimed a monopoly in the world of healing and persecuted uncertified practitioners (now labeled miraculous medics, empiricists, and "charlatans") in the courts.

Recent studies in the history of medicine show how rapidly this process of medicalization took place and how overwhelming it was.[21] While eleventh- and even twelfth-century documents do not reveal the presence of any significant medical services, evidence from around the year 1300 shows the development of patterns similar to those current in the indus-

trialized countries of the West today, at least in terms of the numbers of practitioners in a given population. Recent investigation reveals medieval doctor-patient ratios of 1:500 or in some cases even fewer patients per doctor. Such high ratios were found not only in Florence, the great metropolis of the West,[22] but also in regional agricultural centers like Manosque or Salon de Provence. Research in the archives of York in northern England has also revealed similar numbers.[23] The argument against these numbers is that doctors had to provide services to people in the countryside as well as in the city, thus increasing the overall ratio of doctors to patients. While admitting such an argument for the moment, we may still safely conclude that in absolute numbers regions such as Provence, Catalonia, and parts of southern Italy had hundreds of doctors practicing both in the towns and in the countryside, offering help to rich and poor alike. Furthermore, it becomes clear that even these elevated numbers were deemed insufficient by contemporaries who believed society in dire need of even broader medical services.

Many fourteenth- and fifteenth-century documents complain of this real or presumed scarcity. "At present there are very few experts in the aforesaid [medical] arts who reside in the Dauphiné," declares the governor in 1370.[24] He goes on to say that this scarcity "causes a lot of damage to the inhabitants so that all kinds of sufferings are experienced daily." In 1359 and in 1384 the counsel for the Italian city of Pistoia could not have expressed the necessity better than when he declared: "In the city of Pistoia there are not enough doctors to satisfy the needs of the city."[25] The city councillors of Marseilles employed similar language. There too we hear about "the urgent necessity" for doctors. When in 1476 the council of that city seemed to be hesitant about hiring *magister* Vitalis, the impatient doctor, with the help of a friend, issued an ultimatum. His bargaining position was sufficiently strong to compel the city to reach a decision more quickly.[26] In 1352 in Valencia the lord of Nules described the shortage in a plea to King Pedro IV: "In the town of Nules and in your other towns and villages there is no physician or surgeon or other skilled person from

whom you and the inhabitants of these towns and villages could get help and assistance and medicines for sickness and other afflictions."[27] In 1350 in Xativa, another Valencian city, the local authorities also lamented that the "abundance of physicians and surgeons that used to be found in the city of Xativa and other large cities is now so diminished that it is scarcely possible to find a single surgeon here."[28] Finally, in Barcelona around 1350 there is even a question of forcing a doctor to stay in the city. In response to Benvenisti Ismael's wish to leave the city, a certain Pera Folquet, presumably a royal official, wrote to the queen asking her to seek an order from the king to prohibit the doctor from leaving.[29]

Faculties of medicine clearly did not turn out sufficient numbers of graduates. Far from it. A recent study quotes surprisingly low numbers.[30] A university metropolis such as Bologna conferred only sixty-five degrees in medicine and one in surgery in the fifteen years between 1419 and 1434. The output of Padua was equally poor: a mere four in 1407, eight in 1434, and nine in 1450. Other universities had even poorer results. Turin could boast only thirteen graduates for the thirty-six years between 1426 and 1462, while Tübingen gave thirty-five doctorates in medicine between 1477 and 1534. We do not have numbers for earlier periods, but the situation must have been just as bad. Certainly the demand was greater than the supply.

The principal reason for this scarcity of physicians must be related to the price of a university education. Such training would have been beyond the reach of most people, according to a document issued on May 15, 1339, by Pope Benedict XII, describing the expenses of a year of study. According to this estimate done by the papal administration at Avignon, a student would spend between thirty-five and forty pounds "for living, clothing, shoes, books and for whatever other necessities he may have." Similarly large sums (for example, thirty florins) are recorded for the fifteenth century in Italian universities such as Siena, Bologna, and Florence.[31] Such a sum represents the yearly salary of municipal doctors in the south of France or in Italy (as we shall see in chapter 6 below). While the papal estimate seems high, if the order of magnitude is

right the sums are still prohibitive. Most families could not have dreamed of putting aside such amounts for a period of four or five years.

Church Opposition to the Clerical Practice of Medicine

Only the church could afford to educate enough clerics to satisfy society's need for medical practitioners. But the church itself soon complained that clerics' talents were being diverted. During the twelfth century the attitude of church authorities turned negative, or at least defensive.[32] Starting in the 1130s conciliar legislation—regional for the most part, but also general—reveals the defection of clerics to the secular world. In 1130 the Council of Clermont, the first to express such worries, had already identified medicine and law in its prohibitions. "We understand that an evil and detestable habit has taken root, one according to which monks and regular canons, after having received the habit and made profession [of faith], engage in the study of jurisprudence and medicine, despite the rule of Saints Benedict and Augustine: and this they do for the sake of temporal gain," declared the alarmed prelates.[33] The undisciplined clerics were threatened therefore with expulsion and their superiors with being stripped of their honors for knowingly tolerating such "enormity." The Clermont canon was adopted word for word by the Council of Reims in 1139. In the same year the Second Lateran Council repeated it and reminded the clerics that they were supposed to engage in the "cure of souls."[34] The prohibiting canon was subsequently incorporated into the conciliar decisions of Montpellier (1162), Tours (1173), Montpellier (1195), and Paris (1212).[35]

How effective were these decisions? Professor Darrel W. Amundsen is probably right in concluding that the canons had little lasting effect and that, in any event, their fire was aimed only at monks and canons regular, not at secular clerics who did not withdraw from society.[36] Moreover, we note that no objection in principle (such as man's tampering with God's

creation) is ever raised in these conciliar decisions. The church was simply concerned about losing the services of some of its members. And the pressure on the church came not only via the medical profession but also, as the legislation of the 1130s repeats again and again, from the legal one. In addition, educated priests were much in demand in expanding secular administrations. In many instances the church's prohibitive legislation omits medicine altogether and focuses on these other professions. Thus, the Third Lateran (1179) and the Paris council of 1208 single out the profession of lawyers (*advocatus*) in secular courts. This is also the case in Narbonne (1227), London (1268), Avignon (1279), and the Fourth Lateran (1215).[37] As early as 1139 in Reims, St. Bernard denounced the study of Roman law, and the councils of Clermont (1130) and Tours (1163) issued prohibitions against its study.[38] Rouen (1189) was concerned with clerics becoming provosts, sheriffs, and farmers in villages, while Oxford (1222) further enriches our evidence by noting the possibility of churchmen becoming bailiffs and administrators through the levy of taxes (*tallia*).[39] Tarragona (1329) sums up almost two hundred years of repeated criticism of clerics in public positions: "We state and order that those responsible for the cure of the souls . . . shall not assume public office, neither bailiwicks nor vicaries of secular persons. Rather they should keep continuously their personal residence in churches, as is due."[40]

The continuous "antimedical" legislation was not entirely crowned with success. As has happened so often in its history, the church had to be satisfied with partial victory. One can easily encounter regular clerics who were also doctors and discover practitioners even at the highest possible levels of the ecclesiastical hierarchy. One well-known example is Pope John XXI (d. 1277), who, when still called Petrus Hispanus, studied medicine in Siena and Paris and became the author of a most popular medical compendium, the *Tesaurus pauperum*.[41] Less well known yet still high in the church's hierarchy were John XXI's professional contemporaries, Andreas Abalat, bishop of Valencia (1248–1276), and Theodoric, bishop of Bari and later of Ravenna, who wrote an important book on surgery.[42] The list must also include the name of Gaufré Isnard, bishop of

Cavaillon in the Comtat Venaissin (1330–1333), who served as a personal doctor to Pope John XXII.[43] In fact, the names of no less than twenty such "medical" prelates are known from the medieval French records. To these may be added the names of many other clerics who were not as highly ranked in the hierarchy.[44] Danielle Jacquart, calculating from data assembled by Ernst Wickersheimer, found that, between 1350 and 1399, clerics represented 11.3 percent of the medical personnel practicing in France, while between 1300 and 1399 no less than 31.9 percent of students benefited from clerical subventions.[45] Jacquart even talks about a possible "clericalization" of the medical profession around this time. Yet we must insist that this "clericalization" happened not through any encouragement on the part of the church but rather through the blatant defiance of its canons. The numbers would possibly have been much higher had the hierarchy not made efforts to keep them down.

Did this negative stance facilitate the entry of Jews into the profession? Unfortunately, there is no way of estimating the weight of these ecclesiastical policies of restraint, especially since they were not followed to the letter. Nevertheless, we can suggest that while Christian society experienced difficulties in drafting doctors, the church did not respond willingly to the outcry. The entry of Jews into the profession, which may have been the result of this relative standstill, certainly took place under these conditions.

The Opening: The Entry of Jews into the Profession

Jews in the medieval West were unprepared for these new needs for medical services. A long and continuous tradition of Jewish medical science or practice did not exist. In fact, there was almost no medical literature that might have been called "Jewish," that is, written for Jewish doctors in their language and based on a particular Jewish experience or doctrine. The late Salo W. Baron observed years ago that even Hellenistic Jewish culture, which might have been expected to be

preoccupied with medicine, failed to produce Jewish authors in this field.[46] The Bible and the Talmud, although they have much to say about human and animal anatomy, hygiene, and prophylactic healing and identify specific diseases such as hemophilia, rabies, and gout, do not present this information as part of a systematic medical science. No general ancient Hebrew medical documents existed.[47] This was already understood by the Jewish religious leaders, the *Ge'onim* of Babylonia. In the tenth century A.D. one of them warned the Jews not to rely on the medical ideas expressed in Talmudic literature. "One cannot rely on these remedies because we do not know how they cure." Or, as Rabbi Sherira Ga'on (ca. 906–1006), one of the last *Ge'onim* and himself a chronographer, put it: "Our masters were not physicians."[48]

The only possible exception was the famous medical compendium *Sefer Asaph*, also known as *Sefer Refuoth* ("Book of Medicines"), which, according to some scholars, was composed in Palestine in the late antiquity (third to fifth centuries A.D.).[49] This book was known in southern Italy in the tenth century and was reedited (or even possibly composed) by the southern Italian doctor Shabetai Donolo (913–982).[50] Together the *Sefer ha-Yakar*, another of Donolo's works, known also as *Sefer Mirkahot* ("Book of Remedies"), an antidotarium of 120 drugs based mostly on Greek pharmacology, and *Sepher Asaph* were the most important of the few original scientific medical treatises written in Hebrew and available to medieval Jews.[51] This poverty was recognized. As late as 1250 a Jewish translator into Hebrew, Salomon ben Abraham ibn David, could not help but lament how few medical books were available in Hebrew to Jewish intellectuals.[52] The astronomer Jacob ben Machir, a contemporary of Salomon, complained of this lack as well. "In the past," he maintained, there were proper Jewish medical books, but "the wisdom of our sages was lost . . . and [now] we must seek it from the sages of the Nations."[53]

Nonetheless, Jews were active as doctors in the Islamic world.[54] One of them, Isaac Judeus, an older contemporary of Donolo, whose full name was Isaac ibn Sulaiman al Isra'ili (d. 959) of Cairo and Kairawan, was prominent in his time

and was the teacher of two other famous doctors, Dūnash ben Tamim and possibly Hasdai ben Shaprut. Isaac's medical work, especially his treatise on fevers and urine, composed in Arabic, formed part of the university curriculum in the medieval and Renaissance world.

But with Isaac Israeli in the mid-tenth century we have in all probability just the beginning of the Jewish medical tradition in Arab lands. Françoise Micheau's recent analysis of the information about doctors provided by the Arabic writer and biographer Ibn-al-Qifti (d. 1248) in his *History of Learned Men* reveals that there were only 17 Jews among the 124 doctors listed for the five hundred years between 750 and 1230.[55] While Jews were among the first-known doctors in the early Islamic empire, and Ibn-al-Qifti gives the names of three of them, no Jewish name is recorded for the hundred years between 950 and 1050 and only three out of seventeen doctors in the twelfth century are Jewish. By contrast, almost half of the doctors known to al-Qifti—52 out of 124—were Christian. Micheau's observations, although based on evidence provided by only one thirteenth-century author, have support from other, earlier important sources. Jāḥiẓ, a ninth-century Arab writer, described contemporary Jews as ignorant obscurantists, "dyers, tanners, cuppers, butchers, cobblers."[56] At the end of the tenth century the Arab geographer al-Muquaddasi noticed that in his time most doctors in Jerusalem were Christians while Jews were preponderantly money changers as well as manual laborers, dyers, and tanners.[57] Modern observers have noticed the absence of Jews among the doctors in the hospital Adhud founded in Baghdad in the year 987. Salo Baron attributes this absence to mere chance, but Max Meyerhof has another explanation: There were simply not many qualified practitioners among the Jews at that time. It seems to me that his explanation carries the day in this scholarly controversy.[58]

Meyerhof, who left no stone unturned in his search for Jewish doctors in the Middle East, noticed that the eleventh century marked a new era in the history of the Jewish medical profession and that these changes gained even greater momentum in the twelfth century.[59] Of the forty-four Middle Eastern Jewish doctors whose biographies Meyerhof was able to trace,

18 (more than 40 percent) were contemporaries of Maimonides (1135–1204). Research on Jewish doctors in Moslem Seville yielded similar results for the same period.[60] It is thus possible that a process of increasing the number of physicians took place in the Middle East, and in Arab lands in general, following a similar pattern to the one described for the medieval West, but that it occurred one or two hundred years earlier. Such a hypothesis would explain the sudden appearance of great numbers of Jewish doctors in the Islamic sources for the late twelfth century.

The Jewish doctors of the Islamic world, of course, had no linguistic obstacles to separate them from the necessary books. Arabic, the language of science, was their language and provided them with indirect access to the Greek medical classics in translation. Indeed, inventories of libraries found in the huge depository of documents (the *Geniza*) discovered in the Ben Ezra synagogue in Cairo show how well integrated Jewish doctors were into the scientific community. For example, a Jew's library sold in Cairo in 1190 contained 33 of Galen's works translated into Arabic among the 102 pieces inventoried. Other libraries contained medical books by authors such as Averroës, Avicenna, Hippocrates, and al-Razi (Razes).[61]

As we are about to see, on the eve of the massive medicalization of society in Western Europe at the beginning of the thirteenth century, Jews compensated for the lack of a genuine Hebrew medical tradition by relying on their brethren in the Moslem world who had already entered the world of medicine. Jewish immigrants from Arab lands brought their knowledge to Western Europe and other Jews benefited from it. One such individual was Judah ben Saul ibn Tibbon from Granada, the "physician," as the Jewish traveler Benjamin of Tudela (ca. 1165) called him, who became a representative of Arabic scholarship in the south of France in the second half of the twelfth century (see chapter 3). He and other émigrés soon channeled their knowledge of Arabic into the translating of philosophical and then scientific works into Hebrew, thus making the medical literature accessible to Jews of Western Europe.

2

The Making of the
Jewish Doctor

Where were Jewish doctors trained? How did they manage to acquire knowledge and proficiency when generally denied access to university education? How did they obtain proper credentials when the medical profession became subject to severe control and strict licensing procedures in the thirteenth century?

Supervision of the Medical Profession and Licensing Procedures

By the turn of the fourteenth century, and in many instances even before 1250, doctors had to obtain a license (*licentia practicandi*) in order to practice. In principle there was no way around this requirement. The civil authorities saw it as their duty to ensure that only qualified individuals who had passed the appropriate examinations became members of the profession. This procedural rigidity was yet another sign of what I have labeled the medicalization of society.

The first known Western European regulation comes from the year 1140 in the kingdom of Sicily, where King Roger II established the need for such an examination in the Assizes of

Ariano.[1] Whether he was influenced by earlier legislation in the Islamic world is still an open question.[2] This legislation, however, seems to have been premature, for nothing like it appears in any other twelfth-century legislation. Similar decrees were not enacted until a hundred years later, again in Sicily and then in many other regions of Mediterranean Europe. In 1231 the emperor Frederick II in his *Liber augustalis* issued elaborate legislation dealing with the content of medical studies; he even established a list of books for the candidates.[3] Frederick's legislation proved to set more of a precedent. Less than a generation later Count Charles of Anjou enacted similar legislation when he took power in southern Italy and Sicily from the last of the Hohenstaufen. A regulation he issued on July 12, 1296, for the county of Provence, stated: "We forbid anyone, of whatever condition or status he may be, to dare and practice medicine or surgery unless . . . his expertise and preparedness in the area are established beforehand."[4] Similarly in Florence in 1310 city legislation established that no doctor could exercise his art unless he was examined.[5] Detailed legislation was enacted in 1329 in the kingdom of Valencia,[6] while in 1363 similar detailed provisions can be found in the legislation of the Cortes of Monzón, Aragon.[7]

Many medieval governments applied these licensing regulations to the letter. Hundreds of contemporary licenses witness governmental activity in favor of candidates who prepared themselves for examinations and passed them successfully. Evidence also survives of examination failures. The first of three examples comes from Venice, where a municipal deliberation, dated March 21, 1320, reveals that the experts declared master Menego Sancte Fusce unsatisfactory.[8] Notwithstanding this failure, he was permitted to practice. The second is dated 1334 and concerns a Valencian citizen named Jucine Lama.[9] He presented himself for examination that year, but was neither approved by the examiners nor given a license to practice medicine in the city because "he gave back nonsense and inanities to the questions put to him by the examiners and was held to be incompetent." The third failure, a Castilian Jewish practitioner named Rabbi Salomon Abenbila, who was

living in Ocaña, was less fortunate. Sometime in the second half of the fifteenth century he was declared "insufficient" by his examiner Goncalo Días and ordered to stop all practice immediately.[10]

Jews were not expressly mentioned in most legislation but were certainly expected to obey the rulings. Their inclusion is reflected not only in the many Jewish candidates who actually took the examinations but also by statements from the authorities. Thus, just a few weeks after the proclamation of general regulatory legislation in Montpellier in July 1272, King James I of Aragon issued another declaration making it clear that Jews too had to pass examinations.[11] In Paris a year earlier (1271) the faculty of medicine engaged in the first in a series of efforts to assure a monopoly for its members and graduates and to eliminate from the city those deemed unqualified empiricists. Although the document is formulated in very general terms, the faculty in all probability had Jewish practitioners in mind also. In any event, the document concludes with a direct reference: "No Jew or Jewess may presume to operate surgically or medicinally on any person of the Christian faith."[12] Like all other doctors Jews had thus to appear before a licensing agency.[13] And if, as was the case in Florence, a doctor also had to become a member of the Doctors' Guild, inscribe himself in the "matricula dicte artis," and pay the appropriate fees, Jews would follow the rule. This is shown in the case of Salomon ben Abraham Avigdor in 1412 and in other Florentine cases discovered by Ladislao Münster and Mirko Malavolti.[14]

We know a considerable amount today about the individuals who went through this purgatory and obtained *licentia practicandi*. Scholars have had no difficulty in finding such information in southern European archives in Italy, Spain, and the south of France. The Sicilian archives are particularly fruitful in this respect. The brothers Lagumina in the last century discovered dozens of documents for the last 130 years of Jewish presence on the island; they did not publish all of the evidence in their *diplomatarium* but were content to provide just short notes about most of the documents.[15] The first of these

Sicilian licenses dates to February 28, 1363, and was issued for the master Matheus Sacducinus Judeus. The last document is dated May 18, 1492, very close to the date of the expulsion of the Jews. In some years, for instance, in 1375, there is evidence that four or even five licenses were issued in Sicily. The Lagumina records for other years, however, contain no reference to licenses, perhaps because the documents had disappeared.

As for examiners, the Sicilian documentation reveals a clear preponderance of Christian doctors in this role. Such names as Agostino di Vara, Agostino Casamassima, Raymundus de Ripa, or Leonardo Salvacoxa certainly did not belong to Jews. Occasionally, however, a Jewish doctor did certify a coreligionist. This was the case with Joseph (ms.: Iocep) Bonafilia, a Catalan Jew and doctor to the royal court who conferred diplomas on two other Jews in 1396 and 1398. A Joseph Abenafia (Iocep Abanassia), who may have been the same person, carried out a similar function in 1402 and 1403.[16] But it is certain that the authorities in Sicily did not make a point of having a Jew serve on his coreligionist's committee. This was not the case, however, in Aragon, where explicit legislation in this respect existed in the Cortes of Monzón for 1363. The relevant document reads as follows: "Jewish and Saracen physicians should be examined by physicians of their own law or sect, if any are available. One Christian physician should nevertheless assist in their examination. In the absence of physicians of their own law and religion, they shall be examined by two Christian physicians."[17] And in fact whenever information has survived about the composition of the examining committee in Aragon, it is evident that the body was never composed of Jews alone. To quote two recently discovered examples: In 1346 the committee that granted a license to Jaffudà Abenvives was composed of Pere Ros d'Orsins, a Christian, and El'azar Abenardut (spelled here "Alatzar Avinardut"), a Jew. Two generations later, when Ferrarius Saladi obtained his license in 1395, a committee composed of one Jewish and one Christian doctor issued the permission.[18] We even know of one case in which the jury, which was examining Davinus

Bonet Boujorn in June 1390 in Perpignan, included not a single Jewish specialist but only two Christian professors of the local university.[19]

Another licensing agency found in documents from Aragon and Valencia as well as from southern Italy and Sicily is that of the *protomedicus*. Possibly modeled on Arabic and Greek precedent, these *protomedici* (*alcalde e examinador major*) had the power not only to issue licenses but also to examine practicing doctors and disqualify them if they were found to be inept.[20] At least five such doctors entitled *protomedicus* worked in Sicily in the first half of the fifteenth century. Their role, at least according to the documents assembled by the brothers Lagumina, was limited only to granting licenses. One *protomedicus*, Master Pietro d'Alessandro, was prominent for almost thirty years between 1421 and 1449.[21] At the beginning he was called *vice protomedico*, but from 1425 onward he carried the full title. His signature appears on over thirty permissions granted in favor of Jewish doctors.

Protomedici appear also in documents from Aragon, but there they also examined practicing doctors. Thus, in May 1400 a *bachillar en arts y medicina* named Domingo Polo engaged in an examining campaign throughout the kingdom of Aragon in which he disqualified many practitioners, "physicians as well as surgeons," among them several Jews.[22] On December 28, 1421, in Murcia a *protomedicus* named Diego Rodrigues, who was called *alcalde examinador mayor de todos los cururgianos en todos los regnos et senorio del dicho rey*, appointed a delegate, also a *bachiller*, for the bishoprics of Toledo, Jaen, Cartagena, and Cuenca and empowered him to supervise medical activity there.[23]

Jews sometimes acted as *protomedici*. For example, in July 1351 Master Bonjuda (Bonjuha) Carbit, a Jewish surgeon, was given license to examine practitioners in whatever city he might be.[24] He was expected to act, however, along with one of the best local doctors and to denounce to the royal authorities those who had jeopardized the lives of the population by their lack of knowledge. Documents from Valencia dating from the 1370s to the 1390s show Omār (Humer) Tawil, also a Jew, acting as *protomedicus* and granting licenses to some of

his coreligionists.[25] But he was not the only one holding this office in Valencia at the time. A Christian physician, Petrus Caveti, also acted in such a capacity. Two documents, one from 1332 and the other from 1338, show Caveti conferring licenses on two Jewish candidates, Salomon Caravida and Vitalis Habib (Abib).[26]

At times it is possible to discern the considerations that guided these licensing boards. Raffaele Calvanico, an Italian scholar who worked at the Neapolitan Angevin archives before their destruction during World War II, discovered approximately 3,600 licenses relating to the region of Naples and dating from the short period between 1273 and 1345; this collection constitutes our most copious source of information about licensing anywhere.[27] The material makes it evident that not all doctors had the same level of training and consequently did not receive the same type of license. Committees had to accept people of limited abilities. In many cases, a candidate's education did not consist of any theoretical studies but was acquired through apprenticeship.[28] Some Neapolitan candidates were designated "simpletons" and "illiterates" by the committees, but they nonetheless received their permits as a result of their experience and practical capabilities. One license states that the candidate, Francisca, wife of Matheus Romani, was considered by the board "tamquam idiota, sufficiens est inventa," while another describes the female candidate Polisena de Troya as "perita et ydiota."[29] Similarly, a male surgeon, Roberto da Borello, "surgeon," "expert," is nevertheless labeled "ydiota," while one of his colleagues, Andrea Barbara, is described simply as "illiteratus."[30] Many of these people worried the committee because of their lack of theoretical knowledge (*theorica*) but they were still considered and approved because of their experience.[31] Incidentally, the reverse predicament faced a committee in Valencia which examined the Jewish candidate Isaac (Icach) Gabriel and found that he had no practical experience. "We found him introduced to the principles of the science of physics, yet he did not practice it with patients for long enough a time."[32]

Such candidates did not receive a full license, and in many instances they had to be content with limited medical capacity.

In fact, many Neapolitan licenses restricted the functions of the doctor to healing "fractures and dislocations of human bones," to extracting "stone," and to curing "simple" wounds.[33] Others gave permission for the practice of ophthalmology or the treatment of "hernia of the intestines and the extraction of the stone."[34] In Barcelona Vitalis Habib (Abib) had to accept another type of limited capacity. His committee awarded him his license on October 1, 1344, on condition that he showed other doctors every medicine he intended to administer and explained his reasons for using it.[35] In Aragon a few years later Vidal Aron, who did not do too well in his examination, was warned by his board of two examiners, one of them the Jewish doctor Joseph (Jucef) Abenardut, not to treat Christian patients for the next three years without being accompanied by a Christian doctor.[36] Isma'el (Hizmel) Morcas was subject to another type of limitation to his license in 1378. When seeing patients he had to be accompanied by a senior practitioner, "competent and accomplished in the speculative [part of medicine]" (*abte et antich en speculativa*).[37] In a similar situation in Avignon in 1460, permission was issued to a man who demonstrated more strength in practice than in theory; it was made clear that he would always have to consult with a physician when practicing.[38] These young men should have still considered themselves lucky, since some of their fellow candidates were denied licenses altogether.

Turning to the question of law enforcement and the actual control exercised by the authorities in prosecuting unlicensed practitioners, a handsome file of documents exists to testify to alertness and close surveillance. In Valencia, for example, the legislation of 1329 was at work within three years. A recent study shows that three "empirics" were brought to trial between 1332 and 1338. One of them, Ramon Salena, was an apothecary in the city of Borriana.[39] The trials against two unlicensed women, Clarissa of Rouen and Jacoba (Jacqueline) Felicie de Alamania, in 1311–1312 and 1322, respectively, are well known to historians of the University of Paris.[40] The faculty of medicine brought the women to court with the aim of ousting them from the profession. In the south of France, probably in 1330, the Jewish woman Mayrona was fined forty

shillings for practicing in the village of Bayons in northern Provence in defiance of the constitution according to which "nobody should practice unless he was approved by experts in such matters."[41]

Further evidence comes from Spanish archives. In Jativa (Valencia) a Moslem named Ahmad (Hamet) was brought to court about this time in the fourteenth century for having practiced "for three years," "although he had not been examined in the said art as should be done according to the law."[42] In the mid-fourteenth century a similar fate befell three Valencian Jews: Isaac (Icaach) Alcacani, Joseph (Yucef) Marcho, and Moses Brossa.[43] Another Catalonian Jew found himself in even worse shape: the "empiric" Moses de Portal of Camprodon is reported in 1368 as having been thrown in jail.[44]

There is, however, reason to doubt whether the authorities were always as alert and decisive as these documents suggest. We have just observed that the Valencian Moslem Hamet practiced for three years before the authorities acted.[45] Jacqueline Felicie, as the witnesses in her trial testified, practiced extensively in Paris and her activities were probably not a well-kept secret at the time. The authorities may have shown leniency or flexibility until a serious accident or failure occurred or until a formal complaint pressed them to put the legal machinery into motion. This was no doubt the case with Michael Aucemont, who around the year 1310 engaged in a relatively daring (and unsuccessful) operation on the reproductive member of a male patient.[46] When called before the court of Manosque, he admitted his ignorance and his illiteracy. Asked if he had treated other people in the city, he answered in the affirmative and even gave one name. Still, the relatively high fine of forty shillings decreed by the judge probably had more to do with his failure in this particular operation than with his history of unlawful activity.

Since licensing agencies often took experience into consideration when granting permission to practice, it is understandable that while gaining experience individuals often found themselves in an area that bordered on the illegitimate and thus left them open to prosecution by the authorities. But how, otherwise, could many of them gain experience? Women, to

whom institutions of learning were closed and who encountered many difficulties in leaving home to study with a master, found themselves in a particularly delicate situation. Many documents suggest that they were harassed with singular zeal. The cases of Clarissa and Jacqueline of Paris and Mayrona of Bayons have already been noted. A recent study by Angelina García[47] describes the cases of four other women—Na Benvenguda (also called "La maestra"), Na Blanca, Na Bonfilia "the wife of Berberch," and Jamila—that came before the court of Valencia in the last years of the fourteenth century. Jamila in particular was warned not to "interfere" any more in the medical profession. In 1399 Carinyea, another Jewish woman, was prosecuted severely, receiving a fine of twenty florins.[48] These "empiricists" or "informal" practitioners, however, were not always lost forever to the profession. Their experience and proficiency may well have impressed the board of specialists at one time or another. It may even have been possible for a condemned "charlatan" to "cleanse" himself or herself and finally become legitimate. I wonder, for example, if Mayrona of Bayons is not the same person as Mayrona of Manosque, who is described in dozens of documents in the year 1342, always labeled *fisica*.[49]

We have seen that such licensing boards were sensitive to the kind of knowledge candidates possessed and their proficiency in *theorica*. Any candidate's chance of success no doubt improved if he could boast good schooling or present references from a great master under whom he had studied. Yet where could Jewish candidates obtain such preparation around the year 1300?

Private Medical Education: The Masters and the Students

Is it possible that medicine was taught alongside traditional rabbinic studies in any of the Jewish academies (*yeshivot*) that flourished in the Middle Ages? I am skeptical about such a possibility and have so far found no evidence to sustain it. But some years ago Mordechai Breuer, today's leading

specialist in the history of Jewish medieval academies, called my attention to Joseph Gallouf Yeshu'ah, rabbi of Saragossa in the mid-fifteenth century, who was described by his enemy Shlomo Bonfed as someone who taught not only Talmud and rabbinics but also astronomy, physics, and medicine.[50] But did Joseph Yeshu'ah teach all disciplines at the same place and the same time? Professor Breuer recently informed me in a private letter that new evidence has strengthened his convictions about medical education in the *yeshiva*. I must therefore leave this important question in abeyance until my colleague has completed his study. For the present, I can do no more than state my belief that for the greater part of the period under discussion young Jewish women and men received their medical training privately, mainly on a one-to-one basis, not in any institution of higher learning.

In many cases the Jewish family provided the framework in which learning took place. "Come study medicine under my guidance," suggested a father to his son in a Hebrew *exemplum* composed in Germany around the year 1200.[51] The very existence of Jewish medical dynasties in which the profession passed from father to son for generations is yet another indication of the importance of the family in this respect. Historians have no difficulty in discovering such Jewish dynasties, as a study of the south of France by Isaac Alteras has shown.[52] (One such dynasty, the Abenardut of Aragon, is discussed below in chapter 3.)

Echoes of master-teacher relationships within the family are also in evidence from marriage arrangements that included an undertaking by a father-in-law to teach medicine to the young groom. Two contracts from Provence, enacted almost at the same time, reveal this kind of arrangement. In the first, concluded in Marseilles on March 7, 1431, Moses Bonsegnor, physician and surgeon, father of the bride Mandina, promised the family of his future son-in-law, Bonjuda (Bonjuas) Durant, that he would teach him one or both sciences "free of charge, for a whole year," if, as the contract specifics, the young man was interested in learning them.[53] In the second contract, enacted in Aix-en-Provence on November 1, 1432, less than two years later, Master Crescas Creyssent (Creysse), who gave away his daughter Bellete to a certain Boniaquet

Durand, promised without any time limitation to teach the young man "all the sciences that he acquired" and especially medicine.[54]

Those who could not rely on family had to pay for their education. For the satirist and social critic Kalonymos ben Kalonymos (d. after 1329), a typical Jewish doctor was someone who studied under a famous doctor and had to pay for his education. Years later, when he charged his patients exorbitant sums, the doctor could justify his actions by saying: "I was paying then and you have to pay me now. My teacher did not teach me for free."[55] Several documents reveal the financial dimension of such private teaching. A notarial contract, issued at Avignon on October 11, 1486, established the following relationship between Master Joseph Leon of Cavaillon and his student Mordecai (Mordecassius) Astruc Abraham.[56] During a two-year period the master surgeon hoped to teach his student sufficient to enable him to present himself for examination and obtain a license. A tuition fee of twenty-five florins was stipulated, fifteen of which were payable immediately and the other ten only after young Mordecai successfully obtained his license. Also at Avignon, but fifteen years earlier, two Jewish surgeons, Joseph (Josse) Farrusol and Jacob Leon, undertook to teach their art to the Jew, Thomas of Basel.[57] The books of Lanfranc, and of Gui de Chauliac, all medical classics, are specifically mentioned in this contract; Thomas would have to be taught all of them within a year. The surgeons demanded a fee of thirty scudi, to be paid at the end of the period. In yet another agreement the teacher's reward was to be not money but medical books: Astruch Rimoch, a doctor in the Catalonian city of Fraga, was promised a series of books—Avicenna, al-Zahrawi, "Ipocrates cum glossa Galieni," as well as the code of Maimonides—as remuneration for teaching "medical art" to Joseph (Jucef) Avendita, a Jew of Monson. The deal ultimately soured and Joseph brought the doctor to court sometime before August 23, 1381.[58] Finally, in the earliest and best known of these teacher-student contracts from Marseilles, dated August 28, 1326, we see Sara of Saint-Gilles accepting Salvetus de Burgenovo of Salon as a student in order to teach him "the art of medicine and physics." Salvetus must

already have been in the final stages of his education, since the contract suggests a study period of only six months. Instead of receiving a salary or other payments, Salvetus agreed that all the income he would make as an assistant doctor during this period would go to his teacher.[59]

Private education thus emerges as the most common method of training Jewish doctors. Such education was considered a family responsibility and was carried out within its framework. It is even possible that in some cases a few families agreed to hire a teacher who would handle their children as a group. "In Marseilles in the middle of the fifteenth century there seems to have been something in the nature of a Jewish medical school," writes Cecil Roth. His source is a notarial deed issued in Marseilles on September 19, 1443, discovered and interpreted by Dr. L. Barthélemy in a medical context in his history of the doctors of Marseilles in the Middle Ages.[60] The deed describes four Jewish families who hired the master Salomon Gerundini to teach a class of five young men, called *pueri* or *liberi* in this Latin text. These were the two children of Vitalis Cohen, the son of Abraham Astrugii, the son of Ferrerius Marvani, and the son-in-law of Vitalis Amelhuti, whose name was Joseph Cohen. The contract, for a period of one year, promised the master an income of no less than forty-eight florins. Yet was it medicine that he was expected to teach? To my great regret, a close look at at the text does not allow such an interpretation. The words *medicina* or *chirurgia* are totally missing. *Sciencia* is there, but it refers to the master's knowledge, referring to "knowledge" and "expertise in Hebrew letters and in Jewish law." These were the subjects Salomon Gerundini taught in his small class in the year commencing September 19, 1443. It is not impossible that an identical model was employed in medical instruction as well, but so far we have no formal proof.

Similarly, the only known project involving the creation of a Jewish university (*studium generale*) does not make clear that the teaching of medicine was intended, although the language does not exclude this possibility. The document in question is a charter granted to the Jews of Sicily by the king on January 17, 1466.[61] Jews were permitted to create a *studium generale* on

the island and to hire "doctors, experts in law, and masters" to teach there. The document, however, makes no explicit mention of medicine or surgery, and the phrase "whatever approved sciences" ("aprobatas sciencias quascumque") does not necessarily refer to natural sciences. The mention of "experts in law" among the professional personnel of the *studium* may indicate that this institute was intended to teach rabbinics and that here, as in other cases, *studium* is the simple equivalent of the Hebrew *yeshiva*.[62]

Were the Jewish communities willing to help young medical candidates by offering them support or at least exonerating them from communal charges? This may have been the case in the small Catalan city of Cervera, which in 1323 issued legislation exempting all young people from taxation until they reached the age of sixteen.[63] In the case of students, the limit was extended to twenty-three years of age, or as they put it: "those who do not study or pursue literary studies, down to the age of sixteen . . . while those who learn and study— until they reach the age of twenty-three." The word *medicine*, however, is absent from the document. It may or may not have been in the legislators' minds when they talked about "learning."

We can be more affirmative about tax exemption for medical students in the communities of Sicily. A document enacted on May 13, 1413, on behalf of the medical student Moses Bonavogla of Messina, alleges that it is customary in this community to exempt from all taxes those who pursue the study of medicine.[64] In this particular document, the only one of its kind published by the brothers Lagumina, King Ferdinand assures us that he complied with the customary legislation when granting Moses' request and exonerating him from the poll tax (*gisia*) as well as from all other impositions the Jewish community had to carry. Yet can we be sure that this report about medical students and Jewish customary law in Messina is accurate? Did Moses inform the royal chancery properly? The only certainty is that Moses believed that as a student of medicine he was entitled to the traditional exemption Jewish communities granted to rabbinical students (*talmidé ḥachamim* as they are called in Hebrew). These exemptions seem to be as

far as Jewish communities were willing to go. The student and his family were otherwise left on their own in their quest for medical education.

Jewish Students in the Faculties of Medicine

For most of the High Middle Ages neither Jews nor women were admitted to universities. Nonetheless, recent research into the history of Montpellier and its university includes discussion of Jews among the founders of this famous faculty of medicine. Jacob ben Machir, the last great Tibbonide (d. ca. 1307), has even been made the "magister regens" of the faculty.[65] In addition, at least three of the first twenty-two doctors presumed to have practiced in Montpellier in the twelfth century have Hebrew names. These are Isaac ben Abraham and Meschulam and Shem Tov ben Isaac. Although their names are engraved in marble at the entry to the university, Ernest Wickersheimer has shown conclusively that none of these claims, whether for Jacob ben Machir or for any of the other three, has any substantiation in the medieval documents.[66] No text, either in Hebrew or Latin, supports the claim that any of the Jewish scholars named ever taught or even studied at the university. The famous charter that Count Guillem gave to the scholars of Montpellier in 1181 and that is often quoted as proof of liberality and tolerance has been mistakenly read in an anachronistic context of religious toleration. Guillem said: "I wish . . . that all persons whoever they are and wherever they hail from could hold school of physics in Montpellier without hindrance." But Guillem does not have religion or ethnicity in mind. His charter was in fact issued in order to combat monopolies by competing masters seeking to keep students and income for themselves alone.[67] As for Jacob ben Machir, he and some Jewish scholars around him did indeed maintain contacts and exchanges with professors at the university around the year 1300.[68] Jacob knew Bernard Gordon, author of many influential medical treatises; he maintained contacts with Armengaud Blaise, who translated medical writings from Hebrew to Latin. It is most probable that he

also knew Arnold of Villanova, then the most eminent professor of the faculty. He shared with them common interest in astrology and medicine and helped them to translate scientific works from the Arabic. But no document indicates that Jacob ever actually participated in any aspect of university life or that he or any other of his Jewish contemporaries had any wish to do so.

In the second half of the fourteenth century, however, Jewish students show greater interest in the university of Montpellier. Unfortunately, the earliest evidence for such interest is simply incorrect. In a list of the Jews of Avignon for the year 1358 a certain Cresconus de Sancto Paulo is reported as bearing a university title from Montpellier, which would have made him the first Jewish graduate of this institution.[69] But examination of the original, well-preserved parchment in the archives of Avignon (penta 32, pièce 34) reveals only the title *magister* after the man's name; the words "in medicina de Montepessulano" are missing. Moreover, Cresconus was in my opinion not a physician; the title *magister* belonged to the next Jew on the list, Jacob de Villanova.

Nonetheless, Jewish interest in Montpellier's faculty can be shown clearly in a short Hebrew medical treatise labeled *Be'er la-ḥai* (The Well of the Living One," Gen. 16:14) composed in 1370 by Isaac Todrosi, who was then living in Carpentras, not too far from the citadel of learning, and who in 1367 served as one of the secretaries of his community.[70] In his book Todrosi never refers to studies in Montpellier or even to visits to the university, yet he displayed an interest in what was happening there and expressed unrestricted admiration for its master. For instance, Todrosi had been shown by "one of his friends" a new *regimen sanitatis* recently composed by the then chancellor of the university, Jean Jacme. He also knew of the other great man of the time, Jacme's rival, Jean de Tornamira, and had been shown a treatment developed by him. I should add that Tornamira served as a doctor to the pope at Avignon in 1370 and resided in that city, which is very close to Carpentras. For Todrosi, Tornamira was not simply another doctor but rather "the most eminent among the doctors of our times who holds the most distinguished chair [in the university]." Jacme

was treated by Isaac Todrosi with even more reverence: "Doctor, great scholar, among the great experts God even created in any country."[71]

Abraham Avigdor of Arles is the first Provençal Jew to state expressly that he was in Montpellier and studied at its university, which he labeled in Hebrew *yeshiva*.[72] A translator of medical works from Latin to Hebrew and the author of original works in philosophy and logic, Abraham shares with Todrosi his admiration of Montpellier and its professor. Unlike Todrosi, however, Avigdor himself actually attended the university. He refers to this fact, albeit casually, in three prefaces to translations. In what appears to be the earliest of the three, a translation of Gerard de Solo's treatise on fevers, completed in 1379, Avigdor already speaks in the past tense about his stay at Montpellier. The book, he says, came into his hands "when I went up on the mountain [reference to the city] in order to study medical sciences in the distinguished academy of Montpellier." Similarly, two years later, he informs his readers that he found Arnold of Villanova's work on digestive and purgative medicines "when I attended the academy of Montpellier." Abraham elaborates a bit in his third assertion, which prefaces his translation of Bernard Gordon's work *Introduction to the Practice*. There he speaks about his juvenile ambition to be called "master" ("*rav*" in Hebrew) and how he went on to make his dream come true: "I went up on the mountain therefore, that is to say, the city of Montpellier, in order to study the science of medicine from the mouth of the Christian scientists and erudites."[73]

Abraham arouses our curiosity without satisfying our desire for details. He does not give us dates or tell us about the conditions of his studies. We do not know if he obtained the title *magister in medicina*. We ask ourselves: Did he meet other Jewish students? Was his Jewishness an issue? In one of the prefaces he speaks of "friends," probably Christian friends who showed him Gerard Solo's book, but it is not at all certain that friendliness would be the only sentiment a Jewish student would experience there. Judging by evidence from Perpignan, the closest university to Montpellier, the opposite was closer to the truth. A proposal made around 1390 to the university

council sought to revive regulations excluding Jews and other foreigners from the institution. The text reads thus: "Also let a statute be made anew that no one of an alien sect, such as a Jew or Saracen, or anyone else of whatever alien sect he may be, be given instruction by any doctor, master, licentiate, bachelor, scholar, publicly or privately in grammar, logic, philosophy, medicine, or law or other science. And let a good penalty be included as shall have seemed best, so that it may be the better observed."[74] Abraham too may have experienced hostility but did not report it in his brief references.

Our third informant, Leon Joseph of Carcassonne, makes up for the laconic tongue of his contemporary, Abraham Avigdor.[75] Leon Joseph was originally from Perpignan, where he settled in 1372. He studied in Montpellier during the time when Jean of Tornamira was *magister regens* for the second time, that is, between 1384 and 1394. Then he returned to Perpignan, perhaps with the general expulsion of the Jews from France in 1394. He became active in communal affairs and as a doctor. The notarial documents of the city call him *medicus* and *phisicus*.[76] But after he converted to Christianity at the end of his life, sometime between 1414 and 1418, the documents mention his university title. In his new personality he now appears on April 28, 1416, as "Leonardus Benedicti magister in medicina." How should this change in title be interpreted? Were Jews at this time not entitled to this distinction? Did one have to convert in order to obtain it? I can do little more than raise the possibility that this was the case.

Leon Joseph's report, which is in the introduction to his translation of Gerard de Solo's commentary on Razes's *Almansouri*, is particularly long; it has almost two thousand words.[77] He is very personal and talkative and clearly greatly admired the university, which he attended for some time. He was not the only Jewish student around, which emerges indirectly from his comments, but his status at the institution was precarious and dependent on the good will of the chancellor, "Tornamira . . . who used to sustain the Jewish students in all his might." Leon Joseph assures us that he knew personally the great man "who was the head of all scholars of Montpellier, who on their part were subject to his control." Luckily

for Leon Joseph and for the other Jewish students, the tolerant Tornamira was in power and able to counterbalance animosity from other professors. And animosity there was. About this time the scholars of Montpellier, Leon Joseph informs us, issued a hostile decree similar to the one suggested in Perpignan, which was intended to prevent Jewish access to Latin medical works.[78] As he put it: "The scholars of Montpellier would excommunicate and put under ban whoever would sell books to non-Christians." It is therefore not at all clear what Leon Joseph's status as a student was and whether he had any right, on completion of his studies, to the official university title.

All three Hebrew reports express admiration for the university and its professors. Even if some of this praise can be ascribed to a marketing motivation (Leon Joseph wanted to make his readers aware of the importance of Solo's book, its difficulty, and, indeed, its expense), his story nonetheless contains much appreciation and adulation. This is in a way surprising, for at this time Montpellier did not enjoy a reputation in the region and was greatly criticized by students. About the year 1390 the students presented grievances to the city council, complaining about professors who charged too much money to students presenting themselves for examinations and about the mass desertion (*depopulatio*) of pupils who now preferred other *studia* to their own.[79] In 1373 an inhabitant of the coastal city of Hyères in eastern Provence, Antonin son of Foulque Jourdan, expressed his wish to study medicine; he specified that he wished "to go to Perpignan where, so it is said, there are the best and most experienced doctors."[80] In 1379 the possible abandonment of Montpellier altogether had become common knowledge. The councillors of the city of Orange spoke of taking advantage of this decline to move the *studium* to their own city.[81] "Prince," they suggested to the lord of Orange in the session of November 30, 1379, "as the university moves out of Montpellier why don't you make an effort to have it." Little wonder that such pressure prompted Tornamira to show liberality toward Jewish students. And for Jews this presented a wonderful opportunity to obtain the much desired title *magister in medicina*.

Evidence from Italy also confirms the appearance of Jews in the Christian universities. To be sure, no witness like Leon Joseph exists to describe peninsular studies. The most we have is a short notice by a practically unknown Jewish philosopher named Judah Cohen. In a commentary on Averroës' paraphrase of the *Organon*, Judah reminisced briefly about the time he spent studying in the "circle" in Bologna and about a question that was asked of Nicolo di Fava, "the great teacher, rector [probably] of the academy [*Sar ha-yeshivah* in Hebrew]."[82] According to the records of Bologna, Nicolo di Fava taught natural philosophy and medicine between 1406 and 1439, the year of his death, so Judah must therefore have studied there at some time between these dates.[83]

Judah was not the first Jewish student who attended an Italian university or even Bologna. More than fifty years before the earliest possible date that Judah could have attended university, two Jewish men approached the great professor of civil law Bartolo Sassoferrato (1314–1357), claiming the right to be invested with the *laurea*, a university doctorate, which would enable them, among other things, to teach students. Bartolo refused.[84] Referring to the Theodosian code (c.1.9.18), which excluded Jews from "all administrations and dignities," Bartolo claimed that the doctorate was a "dignitas" and thus out of reach for them. He added to this statement the observation that "doctors have ordinary jurisdiction over their students," a situation entirely unacceptable in the framework of Jewish-Christian relations. "I say that Jews who study here cannot obtain the honor of doctorate," states the lawyer, assuring us that Jews were indeed studying there around the 1340s. On two occasions Bartolo is even more specific. The first instance is when he mentions a Jewish student aspiring to the doctorate "this year." The second is when he asserts, "I have said last year to two Jews who were [perfectly] sufficient scholars in medicine that in no way will they get the doctorate as a doctorate is a 'dignity.'" We shall see below how Jews ultimately managed to obtain this dignity. For now it is enough to know that students and candidates of Jewish origin somehow obtained entry into the university of Bologna in the mid-fourteenth century.

Bartolo Sassoferrato does not mention the names of any of the applicants he had to reject. Not until the last quarter of the fourteenth century and the first quarter of the fifteenth are such Jewish students identified by name. The late Réjane Brondy discovered in the municipal archives of Chambéry in Savoy the name of a Jew, the master Isaac, who is referred to in 1396 or 1397 as graduate (*licenciatus*) of the university of Pavia. He may already have been in service there in 1383.[85] The Sicilian student mentioned earlier, Moses Bonavogla of Messina, appears in Padua in 1416. The brothers Lagumina discovered a recommendation written on his behalf in June of that year by John, brother of King Alphonso, to the rectors of the university.[86] Notwithstanding the presence of a Jewish student at this university in 1409,[87] Moses deemed it advisable to solicit royal intervention in order to gain entrance there.

Italian Jews did not abandon their ambitions to acquire the *laurea*. With the support of the papacy, three of them managed to obtain it in the year 1406. The three were Elia di Sabbato da Fermo, Moses of Tivoli, and a certain Moses of Spain. The papal document states that all three received it as a token of recognition for the services they had rendered and were about to render the Holy See.[88] Yet another Jewish doctor, Guillelmo, son of Isaiah of Urbino, received the *laurea* in 1426. An extraordinary document exists for this case, explaining how the "dignitas" was conferred on him, a Jew, and what it entitled him to do.[89] It states first that Guillelmo, whose Hebrew name must have been Benjamin, had studied at the universities of Bologna, Padua, and Siena. His doctorate would entitle him to "read, teach, dispute [and] interpret" at an institution of higher learning, and he would be able to occupy a cathedral chair at the three universities where he studied. It goes without saying that on the occasion of the celebration he received all the usual university *insignia*—a closed book, a ring, and a *biretus*, the appropriate hat. In principle, the *laurea* celebration should have been held in the city's cathedral and administered by dignitaries of the church.[90] But as the candidate this time was Jewish, the university authorities found a way to circumvent the custom. The local bishop was represented by the chancellor of the university who also

happened to be a cleric. And the celebration took place in one of the halls of the university instead of in the cathedral.

Did Guillelmo and the other early Jewish *laureati* actually teach at any of the Italian universities? Two documents suggest that this might have been the case, but both in fact are suspect. The first, dated 1417 or perhaps 1413, comes from the Umbrian city of Perugia and has only recently been brought to the attention of scholarship.[91] It is a page from the municipality's register of payments and expenditures recording the salaries of judges (*judices*) and professors (*doctores*) of the city. One of the individuals listed is Master Musetus Hebreus. As this Moses could not possibly have been a judge, we conclude that he was one of the professors. A quick glance at the title page of the manuscript, however, shows that the words "et magistri" were inserted later above the line to the title of the page.[92] This changes everything since we now have judges, professors, and masters, the last certainly referring to physicians. Thus Moses (Musetus) was probably a physician and we are left with nothing to prove that he was a professor at the local *studium*.

The second document is even more problematic, and it needed Ladislao Münster's insight and hard work to demonstrate how misleading it could be.[93] Although this piece of evidence from the late 1520s exceeds the chronological boundaries of this study, its content merits comment. In March 1528 the senate of the university in Bologna decided to award the Jewish doctor Jacob Mantino a salary of four hundred pounds as an honorarium for his teaching in the local archigymnasium. As Professor Münster discovered in the university account book for April of that year, Mantino was indeed awarded the sum in question. Could there be any doubt that he actually stood, or sat, before his students and taught them that year? The answer is yes. For a search in the later account books of the university failed to reveal the name of the Jewish doctor. He probably did not even reside in the city between 1528 and 1530. What the records do show, or rather conceal, as Professor Münster demonstrates, is the way in which Pope Clement VII, who owed the sum to Mantino, found a way of reimburs-

ing the physician. He did it by putting the sum through the payroll of the university.

One is therefore entitled to suspect whether Guillelmo of Urbino, Moses of Tivoli, or Elia di Sabbato da Fermo, all named *laureati* as we have just seen, were really able to benefit from their diplomas and actually teach at any universities. We are perhaps on much safer ground in considering the titles honorary ones. The Jewish doctors wanted to obtain them because they signified appreciation and official endorsement of their knowledge and skill. Moreover, such recognition enabled them to aspire to much higher fees.

The foundations laid by the fourteenth- and early fifteenth-century Italian Jewish students proved solid. Padua, at least, became a haven for such students, who continued to flock there from all corners of the Jewish world. This was not the case with Montpellier, where the general expulsion of the Jews in 1394 ended the brief experiment of allowing these non-Christian students to enjoy the teaching there. Probably not until the later part of the nineteenth century would Jews be present there once more. But even in the two generations following the Black Death of 1348, the contribution of Montpellier, and for that matter of the Italian universities, to the making of Jewish doctors was at best minor. The majority of Jewish doctors had to study privately and received no university training. In their quest to obtain the proper medical education they had to rely on their own resources. They were forced to develop an entire medical and scientific library. This they did with much energy, using the Hebrew language as their language of study.

3

The Hebrew
Medical Library

The primary task in Jewish medical education was to build up a "Jewish" medical library. The books had to be chosen purposefully and with care so as to include all works mandated by the examination boards for a legitimate medical education. Civil and university authorities made a point of specifying the works candidates were to master in order to pass licensing examinations.

Required Bibliography: Examinations

In Salerno as early as the time of Master Maurus, around 1170, a program was established which used six medical books.[1] A hundred years later when Charles of Anjou became lord of southern Italy, his legislation shows that he worried not only about examination formalities but also about the bibliography candidates had to master.[2] In Paris in 1272 and in Montpellier in 1309 and later in 1340 elaborate *curricula* were conceived and the titles of the required books spelled out. Among the authors were Arabic writers and Greek writers translated from Arabic such as Galen, Ḥunayn ibn Isḥāq, Avicenna, and Isaac Israeli among others. Jews had to find ways of obtaining these books.[3]

A document from Montpellier, dated September 5, 1307,

shows that as part of their examination candidates were asked to perform a *lectio* of a medical text, a technical reading that entailed the explanation of phrases and terms and a general exegesis.[4] Jews too had to become accustomed to using these techniques. The following description is given about the examination of Salomon Avigdor, probably Abraham's son, which took place in Arles in May 1402. Examined by a board of four doctors, one of them Christian, Salomon answered

> in a high and clear voice, with all reverence. First, he elegantly set out his introduction or poem and then put forward his problem in the manner of discussion, expanding the subject in the accustomed manner and intimating that he was prepared to support or to defend it against any opponent as far as his sense, knowledge, and discretion would permit. He stated, moreover, many arguments and in support thereof adduced texts and glossaries out of books, institutes, and canons of the most learned doctors.[5]

Medical texts were naturally the focal point of such examinations, but auxiliary disciplines also had a place. The authorities wanted doctors to show proficiency in logic or metaphysics and, as the fourteenth century progressed, in astrology. The connection between logic and medicine was deemed so natural that in his 1231 legislation the emperor Frederick II made studying this discipline for three years a prerequisite for the study of medicine.[6] Astrology was a less obvious requirement and the subject had its supporters and its critics. The fourteenth-century thinker Cecho de Ascoli, who warned against the practice of medicine without considering the celestial conditions, had to pay with his life for his heretical convictions.[7] But he certainly was not the only one to promote astrology. In 1318 his contemporaries Taddeo of Parma and Arnold of Villanova each composed treatises on astrology for medical students.[8] Their ideas became more and more accepted over time, so that Jewish doctors could not disregard the subject if they wished to be licensed. A report exists to the effect that Bendit Çaravida, when examined on March 22, 1386, had to answer "not only in the art of medicine and physics but also in metaphysics, in natural sciences, and in some

part of astrology."[9] While Samuel Aventuriel (probably Aven-
çuriel), when examined in Murcia in January 1428, was found
knowledgeable "in the arts of logics, philosophy, and medicine" only,[10] another Murcian Jewish doctor, Leon, who informed the city council about his education in 1449, boasted of
his capacity "in logic, in the art of medicine which I practice,
as well as in philosophy and in astrology."[11]

It is almost certain that examinations were conducted in the
regional vernacular, which served as a vehicle of communication between all the committee members, both Jews and
Christians, and the candidate. The books studied, however,
were not written in that language. Christian students had to
know Latin, and Jewish students (those who did not attend
universities; see chap. 2) learned their profession mostly in
Hebrew. In most instances, the examining boards seem to have
been indifferent to the question of language as long as the
candidate knew his subject matter. And yet a sensitivity to this
issue of the language of education is expressed in Venice in
1344.[12] Giovanni (or Guillelmo), son of Mognezio of Rome, a
converted Jew, was examined and accepted into the college of
doctors, notwithstanding the jury's knowledge that he had
studied entirely from Hebrew texts.

Hebrew: The Language of Medical Instruction

The history of the Hebrew language and its service to
Jewish medicine during the High and Late Middle Ages is in
essence the story of the effort to translate a complete scientific
library from Arabic to Hebrew and later, perhaps to a lesser
extent, from Latin to Hebrew.[13] This activity forms yet
another chapter in the cultural history of the medieval West, a
history in which Greek scientific culture was transmitted to
Europe. Recounting the story of translation to Hebrew from
the perspective of Jewish medicine has the advantage of expos-
ing the motivations and even the economic interests of those
scholars who undertook translations and revealing the trouble
they were willing to take to achieve their aims.

The reception of Greek science by Islam dates to the flourishing of Islamic culture in the Middle East in the second half of the eighth century and throughout the ninth. A colossal amount of translation into Arabic, amounting to a planned and systematized project, took place.[14] The major figure in the story is the Nestorian doctor Ḥunayn ibn Isḥāq (808–873), who, together with his disciples, mostly members of his family, translated dozens of scientific works in philosophy, mathematics, and astronomy either directly from Greek or through the intermediary of Syriac. In medicine alone Ḥunayn translated no less than ninety-five Galenic books into Syriac and another thirty into Arabic.[15]

While the Moslem world was ready for this infusion of Greek scientific culture and actually required it, the medieval West, at this time sinking into the shadowy "first feudal age," showed little interest and was not ready for the challenge. Western interest in the scientific legacy of the Greeks only truly developed at the beginning of the eleventh century. Gerbert of Aurillac (ca. 945–1003), later Pope Sylvester II, went to Catalonia as early as 967 in search of Arabic learning. Gerbert was perhaps ahead of his time, but not too much so, for just fifty years after his visit to Catalonia we find scholars in southern Italy engaged in a project to translate Greek works into Latin.[16] Aleksander Birkenmajer and Marie-Thérèse d'Alverny both emphasize this first wave of direct translation from the Greek lest we be blinded by the more famous wave of twelfth-century translation from the Arabic.[17] This early enterprise began in Salerno and Montecassino, where Constantine Africanus (ca. 1015–1087), a convert to Christianity, translated dozens of scientific works from Arabic to Latin.[18] In 1140 the impetus moved to Toledo, under the leadership of the Western Arabist Gerhard of Cremona (1114–1187), who undertook a project similar to that led by Ḥunein some three hundred years earlier.[19]

Jews were very much involved in this effort of transmission through translation. As part of Islamic civilization in Spain, many Jews knew Arabic and possessed Arabic books. As late as the year 1302, when a faculty of medicine was created in Lérida, Aragon, a royal decree presupposed that Arabic books

could be found among the city's Jewish community. The local administration was therefore ordered to make the Jews lend their books to the new Leridan professor, Guillem Jaubert of Béziers.[20] There is evidence that even beyond this date Arabic was used by Jewish doctors in Aragon. The Bibliothèque Nationale in Paris has in its collection a handbook in pharmacology compiled by (or for) Moses ibn Ardut of Huesca around the year 1350 (ms. héb. 1082) as well as a fourteenth-century compendium of medical treatises by Hippocrates, Galen, and Maimonides written in Hebrew letters but in the Arabic language.[21]

Jews may have taken part in translating from Arabic at a relatively early date. José María Millás Vallicrosa believed that Jews were already translating Arabic works into Latin as early as the tenth century.[22] Certainly by the beginning of the twelfth century their presence on the scene was obvious. In the 1140s Abraham bar Hiya of Barcelona, an astronomer and mathematician of great merit, is known to have collaborated with Plato of Tivoli in such translations.[23] Abraham ibn David, ("Avendaut"), a young contemporary who was a historian and philosopher, was active at the translation center in Toledo, where the central figure was Gerhard of Cremona.[24] It is also possible that the documents we possess today do not provide a complete picture of the place Abraham (himself of Andalusian origin) held in the story of translation. The same is probably true of another Jew, Moses, a convert to Christianity who assumed the name Petrus Alphonsi. With his knowledge of Arabic, he too may have played a much bigger role in this stage of Western cultural development than we know today.[25]

Interest in translation did not diminish in the thirteenth century, and Jews were once again invited to participate in the process of transmission. In southern Italy in the 1230s Jacob Anatoli, one of the Tibbonides, was invited to Palermo and Naples to the scholarly court of the emperor Frederick II.[26] In later years Jewish translators such as Moses of Palermo and Faraj of Agrigento were active under the rule of the Angevins. In Spain at the initiative of King Alfonso X (the Wise) Toledo engaged in a second wave of translations in the middle of the century.[27] Judah ben Moses ("al-Cohen," "el menor"),

Yehuda ben Salomon ("Ibn Mosca"), Abraham al-Faquim ("Ibn Wakar"), Samuel ha-Levi, and Isaac ha-Ḥazan ben Sid (known also as "Cag" or "Rabicag Aben Cayut") played perhaps an even greater role here than some of their coreligionists had done a century earlier. They translated works on astronomy and astrology into the vernacular and built astronomical instruments. Later in the thirteenth and at the beginning of the fourteenth centuries we find Arabists like Judah Bonsenior in Catalonia and Kalonymos ben Kalonymos of Arles still active as translators in the court of Naples.[28] As the fourteenth century progressed, however, Jewish contributions to the effort of the translation diminished until they practically ceased.

At the same time as Jewish scholars were translating Arabic works into Latin or the vernacular, others were rendering scientific works into Hebrew. Some even undertook both. This insistence on maintaining Hebrew as a language of science was in part a result of a certain tradition, even if a very recent one, of translating philosophical works from the Arabic into Hebrew.[29] These early translations were carried out in the south of France and were sponsored by the Talmudic scholar Meshulam ben Jacob of Lunel, who as a wealthy man found ways to finance this enterprise.[30] He and the people around him were interested principally in the works of the great Jewish philosophers originally written in Arabic. In the third quarter of the twelfth century Meshulam persuaded immigrant intellectuals of Andalusian extraction, contemporaries of Abraham ibn David of Toledo, to translate these classics of Jewish philosophy into Hebrew. At times parallel translations to the Hebrew were solicited, manifestly in order to check one against the other. Thus Saʿadiah's work and those of Baḥya ibn Pakuda, Judah (Yehudah) ha-Levi, and Maimonides were translated twice.[31] Joseph ibn Zabara, Joseph and David Kimḥi, Judah al-Ḥarizi, and especially Judah ibn Tibbon and his son Samuel, all Andalusians, took part in the project. Meshulam thus created a "school" of translators in Lunel and its surrounding cities; his role was similar to that of Raymond de la Sauvetat (1125–1152), archbishop of Toledo, and his successor, archbishop Jean (1152–1166), who two generations

earlier had patronized the important school of translators in his city.[32] By 1200 the *Guide for the Perplexed*, the major Jewish philosophical work of the Middle Ages, had been translated twice into Hebrew; its author, Moses Maimonides, was still living. He was in contact through letters with the translator Samuel ibn Tibbon and actually helped in translating the treatises into Hebrew.[33] In the ensuing years a "Maimonidean myth," founded on fact, to be sure, would govern Jewish spirits in southern Europe, and young Jewish intellectuals, the future physicians, would see in him an exemplary figure, a hero whose intellectual posture and career should be emulated.[34]

The direction of translation to Hebrew changed in the beginning of the thirteenth century. Arabic and other non-Jewish authors now received consideration, and attention turned to specialized, technical works rather than general philosophies. In Béziers in 1199 Samuel ibn Tibbon translated Galen's *Microtegni* with a commentary by 'Ali ibn Ridhwān.[35] Fourteen years later, while returning from a visit to Egypt, he completed his translation of Aristotle's treatise *Meteorologica*. He did so, he reports, between the islands of Lampedusa and Pantelleria.[36] Samuel's successors were three members of his own family: Jacob Anatoli, Jacob ben Machir, and, especially, Moses ibn Tibbon, Samuel's son.[37] They all became involved in translating specialized scientific treatises. Moses, Samuel's son, the most prolific of all three translators, translated into Hebrew medical works by Galen, Avicenna, Razes, and Averroës, along with many others.[38] One reason he engaged in such technical and uninspiring works (even his translations of Maimonides were of the master's medical treatises rather than his theological or political works) must obviously have been the demand for this literature. What is more, in the 1250s the contemporary professional Jewish world was apparently able to remunerate the translator for his effort.

The Economics of Translation

Financial reward and "supply and demand" certainly played a role in the history of these translations. By the 1250s

material compensation for professional effort was an accepted norm, and there is no reason to exclude translators from this social reality. Documents that have surfaced here and there in Mediterranean archives certainly reveal that remuneration was a motivation for undertaking translations. This is clearly stated in a contract enacted on March 2, 1296, at the demand of Vitalis Benvenist de Porta. He was about to translate "from Arabic to Roman language, certain books of medicine" that the Aragonese monarch considered "very much necessary for us." Benvenist was to be paid two shillings a day by the bailiff of Barcelona for the period of the translation. He would also be provided with paper and suitable clothing. On his part, the translator undertook to deliver, once a month, all the "quaternos" he had translated.[39]

The best-documented case study in this matter is that of Faraj (Mose), son of Salim, of Agrigento, who worked for the Angevin court between 1278 and 1282. Recent scholarship has raised the possibility that he might have been the philosopher Moses ben Salomon of Salerno, but this is impossible since, according to the philosopher's tombstone, Moses died on 15 Shvat, 5039 (30 January 1279) while Faraj was still active three years after that date.[40] His name, also transcribed in the documents as "Farasius," "Farragut," or "Farresche," indicates an Arabic-speaking country of origin for himself or his immediate family.[41] In a short period of three years Faraj translated at least three medical works into Latin. The first was Razes's very important medical encyclopedia al-Hawi (Liber continens), which he translated between February 2, 1278, and February 13, 1279. The second was a pseudo-Galenic treatise, labeled in some manuscripts Liber de medicis expertis and in others De expositionibus vocabulorum seu sinonimorum simplicis medicine, which Steinschneider believed to be part of the Liber continens. We know that he started to work on this in October 1280, but no date of completion is given. The third work was a treatise in pathology written by Abu 'Ali ibn Ghazāla called Tacuynus or Tacuini aegritudinum morborum corporis, which he finished translating on March 2, 1281.[42]

The rich archives of the Angevins of Naples, before their destruction in World War II, allowed the German-Jewish

scholar Willy Cohn to investigate the financial conditions
under which Faraj worked.[43] It becomes clear that Faraj and
his colleagues expected to be remunerated for each stage of
their work: for translating, copying, even proofreading. Cohn
discovered that when translating Razes, Faraj was entitled to a
daily allowance of one and a half gold tari (seven and a half
tari made one gold karlin) and that when he had accomplished
his task he was awarded a gift: "two cases, good, and of big
size" which were delivered to Castel Nuovo, where he probably lived at the time. In 1282 Faraj and a man called "Cinus"
read galley proofs of two copies of the *Tacuinus*. For this
proofreading, which required twenty days of work, he did not
receive more than twelve tari. In another document dated
April 3, 1278, Count Charles of Anjou ordered that the Jew
"Faresche" be given three ounces of gold, no doubt in connection with his work. Another person, "Moises Li Juif tras-
lateur," is rewarded on this occasion with two ounces, equal to
ten florins, for translating the pseudo-Hippocratic *Liber de
curationibus infirmitatum equorum*.[44]

Documents concerning other translators, while not as informative as the ones we have just examined, nevertheless
confirm that remuneration was standard in this period. Thus in
Aragon in 1313 Judah (Jafuda) Bonsenior received the sum of
a thousand shillings for translating a medical work. The title of
the work is not easily deciphered in the manuscript. Some
scholars suggest that it may have been the famous *al-Zahrawi*,
known in Arabic as the *Kitāb al-Taṣrif*.[45] This identification
may be doubted not so much on paleographic grounds but because the sum paid seems far too modest for a book like *al-
Zahrawi*, one of the most voluminous in the Arabic medical
library.

Another model of remuneration, this time without the support of a patron, appears in 1316 in connection with a Hebrew
translation of the *Kitāb al-Taṣrif*, or *al-Zahrawi* as it was
commonly known.[46] Composed in Andalusia by Abu-Qāsim
Khalaf ibn 'Abbas al-Zahrāwī ("Abulcasis"), this classic encyclopedia of medicine and surgery in thirty books, was first translated into Hebrew in the thirteenth century in Marseilles by a
translator whose name was Shem Tov ben Isaac of Tortosa

(1198–d. after 1264).[47] Shem Tov explained in his introduction that he completed a first version of the translation in the years 1254–1258 and then revised it in 1261;[48] he also expressed the hope that his work would serve as his monument to posterity since (like the famous Isaac Israeli to whom a similar statement was attributed[49]) he had no heir to carry his name. But Shem Tov must have had some family in Marseilles. In 1280 a man named Abraham of Tortosa ("Tortuensis") was working, along with Simon of Genoa, on a translation of parts of the al-Zahrawi into Latin, perhaps from Hebrew.[50] Furthermore, in our 1316 model contract concerning the al-Zahrawi the name of the book's owner was given as "Mossonus [i.e., Moses] son of master Abraham." "Master Abraham" is possibly the Abraham "Tortuensis" mentioned earlier.[51]

Let us turn our attention to this private contract of 1316 arranging for the copying of one exemplar of the al-Zahrawi. In essence this document is a model for private remuneration to translators and also, quite unexpectedly, to their heirs. In other words, this is an early experiment in securing a translator's copyright. In addition to receiving payment, the al-Zahrawi's owner wanted the circulation of the book to be restricted and limited. He therefore asked the man who wanted the copy, a doctor from Avignon named Bonfil, to execute the copying personally. The Avignon doctor was also to assure the owner that he would not let this new copy be copied by a third party and to promise that after his death if he did not have a male heir interested in medicine, the exemplar he himself had copied would be given back to Moses or, presumably, to his family. All copying had to be completed within a year. A handsome sum of twenty florins was requested as remuneration. All this, we must remember, was required by someone who belonged to the generation of the original translator's grandchildren. In other words, more than fifty years after its completion, the translation remained an economic asset within the family of the man who originally expended his time, effort, and knowledge on the work.

This Hebrew translation of the al-Zahrawi is well known today. Several copies, some of them magnificently illustrated, are preserved in depositories of Hebrew manuscripts, for

example, in Oxford or Paris. One of these manuscripts was completed as early as 1269, only a few years after Shem Tov finished his revision of the translation.[52] The copy was done in the city of Trets, close to Marseilles, and it is possible that the local Jewish doctor who ordered it knew Shem Tov personally and obtained the copy directly from him. We have contemporary information (in a recently published Hebrew letter) about how personalized such medieval relationships were and how doctors set about acquiring books that interested them.[53] This is a letter that the famous Italian philosopher Hillel ben Samuel of Verona (ca. 1220–1295) wrote to his friend Isaac, known as Master Gaio, the pope's doctor, in which he asked for two medical treatises by Maimonides, his commentary on Hippocrates' *Aphorisms* and his own *Aphorisms*, translated into Hebrew by Nathan ha-Me'ati and known as *The Chapters of Moses* (*Pirke Moshe*). Hillel already possessed the Latin translation of Hippocrates by Constantine the African as well as a commentary by Burgundius of Pisa; he still wanted to have the Maimonidean commentary in order to resolve the "hundred" queries he had. "Do not care about the cost," writes Hillel to his friend, "and make a scribe copy them . . . and I shall immediately send you the scribe's salary and [the price of] the paper and the corrections, as much as demanded. Even if it turns out to be a substantial expenditure it will become smaller [in my mind] when considering how much I love them [the books]." The short letter ends with a sentence somewhat difficult to decipher completely but whose sense is still understandable: perhaps Master Gaio would be willing to offer the undertaking first to the "grandson of R. Nathan," possibly the translator ha-Me'ati. If the grandson refused the task, Isaac could hire whomever he chose.

To find three generations of the ha-Me'ati family involved in translating and copying medical works recalls the *al-Zahrawi* of Marseilles and the arrangements surrounding it.[54] We do not have any information about the economic arrangements that lay behind this enterprise, but they must have existed. Nathan and his son Salomon translated such works as Maimonides' medical aphorisms and Galen's commentary on Hippocrates' treatise on airs, waters, and places,[55] not to mention

Avicenna's monumental *Canon of Medicine*. Surely they expected that both they and their descendants would be remunerated for their efforts.

Like most of these translators, Nathan ha-Me'ati and his son Salomon are today little more than names. We are content if we are able to be relatively certain about where and when they were working. The same is true of most other translators. An exception is Kalonymos ben Kalonymos of Arles, who left not only numerous translations, all carried out in the first quarter of the fourteenth century, but also some original work.[56] The most important of these are two long personal letters, one written in 1305 when he ran away to Barcelona in the hope of increasing and deepening his knowledge of Arabic, the other written in 1314 or 1324 when he was in Naples, helping with translations at the court of King Robert "the Wise."[57] Kalonymos is also the author of a polemical letter against his contemporary, the philosopher Joseph ibn Kaspi, and is appreciated in the history of Hebrew letters for his book of social critique, *Touchstone*.[58] Between 1307 and 1308 Kalonymos translated 'Ali ibn Ridwān's *Colonne des Racines*, Galen's *De clysteriis* (*On clysters and Colic*), and Galen's *Venesection* for the use of Jewish doctors. He also translated Averroës' commentaries on Aristotle's *Topics*, *Sophistics*, and *Metaphysics* as well as many other scientific works.[59] His name came to royal attention and he was in Naples at least once, for he sent his family quite a depressed letter from there. Yet his status in life must have been high, precisely because of his success at court. Immanuel of Rome, in a letter addressed to Kalonymos's family in Arles, talks about Kalonymos's notoriety, his prestige, and his success, all resulting from his service as a translator.[60] Intervening on behalf of the Jews of Rome, Kalonymos was able to obtain a royal privilege for them and thus apparently to annul hostile measures contemplated against them by the Inquisition. We do not have details about this political intervention, but the sixteenth-century historian Salomon ibn Verga also knew that King Robert intervened on behalf of the Jews of Rome, who were threatened by the pope with expulsion.[61] Kalonymos enjoyed not only prestige but also some wealth toward the end of his life. An entry in the payroll of the Angevin

administration for the year 1329, the last time we hear of him, states that the royal bailiff of Arles allocated the annual sum of six ounces of gold, the equivalent of thirty florins, to "Master 'Calo' . . . for the translation of certain books and for other services."[62] That a scholar could hope for such a spectacular career and for such handsome remuneration in the first quarter of the fourteenth century indicates how viable the translations market was at the time and how prepared people were to invest in medical education.

Building the Hebrew Medical Library: Strategy and Timing

The translators' task was to supply medical works and treatises in auxiliary sciences for the use of the ever growing number of practitioners. By 1400 all the most important medical books known to the Arabs and also many of the more recent Latin medical treatises composed in medieval universities and elsewhere had been translated into Hebrew. All these works had to be translated for Jews to study and to practice in accordance with the standards of the time. What is less clear is the individual translator's reason for working on one specific book rather than another at any given date. Was the choice arbitrary? Did it depend on the translator's professional or economic interests? Did the availability of an Arabic or Latin manuscript make the difference? Or should we look rather for developments within the profession?

We shall probably never have firm answers to these questions for most of the treatises translated during our period because we simply lack the documents. There is one book, however, for which we can attempt an answer. This is Avicenna's *Canon of Medicine*, the most important medical book in the High Middle Ages and certainly the most influential. This great *summa* of Greco-Arabic medicine in five parts (the human body, ailments and their treatments, materia medica, pathology, and fevers and their accidents) was composed by Avicenna (980–1038), the greatest Arabic physician of the Middle Ages.[63] The *Canon*, whole or in part, was trans-

lated into Hebrew several times.[64] First, Nathan ben Eli'ezer
ha-Me'ati translated all five parts in Rome, an enterprise that
took some years to accomplish and was completed in 1279. A
few years later, probably also in Italy, a famous translator and
thinker of Catalan origin, Zeraḥiah ben Shealtiel Ḥen (Graçian)
(1217–1294), translated books 2 and 3 of the *Canon* on their
own. Finally in 1402 Joseph ben Joshua ha-Lorki undertook a
revision of Nathan ha-Me'ati's translation of the first two
books. These, however, were not the only translations made.
A recent and comprehensive study of the Hebrew manuscripts
of the *Canon* noticed that other translations existed, made by
translators whose names are not known. The *Canon*, quite expectedly, became the most popular book in the Jewish medical
library.[65] Benjamin Richler described more than a hundred
codexes, more than any other medical work preserved in
today's libraries or museums. To facilitate the *Canon*'s use, one
of the greatest Jewish physicians of the Middle Ages, Jeda'iah
ha-Penini (ca. 1270–ca. 1340), composed a commentary in
about 1300.[66] He was followed by others, at least thirty and
perhaps more, as Moritz Steinschneider's list shows.[67] It must
be added that the *Canon* was one of the rare medical works
printed in the sixteenth century and was still being used as late
as the eighteenth century by a Persian Jewish doctor, as the
copy preserved at the Houghton Library of Harvard University shows.

While Avicenna's *Canon* was translated into Hebrew in
1279, it had been translated into Latin a hundred years or
more earlier, at the latest in 1187. In fact, this translation was
one of the first projects Gerhard of Cremona undertook in
Toledo.[68] How, therefore, can this hiatus of one hundred
years between the Hebrew and the Latin be explained? Why
were the Jews so slow to translate it? Why did translators prefer to concentrate their efforts on other works, such as the *al-
Zahrawi*, before turning to the *Canon*? Did they not feel dis-
advantaged in comparison with their Christian competitors?
Recent studies indicate that this delay did not in fact constitute
any handicap to the Jewish medical profession and that,
moreover, the timing of the translation into Hebrew was
perfect. Several scholars[69] have pointed out that medical

faculties took no interest in the *Canon* until the second half of the thirteenth century. This interest began in Paris and reached Montpellier in the 1280s and Bologna and Siena around the same time. The *Canon's* reception in Montpellier was, however, neither easy nor self-evident. While Bernard Gordon, one of the two major professors, pushed very hard for Avicenna's work to become part of the official curriculum, the other professor, Arnold of Villanova, preferred to promote Razes's *Liber continens*, which was translated into Latin in the late 1270s.[70] In any event, only one hundred years after Gerhard of Cremona translated the *Canon* into Latin did it became relevant to scholars. For almost an entire century the work remained buried, like dead wood, on the shelves. It is no wonder that between 1170 and 1270 Jews did not feel compelled to translate it. With the emergence of the "New Galenism" in the 1280s, when Avicenna's work was expected to increase understanding of Galen, Jewish translators were quick to react and, as we have seen, did so quite energetically.

Similarly, the motives for translation of what may be called auxiliary sciences and for preparation of commentaries by Jewish intellectuals are not difficult to discern. As noted, a doctor was expected to be educated in these sciences as well.[71] Consequently, translators went beyond physiology, dietetics, and therapy and looked for works in logic, metaphysics, mathematics, astronomy, or astrology, in addition to those in botany, biology, and zoology.[72] Jewish doctors knew the entire "corpus Aristotelicum," although mainly through Averroës' elaboration. Moses ibn Tibbon and his relative Jacob Anatoli worked on Averroës' commentaries on the *Organon*, the collection of Aristotle's eight treatises on logic.[73] This was presented to Hebrew-reading intellectuals along with a translation of Porphyrius's *Isagoga*, which formed an introduction to the *Organon*.[74] Scholars of the caliber of Levi ben Gershon— Gersonides—(1288–1342) and his contemporary Jeda'iah ha-Penini and later Abraham Avigdor and Judah Cohen also wrote Hebrew commentaries to facilitate the study of these treatises on logic.[75] Aristotle's writings were now physically incorporated into the Hebrew heritage and young men were exposed to his *Phisics, De generatione et corruptione, Historia*

animalium, De caelo, and *Meteora.* Original scientific works by Arab scholars were not neglected either.[76] In addition to Averroës' commentaries on Aristotle, translators also spent time on the works of Costa ben Luca, Avicenna, or al-Btaljusi.[77] Studies in geometry, arithmetic, and optics received attention. When astrology became legitimate, or even indispensable, in Montpellier, such men as Jacob ben Machir ensured that relevant treatises, such as Ibn al-Shaffar's work on the making of the astrolabe, found their way into the Hebrew library.[78]

Encyclopedias and introductory compendia facilitated studies and introduced young men to the sciences. In the thirteenth century three Hebrew authors made significant contributions in this respect. The first, Gershon ben Salomon of Arles, who was possibly Gersonides' father, wrote a three-part work, *Gates of Heaven,* which was a detailed presentation of the natural sciences, astronomy, and theology.[79] The chapters concerned with anatomy and physiology and those where the author presented his own clinical observations were especially interesting to medical students. The second author, Judah ben Salomon ha-Cohen ibn Matka of Toledo, was probably active in the scholarly court of King Alphonso X. His fame as a scholar reached the emperor Frederick II, who exchanged letters with him for more than ten years and finally invited him to visit Tuscany.[80] Judah produced an introductory work similar to that of Gershon ben Salomon, written first in Arabic and then translated into Hebrew under the title *Midrash ha-Hochmah.*[81] The third author was Shem Tov Falaquera (ca. 1225–ca. 1295), a member of a well-known Navarese family. His introduction to the sciences took the form of a story, *Maqama,* and was entitled *Reshit Hokhmah* (Initiation to Sciences).[82] In 1314, Kalonymos ben Kalonymos of Arles found it opportune to translate Alfarābi's *Classification of Sciences* and his letter concerning the order of learning.[83] Incidentally, Falaquera's *Maqama* includes his translation of Alfarābi's *Classification.*

Arabic scientific works seem to have furnished the essential Jewish medical arsenal. Until the first quarter of the fourteenth century and even later, Jews turned to this source for

materials. Beginning in the last quarter of the thirteenth century, however, a new trend gained momentum among translators as Jews turned to Latin and to books written in Latin in their quest for medical and scientific inspiration. J. L. Teicher in a famous study suggested that a prototype of this trend can be detected in Catalonia as early as the mid-twelfth century.[84] But this early example had no lasting influence and the trend did not come into full view until the second half of the thirteenth century. Moritz Steinschneider has shown that in the south of France about 1250 Salomon ben Moses of Melgueil translated Avicenna's *De caelo et mundo* as well as *De somno et vigilia* from Latin, not Arabic.[85] But it was in Italy, where Jews had no difficulty in learning Latin, that we first notice a concentrated effort to translate from that language. Judah ben Moses ben Daniel Romano (1292–1350), the brother of Immanuel, translated works by Aegidius Romanus, Albertus Magnus, and Thomas Aquinas, among others, an effort that incidentally had little influence on the later history of Jewish literature or philosophy.[86] Hillel of Verona, the only Jewish thinker who appears to have taken these translations into account in his own philosophical work *Tagmulé ha-Nefesh* (Book of the Rewards of the Soul), translated Bruno di Lungoburgo's work on surgery and 'Ali ibn Ridwān's commentary on Galen's *Tegni* from Latin to Hebrew.[87] Jacob ben Elia, a Provençal working in the city of Venice, became friendly with a local scholar, Patarinus, and with his help translated another medical treatise by Ibn Zohr from Latin to Hebrew.[88] About 1300 another Provençal, Jacob ben Machir, enjoyed close scientific relationships with the professors of Montpellier.[89] It is perhaps possible at his instigation that between 1299 and 1300 the otherwise unknown Jacob ben Joseph ha-Levi (Jacob of Alesto) translated some works by Arnold of Villanova, who was then a professor in the faculty at Montpellier.[90] Ben Machir himself translated Arnold's *Regimen sanitatis* (*Arnaldina*) into Hebrew sometime before 1306, but his work was lost in the confusion resulting from the expulsion of the Jews from France in that year. Another translation was made about twenty years later by Israel Caslari (1322), who in his introduction tells the story of the lost manuscript.[91]

But it was in the last quarter of the fourteenth century that the quality of these translations reached its peak. Hebrew scholars like Abraham Avigdor or Jekuthiel ben Salomon of Narbonne, who were themselves students at Montpellier, translated into Hebrew the works of the great masters of Montpellier: Bernard Gordon's *Lilium medicine*, Gui de Chauilac's *Great surgery*, and, of course, the work of Arnold of Villanova.[92] In addition, the works of the acting masters of the faculty, such as Jean Jacme and Jean of Tornamira, were incorporated into the Hebrew library.[93] These late fourteenth-century translators had a much more difficult task than did their predecessors. The unwillingness of those in the university world to allow Jews to have copies of such treatises meant translators had to go to much more trouble and expense in order to obtain them. Leon Joseph of Carcassonne may have exaggerated his description of the troubles he himself experienced (see pp. 30–31 above) in order to make his translation of Gerhard de Solo more appreciated by customers. The general tenor of his testimony, however, leaves little room for doubt that he did indeed have problems.[94] Moreover, he complained that Jewish doctors of his time did not consider medicine a science, so they did not invest time in studying it or in expanding their knowledge. As he rightly observed, the Jews, having exhausted Arabic sources and not having developed a significant literature of their own, were now at the mercy of their Christian colleagues for enriching their library.

Leon Joseph's complaint about the lack of original Jewish work is in principle justified. In the High or Late middle ages no Jewish doctors composed major medical treatises equivalent to the *summae* of Arnold of Villanova or Bernard Gordon. The most important treatise in practical gynecology, *Sefer ha-Toledet*, for example, has its origin in the *Gynaïkea*, written in Greek by Soranos of Ephesus and translated to the Latin sometime in the sixth century by a certain "Muscio." Its translation into Hebrew must have taken place in the thirteenth century in the south of France.[95] Ron Barkaï, who recently published the treatise, reminds us also that another medical book in Hebrew, *Balsam of the Body* (Zeri ha-Guf) by Nathan Falaquera, which has no less than 167 folios in the

Ambrosiana Library in Milan (ms. no. 99) and 203 folios in the Bibliothèque Nationale in Paris (ms. no. 1192, incomplete), borrows essentially from Arab authors. Falaquera himself acknowledges his indebtedness.[96] Nevertheless, there was some creativity, although very rarely noted by modern scholars. It was genuinely Jewish in that it was written in Hebrew and intended for the use of Jewish practitioners. The miscellaneous collections of short medical treatises in the Bodleian Library in Oxford or the Ambrosiana in Milan include notices by doctors like Sheshet Benvenisti, Salamias Davin of Lunel, Moses ben Ardut, Isaac de Lates, or even Gersonides or the still unidentified Jacob ha-Levi of Alès.[97] After 1348, when Jews were accused of initiating the plague, some Jewish writers composed original works, like Abraham Caslari's *Pestilential Fevers*, which put forward medical explanations for the spread of the disease.[98] These were isolated efforts, however, and did not amount to a genuine medical tradition. Symptomatic of the decline of medical creativity among the Jews is the fact that the most prolific Jewish medical writer of that time was Moses ben Isaac ibn Waqār, who flourished in the beginning of the fifteenth century.[99] He wrote at least four medical treatises: *'Ezer ha-Beri'ut* (Assistance to Health), *Mekor Hayyim* (Origin of Life), *Milhamot ha-Refu'ah* (The Wars of Medicine), and one whose title is unknown (the manuscript is preserved in the library in the city of Munich). As far as we know, none of his works had much impact on the history of medicine.

We have reached the point where we are entitled to draw some conclusions concerning the system of medical education developed by the Jews of the High and Late Middle Ages. The first concerns educational facilities. Jews, unable for most of the period to gain access to universities, and initially probably uninterested, had to rely on private initiative or family relationships in order to prepare for examinations so that they could be certified by civil authorities. Second, Jews had the primary task of investing talent, money, and effort in translating an entire medical library into Hebrew, mostly from Arabic, in order to acquire knowledge of what were considered the medical classics of the time. Nonetheless, they achieved their

aim. The medieval Hebrew library was probably richer in volumes than the one that exists today in Israel, where four universities teach medicine in Hebrew but use English textbooks. Much of the vitality of which medieval Jewish medicine boasted resulted from direct access to the rich literature in Arabic. But Jewish doctors found themselves in difficulty once these sources were exhausted and they had to turn to works in Latin.

Many Jewish doctors enjoyed considerable success and were at the service of monarchs, princes, and prelates. But we should not infer any universal appreciation for the products of the Jewish educational system; it had its critics as well. Around 1426, for example, in Pernes in the Comtat Venaissin, the municipality and the governors of the county insisted on examining all Jewish doctors, no doubt in order to weed out the incompetents.[100] Some twenty-five years later in the city of Burgos, Castille, a graduate of a university was hired as a municipal doctor to join an existing group of colleagues, most of them Jewish. One of his first tasks was to make his colleagues appear before him and be examined "a dar razon de sus oficios."[101]

The titles that Jews generally carried—*medicus, phisicus, chirurgicus*—were undoubtedly legally valid. But a university graduate holding a title like *magister in medicina* or even *bacellarius in medicina* enjoyed immediate seniority over all *phisici* and *medici* around him. When Peter the Ceremonious (1336–1387), king of Aragon, organized the medical services of his palace in 1344, he also established a hierarchy for the two doctors in his service. If both had equal titles, the one who was hired first would become the senior. But if only one of them happened to have a university degree, he was then automatically awarded leadership.[102] It is hardly surprising then that in the late fourteenth century Jews tried to gain admittance to universities and to obtain the desired degrees. Yet those who did not succeed still had a chance in the profession. Skill, success, and reputation were well remunerated and were not out of reach for other practitioners, even if they were Jewish.

4

Reputation: Brilliant Medical Careers

Some Jewish doctors in the Middle Ages enjoyed spectacular success. Their careers as revealed in medieval documents outshine similar success stories of Jewish practitioners in Wilhelmine Germany or in the United States of America today. When we remember that these physicians and surgeons followed a religion that was considered the arch-enemy of the governing one and that they belonged to a social group simultaneously feared and despised, their achievement becomes even more remarkable. "Success" in this particular context does not merely mean professional recognition or monetary compensation. It also means prestige and high position. We can chronicle dozens of Jewish doctors who found their way into the service of kings and princes and were employed by barons, counts, and prelates. As a result, in many instances they became intimate with the sources of power in society. At times they were privy to state secrets, entrusted with diplomatic missions, and even consulted in policy-making. They were entitled to rights and privileges most people did not enjoy and they were sometimes able to help their brethren in distress. Other Jews, whether living in the vicinity or in distant countries, knew of these doctors of great repute and were proud of them. The "royal" doctors became the heroes of Jewish society, the equivalent of modern role models, and the myth of their success inspired young people to fol-

low the same path. Thus, around the year 1200 the fame of the doctor and courtier Sheshet of Barcelona spread as far as the Rhine valley. A German Jew, Salomon ben Ḥanan'el, traveled all the way from Mainz to the city of Barcelona in Catalonia so that the great master could operate on him.[1] In 1180 or 1190 in Lunel in southern France, Sheshet was invoked by Judah ibn Tibbon in a letter to his son Samuel as an example to the young man to encourage him to widen and improve his command of the Arabic language. Judah's letters to his son show clearly that the study of Arabic created opportunities for Jews in a society that was otherwise not very accommodating.[2] We may assume that parents made an effort to discover medical talent in their children and cultivate them in the same way that later generations evoked and encouraged an aptitude for music and mathematics.

The documentation for these Jewish medical successes is abundant. As these prominent doctors moved in the highest levels of society, the chanceries of the magnates, especially the crown of Aragon, preserved numerous records of their activities. Dozens of letters inviting Jewish doctors—always urgently—to help an ailing member of the family are accompanied by hundreds of orders issued to the treasury and other agencies regarding their remuneration. On occasion members of the princely class wrote to each other about their doctors, recommending them or begging that they be sent to their courts to assist in a crisis. As a result, the careers of some practitioners are quite handsomely illustrated, providing the most detailed biographies of any Jews living in the Middle Ages. It is therefore tempting to investigate the attitudes of these powerful clients toward their Jewish practitioners and the particular system of remuneration and compensation.

Doctors in Princely Courts

It was nothing new for Jewish doctors to become part of a princely retinue in Spain during the Reconquista. Under Moslem rule, both in the East and in the West, Jewish doctors

found their way to these courts as early as the tenth century. The well-known examples of Ḥasdai ibn Shaprut,[3] Isaac Israeli, and Moses Maimonides[4] and the less well-known one of Joseph ben Isaac ibn Bilkirish at the court of the sultan of Saragossa (ca. 1100)[5] are just a few of dozens known today. What makes the epoch of the Spanish Reconquista a fascinating subject for study is the abundance of documents that illuminate these court doctors. We know the conditions under which the doctors worked, their relationships with rulers, and their remuneration. To quote a typical example: Master Joseph (Juceff) Cavaller of Cervera spent forty-one days at the castle of the seigneur of Bellvehí caring for Lady Beatrice in what turned out to be her last illness.[6] His salary was two florins per day. A Christian doctor who spent only twenty days there was paid the same daily fee.

Jews were not the only doctors in such princely courts. The Jewish doctor was usually one of many and was invited to join an existing group, described as "the college of our doctors." It was not even unusual to have several Jews concurrently in the medical cohort (*consortium*) of a ruler. Joachim Miret y Sans found no fewer than 11 Jews—and only 6 Christians—serving in the 1330s as royal doctors of King Pedro IV of Aragon.[7] Nonetheless, Jews did not necessarily constitute a majority in such a college. Only 38, or at most 40, of the 323 thirteenth- and fifteenth-century practitioners listed by Ramón Jordí y González were Jewish.[8]

A "royal" doctor would very often be referred to not as *medicus* or *phisicus* but rather as *alfaquim* or, in Latinized form, *alfaquimus*. In the Middle East there is no difficulty in understanding the term. S. D. Goitein showed that the name was derived from the Arabic *ḥakīm*, "the physician" or even "the scholar."[9] In Reconquista Spain, however, the institutional dimensions of the profession are somewhat more awkward to define. David Romano has shown in a remarkable series of studies that the *alfaquim* in Spain was seen not only as a doctor but also as an interpreter to the court.[10] Historians today are rightly perplexed by this combination of medical, diplomatic, and linguistic skills in the person of the *alfaquim*. But such a two-headed profession must have been considered quite

normal in a period where doctors almost naturally became part of the policymaking establishment, serving as confidants and trusted envoys to the rulers. It would take much more knowledge than we possess today to establish which of the two functions was more predominant in the life of an *alfaquim*. David Romano, who studied the careers of the cousins Abenmenasse, two prominent *alfaquimi* in Aragon serving at the court of King Pedro the Great in the 1280s, noted that they were involved in political missions or in tax collection but rarely in medical care.[11] One of the cousins, Samuel, is referred to as "Alfaquimus et fisicus noster" as if to suggest a separation between the two functions. The many other *alfaquimi* found in the documents published by Baer, Régné, and, earlier, by Miret y Sans and Schwab do not help to explain the problem.

To be labeled *alfaquimus* was to be recognized as having special status in the royal retinue. There was another way rulers expressed the official status of a Jewish doctor in their court. Royal letters declared him a *familiaris* or even *domesticus*. Jews were not the only people so labeled and the appellation was not conferred only on members of the medical profession. Many individuals, such as diplomats, goldsmiths, or even jugglers, who came close to the ruler were declared *familiares* at one point or another.[12] The point is that Jewish doctors also became *familiares*.

We know about these Jewish *familiares* not only because the princes were careful to mention that status but also because the chanceries issued special letters making that status official. A document dated April 8, 1399, announced that Bonsenior Hasdai (Azday), "master in medicine," is received "by the tenure of the present letter as our doctor and *familiares*."[13] Almost sixty years earlier, in April 1338, a similar writ was issued concerning Master Isaac Meir (Ycach Mayr), a Jew of Fraga,[14] and in 1353 and 1373 the names of two other doctors, Aaron Cohen of Jajora and Benveniste Samuel of Barcelona, were added to the list of these fortunate *familiares*.[15] In the case of Benveniste the chancery insisted that he be granted the status "because of his aptitude in sciences and the elegance of his manners."

It is impossible to define the terms *familiaris* or *domesticus* or enumerate the attendant privileges and special rights. We can only glean indications from the documents. The chancery of the count of Provence, when conferring the rank of *familiaris* on the master Bendit Ḥayyim (Ahim) of Arles on January 4, 1369, exclaimed: "We wish that henceforward the said Benedictus should enjoy, like all of our other *familiares* . . . in all the honors, privileges, prerogatives, immunities, liberties, and favors."[16] Queen Johanna of Naples employed almost exactly the same language when in a special document issued in August 1426 she created Master Salomon of Anagni one of the "consortium of doctors."[17] Similarly, even a verbose declaration issued by the chancery of the duchy of Milan forty-one years later on August 12, 1467, in favor of the master Guillelmo Portaleone failed to rise above the level of generalities and give any concrete information about what becoming *familiaris* really meant.[18] The popes too declared some of their Jewish doctors *familiares*. In the official letters of nomination they insisted that this designation was done in accordance with the authority of "saints Peter and Paul," but otherwise their statements remain in the realm of generalities.[19] Fluid and undefined as the status *familiaris* was, all men of account seem to have sought the distinction and been proud of having obtained it. For Jewish doctors this appellation meant recognition, an outward sign of success.

A Successful Medical Dynasty: The Abenardut

Perhaps the best way to understand what it meant to become a royal doctor, *alfaquim*, *domesticus*, or *familiaris* is to follow the careers of some of the doctors who successfully reached the princely courts. The best documented case in Reconquista Spain is that of the Abenardut family (originally probably "ibn Ardut," "Ardus," or the like), and particularly one of its members, El'azar (also spelled in the documents "Alazar," "Aliazar," "Altazar," and "Alazarus"), who was active in the first half of the fourteenth century and referred to

himself in a Latin document of 1330 as "physician to the most illustrious Lord King Alphonso."[20] Two well-known Spanish scholars who undertook collaborative research on the registers of the crown of Aragon were able to establish a rich file about El'azar and his family.[21] Some years later other students of medieval medicine, notably Michael McVaugh and José Ríus Serra, were able to add significantly to this body of knowledge.[22]

El'azar was a royal doctor but not *the* royal doctor. By no means was he the only royal doctor or even the head of the college. In fact, he did not attend court permanently or regularly follow it on its travels around the realm. He did not even live in one of the three capitals, Barcelona, Valencia, or Saragossa, but for the greater part of his life probably kept his household in Huesca, his family's native city. For El'azar being a royal doctor meant, on the one hand, enjoying the prestige and the privileges the title carried and, on the other hand, putting himself at the disposal of the court in cases of urgency. He received written orders and was expected to follow them. On August 29, 1337, for instance, the monarch ordered El'azar to present himself in Saragossa within five days to take care of the daughter of a royal counselor, Miguel Pedro Capata.[23] Two years earlier, in 1335, El'azar had treated the king for a fractured leg, and in 1344 he was seconded to the service of the archbishop of Saragossa for a period of a month, or longer, as necessary.[24] His task was to care for both the prelate and the infanta Yolanda, wife of Leopold do Luna. As a royal physician El'azar was also expected to be at King Pedro's side during military expeditions. Thus, during the war that was waged in 1343 against the kingdom of Majorca he accompanied Pedro to the island itself and to the county of Roussillon on the mainland.[25]

The military aspect of the office of royal doctor certainly deserves more attention. Jewish doctors were not exempted from this obligation and, as we have seen, El'azar had already been invited to take part in the campaigns of 1333 and 1334. His father had participated in the conquest of the county of Cerdagne in 1323–1324 and lost his life there.[26] Another Jewish physician, Azariah Abenjacob, also participated in this

campaign.[27] In Murcia, one corner of the Iberian peninsula, Doctor Joseph (Yucaf) Axaques participated in the 1407 campaign against Granada.[28] We know of his presence from a document recording his compensation of 300 maravedi. In 1421 another Murcian Jew, Moses Meir (Mayer), found himself in the army camp, acting as a military surgeon.[29] Participation in warfare and its perils no doubt only strengthened the bonds of trust and confidence between doctor and ruler.

These glimpses of Abenardut's activity are no more than bits and pieces rescued from oblivion by the luck of the archives. In real life El'azar Abenardut's service to the crown must have been much more eventful and much more frequent, for the familiar and appreciative language the monarch employs when writing to him and the delicate and arduous political missions he handled reveal the trust and confidence bestowed on him. Some of the expressions the monarch used include "our domestic" and "our doctor," and the king remarked on the "services extended by him to us quickly and effectively."[30] As for El'azar's diplomatic activity, we know that in 1331 he was sent on a secret mission to Tarragona.[31] The monarch assured the receivers of the letters El'azar carried that the oral message the Jewish doctor conveyed was authentic. Two years later Abenardut was on the road again, carrying a royal message to the Knights of St. John in Catalonia. This time the emergency concerned preparations by the Moslem kingdom of Granada to attack Valencia.

The trust El'azar Abenardut enjoyed is even more apparent when he was involved in settling disputes between Jews, both as individuals and as a community, and their monarch. In 1333 there was a misunderstanding between the king and the great financier Isma'el Ablites, then one of the richest Jews in Aragon. King Pedro appointed El'azar as his negotiator and delegated unlimited powers of representation.[32] Five years earlier, in 1328, when thirty thousand shillings had to be raised among the Jews of Aragon on the occasion of the marriage of the king's daughter, the committee established to raise this extraordinary tax consisted of two Christian officials of the treasury together with El'azar Abenardut.[33]

Some of our documents show how El'azar exerted power

and influence in the court. When his brother Salomon suffered financial troubles around the year 1328 and his property was about to be confiscated, the doctor intervened and persuaded the monarch to impose on Salomon a light and reasonable program of payments.[34] Around 1336 we see the physician again trying to smooth things out for a group of six Jews from Huesca who had allegedly assaulted a Moslem, a subject of the count of Urgell. The name of Abenardut's son Joseph appears among the accused.[35] Finally, a document dated 1332 shows him extending help to the Jews of the small county of Ampuries in Catalonia. A royal letter written at Abenardut's instigation urged the count of Ampuries to treat his Jews "rightfully and with compassion [*misericorditer*]."[36]

As for remuneration, we learn that El'azar was granted an annual income of a thousand shillings in 1326; the sum was confirmed in 1328, in 1333, and again in 1340.[37] But this rather modest grant constituted only part of the physician's income. In 1326 he was already assigned, also by royal writ, all income generated by the notarial office (*escribania*) handling Jewish deeds in his home city of Huesca. This income too was confirmed in 1328 and 1340.[38] In 1332 the king made Abenardut judge of appeals for all the Jews of Aragon, an appointment held until then by the Jew Bahya (Baffiel) Constantini and one that must have generated considerable income.[39] Indeed, when El'azar served as arbitrator in Saragossa three years earlier, he was paid for his work.[40] In 1333 he appeared as an arbitrator in a family conflict in Montclus concerning the distribution of an inheritance.[41] His new job as judge of appeals made his selection for this mediatory task natural.

Other royal remuneration involved tax exemptions. In 1336 Abenardut received an exemption, valid for seven consecutive years, from all taxes on Jews.[42] In the 1330s (a probable date) another example of tax exemption is mentioned. Neither the physician nor any other member of his family was to be taxed more than nine shillings on any five hundred shillings of assessed fortune by the community.[43] In 1340 Abenardut and his family were declared "free men" (*francos*), which meant that they were exempt from all Jewish taxation. When in that same year King Pedro revoked all privileges awarded to Jews by

himself or his predecessors, El'azar Abenardut received a special exemption.[44] We notice also that when the doctor's daughter married in 1322, the monarch awarded him a thousand solidi.[45] This, by the way, may have been a customary gesture. In Sicily in 1440, when the Jewish doctor Moses Bonavogla of Messina celebrated a similar family occasion, the king gracefully offered a hundred ducati as a gift.[46]

El'azar Abenardut was a member of a medical family whose activities can be traced for more than two hundred years. The first Abenardut physician we know about was Salomon Avenardusi, referred to as *medicus* and as *alfaquim*, who was in King Sancho of Navarre's retinue in 1178.[47] The last members of the family known to us appear in documents dated 1472 and 1481.[48] In 1350 and 1360 there were two doctors Joseph (Jucef) Avenarduç, one of them possibly El'azar's brother, the other certainly his son,[49] while Joseph (Juce) Abin Ardut and Hayyim Abin Ardut appear in our documents in 1398, when both received their licenses. In 1415 another doctor El'azar Abin Ardut dictated his last will in Huesca.[50] They may all have had as colorful and exciting careers as the famous El'azar enjoyed in the 1320s and 1330s, but their cases are not as well documented as his. It is particularly unfortunate that so little is known about Moses Abenardut, El'azar's father. We have mentioned previously that he was already in the service of the king in 1323, when he participated as a military doctor in the Cerdegne campaign led by the heir to the crown, don Alphonso, against the kingdom of Majorca. He lost his life there.[51] Years later his service and sacrifice were remembered and recorded in official letters. It is probably safe to assume that it was Moses who introduced El'azar to the royal court and launched his brilliant career.

Luminaries: Jewish Doctors of International Repute

The name of a physician of Abenardut's caliber must have been known beyond the borders of Aragon, and indeed beyond the Iberian peninsula. The Provençal philosopher

Joseph ibn Kaspi states that on his visit to the island of Majorca he enjoyed the hospitality of "the distinguished scholar, the doctor El'azar ben Ardut the priest [*ha-Cohen*]." Kaspi apparently expected his readership to know who the great man was.[52] More formal proof of international repute does exist, however, in the cases of other Jewish physicians. Such information permits us to measure the extent of the reputation some attained and the ways in which they were appreciated. The archives of monarchs and dukes, bishops and indeed even popes, contain letters concerning the health problems, anxieties, and fears of these magnates. So abundant is the documentation for Aragon at the end of the fourteenth century that a modern historian of medicine, Joseph María Roca, was able to write several books based principally on the exchange of letters between King Juan 1 and his family regarding their health.[53] Our information is not confined to this rich series of registers in the Aragonese chancellery. The archives of England, France, and the recently published ones from the duchy of Milan all contain information about Jewish medical luminaries and the ways in which the great people of the world tried to enlist them in their services.

The most passionate of these letters comes, as might be expected, from the archives of Aragon. It is undated, but must be from the year 1349; it was written by none other than the queen of Navarre, Johanna, daughter of the king of France. Having fallen sick, she ordered the Jewish doctor Salomon of Tudela to come to France, where she was staying, and attend her bed. The doctor refused and even managed to escape to the lands of the king of Castile. No reason is given for his refusal. In her letter to the king of Castile Johanna begs him to compel the Jewish doctor to change his mind. She describes Master Salomon as "a very good doctor" who in the past performed "many and beautiful cures in Navarre" and expresses her belief that he would be able to provide her with a swift cure. She then adds, "We in similar circumstances would have sent one of our children [as hostage] were we to know that that could ameliorate your health."[54]

Why did the doctor refuse to go to France? Did he fear for his freedom? A clue may be found in a similar "medical" letter

written by Gaucelin of Lunel on May 23, 1253, to Count Alphonse of Poitiers, brother of Louis IX of France, one of the mightiest men in Europe at the time. Alphonse, who suffered from an eye disease, had heard about a Jewish specialist from Aragon named Abraham ("Habrahym" in our document) who happened to be in the south of France on nonmedical business. He asked Robert Gaucelin, lord of the tiny seigneurie of Lunel near Montpellier, to contact the specialist on his behalf. This was done immediately, and within two days Gaucelin sent a response. If the prince was still able "to distinguish one small object from among others within a given small space" he could "on peril of his head" deliver him from his ailment. But the Jewish doctor, who was also a very rich merchant, had other concerns. He would not commit himself unless his personal safety and freedom were secured. Afraid "lest you wish to detain him with yourself against his will," the doctor even dictated the substance of "letters patent for his safe conduct" required from the prince. Abraham's worries were neither imaginary nor overcautious. In his wish to please the great prince, Robert Gaucelin had stated his intention of kidnapping the doctor twice in this one short letter, the only document surviving today. "We think of demanding his coming despite himself," Gaucelin wrote.[55]

Safe conduct and personal security are at the center of yet another case concerning a renowned Jewish physician. This time the scene shifts north to England and the Low Countries. A letter dated to the year 1280 exposes another Jewish physician's fame and concern for safety. The doctor, Master Elia of London, or as he is known in Hebrew, Eliahu ben Menahem, the leading figure in English Jewry in his time, was asked to render himself to Flanders. He had for some time been successfully solicited by the court of Flanders to offer help to Prince John of Hainault. Through a courier Elia had sent the prince medicines that had been effective. Master Elia wrote about this matter in a letter in French to Robert Brunell, the chancellor of England. The court in Flanders was now insisting that the physician come in person, and for this reason Elia was requesting a safe conduct. Indeed, the appeal for this document is the most interesting of the three documents in this file.[56]

The perils of such medical expeditions are more clearly illustrated in the case of another thirteenth-century celebrity, the oculist master Vidal Espeçero of Monson in Aragon. In about 1284 he was asked to come to treat the wife of the nobleman Bernardo de Mauleone. En route he was kidnapped by a certain Pedro de Arey, the man who had solicited him to undertake the journey, and held for ransom at the castle of Monfulco. Although Espeçero had been traveling along the king's highway and his journey was secured by a safe conduct, his captor was demanding the sum of 150 pounds for his freedom. King Pedro himself reported this incident, on August 3, 1284.[57]

Even if these doctors appear hesitant and cautious in these documents, they were proud of their fame. Elia of London, for example, had difficulty containing his feelings in a letter when he wrote that "my name is known much in distant lands," but he immediately added the expected qualifying phrase, "more than its true value, which is nought." The physicians' patrons, whether the king of England or of Castile, did not fail to realize that they could gain some political profit from the reputation of these doctors. That the princes were asked, even begged, to send their own specialists gave them some advantage in the political game they were playing. This probably never became a major diplomatic asset for the rulers, but it was an asset nevertheless. The name of Master Judah Mosconi, for example, appears in such a context in a letter from the king of Majorca to the Moslem emir of Algeria in the mid-fourteenth century. The Christian king, who highly recommended the Jewish physician, was no doubt expecting some political reward.[58]

A blatant example of politics mingling with medicine appears in a report dated January 3, 1473, which the Milanese ambassador to the court of Savoy makes to the duke of Milan about the activities of a Jewish doctor, Master Jacob.[59] The report illustrates the pressures the political establishment could exert on such a specialist. Jacob had been asked to undertake a trip to Savoy and the ambassador had had to work hard to persuade the reluctant physician to go. Having arrived in Chambéry, Jacob had no difficulty in carrying out his assign-

ment, relieving the duchess Oliveta of pain in her legs. Then a complication arose. Oliveta's son, young Filibert, suffered "da quilla picola ancitura [*antitora*? i.e., "wound"]" and she wanted Jacob to treat him as well. The Jewish doctor balked. In order to cure Jacob he needed certain herbs and flowers that only grew in springtime; it was January then, the most bitter period of Savoy's winter. In the doctor's judgment, the chemicals, powders, and lotions that could have been used for ordinary people were out of the question because of the prince's delicate complexion. He proposed therefore to postpone all treatment until April or May. Oliveta called on the ambassador to exert pressure on the doctor to start treatment immediately. If the diplomat's report is reliable, he too rejected the duchess's demands: "Illustrious Madame, I am of a contrary opinion." Other doctors then agreed to start the treatment. Recording this account, the ambassador declared himself content that he had supported his doctor because the ultimate deterioration in the prince's condition vindicated Jacob's point of view. In his report the ambassador wanted the duke of Milan to know the entire truth "about this Jew" (*da questo ebreo*). But this may have not been the end of the story, for on that same day in January Master Jacob received twenty ducats from the princely treasury.[60] If this payment was not his remuneration for treating the duchess, he may well have carried out the young man's treatment after all.

Elia di Sabbato da Fermo was no doubt the most illustrious of international Jewish physicians in the fifteenth century.[61] He too must have been exposed to similar hard choices and pressures during his long and colorful career, yet perhaps typically the documents never show him in such difficult situations. Rather, they testify to a long, brilliant, and most successful career. He is the best-known doctor of the Late Middle Ages, probably because he practiced for more than fifty years and because his international renown far exceeded that of any of his colleagues. In one of the dozens of documents that testify to Elia's fame, a sick inhabitant of Ferrara addressed a petition to the duke of Milan and declared that in the whole of Italy there were only three doctors who could help him: Master Venanzo Camerino, Isaac of Cremona (another Jewish doc-

tor), and Master Elia.[62] There is as yet no way of explaining Elia's great professional success. In Hebrew letters his greatest achievement seems to have been the ordering of scientific works. One example is manuscript 933 at the Bibliothèque Nationale in Paris, a compendium of Averroës' commentaries to some Aristotelian works, sponsored by Elia's son Benjamin in the spring of 1448.[63] But apparently this lack of originality did not stop Elia's contemporaries from admiring him. In the compendium by Averroës, Elia is referred to as "light of the exile," "head of the doctors." Non-Jewish sources refer to him as "egregio et famosissimo." No dignity or honor seems to have been too high for him. He was one of the first European Jews to have been knighted (by the duke of Milan) and to have thus obtained the title *miles*.[64] In 1405, along with two other Jewish doctors, he received the status of Roman citizen (*civis romanus*).[65] Three years later a rival and a most distinguished colleague named Moses of Tivoli was forced to leave Rome and settle in Naples "because of envy, for he was a better doctor than the aforesaid Elia."[66] Thereafter, Elia was made doctor and *familiaris* to Pope Martin V, a distinction that enraged the canonist Giovanni di Anagni, who argued that a Jew could not serve as a doctor to the pope.[67] While other Jewish physicians had to be satisfied with a title *medicus* or *phisicus*, Elia, probably a graduate of Bologna, was "artium et medicine doctor." We have seen him (see p. 33 above) obtaining the laurea at the instigation of the pope. Privileges and favors were bestowed on him throughout his life.

Although Elia was still active in the early 1460s, he enjoyed international fame as much as fifty years earlier. In 1410 he was invited to England to attend King Henry IV.[68] On his way there he passed through the city of Basel and on August 6 received permission to stay in the city for three months.[69] In December "Magister Helia Sabot Hebrewe de Boleyne la Grase" and his retinue of ten people were issued with an English safe conduct, but Elia does not seem to have spent much time on the island. Just a few months later he was in France, traveling to Bruges on the orders of the duke of Burgundy, Jean sans Peur, "for certain secret business."[70] Back in Italy, despite suspicions raised against him in about 1424, resulting in his

temporary imprisonment,[71] Elia was appointed doctor to popes Martin V and Eugenius IV and was sent on a secret diplomatic mission to the port city of Ragusa on the Dalmatian coast, where he spent some time between 1427 and 1430.[72] Once again he appears to have been in the service of the Holy See. He was still serving the pope in 1435 when he was invited to Milan, a city that did not allow Jews within its confines, and he became the duke's personal physician.[73] In 1436 Elia and a group of his relatives obtained permission to embark on a trip to the Holy Land at a time when such pilgrimages were formally forbidden to any Jew.[74] His appointment to Milan, incidentally, was not his last. A document date October 9, 1445, reported that Elia was in Ferrara, probably tending to the duke.[75]

Royal Favors Bestowed on Doctors

Court physicians like Elia di Sabbato or El'azar Abenardut were not only famous, they were presumably also rich. Although we have little knowledge of the finances of any of these doctors, it stands to reason that royal and noble patients did not consider any fee too high for a cure. Nonetheless, the payments from the courts themselves almost always appear unimpressive. El'azar was remunerated, as we have seen, with a thousand shillings (equal to fifty pounds) a year, while in his time Elia was entitled to twenty ducats, a sum that was raised to thirty when he was sent abroad to Ragusa.[76] Such sums certainly did not correspond to the reputation of these men.

A recent study has looked at the question of the remuneration of royal physicians to the crown of Aragon around the year 1300.[77] The hundreds of documents examined reveal long delays in reimbursement to physicians. The picture that emerges from these documents is one of a monarch who was poor, who was always overspending, and whose treasury was practically empty. Under such circumstances the monarch in Aragon, no doubt like other European rulers, had to find other ways of fulfilling his obligations. The monarchs did so mostly by assigning physicians income in the form of feudal rights and rev-

enues due to the rulers themselves as well as by exempting them from many onerous impositions and taxes. Another way was to reward the *familiares* with a variety of privileges of symbolic value. The Catalan scholar Luis Comenge was able to draw up a handsome list of such royal grants, concessions, and dispensations to which doctors and other *familiares* were entitled.[78]

What was true for doctors in general was also true for their Jewish colleagues. But while Christian physicians like Bartolomeu de Vernet or Pere Molinet, for example, would be assigned the "general" right to exploit vineyards or fields belonging to the monarch,[79] Jewish doctors usually seem to have been assigned rights, favors, and exemptions that had a "Jewish" origin or that were particularly desired by Jews. The most valuable privilege seems to have been the appointment as supreme judge over the Jews of the realm, but the most commonly awarded grant was that exempting the favorite from the taxes normally imposed on other Jews. Between these two distinctions a whole series of rights and privileges was created, for instance, the exemption from the obligation to wear a special Jewish sign. Of course, all these rights and privileges were not only awarded to doctors; other Jewish *familiares* also enjoyed them. Doctors, however, were part of this privileged class.

The office of supreme judge of the Jews, also called in Spain *rav major*, seems to have been at the top of the hierarchy. The late Professor Salo W. Baron decided that the office must have been inspired by that of the head of the Jewish diaspora (the exilarch) in the Middle East in late antiquity and the Early Middle Ages. The exilarch's office consisted "in having responsibility both for the revenue due to the state by the Jews and for the orderly management of Jewish communities." "He appointed seven overseers [judges] . . . [and] . . . passed final judgment in all civil litigation among Jews."[80] It should be noted that his counterpart in the Moslem communities in Spain, the *alcalde major*, had similar responsibilities.[81] According to a document of 1414 from Sicily, then under Aragonese rule, Master David of Marseilles "fisicus," the Jewish supreme judge, was expected to render justice to his coreli-

gionists in all matters civil or ceremonial, which, according to "their nature," had to be decided according to the "law . . . of the Jews," matters in which the ordinary system of justice had no claim to exclusivity. Yet the supreme judge was warned not to "intervene" in other cases.[82] From his title, *assasore*, we may perhaps deduce that his duties also included imposing the annual taxes and other impositions Jews of the principality had to pay. The Sicilian document also mentions "salaries, primes, and emoluments" resulting from the position, but that is all that it says about the financial side of the office. For the most part the office appears in the documents as a position of utmost authority, power, and honor. We notice that both great doctors held the office in the course of their careers: El'azar Abenardut in Aragon and Elia di Sabbato in the duchy of Milan. Others who held the office included "Moysey medicus de Bonavogla" (who was described earlier in this book as a student) in Sicily,[83] Joseph Orabuena in Navarre, Judah ibn Wakar and Meir Alguades in Castile,[84] and several physicians in Sicily.[85] Secular rulers were not the only ones who took the initiative of appointing a favorite doctor as *rav major*. In 1338 the archbishop of Toledo made his doctor Ḥayyim ha-Levi "rab" over all Jews of his bishopric.[86]

The most common privilege seems to have been exemption from the taxes generally imposed on Jews. No doctor for whom significant documentation survives failed to receive this exemption at some stage in his career. We have seen that El'-azar and his family were relieved from the obligation first for a limited period of seven years and then they were declared *francos* in general. Similar information exists for other physicians. Even if we limit ourselves to the findings of Antoni Rubió y Lluch for Catalonia in the fourteenth century, we can quote the names of doctors such as Abraham Hallena (Halleva?) in 1338, Azariah ibn Jacob (Azarias Aben Jacob) in 1320, Bendit Des Logar in 1321, David Abenadcar in 1340, or Saltel Cabrit in 1351, all of whom received tax exemptions.[87] Sometimes the royal exchange of letters is so rich and informative that it even reveals the politicking preparatory to such an exemption. On December 10, 1326, for instance, the *infanta* Maria wrote to her father King Jaime II of Aragon in support

of her physician, Salamon of Calatayud. "He did much service to me and to donna Blancha my daughter," writes the infanta, insisting that he is worth to her "much more" than any taxes he might pay.[88] Writing on January 6, 1391, about Master Junec (Junez) Trigo of Saragossa, Queen Violante of Aragon is even more laudatory. He deserved the exemption not only because of his care of the king, herself, and her daughter, she declared, but also for his altruistic deeds in favor of poor people from whom he could not have hoped to receive any remuneration.[89]

Jewish communities, however, were unhappy about such tax exemptions, for the share of the tax originally assigned to the doctor now had to be paid by the rest. The documents tell us just how unhappy the thirteenth- and fourteenth-century Sicilian Jewish community was with the Busach family of Salerno. Its founding father, Master Busach, received his exemption from the emperor Frederick II as early as 1237. In 1258 the emperor's son confirmed the privilege.[90] We do not know how the Busachs fared under Angevin rule, but once the island was conquered by the Aragonese the family found ways to reconfirm the old text[91] almost fifty years after it had been issued. They still retained the privilege as late as 1325, and the leaders of the Jewish community were still fighting them over it.[92] Documents relating to another Sicilian doctor, Moses Gasendi, and dated February 1476, show the leaders of the community in Palermo struggling in court to revoke his privileges as royal favorite and to make him one of them in all matters concerning taxes.[93] In September of that year when a new tax on wine was imposed on the Jews of Sicily, their leaders took special care to specify that physicians' families were not exempted from it.[94]

Even privileges that did not entail tax exemption probably aroused envy and created discontent in the Jewish community. For instance, from 1215 all Jews had tried to escape the humiliating and even dangerous obligation to wear a special distinguishing sign or a special hat.[95] Doctors and other royal favorites quite easily obtained letters of exemption, which sometimes even contained a justification connected with their profession. "You have to travel on various routes by day

and by night and if you wear on your vest the sign or the roll that Jews have to [wear] on their external vest, you risk being molested by unknowing Christians," wrote the king in a privilege issued on November 18, 1330, to Ezra (Ezdra) Alacar.[96] Samuel de Valencia, "faithful alfaquim," received an identical exemption on April 11, 1284, because he "accompanies the king in his department."[97] Joseph (Jussef) Baron, "medicus" from Saragossa, Moses (Mosse) Constantini, "fisicus," son of Baḥya (Bafiel), Joseph (Jucef) Almujuciel of Lérida who cared for "many of the retenue [families] of our house" are three other doctors exempted from carrying the badge.[98] Other Jews who were unsuccessful in avoiding the stigma no doubt resented it more because of those who were exempted.

Another example of a breach of solidarity was recorded in the city of Játiva, Valencia.[99] The local Jewish community enacted sumptuary laws for its members in order to limit the wearing of luxury clothing. Such enactments were initiated from time to time by both Jewish and non-Jewish communities. In Játiva the king's physician, Samuel, "alfaquim," felt that his role at court should qualify him for exemption. He managed to obtain a royal privilege for himself and for his relatives as well. But the Jewish community responded with new legislation specifically directed toward dissenters like Samuel, forbidding them to wear colored clothing. Samuel approached the infanta and she intervened in his favor. These confrontations are reported in a document issued by the royal chancery on February 10, 1282.

Privilege could also take the form of royal interference in affairs of the Jewish community. An example, a most sensitive one, once again in favor of a doctor, is described in a document issued by the royal chancery on August 16, 1385, concerning the reading of the Torah in the synagogue.[100] We know that around the year 1200 in France and Germany non-Jewish authorities would, at the request of their favorites, compel other Jews to let them read the Torah and roll it, a privilege that many Jews appreciated then as they do today.[101] Information about instances of this strange intervention in Germany is vague and general, but for Aragon, Fritz Baer has discovered precise information about such an intervention on behalf of

Junez Trigo, a surgeon of Saragossa whom the king referred to as "familiar et domestic nuestro." He and his relatives (his "lineage") were empowered to "pray at the tribune of the synagogue and read the law of Moses in the rolls" whenever they wished, notwithstanding the opinion of the rabbi or other Jews.[102]

Doctors sometimes asked their princely patrons for aid in other Jewish communal affairs, principally in matters relating to their participation in the communal council and in their assumption of public functions. When participation in communal leadership was desirable the patron was expected to impose the doctor, or any other favorite, on the community, making him part of the governing board. We have already seen cases when a doctor was made the supreme judge, and such intervention must certainly have occurred with lower-ranking positions at the local level, although no documentation exists. When communal work proved onerous, the doctors requested exemption. The monarchs could at least justify such intervention by "medical" argument, stating that the doctor needed all his time for his practice. On October 13, 1382, the Majorcan physician Abdalhac asked to be excused from the office of *secretarius* and *conciliarius* in his community as well as of that of "messenger" (*nuntius*) and "ambassador."[103] To justify his demand he raised the issue of the time needed to practice his profession. In seeking and obtaining the exemption Abdalhac was treading a path paved by generations of doctors before him. In Saragossa alone we know of three such exemptions for the first quarter of the fourteenth century. On September 2, 1302 Salomon ibn Jacob (Abenjacob) obtained one with help from the municipal council; on July 30, 1303, almost a year afterward, Baron Almelich, another doctor, earned the same privilege, while on October 24, 1324, Rabbi Azariah ibn Jacob and several of his relatives were promised that they would no longer have to serve as scribes and notaries of the community.[104] In Valencia the exemption was awarded twice, in 1314 and again in 1317, to the doctor Omār Tawil (Omer Tahuyl), and on March 8, 1318, it was extended to his son Abraham (Abrahym).[105]

Finally, physicians benefited from a variety of unrelated

favors not necessarily linked to their occupation. A document of January 29, 1302, shows that the Valencian doctor Isma'el Aminorisp, a Jew, had a royal privilege that threatened with a fine of a thousand maravedi anyone who might hit or beat him.[106] It so happened that another Valencian Jew, Joseph (Jucef), son of Salomon Addaran, did in fact attack Isma'el Aminorisp and in addition forcibly took away and burned all privileges the physician carried with him. It is the doctor's complaint that reveals the very existence of this grant. Other doctors asked for privileges in family matters. Spanish Jews, for instance, could contract bigamous marriages in accordance with Jewish law. They nevertheless had to ask special permission from the civil authorities to do so, and it probably cost them money to obtain such a license.[107] Three documents issued by the Aragonese monarchy show Vitalis Almuviçuel, a doctor's son, and the doctors Duran de Cortali and Judah (Jafuda) Bonseniyor dez Cortal obtaining such licenses; the last two received these grants in 1384 and 1373, respectively.[108] Vitalis Almuviçuel, who received the privilege in December 1336, had had no children after fifteen years of marriage;[109] Judah Bonsenior also cited barrenness as a reason for the dispensation.

In December 1330 the doctor Azariah ibn Jacob (Azarias Aben Jacob) of Saragossa sought and obtained royal help in an embarrassing family affair. His niece had been deflowered by a young Jewish man, Bonetus, son of Gento Arziello, and as a result her value on the marriage market had declined significantly: "She cannot get a husband that she could have had before the deflowering [occurred]." The doctor secured a royal writ that obliged the young man, a servant (*famulus*) at the doctor's house, to furnish indemnities.[110]

Doctors also used their influence in matters affecting the Jewish public as a whole. In 1427 when the inquisitor Giovanni da Capistrano engaged in a campaign against the Jews of Naples, a Jewish papal doctor, Salomon d'Anagni, who was also a *familiaris* of the king of Aragon, threatened to leave for Sicily. The result was that Pope Martin V managed to calm the zealot.[111] Such intervention by doctors must have been a fairly common occurrence. Moses Bonavogla, whom we have seen

as a student in 1413 and 1416 (see p. 26) and who made a spectacular career in Sicily in the ensuing thirty years as a royal physician, is seen on two occasions acting on behalf of his brethren. In June 1429 he obtained privileges concerning their commercial activity.[112] In July of 1431 he managed to exempt them from the obligation to attend Christian religious sermons. Jews were thus aware of the political influence doctors could have. This awareness appears even in Hebrew letters. The traveler Benjamin of Tudela (ca. 1165) lamented the oppression under which his coreligionists of Constantinople—capital of Byzantium—were living. He observed, however, that they got some relief because of a certain Salomon, labeled "the Egyptian," who served as the king's physician;[113] three hundred years later the Jewish statesman Don Isaac Abrabanel (1437–1508), discussing issues of Jewish politics with the Italian notable Isaac of Siena, asked at the end of his letter if there were any Jewish doctors in the papal court or whether any cardinals employed such doctors.[114]

That the Jewish community battled over the privileges physicians received (at their expense) does not imply any lack of appreciation for the profession. Quite the contrary. The more successful some of these doctors became, the more they served as models or sources of inspiration to young people. An internationally recognized doctor incurred some risks from his distinction, as the documents show, but the physician also enjoyed fame and influence. Yet the abundance of favors and honors bestowed on these doctors should not necessarily lead us to conclude that Christian society unquestioningly accepted these Jews. If Jews themselves could resent their luckier brethren, Christians could display envy, even hatred.

5

Rejection: Apprehensions about Jewish Doctors

Some elements in medieval society may have recognized and admired Jewish doctors, but there are many surviving testimonies to the uneasiness and apprehension that governed the minds of many. Occasionally these negative feelings translated themselves into accusations and even drove civil and ecclesiastical authorities to legislate against Jewish practitioners. No one forgot that these people were Jewish, and their professional or ethical failures were often projected on the whole Jewish community. The failure of a single doctor could turn into a nightmare for all his brethren.

Failures, Accidents, Incompetence

In the High Middle Ages, as at all times, a physician's career was scarcely an uninterrupted succession of professional victories. Failures and mishaps have always been part of professionals' lives. Court records of the period reveal many such embarrassing moments in practitioners' lives, but such legal cases are not the only source for this particular aspect of medical

life. Doctors themselves remembered such accidents and wrote about them. At the beginning of the fifteenth century, for instance, the surgeon John Arderne in his book of professional recollections, *Fistula in ano*, wrote candidly about his first experience with arsenic, which almost killed two patients he treated with it. Although, as he writes, the mistake happened in the "bigynnyng of my practizing," it left its mark on him for years to come.[1] A more detailed account of a medical disaster was written by Shem Tov of Tortosa, who translated into Hebrew the *al-Zahrawi*, the famous medical encyclopedia. The accident occurred in Marseilles around the year 1260. It was caused by two Christian practitioners and cost the life of a Christian patient. Shem Tov's recollection of the accident must have been written just a short time after the event; it runs as follows:

> A Christian doctor of Montpellier had in his care an important merchant from beyond the seas, who was in a hurry [to leave] the city. The physician prescribed . . . a purgative that included half a drachm of white hellebore. The merchant arrived in Marseilles and handed over the prescription to one of the Christian doctors to prepare [the drug. The doctor] made him drink the purgative drug in the evening, according to the instruction. After a few hours, however, the merchant was seized by a convulsion of vomiting and died immediately, suffocating.[2]

Shem Tov suggested an explanation for the death: "When the vomit came up from the stomach to the esophagus, the purgatory drug followed it and suffocated him." "In my opinion," Shem Tov concluded, "all this happened because both doctors had little knowledge about the [different] qualities the two kinds of hellebore possess."

This short paragraph contains the only surviving record of this particular case, so it is impossible to determine whether Shem Tov obtained his information from colleagues' gossip and rumors or whether the incident provoked a malpractice suit. This second possibility should certainly not be overlooked. Probably by the mid-thirteenth century and certainly by about 1300, doctors had to account for such accidents and pub-

lic authorities made it their business to carry out inquiries and punish practitioners, even if the injured party was not willing to lodge a complaint.[3] About 1276 allegations of malpractice against two English practitioners, Master John of Hexham and Master Semann, resulted in their being sent to jail. Two patients had received too high a dose of medication and had died soon afterward. Information about this case has survived because both doctors managed to escape prison and one of them, Master Semann, was captured and retried.[4] Around 1310, again in England, we encounter the case of Master John of Curnbull whose patient's leg got worse, not better, after treatment. The physician was brought before a jury, which found him guilty and imposed the enormous fine of thirty pounds.[5]

Evidence from another corner of Europe, the city of Barcelona, confirms the impression that prosecution for malpractice was rigorous by the fourteenth century. In July 1364 a Muslim doctor called Durramen had to explain the death of his patient Francisce, the wife of Bernard, whom he had treated for a head injury. He was accused of negligence and was fortunate to be acquitted at his trial.[6] Some thirty or forty years later, in the same city of Barcelona, a female slave (*serva*) became the subject of an inquest led by the governor of Catalonia. The doctor, Petrus Ripoll, alias Casals, was accused of performing a phlebotomy at the wrong time and of introducing an object (*lantenta*) into the patient's mouth "against the advice of other doctors."[7] The verdict in this case has not survived, but the very fact of the trial shows us that late medieval society and its authorities had no intention of considering medical failure an inevitable part of practice.

Just how heated such conflicts with doctors became is amply illustrated in a trial before the court of the city of Orange in the south of France in the fall of 1459.[8] Blanqueta, a Jewish woman from that city, held a fellow Jew, the master Vitalis Salves, responsible for the death of her father. "Incompetence" and "wrongly prepared medicines" were the accusations she made. When the court found Vitalis innocent he retaliated, suing her for the enormous sum of five hundred scudi for the damage she had caused to his reputation. Blanqueta, so he claimed, expressed her accusations "vociferously" in the

presence of many "in the synagogue of women." And, what is
more, she did so on September 8, which that year happened to
be both a Saturday and the Day of Atonement, the most holy
day in the Jewish calendar when worshippers are expected to
forgive and pardon each other.

Many documents discovered in the archives of the crown of
Aragon refer to trials of Jewish doctors, who, like others, were
held accountable and faced prosecution when they were involved in failures. In May 1283 Master Bonastruch Baço was
named responsible for the death of a Jewish patient, whose
name is not given, and the physician was imprisoned. In Vilafranca del Penedés on May 28, 1321, the surgeon Abraham
Carbo had to explain in court the death of a patient named
P[etrus] Amblart.[9] On June 8, 1330, harsh language is employed against a Jewish woman, Mira, who treated a mother
and a daughter, Sancia the wife of Dominicus Amargo and her
twenty-month-old Gracieta, with fatal results. "You made
[them] drink a certain purgative which was supposed to cure
the patients of their infirmities . . . However, because of this
purgative the aforementioned Gracieta died and the said Sancia [the mother] lost a living foetus that she had carried in her
womb for six months."[10] And on January 17, 1338, we hear
about Maria Egidii of Alagón (Valencia) and her intention to
sue Master Mayhl; she accused him of causing the death of her
daughter Romana, who suffered in one of her legs.[11] Fifty
years later in 1388 the Jewish medical woman Na Regina was
in jail in Barcelona. She was imprisoned after the death of a
slave girl named Violante; Na Regina was accused of administering the medicine that caused her death. In the document
describing this incident, the lady practitioner is being set free
by the authorities.[12]

More details are provided for two other legal and police actions involving Jewish doctors. The first occurred again in the
small Catalan city of Vilafranca del Penedés, where in the very
last years of the thirteenth century the Jewish doctor Isaac
Mercadel had to explain the death of one of his patients, a
carpenter. Even though the doctor was acquitted by the local
administrator (the *cort*), this individual succeeded in extorting
from Isaac what seems to be a bribe of 450 solidi, which he

refused to give back. The doctor, however, was uneasy about the affair and refrained from referring to the incident even when the *cort* was finally brought to trial.[13]

The second case occurred in Candia on the Mediterranean island of Crete sometime around the year 1419. Master Judah of Damascus is at the center of a legal drama for allegedly administering an abortive lotion to a Greek woman, who ultimately died. After an autospy had been ordered and Judah declared guilty, he was sentenced to exile from the island. Since he apparently succeeded in hiding or escaping, an announcement was made that all persons extending help to him risked one year of imprisonment and a fine of two hundred hyperpers. Once captured, Judah himself would first lose his right hand, a ceremony that was to take place in front of the deceased woman's house, then he would be hung. This case was first reported by David Jacobi, who discovered it in the archives of Venice. Jacobi also discovered that two years later Judah succeeded in his appeal against this sentence.[14]

The most detailed document relating to a malpractice suit comes from the tribunal of the city of Marseilles in 1390. The doctor, Abraham Bondavin, allegedly treated his patient, a certain Aycardet, with an ointment obtained from garlic and nettles. The patient reacted violently to the treatment. "I am all burnt, I am all burnt!" he screamed as he hurled himself to the floor. "I am all burnt, I am dead! What a traitor this doctor!" ("ieu cremi, ieu su mort, aqueu trahidor de mege"). According to the patient's mother's testimony, his neighbors gave him a bath and saved his life, but the nerve endings of his hands and feet were contracted and paralyzed. Master Abraham defended his treatment, which he had conceived with the help of a non-Jewish practitioner, Raymundus Pibaroti, and spelled out the theoretical grounds for his course of action. He also told the court that the patient had previously been treated by a doctor Vitalis de Lunello, another Jewish practitioner, who cauterized him and extracted no fewer than fifteen bones from his leg. Although Bondavin's lawyer raised some technical legal points in his favor, the physician was found guilty and fined thirty-five pounds.[15]

All of cases considered so far reveal no religious or ethnic

animosity. Terms such as "diabolic" or "demonic" are absent, though they were quite often used in medieval society with reference to Jews. Indeed, these cases against Jewish doctors were treated like all other accident/malpractice cases. Moreover, accused, even convicted, Jewish doctors apparently had fair recourse to appeal. Both Master Abraham Carbo and the female doctor Mira obtained royal pardons in 1330. Bonastruch Baço, who presumably caused the death of a Jewish patient, had all his belongings confiscated but appealed his sentence and obtained a pardon for his case; Na Regina, who was imprisoned in 1338, was ultimately released. The message disclosed by all these cases is thus one of fairness and impartiality. These cases all display apparent indifference to the Jewishness of the doctor.

But our story can have a darker side. Evidence exists simultaneously for impartiality (on the one hand) and for discrimination (on the other). Several documents expose "Jewish" dimensions to cases of medical failure. In his introduction to the Hebrew rendering of the *al-Zahrawi*, Shem Tov of Tortosa described a mishap that took place in Marseilles in the spring of 1261 when an inexperienced Jewish practitioner caused the death of a Christian patient:

> An ignorant, foolish man, a fellow Jew, arrived in the city of Marseilles, claiming to be a physician, although he was [in fact] estranged from that science. Worse, he really had no medical knowledge at all. His patient had been bedridden for a long time, suffering from arthritis, *retet* in Hebrew. In his ignorance [the "doctor"] ordered the root of a certain herb to be boiled and that [the patient] should drink the liquid from it. This ignoramus knew neither the strength nor the properties of this herb, nor that it was potentially harmful. As a result of this treatment, the sick man fell into a coma, lost his memory, and [eventually] lost his mind. His face and eyes turned red, his tongue dry, and his throat parched. Unable to speak or breathe, his body turned cold. Saliva and moisture came out of his mouth and he was unable to control it. That night he died suddenly. The ignoramus rose early the next morning to visit his patient, as doctors do. He found him sleeping deeply, in the torpor of death. Nevertheless, he assured [the patient's] relatives and neighbors that this was the way in which the herb

worked and that [the patient] was merely asleep and would eventually wake up.[16]

So much for the history of this medical fiasco. But our Jewish reporter goes now a step farther, relating the consequences of medical incompetence for the Jewish community of Marseilles as a whole:

> Still [the doctor decided] to go into hiding. When evening came, the bailiff, [ha-shoter] ordered him to present himself before him, otherwise he would be hit with a fine of one hundred marcae. [The "doctor"] left the city, escaping on the second day of the feast of Passover of the year five thousand and twenty one (March 18, 1261). Had it not been for the divine misericord and for the fact that the Christian happened to be a foreigner, we all would have been in great danger on his account.

Another instance in which the Jewish community was affected by a medical mishap comes from the court records of the city of Manosque for the year 1298.[17] Even though parts of the manuscript relating to accidents are hopelessly erased, enough is known to make it clear that in November of that year the Jewish doctor Isaac, son of Resplanda, was charged with performing an abortion that caused the death of the fetus. The physician allegedly administered "poisonous medicaments" to the mother. In his defense the Jewish doctor presented a letter claiming that no death had resulted and that he himself had seen the living baby being carried away from Manosque by the grandmother. For reasons not explained the judge did not accept the doctor's defense. Master Isaac was heavily fined and had to raise the very considerable sum of thirty pounds from his relatives and other members of the community. Moreover, a few words in the otherwise illegible parts of the manuscript suggest that the doctor was also imprisoned. The leaders of the Manosque community, probably out of fear of riots or vengeance, seem to have asked the authorities to keep him in jail but release him from his chains.

Jews seem to have been conscious of the risks the medical profession posed to practitioners. A Hebrew moral treatise, *Sefer ha-Yosher*, written at the end of the Middle Ages, urged

Jewish doctors to avoid any professional adventures for fear of the consequences:

> We Jewish doctors in the diaspora have to possess extraordinary knowledge, for the Christian doctors envy us and challenge us, so that at times we have to provide explanations about our procedures [lit., "science"]. And if they discover any ignorance on our part they say, "He kills gentiles." This is the reason I advise each and every Jew not to [even] touch a gentile if he is not able to answer [the questions of those Christian doctors] in natural sciences.[18]

Suspicions

The cases cited thus far never suggest a premeditated attempt to kill a Christian patient. The most that emerges is a somewhat hysterical reaction to medical failure which affects the whole Jewish community. Such reactions, however, testify to an underlying current of suspicion and fear which governed medieval Jewish-Christian relations as a whole. But there could be even more to it. Jewish physicians were at times suspected of deliberately attempting to poison Christians, and Jewish doctors were particularly the object of such accusations.

A sixteenth-century German writer, Hans Wilhelm Kirchhoff, author of the *Wendunmuth*, provides a perfect example of these fears and animosities. The author, frustrated and indeed terrified by the absurdity that forced Christians to turn to their enemies for medical help, wrote:

> The Jews who pretend to be doctors bring poverty and physical danger to the Christian in need of their medical skill. They believe that they are serving God when they cruelly torture Christians, when they kill them secretly, or when they cheat them. They also teach this to their children and their disciples. While we Christians are such brainless fools that when lives are in danger we turn to our archenemies in order to save [our lives], thus shaming both God and the medicines of righteous Christian doctors.[19]

"Jews nurture much hatred toward Christians" read a "confession" put into the mouth of a Jewish doctor by the tribunal of the Inquisition at Briançon in the Dauphiné in March 1433. The confession continued: ". . . and they have it as part of their customs that their doctors do not heal any [Christian] but rather kill as many of them as they can." This statement was extorted at the height of the witch-hunt from Jean of Saint Nicholas, a converted doctor who was originally from the city of Bari in Apulia and whose Jewish name used to be Abraham. Also accused of necromancy and invocation of the devil, the physician admitted to whatever the inquisitors attributed to him and was sentenced to be burned at the stake. The surviving court records report that even when still in Italy Abraham had administered toxins to at least five people. "He said and admitted that he killed two [Christians] in the kingdom of Apulia, administering them powder obtained from a toxic herb called in the Apulian language *saragalla*," the document specifies, alleging also that a third person named Anthonius, the son of Benedictus Mourley, was treated with a syrup extracted from this same toxin. To compound matters, the doctor accompanied his treatment with a charm in Hebrew: "In the name of Satan and so many other devils, kill him."[20]

Documents from the neighboring county of Savoy describe another incident with a Jewish "doctor and sorcerer" at its center. In 1466 a doctor named Rufus Lentilosus allegedly asked one of his patients to dig up the skull of a dead Christian. After pulverizing it, Lentilosus prepared a lotion for the man, but the balm was of no help.[21] It is interesting that almost three hundred years earlier Joseph ibn Zabara, a Hebrew writer from Spain, knew that non-Jews said that the "Jews open our graves and take out the bones of our dead people, burn them, and then prepare medicines and sorcery out of them."[22] These fifteenth-century incidents in the Briançonnais and Savoy must be understood in the context of the witch-hunts taking place in these regions around this time.[23]

A few years before this inquisitorial procedure took place in the Dauphiné, another fifteenth-century Jewish doctor lost his life as a result of a similar accusation. His name was Moses Rimos and the drama of which he was part took place in Pa-

lermo, Sicily, around the year 1430. This time the source of information is not a court protocol or a judiciary sentence but a Hebrew elegy Rimos wrote on the eve of his execution. He hoped to smuggle out the lamentation and begged his readers to copy it and send it in all directions "until it reaches my desolated relatives." "Know, o my friends, that I am not slain for some dire offense that I have committed," he protested. "Deadly poison, they assert, I planned to be put in the dregs of the cups of trembling, for gentiles who died: I was not guilty. They have crushed out my life on this false charge." Another Hebrew document records that the twenty-four-year-old was executed and buried "out of the town, under the wall."[24]

A generation earlier toxins, poisons, and the intention to kill were also at the heart of a trial that ended the life of a Jewish doctor in Florence. He was only involved indirectly in the murder itself; it was claimed that he supplied a Christian woman with the poisons to kill her husband. The court found him guilty of complicity in the murder and he was executed in 1404.[25] It is not known whether this was also the destiny of a French surgeon named David "the Young" in 1317. He was accused of having poisoned several persons, in particular a priest who had lent him one hundred pounds. The bailiff of the Vermandois in northern France was instructed to follow the case. Another Jew, Abraham was accused of complicity, and the authorities initiated an inquiry against him as well.[26]

This fear of poisoning by Jewish doctors was not limited merely to popular belief or to zealous inquisitors. We find additional proof of such fears in church legislation and in laws promulgated by secular princes. The famous Castilian code *Las Siete Partidas* enacted precautions against such poisoning: "We prohibit any Christian from receiving medicines or cathartics made by a Jew, although he may obtain it on advice of a knowledgeable Jew as long as it is prepared by a Christian fully aware of its content."[27] In April 1397 Queen Maria of Aragon found it opportune on her part to pass legislation against Jewish physicians "because these perfidious Jews are thirsty for Christian blood, as enemies would be, and it is dangerous for Christians to obtain any medical help from Jew-

ish doctors, when they are sick." While she repeated the legislation of the *Las Siete Partidas* in substance, she found ways of sharpening its expression: "We ordain and establish that no Jew, in any case of a Christian's infirmity, should dare to exercise his office of medicine unless a Christian doctor will take part in the cure."[28] A punishment consisting of imprisonment and a fine of ten pounds was also decreed in order to deter transgression of the law. This was not the first time that such allegations received the force of law on Spanish soil. Church councils of Valladolid (1322) and Salamanca (1335) had warned believers against Jewish doctors who "under the guide of medicine . . . kill the Christian people when administering medicaments to them."[29] It was also for fear of poisoning that Provençal legislation about 1349–1350, shortly after the Black Death, stated that "a Jewish surgeon has to taste from the wine given to sick ones to consume in order to stop their overfeebleness." Knowing that a Jew might evade this stipulation for religious reasons, claiming that the wine was not "kosher," the text immediately continued: "notwithstanding your custom not to drink with Christians a [custom] which your law and your Jewish scriptures oblige you to follow."[30]

These suspicions may be behind the fact that Jews did not play any important role in pharmacy. They are rarely seen as pharmacists, but when they are, they seem to be engaged in the profession in defiance of both the legislation and the custom of the land. For example, a document from the island of Majorca, dated May 1, 1320, describes "several Jews" acting as apothecaries (*operatoria apotecarie*) on the island; it hastens to add that the local bishop protested this activity, pointing out to King Sancho its illegality. In the same vein, we note a royal privilege issued in Barcelona on July 5, 1325, in favor of Vital Sahon, a Jewish pharmacist, making him an exception to the rule excluding Jews from the profession. King Jaime II of Aragon also made it a condition that the pharmacist should serve only Jews, not Christians.[31]

Jewish doctors were also frequently suspected of sexual misconduct, especially with their female Christian patients. In conciliar decisions the prelates of the church circumvented the embarrassing subject, only mentioning in general terms "scan-

dal" and "abuse." But there is no doubt that sexual misconduct was on their minds. The participants of the synod of Avignon (1337) circled the issue, talking about Jewish medical practices that "bring about too much familiarity and conversations between Christians and Jews, which, in their turn are incentives to many nefarious crimes that seem to be perpetrated." The prelates are just as vague in the following sentence, but it is very clear that they have sex in mind when they write: "It may well be that they set the scene for other worse crimes in the future, unless the right measures are taken to prevent such things from happening."[32]

As we might expect, court records are more straightforward about sexual misconduct allegations. This is shown in evidence from the archives of the duchy of Milan for the 1460s and 1470s, recently published by Shlomo Simonsohn. A document dated September 27, 1470, describes how the physician Master Vitalis was in custody, his property having been confiscated, after he was accused of having attempted to seduce one of his female patients. About two weeks later the duke, who took a personal interest in the case, was informed that the charges were not proven and that Vitalis's father, also a doctor, had complained officially about these false accusations.[33] A similar complaint concerning an identical accusation was made against Master Angelo two years earlier, but in his case we do not know the court's verdict. Another interesting case is that of the master Angelo of Cesena, who was practicing in Gravedona. Sometime around March 1464 he actually fled the town for fear of punishment, having allegedly fornicated with a Christian woman. But the people of Gravedona, who needed his medical services, intervened on his behalf. They brought forward new evidence in which the woman retracted her former testimony. The popular pressure had successful results: some five months later the duke released the Jewish doctor from punishment and also declared Angelo free to settle in the city again.[34]

An embarrassing sexual scandal is described in the court registers of Manosque for 1340. If we take what is registered on the four folios of the court register at face value, there is no doubt about the doctor's guilt. It seems that Master Crescas of

Nimes, also called Crescas of Mirabeau, made advances to a woman named Alexia from the first time he was consulted to treat her sick daughter and then later herself. He apparently took advantage of the poor widow because she could not afford the necessary medicine. The doctor became more and more insistent, and when they were alone in her room he made his intentions explicit. The woman succeeded in persuading him to postpone the rendezvous until the next day and in the meantime informed the authorities. The next day two agents of the court were hidden behind a curtain. At the height of the encounter, they burst into the room. Crescas at first denied the accusation and then threw himself on the mercy of the court. He was sentenced to "lose his member," a punishment imposed on similar occasions.[35] Rodrigue Lavoie, who published the proceedings of this trial, believes that the cruel operation was not in fact carried out and that Crescas succeeded in having his punishment commuted to a fine.[36]

Jewish doctors, we must note, were not the only ones suspected of taking advantage of their female patients, nor were they the only ones brought to trial for such actions. To give just one example, from the same city of Manosque about ten years earlier, the surgeon Anthonius Ymberti was accused of having had sex with Douceta, the daughter of Raymundus Martini, one of his clients.[37] Future researches in archives of the Mediterranean countries will probably yield information about Christian, Moslem, and especially Jewish doctors, the last because of the society's greater sensitivity to that group. As today, governing classes found the alleged sexual exploits of their rivals, whom they regarded as inferiors, particularly infuriating, somehow infringing their own sense of honor and dignity. Medieval suspicions here added yet another brick to the existing wall of animosity.

Ecclesiastical and Secular Legislation against Jewish Doctors

Opposition to Jewish doctors did not remain purely a subject of popular sentiment or outrage. As the thirteenth

century progressed, public authorities, both ecclesiastical and secular, took action, promulgating special legislation intended to curtail and even eliminate Jewish participation in the medical profession. So far, we have seen but a few instances. Conciliar decisions of the twelfth century have nothing to say about Jewish doctors, probably because of the backward state of medicine in that century and the lack of involvement of Jews in the profession. Even the Fourth Lateran Council of 1215, which left no stone unturned in its anti-Jewish legislation, said nothing about doctors.[38] Specific legislation concerning physicians appeared only in the 1230s and in the beginning remained brief and laconic. In 1227 the synod of Treves, the first to face the issue of Jews in medicine, briefly enjoined "temporal lords" to ensure that no Jew offered help or medicines to Christians.[39] "All Christians who, when sick, put themselves in the care of Jews will be excommunicated," declared the synod of Albi in 1254, and this proscription was repeated verbatim at the next synod of Albi, also held in 1254.[40] Later councils, after repeating Lateran legislation obliging Jews to wear special badges, among other injunctions, then generally added a short statement curtailing the activities of Jewish doctors.

These early thirteenth-century ordinances give no reason for their prohibitions, but the church may have been worried that Jewish practitioners might prevent dying Christians from receiving the last sacraments. Not until the fourteenth century was this reason spelled out clearly. It appears in Provençal legislation of 1306 (which will be discussed more fully below, see p. 93) and it even forms part of a *Licentia practicandi* given that year to David of Arles, a Jewish doctor. David was forbidden to "dare" approach the sickbed of a Christian unless the person had already confessed and received the *corpus Christi*.[41] In 1341 the synod of Avignon referred to this delicate issue, and about 1350 the diocesan synod of Barcelona repeated legislation first enacted there in 1311.[42] In Murcia in 1419 a complaint was made that Jewish doctors intentionally failed to tell Christians the real gravity of their condition in order to prevent them "from making their last ordinances." On April 4, 1432, Pope Eugenius IV accepted a petition sub-

mitted by a Christian doctor, Johanes de Cava, which attempted to remedy this situation in southern Italy.[43]

The constitutions of church and state became much more aggressive in the fourteenth century. Leaving aside the question of whether the *corpus Christi* was administered, the council of Valladolid in 1322 censured Jews and Saracens who "under guise of medicine, surgery, or apothecary commit treachery with much ardor and kill Christian folk when administering medicine to them."[44] On that occasion the prelates also observed the negligence displayed hitherto and urged ecclesiastics to make more use of church censures in order to enforce the law. In 1335 this statement was repeated word for word at Salamanca, the prelates also adding comments about "scandal, abuse, and malice" of the infidels. Christian patients were threatened with excommunication and with being deprived of the right to enter a church.[45]

The best-developed legislation against Jewish doctors is to be found in the proceedings of the council of Avignon in 1337.

> We establish and ordain that no Christian from our provinces, cities, and diocese of whatever status, condition, or dignity he may be, should approach and ask, or make us ask, any Jewish physician or surgeon for any medicine, medicament, or cure to be received from him. Neither should he dare to accept for himself, or through an intermediary person, any medicine, counsel, or cure coming from a Jew, or spontaneously sent by one, however excellent it may be, unless imminent danger to the patient exists and it is impossible to appeal conveniently to Christian doctors or surgeons. We equally forbid Jews of both sexes to become in any way involved in the cure of Christian patients' infirmities. Whoever will violate this decree, if Jew, the communion with the faithful will be taken from him. A Christian, however, will be punished according to the decision of his superior.[46]

Secular legislation was at times even more stringent. In 1310 the constitution promulgated by Frederick III in Messina, Sicily, against Jews and Saracens spelled out punishment for both doctors and patients. The Jew would be imprisoned for no less than a year on a miserable diet of bread and water; the

Christian would be subject to identical treatment but for a period of three months only. The Sicilian legislation also decreed that whatever salaries and remuneration the Jewish doctor might have received should be confiscated and distributed to the poor. The preamble contains the following argument justifying these draconian measures: "We cannot have faith in those who do not have any faith, nor can those who betrayed their Lord be faithful to others."[47]

The legislation promulgated by Count Charles II of Provence on May 6, 1306, was equally aggressive in tone and content. Charles's intention was to do away with Jewish practitioners altogether. To this end, he issued the following edict:

> We order that no one, when stricken by a sickness, should turn to a Jewish doctor or any other infidel or get from him, or through his counsel, any medicine. Neither, in the future, will any license to practice among the faithful be awarded to any Jew by the seneschal or any other official. And if [a license] was awarded to anyone before this date we revoke it and declare it not valid. A Jew called upon [by a Christian] will pay a fine of ten pounds of the new money [*reforsas*] if he tends him against the [tenets] of the present ordinance. If he refuses to pay it, we order his body to be scourged. As for the faithful [Christian] who called upon him, he will be punished according to the decision of the judge under whose jurisdiction he lives.[48]

The Ineffectiveness of Legislation

Was this legislation effective? Answers emerge when we note that the draconian Provençal legislation of 1306 was revoked only a few months after it was made public. In addition, the Avignonnaise ordinances of 1337 were revoked and suspended four years later by a synod assembled in the same city.[49] This 1341 synod of Avignon did not use vague language or resort to sophistries to conceal the change in policies. On the contrary, it justified the suspension in clear terms, remarking that changes in conditions required changes in attitudes. Justifications like "public utility," "urgent necessity," "scarcity

of Christian doctors" were brought forward. It would have been "irresponsible" not to revoke the previous constitution. Simply put, society was not ready to reject the Jewish doctor.

That churchmen themselves continued to call on Jewish doctors must have been particularly demoralizing for the initiators of anti-Jewish legislation. There is practically no limit to the evidence available about links between Jewish doctors and members of the clergy at all levels of the hierarchy. The daily behavior of popes and bishops, convents and monasteries, contributed to nullifying discriminatory legislation. Only Hebrew sources claim that Master Gaio the Jew (Isaac ben Mordecai) served as the personal doctor of Pope Nicholas IV (d. 1292).[50] But in the case of other late medieval and Renaissance popes, the presence of Jewish physicians is formally recognized in Latin documents issued by the papal chancery. In fact, according to lists established by Fausto Garofalo, there were few late medieval and Renaissance popes who did not have Jewish doctors in their service.[51] Pope Boniface IX (d. 1404) had two Jewish doctors. One, Angelo Manuelis, was declared *familiaris* on July 1, 1392; the other, Salomon de Matasia de Sabauducio, attained the same dignity several months later on October 23 of the same year.[52] A few years later Salomon's status was confirmed by Pope Innocent VII (d. 1406) while that of Angelo was confirmed by Pope John XXIII (d. 1415).[53]

The picture is no different at the episcopal level. In 1398 a powerful prelate like Pedro Tenorio, archbishop of Toledo, had Master Ḥayyim ha-Levi in his services, while in 1443 Nicholay, archbishop of Avignon, could count on Bonsenior Vitalis.[54] The same Bonsenior also appears to have been at the service of the archbishop of Aix, not far from Avignon. In 1450 another archbishop of Aix, Robert Damiani, engaged Master Crescas Creysse.[55] In Arles the accounts of the archbishop's treasury for 1421 show Moses de Roquemart serving as his doctor.[56] Further north, in Treves, Germany, in 1354 the Jewish doctor Vitalis was connected with the episcopal see, while in 1386 the saintly cardinal Pierre of Luxembourg had in his service a Jewish master whose name was also Vitalis.[57]

Lower-ranking clergy also ignored much of the anti-Jewish

legislation. In Toledo in the time of Archbishop Pedro Tenorio, the local monastery had on its payroll two Jewish doctors, Joseph (Yucaf) and Abraham.[58] The former received 333 maravedi per year, the latter only 200. Also in the late fourteenth century the cathedral of Notre Dame de Nazareth of Orange in southern France had Master Isaac (Ysaquus) Ysaqui, *fisicus*, performing these tasks.[59] In neighboring Avignon the convent of the Cordeliers is on record as employing Abraham of Carcassonne as its doctor in 1374 and then Master Durandus Tamani, who was also Jewish, in 1420.[60] The accounts of the convent of the Dominicans in Aix for 1423–1424 contain the names of Bonsenior Vitalis, Master Crescas, and Master Salomon,[61] all of whom have been mentioned serving elsewhere. It is also noteworthy that the accounts of the hospital of St. Esprit in Marseilles in 1333 show the Jewish doctor Salomon of Salerno treating three members of the staff, sisters Duceline and Quasens and brother Petit.[62] These accounts from Marseilles also show Jews in the service of the hospital throughout the fourteenth and the first half of the fifteenth centuries. Finally, in one of the first experimental universities in Provence, the *studium* established in 1365 by Pope Urban V, the administration engaged Master Dieulosal, a Jewish doctor, to treat the students.[63]

These Christian authorities and institutions knew very well the letter and spirit of the laws they were transgressing. The complaint of Arnold of Villanova in a letter to King Frederick III of Sicily reveals how frustrated many early fourteenth-century church dignitaries must have been. According to Arnold there was not even one convent where Jews were not hired. "We see that the custom is for no other physician to enter cloisters unless he is Jewish, such is the case not only of cloisters for men but for women as well."[64] Around 1470, when the Cabildo Catedral de Cartazena in Murcia replaced its Jewish doctor with a Christian named Martin Jaimes, the group was careful to remind itself that "it will be preferable to have a Christian than a Jew."[65] We hear similar sentiments in a monastery in Burgos a few years earlier in 1464: Rabbi Samuel (Simuel) was hired as a physician to the institution and his salary was established at a thousand maravedi for a year,

notwithstanding that some monks reminded the others about church prohibitions in this respect.[66] In the second half of the fifteenth century Alonso de Spina, a formidable enemy of the Jews, vehemently attacked prelates who in their relationships with Jewish doctors "let the devil enter their homes."[67]

Times changed and attitudes changed with them. Fifteenth-century Western Europe, which faced the abyss in terms of population growth and economic activity ("the waning of the Middle Ages"), also witnessed a worsening in the attitude toward Jews. What was a cry in the wilderness at the beginning of the fourteenth century when Arnold of Villanova made his complaint made sense to people at the end of the fifteenth century when Alonso de Spina rallied public sentiment against Jews. In Italy in the second half of the fifteenth century, preaching against Jews by friars of minor orders occurred daily, and all the old legislation of the synods and councils suddenly became relevant. Preachers now made a point of urging municipalities to get rid of Jewish doctors and to annul agreements (*condotta*) they had signed with them. The elders (*anziani*) of Lucca, for instance, heeded the anti-Jewish propaganda and wondered whether they should continue to employ the doctor Samuel, a Jew of Spanish origin. Their religious guide Felino Sandei, to whom they turned for help, did not relieve them of their worries before giving them a lesson in true Christian piety. Sandei, who a few years later was to become bishop of Lucca, reminded them how wrong it was for people who wished to "live religiously" to employ an "enemy of the cross" as their doctor. But as he realized that the *anziani* wanted to continue to employ Samuel, he recommended that the doctor seek a special papal dispensation permitting him to practice among Christians.[68]

The papal dispensation was one solution for municipalities and for Jewish doctors during these harsh times in Italy. A dozen such dispensations issued in favor of individual Jewish doctors can be found in the recently published second volume of Shlomo Simonsohn's monumental *Apostolic See and the Jews*.[69] The first two dispensations were issued in 1426 and 1427, and the last one, which was the last of Pope Pius II's proclamations, was given in 1464.[70] This last license was

awarded to Doctor Benjamin (Guillelmo) Salamonis in the city of Massa and explicitly mentioned the propaganda of preachers who assured their listeners that to call on a Jewish doctor "cannot be done without committing a sin."

Papal dispensations seem to have become most common in the 1450s. But obtaining one was not a mere formality. The documents extant display no single formula but differ from one another in language and even in content. Two of them express the hope that daily contact with the faithful will show the Jewish doctor the right way to salvation.[71] Three of the documents remind the Jewish practitioners that they have to allow their Christian patients to receive the last sacraments; in one of these three documents the practitioner is even expected to enjoin them to do so.[72] It is taken for granted that all legislation, synodal and conciliar as well as secular and municipal, is valid[73] and that papal licenses constituted an exception to the rule and were but temporary dispensations. In fact, the first license we have discovered, that of 1426, granted a dispensation for a period of five years only.

The records of the municipality of Fabriano for the year 1455 reveal the case of a Jewish doctor who had a difficult time obtaining such a papal document. The unfortunate unnamed physician had trouble from the very beginning. The people of Fabriano were so uneasy about him that even after he was hired, around the month of June, they decided in council by a vote of 23 to 3 to look for a Christian physician "because many refuse to be treated by the Hebrew doctor." Pressure was put on the Jew, who continued to practice in the meantime, to obtain a papal dispensation (*bolla*). The matter was raised in a communal meeting on September 16 and then twice in meetings during November. Finally, at the meeting of December 10, 1455, the physician was given less than three weeks to settle the issue and was expected to present the document at the end of that very month. The Jew ultimately obtained his dispensation on January 4, but this was too late and he lost his position.[74]

Even if a Jewish practitioner obtained a dispensation within the required time, this did not constitute real assurance of employment. Evidence from the region of Umbria shows that

doctors armed with dispensations were still fired by municipalities. Daniel da Castro, who was employed in Narni and in Bagnoregio before establishing himself in the city of Amelia in 1478, brought with him a papal dispensation acquired almost twenty years earlier. But the preaching in the church against him became so aggressive that the municipality had to establish a citizen's committee to examine the suspicions about the "professional insufficiency of the Hebrew." He was fired in 1479, although he did receive some compensation for breach of contract.[75] About five years earlier, in Assisi, Master Elia, a Jewish doctor, presented the municipality with the necessary document. When hiring him, the councillors expressed the wish, which seems by then to have become a formality, that through practice among a Christian flock the Jew will see the "light of truth." But the propaganda against his employment became vicious. Elia applied for and obtained a new papal dispensation, but his efforts were in vain. He had to tender his resignation, which for a medieval Jewish doctor made a unique statement: "He does not intend to go on taking your money as he has understood that the people do not wish to be treated by him because he is Jewish."[76]

This candid observation by Elia, a most painful one, no doubt, must have been shared by many of his contemporaries in Italy. Part of society did not want to be treated by Jewish doctors precisely because they were Jewish. Such fear, suspicion, and unwillingness manifested themselves, as we have seen, elsewhere as well. People justified this unwillingness by claiming that Jews could poison, bewitch, or seduce Christians or even prevent them from performing Christian duties or receiving Christian rites. There was in addition a psychological reason for this unwillingness, one the documents seldom enunciate: A doctor, by definition, finds himself in a position of command in his relations with patients. At all times and in all places the language of medicine constantly reminds patients that they must "obey" their physician, that they are under his "rule and power."[77] Christians quite naturally found it offensive to their sense of dignity that Jews, "enemies of the Cross," "children of the maidservant," should find themselves

through their medical expertise in a position of dominance. The council of Avignon in 1337, at the zenith of Jewish medical activity, is the only one to make this point, but it does so quite candidly: Jewish doctors should be forbidden from treating Christians, for in such a situation "the servile status of these Jews is inflated and elevated beyond its boundaries [*propter quod eorumdem judeorum servilis status ultra metas erigitur inflatur.*]"[78]

When we consider the overall deterioration in Jewish-Christian relations which historians observe taking place from the end of the first quarter of the thirteenth century—a deterioration marked by fantastic accusations, limitation of moneylending activity, and then expulsion—we are not at all surprised to encounter such strong reactions against Jewish doctors. Jewish doctors, after all, were the one group among their coreligionists who enjoyed continued and extensive contact with the surrounding society, in very direct and intimate ways. Given these general conditions, it is perhaps more surprising that people continued to turn to Jews when in need. The lack of Christian doctors is no doubt a factor in this pragmatic attitude, but we also have to account for contradictory behavior: Christians listened to the preaching against Jews and appreciated it, but they simultaneously resisted and sidestepped the propaganda. Clearly fear and suspicion existed throughout the medieval West, but many people, lay and clerical, found ways to overcome their fears and sought help from the "enemies of the Cross."

6

Jewish Doctors in the Medieval City: Numbers and Status

Doctors as Part of the Social Scenery: Literary Evidence

The rapid medicalization of most sectors of society in the High Middle Ages inevitably made the physician an important figure in the social landscape. It is difficult for the modern historian working with original sources not to encounter these doctors. Notarial contracts and court records reveal both the legal framework regulating medical practice and the arrangements for doctors' remuneration. City council records, mostly from Italy but also from Spain and the south of France, show municipalities engaging practitioners' services for the benefit of all citizens, but particularly the poor. The evidence is so abundant for some cities that with a reasonable amount of confidence we can formulate estimates about how many practitioners were active there at any one time. In other instances, the information about women doctors permits us to make educated guesses about their professional education and the branches of medicine they entered. Hundreds of Jewish doctors appear in these documents. Well-furnished "files" or "life histories" can be established for them, enabling us to trace their activity over a period of many years.

Literature and art in the High Middle Ages also reflect the new dimension of medical services and their spread in society. It is well known that geoffrey Chaucer (d. 1400) could not resist a critical description of a doctor from the social galaxy he painted in the *Canterbury Tales*, and his slightly older contemporary, Giovanni Boccaccio (d. 1375), made room in some of the stories of the *Decameron* for satirical accounts of doctors, including a woman healer.[1] A century earlier the "wiles of the physician" had become a favorite *topos* in the works of Hebrew writers in Spain, Italy, and the Provence. These writers usually ridiculed the doctor for his pompous behavior, his incompetence, and, above all, his cupidity. Three of these Hebrew writers—Judah Alḥarizi, Shem Tov Falaquera, and Kalonymos ben Kalonymos of Arles—distinguished themselves by providing vivid and in many respects realistic portraits of contemporary doctors, even though all three preceded Chaucer and Boccaccio in their satire and wit concerning the medical profession.

Alḥarizi (ca. 1175–1230), who spent much of his time traveling in Moslem Spain and the Middle East, depicts his doctor standing in what appears to be an oriental bazaar, offering his services like any other craftsman or merchant to the people gathered around him. He lists dozens of ailments the doctor is competent to treat, from stomachaches and sterility to poisons and broken legs; in addition, he insists on undertaking both dentistry and ophthalmology. To be sure, this doctor is not a respected physician but a market doctor who eventually apologizes to the author for having been reduced to such status. But this type of practitioner must have existed as a part of the market scenery. Alḥarizi's description also details the professional tools and medicines: flasks and bowls containing ointments and syrups, electuaries and bandages. The most frightening items are the metallic instruments for cauterization and phlebotomy, not to mention the pincers, a "flesh-hook of three teeth" (Samuel 2:13), and of course the very sharp knife "to cut into the flesh."[2]

Shem Tov Falaquera (ca. 1225–1295), writing in Navarre, northern Spain, in the second half of the thirteenth century, depicts his doctor working indoors. He is seen twice, once in

his own study receiving a group of patients and once on a home visit. In his study the doctor is called upon to perform a uroscopy. So many people are present in the room that it is almost a public event. Individual treatment and privacy seem to have been discarded and even Shem Tov Falaquera "joined those who came to [the doctor's] home, each looking for a remedy."

> [The doctor] was sitting on a chair with much dignity and magnificence covered with his ceremonial gown, which he put on to cover his cloak. Each person presented then his flask containing urine. The doctor took them and looked at them and examined their appearance and aspect. He observed the urine's appearance, noting whether or not it was cloudy or if there were any other irregularities about it. To one of his patients he said, "This urine indicates a serious illness of the liver, a weakness of the stomach as well as the constipation of the liver. If it is not dealt with at its very inception it will end fatally."

Falaquera's doctor continues issuing verdicts, some good, some bad:

> And this other flask indicates high and strong health, while that one coldness, its proprietor will be harmed by cold [food]. [The doctor then] announced to one patient that he would recover while to another that he was about to die and all his acquaintances will ask "where is he." To one he said that he would be cured by inducing sweating, while to another he said he would recover through cleaning his bowels, while yet another would recover through bringing out the moisture from his stomach . . . [Shem Tov concludes:] He gave these and similar replies to all those asking for his help.[3]

The description of the house visit is caustic. Our narrator "accompanied him when going to visit a patient. They came to the house of a distinguished person, a trustworthy and honest man who had his daughter on the sickbed. . . . [The doctor] stretched his right hand to her and massaged all parts of her body. Then he uncovered her left arm and felt it with his fingers. Then he meditated a moment, as if pondering, and bringing his thoughts together." The sexual insinuations are pronounced in this section, yet notwithstanding this tone Fala-

quera painted a picture of a typical medical visit that contemporaries must have recognized.

Kalonymos ben Kalonymos (1286–d. after 1329) of Arles also placed his physician indoors, visiting a sick man in his home.[4] While ridiculing the physicians, Kalonymos nevertheless captures in his invective the gist of the practitioner's rhetoric when pronouncing a diagnosis, explaining his medical reasoning, and dictating the mixture of herbs and drugs he wanted the apothecary to prepare. "He is suffering from a large abscess in the brain under the skull. I have diagnosed the case clearly from the pulses of the hand and the chamber pot. The indicators are well known and long established, it's all as clear as day to me." This was what he dictated to the apothecary:

> Take down this recipe: 'Take the herbs stocte and onycha from the land of Hefer and beat them into a powder. Mix them with thistle, briar, some loose earth, resin of a young tree, the root of a broom tree, olive leaves, the blood of a locust, radish peelings, the milk of ten donkeys, a rose, a seed of evildoers, and a touch of malicious gossip. Include all these ingredients, add nothing to them, nor leave anything out.'[5]

Although marked by fantasy ("malicious gossip," "evildoers") and spirited satire, the paragraph nevertheless conveys the way medical rhetoric must have sounded to the uninitiated. Kalonymos is important to us also because he makes room in his piece for a description of the relationship between the doctor and the patient's relatives. He has them pay part of his fee before he starts treatment, and he takes advantage of their ignorance and their fear. Awed, they follow his instructions uncritically, but once the patient dies the doctor finds ways of putting the blame on them.

The most important depiction of medical practices known today is found in a fifteenth-century illuminated manuscript of Avicenna's *Canon* in the university library of Bologna. The doctor, dressed in crimson gown, appears in a dozen or so activities in as many scenes. He is shown as a professor in front of his students and also as a surgeon performing phlebotomy. In one scene he is visiting the herbarium looking for medical

plants while in another he is in an audience, similar to the one described by Shem Tov Falaquera, where everyone is standing before him, awaiting his verdict on the uroscopy (see frontispiece).[6] A woman dressed in a light blue gown is seen leaving the room visibly upset by the verdict she has just heard. The most instructive folio shows the doctor indoors, like Kalonymos's and Shem Tov's practitioners, visiting the sick and surrounded by the patient's relatives. The first of these three scenes shows him taking the pulse while in the second he breaks the sombre news to the relatives. The third scene shows the notary taking down the patient's last will.[7]

Similar scenes to those depicted by Kalonymos and the anonymous illuminator of the Bologna manuscript must have been generally known. Just as a person would not leave the world without leaving some written testimony prepared by a professional notary, his relatives would not let him pass away without seeking medical help, if only as a last resort. Of course rich and poor did not enjoy the same medical services, but the poor, or the relatively poor, did receive some kind of help.

The Number of Jewish and Non-Jewish Doctors

The place of the medical profession in the life of the medieval city has become clearer as a result of findings by scholars who have examined evidence from cities like Paris, Toulouse, Marseilles, Perpignan, Arles, Saragossa, or Aix-en-Provence and cities on the island of Crete. Although the sources vary in depth, two results surfaced: the cities showed unexpectedly large numbers of practitioners and an expectedly large proportion of Jews among them. In the kingdom of Valencia, which had an estimated population of two hundred thousand, there were dozens of practitioners, either physicians or surgeons, in each quarter of the fourteenth century. These are only minimum numbers, so the real numbers may have been much higher. The Valentian archives listed the names of 45 practitioners for the first quarter, 19 of them surgeons. Sixty-two were listed for the period 1326–1350, 18 of whom were

surgeons; 53, of whom 12 were surgeons, appear in the generation following the Black Death. Between 1376 and 1400 the number reached a peak of 97 doctors, 38 of whom were surgeons and the rest physicians.[8]

I have carried out research in the archives of Manosque, a city with a population of about thirty-five hundred, listing every medical practitioner, whether a *medicus fisicus* or a *medicus sirurgicus*, employed there on the eve of the Black Death. Some of these physicians are mentioned only once, which may be a result of deficiencies in the archival materials, while other doctors appear dozens of times. Some doctors' careers can be documented for twenty or thirty years, while almost nothing is known about others. And have we discovered all the practitioners? Did the practitioners whose names appeared only once disappear from the city? This search, in any event, revealed the names of more than 40 practitioners to whom we should ideally add the names of 3 apothecaries, for the years 1250 to 1350. Most of them, 33 in number, appear in the half-century preceding the Black Death. We can thus offer a rough average of a minimum of 7 practitioners for each of these five decades.[9]

In most cases information about physicians assembled in other cities tends to confirm the Manosque statistics. The similarity of findings in this medium-sized city in upper Provence and those for the similar-sized city of Besalú in northern Catalonia is remarkable. Professor Grau i Monserrat was able to cull from fourteenth-century notarial records there the names of 39 practitioners, both surgeons and physicians.[10] He added to that number the names of 10 apothecaries practicing there, all of them Christians since the profession was forbidden to Jews. For the neighboring city of Gerona, which with eight or ten thousand inhabitants was much bigger than Besalú or Manosque, Christian Guilleré discovered the names of no less than 125 medical people, half of them apothecaries.[11] In the rich archives of Perpignan the late Richard W. Emery found the names of 120 physicians living there between 1250 and 1418, of whom 67 were Jewish.[12] In the fifteenth century Saragossa, the capital of Aragon, and somewhat larger than Gerona, also counted at least 65 practitioners.[13]

These numbers are not absolute numbers. At most, they show that substantial numbers of practitioners worked in these places. It is obvious that the documents scrutinized did not reveal the full number of practitioners in some cities. Toulouse, for example, a city five or six times bigger than Manosque, on the eve of the Black Death must have had far more than the 9 practitioners (or even 18, if we add 9 barbers) listed in the archives. The total of 37 in the same city for the twenty years between 1390 and 1410 seems a more realistic number.[14] Marseilles, in the second half of the thirteenth century, only listed the names of 11 practitioners in its archives. But in the first half of the fifteenth century, when the documentation becomes more abundant, the number rose to 38.[15] The figures for the Rhodanian metropolis of Arles are particularly disappointing. Despite his remarkable command of the city's documentation, Louis Stouff was unable to find more than 3 physicians and 1 surgeon listed in the archives for the year 1440, although he had already found 6 for 1407.[16] Between 1400 and 1450 Arles's neighboring city Aix-en-Provence had at least 27 medical persons. Neighboring Orange, half the size of Arles, listed at least 15 physicians and 1 surgeon in the notarial registers for the years between 1310 and 1380.[17] The recently published numbers for Barcelona and Valencia also may not be high enough. In Barcelona we discover just 15 and 19 surgeons and physicians for each of the ten years starting in 1325, while in Valencia city between 20 and 25 names surface.[18] In addition, the records for these two cities also reveal the number of apothecaries and barbers in practice, and these added significantly to the size of the medical corps, yielding a total of 54 in Barcelona in 1328 and 66 in Valencia in 1333.

The average of 7 or so practitioners in Manosque for each of the five decades before 1340 is not at all out of order on closer examination. The information available for several medical careers in Manosque enables us, with the help of a simple histogram, to determine how many doctors were practicing simultaneously in the city in each of the years between 1280 and 1348.[19] Since even in Manosque, a city known for its rich archives, the documentation is spread unevenly over the period, the histogram reveals years for which no more than 4

or 5 practitioners were listed. In other years, however, we find higher numbers, 6 or 7. For the years 1303, 1314–1315, 1321, and 1338 we count 8 *phisici* and *cirurgici*, which in my opinion comes very close to reality. The result is a high doctor-patient ratio, almost 1:450, a ratio remarkably close to that found in the most advanced countries of the world today. Fortunately, the numbers discovered for other cities of the medieval West, in England, Provence and, mainly Italy, validate these findings for Manosque. Cities as far away from each other as Salon in Provence and York in northern England or as close as Empoli and Florence all seem to have had an impressive medical corps with ratios of less than 1:1000.[20] The medical presence in the cities of Western Europe in the High Middle Ages resembles that in modern North America as well as that of the Islamic countries in the eleventh and twelfth centuries. Franz Rosenthal, relying on less abundant documentation than that available for Western Europe, was nevertheless able to calculate a ratio of 1 doctor to 350 people for the great medieval Islamic cities.[21]

Jews figure prominently in these statistics. In Manosque and Besalú up to half of the practitioners, acting both as physicians and surgeons, were Jewish.[22] Recall the 67 Jews among the 120 practitioners in Perpignan. In Saragossa the percentage is a little lower, 24 out of 65, less than 37 percent.[23] On the island of Crete under Venetian rule the number is much higher. Between 1365 and 1397, 20 out of 29 doctors, more than 68 percent, were Jewish. Four out of the 6 Cretan physicians were Jewish and so were 13 out of 20 surgeons whose religion was identifiable.[24] Jewish doctors played no less an impressive role in the city of Marseilles, even if the numbers there were a little lower than those found in Crete. During the hundred years preceding the Black Death, we find 15 Jews in the profession, 5 out of 11 in the half-century ending in 1300 and 10 out of 23 in the second half-century.[25] In the fifty years between 1350 and 1399, 19 out of 35 doctors (54 percent) were Jewish, and in the following fifty years the percentage rose as high as 56 percent, with 20 out of 38 doctors. Only in the last fifty years of Jewish existence in Marseilles, that is, from 1450, does a reversal of this tendency appear; the records for this

period listed 13 Jewish doctors, no more than 37 percent of the 35 practitioners in the city. For Avignon, a city with a large Jewish community in the fourteenth century, the numbers of Christian doctors are not known, so it is impossible to express Jewish participation in the profession in percentages. As for Jews, we have the names of 34 in the fourteenth century and 60 in the fifteenth century.[26]

Clearly Jews were overrepresented in the medical profession. Although they constituted no more than 3 percent to 5 percent (8 percent at the most) of the overall population of these cities, their proportion in medicine was ten times greater than that. Other figures may even show us what percentage of Jewish families earned their livelihood from the medical profession. The 5 practitioners in Manosque worked in a Jewish colony that did not amount to much more than 35 families.[27] If the figures from neighboring Aix are reliable, Marseilles must have had 100 or at the most 150 Jewish households in the late fourteenth century.[28] Nevertheless, 20 individuals gained their livelihood from medicine. In 1491 the historic city of Venosa in Apulia had precisely 38 Jewish households, 6 of which were "medical" ones. Rome had 15 "medical" families among the 100 Jewish ones whose profession can be established.[29]

We may thus conclude that writers like Geoffrey Chaucer were accurate in placing doctors prominently in the social panorama. Doctors existed in such great numbers in Western Europe in the High Middle Ages that it would have been impossible not to take them into account. There were no Jews in England in Chaucer's time since they had been expelled in 1290, but if there had been such a presence, we can safely argue that he would have had to explain why his typical physician was Christian and not Jewish.

Women in the Medical Profession

Kalonymos ben Kalonymos and all the other authors quoted so far took it for granted that male doctors were the typical representatives of the profession. This assumption was true, for in most cases probably 90 percent or more of the doc-

tors were male. But women were also members of the profession. I do not have in mind women who informally practiced
folk medicine but rather women who were listed in the archives as full members of the profession, licensed and approved
by the authorities. Like the men, they merited titles, except
that in their case the notaries employed the feminine form,
magistra, medica, fisica, and *chirurgica.* Dozens of the documents refer to such women doctors.[30] A document of May
1292, which probably contained the names of all the active
doctors in Manosque, listed a Christian woman named Laura
de Digna among the 8 practitioners.[31] A Jewess named Hava
(or Hana) appears in a document in the early 1320s in her
medical capacity.[32] The Manosque Jewess Mayrona (see p. 22
above), widowed in 1341, appears from 1342 in over forty
documents, invariably and consistently styled *phisica.*[33] In fact,
3 other female doctors can be found among the 40 practitioners in Manosque in the mid-fourteenth century. To these
women who practiced in one small city in upper Provence can
be added the names of dozens of other women, many of them
Jewish, who practiced openly and officially in Spain, Italy,
Germany, and elsewhere in Provence.

It is almost certain that none of these women ever attended
university. In any event, none of them bore the official
university title *magistra in medicina.* Women, like most Jews,
had to acquire their education privately and then present
themselves for examination. When any information about a
woman's family situation is available, we gather that invariably
she had a male relative practicing the profession. This may
suggest that the women all acquired their education in the
family context. Hava's husband and son were surgeons, and
Viridimura, a Sicilian Jewish doctor who obtained her license
in 1376, is expressly mentioned in the records as the wife of
Pascal "de medico."[34] Na Bellaire and Na Pla, two medical
women from Lérida, Aragon, who were awarded licenses in
1387, were married to Samuel and Judah, respectively, members of the scholarly Galippapa clan and possibly doctors
themselves.[35] It is not impossible, however, that some women
studied with a female master. A famous document from
Marseilles dated 1326 describes such a woman, Sara of Saint-

Gilles, accepting a male student named Salvetus de Burgonovo in order to teach him medicine.[36] There is reason therefore to suspect that Sara herself and other confirmed women doctors instructed female students as well.

The enormous body of data from Naples detailing licensing procedures in southern Italy reveals two factors that facilitated licensing. One was acquired experience, the other the readiness of authorities to issues partial licenses limiting practitioners to a well-defined medical field. These factors may have made the careers of women candidates easier. For most women professionals we encounter in southern Italy had received a license limited to a single aspect of medicine, for example, "to the cure of wounds and of tumors," or "to the cure of dangerous tumors in the breasts and in the matrix," or, more generally, "to cure sick women."[37] But this was not always the rule. There are no such strings attached to the license *cirurgica* awarded in 1307 to Francisca, a woman of Viesti (*mulier de Vestis*) in southern Italy, and two licenses dating from the last quarter of the fourteenth century do not have limitations.[38] The readiness of authorities in southern Italy to help women enter the profession is demonstrated in a document (now lost) of the year 1404: A woman by the name of Cusina di Filippo wished to be confirmed as a surgeon but was unable to travel to the court of Naples to be examined and take the oath there. A royal decree of May 1, 1404, charged the Jewish doctor Benedetto de Roma, inhabitant of Costenza, with the examination and made arrangements for the taking of the oath in a local court.[39]

It is understandable that female doctors in the Middle Ages were expected to deal first and foremost with the ailments of women. In this respect the licenses awarded women in southern Italy were the most specific: they all included a paragraph justifying the access of women to the medical profession on these grounds. This paragraph, which insists repeatedly, if in a minor tone, on women's demands to be treated by other women and not to be embarrassingly exposed to professionals of the opposite sex, reads:

> Although women should not participate in associations of men,
> from fear of compromising their feminine matronly modesty

whereby they may be blamed for impropriety; nevertheless, by an edict of law, women are allowed to practice medicine without impediment, taking into account that as far as honor and morality are concerned they are better suited to treat sick women than are men.[40]

But women did not limit themselves only to treating women, to gynecology or obstetrics. In Paris Jacqueline Felicie de Alamania had male patients, as her trial in 1321 revealed. Only four of the eight witnesses called were women.[41] One could argue that, because she was unlicensed, working in a semiclandestine manner and probably not charging much, she attracted a larger clientele. Such claims, however, cannot be made more than a century later in Seville in the case of Doña Leal, a Jewish physician.[42] Leal was a licensed physician mentioned in four notarial deeds that she signed with four of her clients, all male, in 1474. She specialized in ophthalmology and maintained an official practice. She appeared to have charged her clients quite high fees, the sums quoted being 300, 800, 1200, and even 4,500 maravedi.

Ophthalmology does appear to have been then a female specialization.[43] Around 1350 Judah, son of Rabbi Asher, the great rabbi of Toledo, reminisced about two women, one Christian, the other Jewish, who had treated his eye disease when he was a child. The Jewish physician successfully saved some of his eyesight and thus enabled him to excel in rabbinics. His invaluable testimony should be quoted in full:

> When I was an infant about three months old, my eyes were affected and were never completely restored. A certain woman tried to cure me when I was about three years of age but she added to my blindness to such an extent that I remained confined to the house for a year, being unable to see the road on which to walk. Then a Jewess, a skilled oculist, appeared on the scene. She treated me for about two months and then died. Had she lived another month, I might have recovered my sight fully. As it was, but for the two months' attention from her, I might never have been able to see at all.[44]

We find women, however, in fields other than ophthalmology. The records from Manosque at the end of 1321 and the beginning of 1322 give information about the female surgeon

Ḥava (or Ḥana) who intervened to rescue a wounded Christian gentleman by the name of Poncius Porcelli.[45] He had been hit in the most intimate organs of his body and the court wanted to know whether Ḥava had actually palpated the wound. Luckily, she could answer in the negative because her son Bonafos had assisted her during the treatment. She merely gave the instructions and assigned the necessary medicines, while her son did the actual handling.

The appearance of female doctors as certified and recognized practitioners is another aspect of the medicalization of society. Here again Jews responded to the challenge and found ways of training and licensing women in medicine.

Doctors Hired by Municipalities

Even before the Black Death of 1348, municipal authorities, particularly in Italy, showed interest in public health and in public hygiene.[46] As early as June 1293, to quote just one example, the famous Taddeo Alderotti negotiated to serve as a municipal doctor in Venice.[47] From fear of contamination and from a sense of responsibility toward the poor, some cities hired municipal doctors whose function was to extend medical help to people who were not able to afford it otherwise.[48] After 1348 and because of the series of epidemics that befell southern Europe in the second half of the fourteenth century, interest in public health increased further and even small cities and villages competed with one another to attract practitioners. Those who were ready to serve were declared municipal doctors.

Municipal councillors were obviously under public pressure to hire such doctors. Witness the general statement of the "urgent need for Jewish doctors who will be living and staying in Marseilles" found in a document dated October 20, 1381. The archives of the Catalan city of Cervera contain an undated document, which must have been written in the fifteenth century, which is nothing less than a petition (*supplicatio*) presented by a group of concerned citizens urging councillors to invite a specific doctor to work in the city. This man was

Abraham Chalom (pronounced Shalom), who was renowned for having dealt successfully with "incurable" diseases. The citizens vouched for his good manners and excellent virtues and were also practical enough to ask their municipality to ensure that the doctor's moving expenses would also be paid.[49]

Similar popular pressure occurred in the case of the municipal doctor in the Italian city of Gravedona. Sometime before August 1464 the doctor, Master Angelo de Cesena, apparently became involved in a romantic affair with a Christian woman and had to flee the city. But the citizens of Gravedona wanted their doctor back. In a written statement they advised the authorities in the duchy that the woman had retracted her testimony and, presumably, withdrawn her accusations. They therefore demanded that Master Angelo be allowed to return. It is even possible (although undocumented) that the citizens exerted pressure on the woman who was at the heart of the affair to retract her accusation.[50]

Municipal doctors' duties do not appear to have followed any single formula. In principle the physician was expected to look after the poor—those who had difficulty paying a doctor privately. Arrangements for fees for medical services varied from place to place. In some cities it was decreed that the doctor would offer one or two free visits and then charge for subsequent ones, whereas elsewhere cities made elaborate arrangements for a sliding scale based on social class. Documents from Murcia in southern Spain, Leon in the far north of the country, and Digne in upper Provence describe the duties of the doctors in very general terms. In Digne we only learn about his "work in visiting the poor sick," while in Murcia, his duty was "to treat the poor and their wounds without payment."[51] Master Shem Tov (Santo), who was hired by the municipality of Leon in 1455, was also expected to treat all sick people without charge, except for the cost of medications.[52] The agreement in Besalú was comprehensive. In 1361 the doctor promised that he would visit all sick people of the city, inspect urine, and establish suitable treatment "and they will not have to remunerate me, unless they are strangers in the city"; in the neighboring Castelló d'Empúries in November 1307 Master Bernat de Berriacho was ready, also free of

charge, to "inspect and judge all urines that will be brought to him by all the inhabitants of this city, will give them advice concerning phlebotomy and diet, and in general will [provide them] with guidance and counsel [regimina] [on their health]." His contract specified, however, "that he will not have to visit the sick."[53]

Other cities gave more precise details, probably because they could not offer the doctor a high enough salary. In the port city of Collioure, near Perpignan, in 1362 the municipality insisted that the first three visits to the poor each month be free; and the doctor was urged to make only a moderate charge for ensuing visits.[54] The council of Chambéry in Savoy agreed with Master Isaac of Annecy in 1396 that he could charge the rich a moderate fee but would ask nothing from the poor.[55] In Pernes, the city in the Comtat Venaissin about which much information is available, society was divided into three groups: the wealthy majores could be charged up to four grossi per visit; the middle group, the communi, paid three grossi; and the poor minores paid only two grossi per visit.[56] For its part, the council of Fabriano in northern Italy insisted on the difference between its own citizens and the peasants of its contado. The doctor, Moses of Rieti, was expected, according to a detailed contract drawn up on July 7, 1458, to treat all citizens of Fabriano free of all charge "however serious their sickness may be." As to contadini and villanos, they too were to be treated free of charge "as much as would be needed," but only if they managed to reach Fabriano on their own. If Master Moses had to travel specially to the countryside, he could charge ten shillings for the first visit and double for any ensuing ones.[57]

Municipalities who could not afford to employ a doctor on a full-time basis were nevertheless expected to provide a limited amount of public medicine. The doctors had to show sufficient flexibility to agree to work on a part-time arrangement and to earn their full salary by wandering from one place to another. This must have happened to Master Salomon, the Jewish municipal doctor to the Valencian city of Castellón, who had to work in the city once a week for a small salary of only four pounds a year.[58] It was certainly the case of Isaac of Carcas-

sonne, who lived in Carpentras and was employed in Pernes in the Comtat Venaissin. The municipality, which could afford to pay him no more than ten florins, secured his services (on August 31, 1450) for two days a week, Monday and Thursday. Isaac agreed to the terms, insisting, however, that he would stay in Pernes only until the late afternoon, "so that he could still go back to Carpentras" in good time.[59] A century earlier in Besalú, whose *jurati* could not afford more than fifteen pounds for remuneration, Master Moses Boaç, who lived in the city, insisted before accepting this offer, on July 9, 1361, that he could be absent from its boundaries for two days a week. Obviously he too was one of the itinerant doctors of this era.[60]

The archives also contain hints about the negotiations that took place between doctors and municipalities. The registers of the Pernes municipal council provide a number of examples. In the late fourteenth century the council wanted to attract Master Astrugus de Marnovilla of Arles to work in the city. On January 9, 1385, the municipality offered to cover his transportation costs, among other things. But it had difficulty settling his salary. The doctor wished to be paid fifty florins, while Pernes was prepared to offer no more than forty. On January 23, 1385, the councillors offered to add to this an annual housing allowance of six florins, which they would pay for the next six years. The doctor's son Salvetus, who represented him, then brought the negotiation to a successful end.[61] In 1430, in response to Master Joseph (Joze) Taurosii's threat to abandon the city, the council allocated an additional four florins to his salary to keep him from leaving the locality. But this must only have been a short-term solution, for in 1439 the city was looking for another doctor. The municipal records for May 11 of that year show a councillor named Monetus Caroli, Jr. charged with the mission of going to the neighboring Carpentras to "talk and conclude with the doctor, Master Vitalis, concerning his coming to this locality and serving in his medical capacity."[62] The negotiations must have been successful, for a month later the registers show that Vitalis was invited to visit the town in order to arrange for "serving and coming for two or three days a week when asked."[63]

If municipalities tried to drive hard bargains, it was because they knew that they could profit from competition among practitioners. Evidence for this hard negotiating can also be found in the municipality records of Pernes for the period 1440–1450. In 1448 Master John, a non-Jew, asked for fifteen florins, but the municipality, wishing to spend less money, succeeded in engaging Elia (Helias) of Narbonne, a Jew, for only eight florins.[64] Two years later, the council discussed a demand of fifteen florins from Master Abraham, a Jew, and once again the men of Pernes had their own way. At first they offered only twelve florins. They then appear to have hired a competitor named Abraham Boniac of Carcassonne for only ten florins.[65] Municipal doctors were obviously expected to respond to market conditions by lowering their prices and adjusting their salary demands.

This discussion of negotiations raises a crucial question concerning Jewish doctors engaged by municipalities. Did they obtain their positions because they were ready to work for less? Did they drive a less hard bargain than their Christian counterparts? Information from Umbrian archives suggests that such was the case.[66] City councillors in the medieval West seem to have had a clear idea of the salary a Jewish doctor should earn. Despite certain differences, such as the percentage of time worked and regional variations, salaries for Jewish physicians show a remarkable consistency. Doctors in municipalities as far apart as Marseilles, Chambéry, Digne, and Perugia, the capital of Umbria, all earned similar amounts. In 1396 both Marseilles and Chambéry had 40 florins for their Jewish municipal doctors in their respective budgets.[67] (By 1403 Marseilles had raised this amount to 50 florins.[68]) In 1433 Digne offered 35 florins, while in 1496 neighboring Forcalquier offered a little more, 36 florins.[69] In 1476 Marseilles allocated to its Jewish doctors no more than 36 florins.[70]

Were these "Jewish" salaries considerably lower than those of Christian practitioners in equal circumstances? The data from Spain, the south of France, and, particularly, Umbria in central Italy suggest that Jewish salaries were in fact lower. For example, for fourteenth-century Umbria, the average Jewish

salary was 25 florins, while for Christians it amounted to 35;[71] in 1383 in Assisi the Jewish surgeon received 12 florins while the Christian surgeon earned three times as much. A Christian *fisicus* named Bartolomeo di Jacopo did much better than both of them, earning 125 florins. The most successful Jewish physicians in the region, Vitale di Salomone and Salomone de Benaventura, did not earn even half as much. In Marseilles in 1406 Jewish doctors earned 40 florins each, while the Christian ones received 100. The 40 florins allocated to Master Crescas in 1397 should be compared with the 100 florins Master John de Granvilla received in 1385.[72] In the same year Granvilla also received a subsidy of 25 florins toward his lodging expenses from Marseilles. In Chambéry in 1396 the Jewish practitioner Isaac had to be content with 40 florins while Denis de Lyra, a Christian, earned double that amount.[73]

Similar, and even greater inequalities are revealed in municipal documents from Spain. In Murcia in the fourteenth century the Jewish doctor Abraham (Abrahim) agreed to work for a symbolic 300 maravedi; we know that Christian doctors were paid 1,000, 3,500, and 4,000 maravedi.[74] In 1476 Jaime de Limiaña, a famous Murcian doctor, was awarded no less than 8,000 maravedi (almost 140 florins), and five years later this salary was raised to 12,000 maravedi (about 200 florins), a very large sum by Western European standards.[75] This inequality in Murcia was not unique in Spain, as can be seen by examining the data from the distant city of Burgos. During the period 1440–1450 the Jewish doctors in that city gained annual salaries of 500, 2,000, and even 3,000 maravedi.[76] In 1447, for example, Mordecai (Mordohay) Monsoniego received 2,000 maravedi as his salary and a further 500 for travel expenses. In 1450, as one of three Jewish municipal doctors, Monsoniego received an even higher salary of 3,000 maravedi. He did very well in comparison with the other two Jewish doctors, Moses Judah and Amos, who were cousins, obviously employed part-time and who received only 500 maravedi each. But there was a fifth doctor in town, a Christian, who was also on the city's payroll and whose returns were entirely different. This man, Master Martin, received 12,000 maravedi, the same amount

Limiaña received in Murcia. This enormous salary was confirmed by a contract assuring him of this income for ten years. Martin's seniority was not only expressed through this huge difference in salary. As a part of his installation in the city, he insisted that he examine all the salaried doctors. He was certainly a university graduate and held the title *magister in medicina*, which may help to explain his overwhelming superiority. But it is not at all certain that all the other Christian doctors mentioned in this section possessed similar academic credentials. Therefore, instead of concluding that Christian doctors insisted on higher stipends because they were university graduates or better educated in some other way, I suggest that as a result of their minority status Jewish practitioners were prepared to work for lower salaries.

7

Private Practice: Doctors and Patients in Daily Encounters

Most of the knowledge we have about the day-to-day activities of medieval medical practitioners, both Jews and non-Jews, comes from legal documents preserved in archive collections. At the time when they were drawn up, these documents established the formal doctor-patient relationship. But these dry records can scarcely reveal the human quality of the relationship, and it is practically impossible to assess how Christian patients felt about treatment by a physician who was Jewish. Remember that people in the High and Late Middle Ages suspected Jews of poisoning their food and drink, desecrating and torturing the holy wafer until it bled, and, even worse, participating in ritual murder of innocent Christian children. Would not such a Christian tremble in horror at the idea of a Jew holding power over the individual's most precious property (in our eyes today), his body? Why then did medieval Christians nevertheless turn to Jews for medical aid? What does all this teach us about the real place of superstition in our lives?

Was There a "Mystique" about Jewish Doctors?

Is it possible that alongside medieval fears and suspicions of Jews there existed a "mystique" about their aptitude for medicine? A series of three modern public opinion polls carried out in France between 1966 and 1978 argue for the theory that such opposing attitudes can exist simultaneously.[1] When asked whether they would like to see a Jew in a governing position, most French respondents expressed reservations. The higher the position, the less acceptable the idea of a Jewish occupant. In 1966, 50 percent of the people did not want to see a Jew as president of the republic. In 1978 the percentage of those who retained negative feelings about this possibility had decreased by 17 percent, but, even then, one third of the French were still uneasy about Jews in power. Yet these same people overwhelmingly endorsed Jewish doctors. In 1966 only 16 percent were not prepared to trust Jews at any time with their own and their children's health. Twelve years later this number had decreased to 7 percent. We may therefore justifiably ask whether a mystique about Jewish doctors existed in French society in the 1960s and 1970s.

I am unable to go beyond statistics and inquire into the psychological motives that shape medieval or modern patient-doctor relationships in general, or with Jewish doctors in particular. Instead I would like to put forward a more general observation concerning people in medical distress: They tend to overlook religious differences. They will not even refrain from asking for miraculous help from a saint who is not of their religion. When a doctor gains a reputation for success, people tend to ignore his religion, even though this religion might otherwise be the source of a negative attitude. This is certainly true today. That it was also true in the Middle Ages can be gathered from the evidence that shows Jews turning to Christian doctors in quest of relief.[2]

Jewish Patients and Christian Doctors

Pious Jews must have been upbraided for recourse to Christian expertise; rabbis were certainly reprimanded by their synods when they sought Christian contacts. Some Jews were horrified by the possibility that nonkosher parts of animals might be used in medicinal syrups and ointments, never forgetting the old injunction of the Mishnah (Avodah Zarah 2b) that "we should not be healed by them." A severe reprimand appears in the introduction to an anonymous Hebrew translation of a medical work by John of Damascus. This anonymous translator may be considered an interested party, trying to promote his Hebrew text; he knew at the same time how to exert pressure on his coreligionists:

> I have seen Jews turning to gentile doctors about their sicknesses and those of their sons and daughters. They accept, uncritically, every [medicine] they [the gentiles] prescribe, without understanding or knowing what it is. These doctors do not distinguish between impure and pure [that is, forbidden and allowed] and in most of their ointments and mixtures they mix all kinds of insects and wine and unclean meat, and they put in tallow and blood. In consequence no Jewish patient escapes soiling and [consuming] the forbidden.[3]

In the middle of the thirteenth century Shem Tov of Tortosa wrote in the same vein. Even while explaining the Jews' recourse to Christian specialists by the lack of Jewish doctors, he was unable to disguise his discontent. "I have noticed that our brethren in these regions lack knowledge in this [medical] art, though they would have liked to possess it, and thus turn daily to Christian doctors, put themselves in their hands, transgressing thus the commandments of the rabbis."[4]

Some testimonies go beyond such general statements and describe actual encounters between Jewish patients and Christian doctors. In a Hebrew exchange of letters of around 1450 a famous rabbi, Zalman of Sankt Goar, informs his relative, Rabbi Liwa (Judah) Landau (d. 1464), the principal of one of the greatest Jewish academies of the time, about a gentile

practitioner in the vicinity of Bern (or, as most scholars suggest, Verona) who succeeded in curing a patient of an ailment that had confined him to his home for twenty years. Zalman heard about the case from Salomon, a French Jew living in Bern who was also treated by the doctor. He also knew that the diet prescribed by the doctor forbade the consumption of garlic, lentils, and the "head of mammals" (the Hebrew here is not clear) for a period of a year and a day. As far as remuneration was concerned, the doctor refused a salary but accepted gifts in accordance with the status of the patient. In return for help, the French Jew Salomon gave the doctor a belt worth four ducats. In an effort to persuade Rabbi Landau to see this practitioner, Zalman tries to allay the latter's fears that the gentile might evoke the names of Christian saints when "uttering charms." The ailing Landau had already declared that he preferred "to live all [his] life with the danger of this sickness and not to be considered wicked, even for an hour, in the eyes of the Lord."[5]

Regardless of all this talk, Jews in distress turned to Christian doctors. In fact, Rabbi Jacob Tam (ca. 1100–1170) and his students in France, the Tosaphists, had to condone such practices. "For phlebotomy we go to Christian masters because they are experts in the art."[6] In June 1262 in Manosque a Jewish man, Barba, was treated by two Christian doctors, Master Jacobus and Master Guillelmus Gausi, probably because the city had no Jewish doctors. We know about the two doctors and the treatment they gave because the Jews died and an inquest took place.[7] In Germany, around the year 1300, we learn of a baby that had suffered a severe hemorrhage following circumcision and whose bleeding continued for three days. There was no way to stop the hemorrhaging until, as a Hebrew report states, they "went to a Christian doctor and bought a plaster which was applied on wounds . . . and he was cured within ten days."[8] None other than Judah, the son of Rabbi Asher ben Yehiel (ca. 1250–1327), one of the greatest rabbinic authorities of his time, was brought by his parents to a Christian woman, an ophthalmologist (see p. 111). A letter from Barcelona dated 1306 reports the case of a Jew, Samuel, who probably had cataracts, who became hopeful when "a Chris-

tian doctor passed here" and assured him, "If you will keep me for a [couple of] days or for ten days, I shall take away the clouds from your eyes and you will be able to see once again, as you used to."[9] In Gerona in 1321 a Jewish patient, Cresques de Turri, who had trouble with his spine, refused to pay a Christian surgeon named Guillem Gueran his fee, claiming that the practitioner had administered the "wrong medicines" (*mala medicamenta*) to him.[10]

Jews were not even strangers to Christians' miraculous medicines. The *Sepher Ḥasidim*, a collection of *exempla* reflecting conditions in the Rhineland around 1200, shows in one of its stories the kind of challenge that successful Christian medicine might create for Jews. A Jewish woman refused to cure her child with the help of Christian holy water, even though she was assured of its curative power, preferring to risk her child's life. She was praised by the authors for having shown such devotion to her religion.[11] But the Ḥasidic author did not deny the possible efficacy of the miraculous cure. A story told at almost exactly the same time about a Jewish woman who sought help from the tomb of St. Thomas Becket has a certain element of truth in it.[12] In May and June 1363, during the canonization process of Dauphine de Puimichel, a Provençal saintly woman, the names of three Jewish doctors— Bonafos, Asher, and Macipus of Manosque—were quoted among those who testified about miracles she had presumably produced.[13] But, of course, this mention does not necessarily mean that the Jews believed in the miracles.

That medieval Jews, members of beleaguered communities, however pious and proud they may have been, with so many coreligionists among the doctors around them, overlooked religious differences and crossed the borders in search of medical aid may help us to understand Christians who did the same thing. Religious piety and social sensitivity notwithstanding, mothers and fathers in their anxiety, and suffering individuals themselves, sought the best help they could obtain. As there were so many Jewish doctors around by the year 1300, some of them possessing good reputations, it is little wonder that in moments of crisis and pain Christians placed their confidence in them.

Patients, Doctors, and the Rule of the Law

Any element of warmth, confidence, or human spontaneity which may have existed in the relationship between doctors and patients is almost entirely suppressed in the medieval notarial contracts and court records extant today. Legal contracts then as today were concerned with, and may even have contributed to, estrangements in relationships rather than good will. The contracting parties were generally trying to protect themselves against all possible claims, and they directed the notary to state their concerns and conditions in the most impersonal language possible. Nonetheless, these court documents have immense value as sources of historical information, if only because they provide objective evidence of the rapid spread of legal awareness among both doctors and patients. Moreover, they enable us at times to extract information concerning the medical challenges doctors had to face, the illnesses and accidents they were expected to cure, and the means and methods they employed in response. These sources, of course, also contain many details about the economics of medieval medical practice, the salaries and the fees solicited.

The contracts that medieval practitioners imposed on their patients resemble both in wording and content similar agreements negotiated by other professionals of the time. The agreement reached in Manosque in August 1310 (see p. 2), where the doctor promised free medical care to his client and to all members of his family in return for an annual payment of four sestarii of wheat, testifies to a practice that must have been quite common even though only one such document surfaces in the archives. At about the same time, Master Astruc Vidal Levi of Besalú, Catalonia, "expert in the art of physics and surgery," received what appears to have been an even better deal. He was to receive six sestarii of wheat, perhaps of lesser quality, for taking care of the family of a certain Pere Galceran of Pinos.[14] Such private medical insurance, as we may call it, must also have existed between Jacob de Baherias, a Jew of Manosque, and the surgeon Bonafos, for such a relationship was formally ended in a document

preserved in a notarial register for the year 1341.[15] In the city of Caltagirone in Sicily a more complex arrangement was discovered. There thirty-three families joined together in February 1461 to secure medical services for themselves from the doctor Abram Sargusia.[16] Just how common such arrangements were can be gathered finally from evidence discovered in the archives of the Catalan city of Castelló d'Empúries. Master Bernat de Berriacho is recorded there promising his services—whenever the intervention of "medical art" be needed—in return for an annual remuneration of ten shillings.[17] Twenty-three such documents were discovered for the years 1307–1308. On December 29, 1307, alone, nine contracts were recorded and three others were added a week later. In the month of May in 1308, eleven other citizens of this small locality established similar relationships with the doctor. That doctors were following patterns that existed in other professions can be deduced, for instance, from a notarial contract in which the Manosque lawyer Isnardus Cusenderii undertook to provide legal counsel for a whole year in return for a lump sum of six florins. It was also agreed that if this client's business obliged him to travel, he would receive the sum of ten shillings per day.[18] Other examples must exist in the archives as well.

Besides such overall medical insurance, doctors' services were also secured as the need arose. In one particularly common arrangement the practitioner received part, perhaps as much as half, of his remuneration at the beginning of his engagement, while the rest was only paid at the end, when there was valid proof that the treatment had been successful.[19] This arrangement too was not peculiar to doctors. The Manosque lawyer Cusenderii also agreed to divide up his remuneration, receiving half of it eight days after signing the agreement, the other half at the completion of the relationship. Dozens of such doctor-patient agreements have been discovered, by Henri Bresc in Sicily, by Noël Coulet in Aix-en-Provence, and by other distinguished scholars who contributed to "Le corps souffrant: Maladies et médications," a special issue of *Razo*, the bulletin of the Center of Medieval Studies at the university of Nice, published in 1984.[20]

Italian scholars as well have found such agreements in their

archives. One of the most detailed contracts with a story of suffering and hope in its background was recently published by Michele Luzzati. It is dated April 7, 1462, and it concerned the Pisan Jewish doctor Bonomo, son of Samuel. His patient, a peasant from the neighboring village of Sant'Andrea named Augustinus Ulivi, was suffering from a serious kind of arthritis in his right knee. The doctor claimed he needed six months to treat it. After the cure, he promised, "Augustinus will be able to stretch his knee as he is able to do with the left one and will be able to walk rightly and normally." The doctor must have been quite sure of his abilities, because he agreed to receive all remuneration at the end of treatment, when his promises had been fulfilled; he was even willing to pay for all medicine from his own pocket. Moreover, as Augustinus had obviously had bad experiences with other doctors and had suffered a great deal, Master Bonomo promised to treat him gently, assuring him that he would use "no iron or fire or cauterization (*roctoro* = *rottura*) but only ointment, cotton, and "sicle" (a term unknown to me).[21]

Similar detailed agreements can also be found in Provençal archives. In 1912 Duranti La Calade published a contract produced in Aix in 1413 in which a surgeon promised his patient to give him back the use of his right hand in return for a payment of thirty florins for his labor and another two florins for medicine.[22] Louis Stouff recently found in Arles a promise signed on July 28, 1448, to stretch the leg (*tibia*) of a local laborer called Johan Maystre to the length of the other one, "so that the said John would be able to walk straight and without the help of a walking stick." A sum of twenty florins was agreed on, with an additional six florins for the medicines required.[23] At times, a doctor whose treatments failed would be asked to repay the advance he had received. On July 12, 1446, Master Bartholet Johannis of Aix found himself confronted with such a demand when he was unable to cure the notary Laurent Ramat for a ruptured hernia. Since another surgeon succeeded in curing Ramat, Bartholet was asked to hand over to his colleague the sum of two and a half florins he had received as an advance.[24]

In all these arrangements the doctors' Jewishness is men-

tioned only accidentally and has no bearing on either the legal content or the wording of the contract. The very existence of these contracts in the notarial materials suggests, first, that the same law applied to practitioners of both religions, and, second, that Jewish doctors knew very well how to use the legal machinery that regulated and protected their activity. They also learned to insist on their rights and do not seem to have been discouraged from acting in matters concerning reimbursement. It is true that in the will of the Jewish doctor Joseph (Josse) de Novis his heirs were required not to pressure "many Christians who owe him for the work he did in his art," but this charitable instruction was given at Joseph's deathbed. This is certainly not the kind of attitude usually found in court records, where the doctor, more often than not, insists on his rights.[25]

Disagreements between doctors and patients took a variety of forms. In one instance a doctor was even murdered by his patient in the heat of a debate over remuneration. This episode is related in a document issued in northern France in 1352 in which the murderer, Baudoin Du Jardin, is given a pardon. The doctor's name was Joseph and the incident occurred during the "Great Mortality," obviously 1348.[26] But this is an exceptional case. It was far more common for doctors of both religions to pursue their clients in court for nonpayment. For example, in 1247, in the then newly conquered Languedoc, when citizens were encouraged to pursue complaints and demands through the agency of French royal officials, the Jewish doctor Master Salomon did not hesitate to make a claim. He demanded that his patient Simon de Mueil be compelled to pay him the ten-pound salary he owed him.[27] In an order of the court of Marseilles dated October 1306, a woman named Maria Compte (also "Comptessa" or "Comtessa") was enjoined to pay her doctor Guillelmus Broche, a Christian, forty shillings "salary for the cure of Maria and her child"; at about this time, also in Marseilles, Master Vitalis, a Jew, could not agree with the relatives of his patient Tolosa, who was also Jewish, about his remuneration. A Latin notarial document completed on March 8, 1305, states that both sides agreed on arbitration and that Master Crescas Vidon was made arbiter.[28]

(We possess the results of similar arbitration a century later in Assisi in 1431 which shows that the doctor Abraham was entitled to a sum of ten pounds.[29] In Valencia in February 1313 the doctor Isma'el Abencrespi, a Jew, took action in court against his patient, a textile merchant named Père Gilabert, who refused to pay the one hundred shillings owed for the physician's effort to cure him of epilepsy, arguing that the church forbade Jewish doctors from handling Christian patients. And finally in 1412 in Majorca we encounter another doctor, Crescas Farussol, in court claiming his salary.[30]

Doctors, both Jews and non-Jews, also appear in court records as claimants in the estates of deceased persons. Kalonymos ben Kalonymos of Arles, in his *Even Bohan* quoted in the previous chapter (see p. 103), has quite an obscure comment according to which the physician receives his money first, "before [the] legal heirs."[31] It is quite possible that in this short sentence we have reference to a legal privilege. A document prepared in the court of Manosque in May 1308 also shows the estate of the deceased being divided among creditors and other claimants. The Jewish doctor Isaac was the first to receive satisfaction from the court. He claimed fifteen shillings "by reason of the cure that he made in the body of the said Andrea [Sulpicii], defunct," while his Christian colleague, Master Raymond, received ten shillings. Another medical person, the local apothecary, received his share, and only then were the names of other claimants and heirs listed.[32] Other documents show Jewish doctors turning directly to the relatives of the deceased person. In Perpignan the name of Master Isaac Cabrit appears in 1409 and again in 1410 in two different lists of payments made by the relatives of various deceased people. In the first he receives only five and a half shillings, while in the second he receives no less than thirty "by reason of the labor which I did in visiting, prescribing medicines in the sickness of the said defunct man."[33] In neighboring Besalú in 1396, a few years earlier, Joseph Moses (Juce Mose) de Çeret claimed the sum of sixteen shillings "for the various visits done by me during the infirmity of the said defunct man."[34] In the case of Joseph (Juceff) Cavalaire (Cavaller), a Jewish doctor of Cervera around 1480, the stakes were much higher. Having

attended the deathbed of Dame Beatriu d'Olia, lady of Olula, for a period of forty-one days, he was paid eighty-two florins, a rate of two florins per day. A Christian doctor, Luis Serena, who stayed only eight days in the castle, was paid at the same rate.[35]

Practitioners also had to be alert to the possibility of failure and to the legal ramifications. In order to be on safe ground, many insisted on obtaining from the sick man or from his relatives a release relieving the physician of any future responsibility.[36] There appears to be no end to the number of such waivers to be found in the archives, both in Italy and elsewhere, in which the doctors declare their patient to be practically dead (*pro corpore mortuo*), that they have no hope for recovery, and that they are willing to try to help but assume no responsibility for the results. To quote only from documents issued on behalf of Jewish doctors, we begin in the first half of the fifteenth century with Master Abraham (Abramo) di Sabatuccio, a doctor in Umbria who protected himself twice in such a manner: The first occasion was in 1434 before treating a serf who suffered a fracture in his head; the second occasion was in 1439 when diagnosing a tumor in the throat of a woman named Evangelista di Francesco.[37] In Sipello, Gaio di Sabatuccio, Abraham's colleague, also required a statement *pro corpore mortuo* before treating a woman cruelly beaten on the head by her husband in an act of jealousy.[38]

Noël Coulet published a detailed summary of three such waivers, only one of which involved Jewish doctors, which were enacted in Provence in the years 1409, 1419, and 1432. In the first two cases the surgeon was expected to deliver a stone from the patient's urinary tract, while in the third the physician treated a grave disturbance in the digestive system.[39] According to documents dated 1423, 1425, and 1475, similar precautions were taken by doctors in Saragossa.[40] But the oldest known example to date comes from Manosque. Enacted November 19, 1313, it concerned both a Jewish doctor and a Jewish patient. The gravely ill patient was Dayot of Segriès, a well-known moneylender who possibly came to the south of France from Anjou, as his name suggests, with other Jews expelled from that county in 1288. The doctor Isaac did not see

much hope for his patient and registered a conditional agreement with a notary, who was summoned for this purpose to the house of Salvetus de Berra, another member of the community, perhaps a relative of the sick man. An examination of other notarial deeds filed a few months later proved that Isaac was right to take such precautions. In these deeds, Dayot's heirs were busy disposing of his estate.[41]

Finally, the evenhandedness of the medieval legal system with respect to Jews can be seen in their status in what we may without hesitation call forensic medicine. From the 1280s onward tribunals in Italy and in Provence started asking more and more frequently for expert medical testimony in cases of injury and violent death.[42] Judges would not render decisions in such cases without consulting one or even several doctors. If the parties involved considered it beneficial to their case, they too would urge the court to call for a medical examination. Indeed, court records in Italy—mostly from Bologna, but from other cities as well—have preserved dozens of examples of such expert advice demanded by the courts. In southern France almost sixty such documents, covering the period from the 1280s to 1348, are preserved in the records of the tribunal of Manosque.[43] They show Jewish practitioners pronouncing medical judgment on their own or together with Christian colleagues, employing identical language and making similar references to the classics of medical literature. When the victim happened to be a Jew and the aggressor a Christian, the Manosque court does not make an issue of the fact. In an inquiry held in July and August 1321 the victim was the Jew Abraham (Abramonus), the aggressor was Hugo Ferrandi, and the medical expert the Jewish surgeon Bonafos.[44] Two years earlier, on July 10, 1319, when the victim was a Christian woman and the accused a Jew, the court once more showed similar lack of bias in recording Master Bonafos's expert testimony.[45] The Jew's expert opinion is recorded plainly and routinely, indicating that it had the same legal value here as in any other situation. This particular expert, the surgeon Bonafos, was one of the Jewish doctors active in the service of the court, and his appearances in court are recorded more often than those of any other doctor. Let us examine more closely the file of docu-

ments on this otherwise unknown small-city practitioner, a file that makes him one of the best-known practitioners of the early fourteenth century.

Master Bonafos: Surgeon in Manosque before 1348

Most doctors referred to in this book appear once or twice in the sources and then disappear from sight, probably forever. Manosque, with its rich archives, provides an exception to this rule. Even though the best-documented personal file, that of Master Bonafos, a Jewish *cirurgicus*, cannot paint a complete picture of his life, we nonetheless have dozens of documents concerning him and his family. He was certainly active in the city throughout the first half of the fourteenth century, mainly in the 1320s–1340s, and he may have well survived 1348. It also becomes clear that he was part of a medical dynasty. His father, Astrugus, who was working in the 1290s and who died in 1306, was a surgeon. Astrugus is sometimes referred to as *cirurgicus*, at other times as *aurificerius* (also *aurielerius*), that is, goldsmith, and in two instances both as surgeon and goldsmith. Bonafos's mother, Hava (perhaps "Hana"; in ms. Fava or Fana), was involved with her son in the treatment of a man at the end of 1321 and the beginning of 1322. Bonafos's son Joseph (Iocep) worked in close connection with his father, as two documents dated 1341 describe.[46]

Bonafos's medical activity is much better reflected in our documents than his personal affairs. Two documents dated 1334 and 1342, respectively, establish contractual relationships between Bonafos and his clients. In a third notarial contract, dated October 21, 1332, a citizen named Raymundus Brunenqus promises the master to hand over to him two and a half sestarii of wheat, which constitutes "the rest of the salary for the cure done in the person of Brunenqus, son of the aforesaid Raymundus."[47] Other documents refer in more detail to Bonafos's medical activity. A text issued around March 1326 records that he had "to extract a large bone" from the

skull of a citizen called Guillelmus Pelicernii, who had been hit with a sword.[48] In October and November of the same year he treated Guillelmus Salvator for at least eighteen days for wounds on his arm, breast, and nape of the neck.[49] An eye wound incurred by Andreas Obrerii at the beginning of 1340 must have been a particularly complicated one. As the judge ordered that the surgeon report daily on the state of the wounded person, we have here quite a detailed description of Bonafos's interventions. At first Bonafos treated the injury with the white of an egg and with cotton to staunch the flow of blood "as teaches the art of surgery to do at the beginning of whatever wound." But when he removed the cotton at the end of the second day to inspect the wound and apply the necessary medicine, the vein hemorrhaged and Bonafos had difficulty controlling the bleeding. On the fifth day he applied red pulver, but as the bleeding continued he decided to cauterize the wound with hot silver. When the court heard about this procedure, the patient was still not well and Bonafos was unable to give a definite prognosis.[50]

Although Bonafos was not the only surgeon in the city and certainly not the only medical practitioner, he must have become almost an institution. On the night of January 3, 1322, when a citizen was wounded in the street, the bystanders hurriedly brought him to Bonafos's house.[51] In another incident, when asked to examine a victim of assault, he asked the court to let him take the man to his home because "this is not the right place for examining him."[52]

In cases of great urgency the court of Manosque would travel to where the wounded person was lying and examine him there. A surgeon would always be requested to be a member of the small group, which was headed by the judge, the bailiff or his lieutenant, and also included a notary and sometimes a court messenger (*nuntius*). Bonafos was consistently a member of these expeditions. In September 1324 he was one of three doctors, the others being Master Raymundus Bodyoni, *physicus*, and Master Raymundus Gaudii, *cirurgicus*, whom the bailiff called on to establish whether a certain Raymundus de Villamuris died from the wounds inflicted on him.[53] In October 1325 and on many other occasions he was

the only physician called on by the court.[54] In one of the first documents of September 25, 1315, he took part in a medico-legal expedition to the synagogue in Manosque to establish the cause of death of Joseph (Iossonus), a foreign Jew.[55] In another instance, on January 13, 1342, he examined, with the help of a small candle, the depth of wounds found on the body of a dead man. He did so in the presence of Guillelmus de Biteris, lieutenant to the bailiff of Manosque, to whom he also quoted the authors of *Ars Cirurgie* in support of his conclusion that the victim, Petrus Gautherii, died as a result of his wounds.[56]

In many of his court appearances when he was called to testify about the condition of an accident victim, Bonafos was one of a larger group of doctors who treated a patient concurrently, a procedure that must have been common practice at the time. In all except one of these cases, his collaborators were non-Jewish physicians and surgeons.[57] Thus such Jewish-Christian collaboration must also have been quite common, at least in Provence. In 1357 in Avignon a woman named Dousselin de Sade was treated by a then-famous physician, Paul de Viterbo, in cooperation with the Jewish doctor Crescas de Caylar, who later became famous as an author.[58] In the city of Apt a few years earlier the group of doctors who gave a woman named Aycelena Guisola no hope of a cure consisted of three Christian doctors and two Jews.[59] Documents from Aix-en-Provence for the first third of the fifteenth century contain several examples of such interfaith medical collaboration. Noël Coulet, for example, sees such cooperation in the committees established in 1446 to examine cases of leprosy. According to documents concerning the Aix-en-Provence doctor Master Astruc of Sestiers, he collaborated with non-Jewish practitioners in at least two of the five healing contracts he signed there at about this time.[60] But no collaboration with Christian doctors is better documented than that of Bonafos. In one of the first surviving texts about him, he is seen in June 1310 traveling with Master Antonius on the highway leading to the neighboring village of Sainte-Tulle. It is practically certain, although the document does not confirm it formally, that the doctors were engaged in a medical expedition.[61] Twelve years

later, in January 1321, Bonafos collaborated with the physician
Petrus Aycardi to treat one Hugo Stephani.[62] Over the years
he also collaborated with the Christians Bertrandus Arduini,
Raymundus Gaudii, and Michael Tartona.[63] Although the
name of Petrus Aycardi appears more often than any other,
this does not necessarily suggest that the two men collaborated
permanently.[64] Rather, it appears that each accident attracted
its own group of doctors. It is therefore probably safe to suggest that during his long years of service in Manosque, Bonafos collaborated with practically every Christian doctor of the
city.

Incidents in Bonafos's life within the Jewish community of
Manosque are reflected in three documents of the city
tribunal.[65] On June 1, 1306, Bonafos was accused of insult by
another Jew, Fossonus Levi. He allegedly reproached Levi for
having a brother who had converted to Christianity, using the
Hebrew word for a convert to Christianity, *meshumad*. Bonafos denied the accusation but admitted to having had a heated
discussion with the man. Just a few weeks later a document of
August 16 refers to a scandal occurring at Bonafos's father's
funeral, which had presumably taken place a short time earlier. A Jew by the name of Tuviah (Thobias) insulted one of
his coreligionists, Jacob, by calling him *mihares*. The Latin
notary who recorded the affair provides a correct interpretation of this Hebrew word (pronounced today *mehares*): "which
Hebrew word is interpreted as rebel against the law."[66] Even if
mehares can have many meanings, at this time it referred to
Jewish intellectuals committed to a scientific, "rationalist" way
of thinking, which created difficulties for them with parts of
the religious tradition. In the third document, dated June
1310, Bonafos (called "Fossonus") appears as a law-abiding
member of the community, accepting the authority of the local
rabbi, the then famous Isaac Cohen de Talardo. This document relates a controversy within the community. For some
reason the rabbi had excommunicated a member of the community, and as a consequence no one was allowed to perform
a circumcision on the offender's baby boy. A dissenter, Moses
Anglicus, volunteered to carry out the operation, but he
caused a hemorrhage that proved fatal. Bonafos figured quite

prominently in the inquiry following the incident, for without the excommunication he would have performed the operation. No punishment was imposed on him or on the rabbi.[67]

Other Economic Activities

Although Master Bonafos is labeled in some of our documents as "goldsmith" (*aurificerius*), none shows him practicing this profession. He was engaged, to some extent at least, in another activity, parallel to that of a surgeon. A notarial register for the years 1312–1315 lists several deeds issued in his favor in which he acted as a moneylender, giving modest sums, fourteen shillings on two occasions, twenty-eight on another, as loans to individuals living in the vicinity of the city, in such places as Volx, Pierrevert, and Montfuron.[68] In the same manner the female physician Mayrona (see p. 109) is shown in a notarial register for 1342 as being involved in more than forty such loans.[69] In fact, Mayrona, *fisica*, never appears in the documents of Manosque in her medical capacity. It would, of course, be a grave mistake to conclude that she did not practice medicine in the city and was instead a moneylender. In all probability the extant evidence is simply misleading.

Nevertheless, such distortion has some advantages, for the chance survival of evidence shows us that doctors were not professionally limited to medicine. Jewish doctors certainly appear combining professional activities. The following examples show that these doctors were following a rather common pattern.[70]

Much evidence of the extramedical activities undertaken by Christian doctors has been discovered in the archives of Marseilles through the tireless work of Louis Barthélemy. In October 1306 we read of a Marseilles doctor, Guillelmus Broche, who demanded forty shillings from his patient Maria Comtessa. In fact, the woman owed him sixty shillings, for the doctor had not only cured her and her child for forty shillings but had also loaned her twenty shillings.[71] In the mid-fourteenth century the doctor Pierre Gamel also ran an office as a notary, while in 1407 and 1414 doctors Etienne Meyer and

Pierre Vincent were directing a school in the city.[72] Pierre Correto of Marseilles had an extraordinary career as a teacher; he held a bachelor's degree in law and also worked as a medical doctor.[73]

But the best-known case of a doctor working in multiple professions is that of Jean Blaise of Marseilles, an exact fourteenth-century contemporary of Master Bonafos of Manosque. Blaise, the nephew of the wife of the illustrious doctor Arnold of Villanova, left a great deal of evidence about his extramedical activity, his commerce, and his property. The most important of these documents, all now in the archives of Marseilles, is an account book written in his own hand.[74] This fifty-two-page inventory, written between the years 1333 and 1337, contains hundreds of entries and reveals Blaise as a prosperous merchant, investor, and financier. His business interests ranged from real-estate ventures such as the exploitation of vineyards and fields to commerce in oil, textiles, leather, coal, and herbs. Considerable sums of money were involved in some of his projects. On one occasion Blaise rented a boat and sent it on a commercial expedition to the port of Manfredonia (in Apulia on the Adriatic coast of Italy), a venture in which he invested over five hundred pounds. Other international undertakings brought him into contact with the islands of Sardinia and Majorca and with the city of Naples. After his death much of his estate went to the Hospital of the Holy Spirit, the most prestigious institution in Marseilles. In his will Blaise requested (like the Jewish physician Joseph de Novis did on his deathbed; see p. 127) that the rectors of this institution forgive people the debts owed him totaling four hundred pounds in all.[75]

Jean Blaise's uncle, Arnold of Villanova, was also active in the world of finance and business, at times probably working in cooperation with his nephew. In Arnold's case the evidence is much less extensive, mainly because practically no notarial registers from Montpellier have survived for his lifetime. But fortunately we do learn from two notarial registers that the famous professor and medical author invested a considerable sum of money, 150 pounds, as stated in a short notice dated November 1294, as a *depositum* to an association of two local

merchants.[76] Arnold's name also surfaces in connection with investments recorded in the archives of Marseilles. Acting though the agency of a certain Arnandus Safabregua, who was also in business with Jean Blaise, Arnold purchased taxation rights (*cens*) as well as some real estate in the city, a transaction described in a group of documents dated from June 1308 to January 1309.[77]

In Manosque at least two documents reflect the extramedical activities of Christian practitioners. In one the surgeon Master Antonius was reported to have taken part in the commerce of almonds. At the end of October 1324 he was charged with trying to sell rotten produce. In his defense Antonius claimed that his wife had merely sprinkled water on the almonds. Nevertheless, the court found Antonius guilty and fined him one hundred shillings. Earlier the same year, on June 16, Petrus Aycardi, another doctor, appeared in court to answer a charge concerning the quality of products he was offering customers. This doctor's interest was not in almonds but in candles, a manufactured product. In court Master Aycardi and his brother Mastinus, a butcher, claimed that their products were of the same quality as those found in other cities in the county, especially around Aix-en-Provence.[78]

In fifteenth-century Italy it was not uncommon for the Jewish doctor of a city to act also as a moneylender. Thus, in the city of Cremona, for example, in 1441, when Isaac, son of Salomon, "phisico and ciroyco," handed Duke Francesco Sforza a document outlining the conditions under which he could stay in the city, only one paragraph, a very general one, dealt with medicine, whereas a long series of regulations was devoted to the doctor's credit operations.[79] Mattathias, son of Salomon (Matassia di Salomne), who had not cared to make such an arrangement with the city of Spoleto when he originally came to serve as its municipal doctor, followed suit in 1443. "I have come to live in Spoleto together with my family with the intention of serving the community with my experience in general medicine as well as in surgery," the doctor wrote to the municipality. "But I have become aware of the fact that it is difficult to make a living and to sustain a wife and children solely with the income from the medical arts. I am therefore

compelled to have recourse to an auxiliary activity and am asking for authorization to exercise it inside the city."[80] In 1418 another doctor, Salomon de Bonaventura, gave up his Umbrian medical practice altogether to devote all his time to his bank, and in 1457 yet another practitioner, Bonavita de Tivoli, resigned from the position of municipal doctor in Assisi to engage only in private practice and to look after his banking interests.[81]

Banking and moneylending were not, however, the only activities doctors considered as sources of additional income. In 1289 in Huesca, Aragon, in return for much appreciated medical services, the Jewish doctor Vidal Abulbaça and an associate were granted a license to open a shop for the commerce in textiles; in the not too distant city of Cervera in 1479 the two doctors Joseph (Jucef) and Samuel Cavaller and their brother rented a watermill on the river.[82]

The late professor Richard W. Emery was not mistaken when he suggested that there were so many doctors and surgeons in Perpignan in the later Middle Ages because some did not practice at all while others did so only on a part-time basis.[83] Still, conditions must have varied in different places at different times. Thus, Master Bonafos, between his regular treatment and emergencies and appearances in court, must have lacked the leisure and even the patience for moneylending. The image of such a busy doctor consumed by his medical activities was familiar to people of the time. Overwork often surfaced as an argument when monarchs wished to release practitioners from time-consuming tasks and obligations. In 1314, for instance, the registers of the crown of Aragon showed two Jewish doctors, Azariah of Saragossa and Omār Tawil (Omerio Tahuyl) of Valencia, gaining exemption with the help of the king from serving as communal officials on the grounds of lack of time,[84] since they were both so much absorbed in visiting the sick and in carrying out their professional duties. In 1471 in the duchy of Milan, when the Jewish doctor Jacob wanted to appoint two other Jews to handle his banking business in the city of Cremona, he gave as his reason his extensive medical practice, which did not leave him time to engage in moneylending. The argument was accepted and the duke

granted permission.[85] A vivid description of how intense and time consuming medical practice could have become is found in a document from Sicily dated February 12, 1396. The doctor Joseph (Iocef) Abenafia, who acted as doctor to the court in Sicily (see p. 17), felt that he should be awarded a license to build a synagogue in his home so that he could save time, "because he spends his time in quest of medical art, as many days and nights as possible. The result of this is that he is almost unable to perform ceremonies and prayers in the synagogue or the mosque of the Jews."[86]

Conclusion

The history of Jewish involvement in the medical profession in the Middle Ages is far from complete. If only the historical geography is to be considered, then the horizons must one day be broadened to include the countries of northern Europe, on one hand, and the Arabic east, on the other. Since Jewish doctors were in many instances close to the sources of power in society, the study of their contribution to Jewish politics also promises to be a most engaging topic of research. Even the task of establishing the place of these Jewish doctors in their communities is not yet half finished. We should be able to follow their marriage patterns and that of their children and define their place in the hierarchy of income and wealth. The positions of power and prestige they secured for themselves within the institutions of the Jewish community should be described and assessed. Considering that these practitioners constituted a well-defined group of intellectuals whose education was based to an important degree on secular foundations, the relations between the rabbinical establishment and the physicians also need further investigation. The place of Jewish doctors in the Jewish religious and cultural world must also be explored. Since many also served as rabbis to their communities, we have to ask how they explained to themselves their permanent intervention in God's creation and in heavenly decisions. What kind of *mentalité* did they develop which enabled them to engage in both religious studies and teachings and in secular practices based on pagan knowledge

and analysis? How much were the legal and religious teachings of rabbis like Moses Nahmanides or Nissim Girondi influenced by their knowledge of natural sciences? With regard to their place in the world of learning, clearer statements must be made about the Jewish contribution to philosophy and its auxiliary sciences and about the limited extent of their medical creativity. Why was so little science produced by Western European Jews in these centuries? Is their belated entry to universities the only reason?

But the information presented in this book does lead to some general conclusions about Jews and the medical profession. The first conclusion is that we now know a good deal about the conditions that brought about their entry into the profession in such great numbers. A comparison with what happened around this time in moneylending, the other major Jewish occupation, is revealing. In the same way that Jews' involvement with usury was a product of the growing demand for credit in all sectors of society, so their entry into medicine was related to the growing demand for medical services. In both instances their progress was facilitated by the church, which adopted a negative stance and was not sensitive enough to the new needs of society. Considering that other professional avenues were closed to Jews, it is not surprising that they leaped at the opportunities in finance and medicine. They found ways of creating the necessary learning tools and they turned Hebrew into the language of medical education. As moneylenders, the doctors also benefited from the reintroduction of Roman law to society and its institutions; their status was well defined by the constitutions of the lands and cities, and their professional activities were protected by law.

European society itself also matured to some extent as its relationship with its Jewish doctors developed. The Christian community seems to have discovered some flexibility within itself along with the capacity to lay aside prejudices and fear. Some municipalities even went out of their way to send emissaries in search of Jewish doctors. Tolerance thus emerges as the child of necessity.

The history that has unfolded in this book goes beyond the story of the emergence of a profession and the services it ren-

dered society. Considered in the framework of the history of the Jews, this account of Jews in medicine acquires an almost symbolic dimension. Since any encounter with medical services is invariably laden with strong emotions—fear, despair, hope, or relief—the history of doctors in general treats a myriad of tense moments. Because of the emotional content of the subject, success and failure are often exaggerated. And what is true for doctors in general is much more so for Jewish physicians. At times they were venerated as authors of miracles; in other moments they were suspected of poisoning their patients or they were sued for malpractice. They were heroic when placed on a pedestal, but badly injured, even broken, when they fell from favor. Anyone who is even slightly familiar with the Jews and their history must recognize how such extremes as these reflect society's ever-changing attitudes toward the children of Israel.

Notes

Chapter 1

1. For Avignon see the classic study of Pierre Pansier, "Les méde cins juifs à Avignon aux XIIIe, XIVe, et XVe siècles," *Janus* 15 (1910): 421–451. For Rome we have numbers in the recent study of Anna Esposito, "Gli ebrei a Roma nella seconda metà del '400 attraverso i protocolli del notaio Giovanni Angelo Amati," *Aspetti e problemi della presenza ebraica nell'Italia centrosettentrionale (secoli XIV e XV)*, 29–125, esp. 72, Quaderni dell'istituto di scienze storiche dell'università di Roma 2 (Rome, 1983).

2. Danielle Jacquart, *Le milieu médical en France du XIIe au XVe siècle* (Geneva and Paris, 1981), 163, 246. The question of numbers of doctors will be discussed in chapter 6 of the present work.

3. In recent years many scholars have discussed the question of the size of Jewish populations. Here I can refer the reader to the most recent and most successful work, that of Juan Carrasco Pérez, "Propietarios judios en la ribera Tudelana de Navarra después de la peste negra (1348–1386): Un aspecto de las relaciones campo-ciudad," in *Concejos y ciudades en la edad media hispánica* (1990), 23–72. See also for the south of France, Édouard Baratier, *La démographie provençale du XIIIe au XVIe siècle* (Paris, 1961), 69–72. For further discussion of this topic, see my chapter 5.

4. See Danielle Jacquart, *Le milieu médical en France*, especially 231 ff.

5. The observation and the quotation are from Luis García-Ballester, "Dietetic and Pharmacological Therapy: A Dilemma among Fourteenth-century Jewish Practitioners in the Montpellier Area," *Clio medica* 22 (1991): 23–37, in particular 27.

6. The document is published in my *Médecine et justice en Pro-*

vence médiévale: Documents de Manosque 1262–1348 (Aix-en-Provence, 1989), 123–124 (doc. no. 29).

7. See above n. 6 and the evidence presented in text below.

8. Much evidence for expert medical testimony is presented in my *Médecine et justice en Provence médiévale*, in the introduction as well as in the documentary section. For Paris see the evidence brought by Danielle Jacquart, *Le milieu médical en France*, 290.

9. For Marseilles see Louis Barthélemy, *Les médecins à Marseille avant et pendant le moyen âge* (Marseilles, 1883), 25. For Paris see Joseph Petit, ed., *Registre des causes civiles de l'officialité épiscopale de Paris (1384–1387)* (Paris, 1919), xxiv n. 2, as well as Danielle Jacquart, *Le milieu médical en France*.

10. See Carlos Carrete Parrondo, *Fontes judaeorum regni Castellae*, vol. 1: *Provincia de Salamanca* (Salamanca, 1981), p. 121, doc. no. 338. It reads: ". . . antel señor don Aluar Peres, rector del Estudio, paresçio el . . . maestro Juan de Léon, e para en prueua de su enfermedad presentó por testigo a Rabí Abrahán, judío, médico, veçino de la . . . çibdad [= Salamanca], e pedió que lo conpeliese a jurar e deponer lo que çerca de su enfermedad sabe. E el señor rector conpeliólo e juró; e jurado e por virtud del . . . juramento, preguntado, dixo que sabe quel . . . maestro Juan de León desdel primero día de enero deste . . . año fasta que començo, a leer estouo doliente de parlesía e que en tal enfermedad e disposiçión que podiera buena mente ne en manera alguna leer su cáthedra de Philosophia moral ni otra letura alguna por quanto estaua priuado del mouimiento de sus mienbros, e avn desde que lee acá, e agora de presente e de aquí adelante ha estado e está e estará según la qualidad de su dolençia en tal disposiçión, que non le conpele leer en manera alguna para su salud e vida; e que sy continúa la letura, que está en grand peligro para tornar a recaer e retornar en la . . . dolençia . . . E luego, el . . . señor rector ouo por prouada la . . . dolençia, en avn a mayor abondamiento tomó juramento del . . . maestro sy sentía en sý estar en la . . . disposiçion que . . . Rabí Abrahán desía, el qual, jurado, dixo que sý."

11. The document, still unpublished, is to be found in the Archives départementales des Bouches-du-Rhône (Marseilles), 396E12(a), fol. 15r—5 August 1325. I hope that my student John Drendel, who brought it to my attention, will publish it in the near future.

12. Henri Bresc, "Documents siciliens," *Razo: Cahiers du centre d'études médiévales de Nice* 4 (1984): 109–114, especially 113.

13. The documents are published in Shatzmiller, *Médecine et justice en Provence médiévale*, 218–220 (doc. no. 74).

14. Archives départementales des Bouches-du-Rhône (Marseilles), 381E373, fols. 30v–31r. It reads: "De Jussono de Posqueriis Judeo. Anno domini millesimo CCCVIIII⁰ XVII kalendas aprilis. Cum Jussonus de Posqueriis judeus civis Massilie detineretur in carcere regio Massilie ad instantiam Amigueti Vincentii ut dicitur; ecce quod propter infirmitatem dicti judei placuit discreto viro domino Raimundo Rostagni judici curie Massilie quod idem judeus per aliquas dies a dicto carcere liberetur sub forma infrascripta, videlicet quia dictus Jussonus promisit et convenit in dicto domino judici et mihi Guillelmo Feraudi notario publico Massilie tamquam publice persone presenti recipienti et stipulanti nomine dicti Amigueti, licet absenti, et pro eo, se dicto Amigueto satisfacere in illo debito quod dictus reperiretur ipsum judeum eidem Amigueto debere juxta cognitionem et voluntatem dicti domini judicis hinc ad decem dies proximos, vel redire in dictum carcerem si contra faceret in aliquo, sub obligatione omnium bonorum suorum presentium et futurorum et sub omni renunciatione et cautela juravit. Ad hoc magister Haron de Posqueriis fisicus habitator civitatis superioris Massilie supponens se quantum ad hec jurisdictioni dicit domini judicis sponte, cum sciat se esse alterius jurisdictionis, precibus et amore dicti Jussoni, constituit et obligavit se dicto domino judici et mihi dicto notario presentibus et stipulantibus nomine dicti Amigueti et pro eo, fidem et proprium et principalem debitorem accipientem et procurantem sub obligatione omnium bonorum suorum presentium et futurorum et sub omni renunciatione et cautela juravit. Actum Massilie in dicta curia in presentia testium Ancelineti Ancelini, Guillelmi Raimundi notarii."

15. For this kind of medical certificate see Antonio [Antoní] Cardoner [i] Planas, *Història de la medicina a la corona d'Aragó (1162–1479)* (Barcelona, 1973), 103–104.

16. The document is described in Noël Coulet, "Documents aixois (première moitié du XVe siècle)," *Razo: Cahiers du centre d'études médiévales de Nice* 4 (1984): 115–125, especially 122.

17. The document is published in Yves Grava, "Pratique médicale en milieu rural: Istres au XVe siècle," *Razo: Cahiers du centre d'études médiévales de Nice* 4 (1984): 95–99.

18. See Noël Coulet, "Documents aixois," 123.

19. Ibid. For more examples, see Françoise Bériac, *Histoire des lépreux au moyen âge: Une société d'exclus* (Paris, 1988), 58–65.

20. Jacques Chiffoleau, *La comptabilité de l'au-delà: Les hommes, la mort, et la religion dans la région d'Avignon à la fin du moyen âge (vers 1320–vers 1480)* (Rome, 1980), 321–323. He insists rightly on this point. See also my comments in "Doctors' Fees and Their Medical Responsibility: Evidence from Notarial and Courts Records," in *Pri-*

vate Acts of the Late Middle Ages, ed. Paolo Brezzi and Egmont Lee (Toronto, 1984), 201-208.

21. I have presented several of these studies in my *Médecine et justice en Provence médiévale,* 18-19, and the relevant notes on 46-47. For further discussion see chapter 7 of this book.

22. Katharine Park, *Doctors and Medicine in Early Renaissance Florence* (Princeton, 1985), 54-58.

23. Robert S. Gottfried, *Doctors and Medicine in Medieval England 1340-1530* (Princeton, 1986), 42-48 and 253.

24. Auguste Prudhomme, "Notes et documents sur les juifs de Dauphiné," *Revue des études juives* 9 (1884): 230-263, esp. 251: "Pauci sunt qui resident presentialiter in patria Dalphinali experti in artibus predictis unde multa dampna personarum e lesiones multimodas cotidie patiuntur."

25. "In civitate Pistorii non existet copia medicorum secundum exigentiam civitatis." Enrico Cotturi, "Medici e medicina a Pistoia nel medioevo," *Incontri pistoiesi di storia arte cultura* 13 (1982): 1-14, esp. 3-4.

26. Adolphe Crémieux, "Les juifs de Marseille au moyen âge," *Revue des études juives* 46 (1903): 1-47, 246-268; 47 (1903): 62-86, 243-261; especially 47:243 (doc. no. 30 of the year 1383), which starts: "attenta urgenti necessitate medicorum judeorum, phisicorum et surigicorum nunc in hac civitate Massilie degentium et habitantium hoc tempore apitisme sive mortalitatis." For the negotiations in 1476 see 47:244 (doc. no. 33).

27. Luis García-Balleste, Michael R. McVaugh, and Agustín Rubio-Vela, *Medical Licensing and Learning in Fourteenth-century Valencia,* Transactions of the American Philosophical Society, vol. 79, no. 6 (Philadelphia, 1989), p. 20.

28. Ibid., 20-21. Additional quotations from Valencian sources are reproduced in this recent and excellent study. A similar complaint ("There are not . . . enough [physicians for us]") is heard from another crusading country, Palestine. See Pierre Dubois, *The Recovery of the Holy Land,* ed. and trans. Walther I. Brandt (New York, 1956), 114 (no. 58), 118-120 (no. 61), and 138 ff. (no. 85).

29. See Fritz Baer, *Die Juden im christlichen Spanien,* 2 vols. (Berlin, 1929-1933), 1:173: "esto pus exellent metege qui sia en aquestas partidas . . . que ha be dell senyor Rey vostre li factas fer mandement de par dell senyor Rey que ell stia uci in Barchinona."

30. Nancy G. Siraisi, *Medieval and Early Renaissance Medicine: An Introduction to Knowledge and Practice* (Chicago and London, 1990), 63-64.

31. For the papal estimate see Giovanni Domenico Mansi, ed.,

Sacrorum conciliorum nova et amplissima collectio, 58 vols. (Florence and Venice, 1759–1798), 25:1006: "tam pro victualibus vestimentis ac calciamentis quam pro libris et quibuscumque necessitatibus aliis eorumdem." For the Italian universities see Katharine Park, *Doctors and Medicine in Early Renaissance Florence* (Princeton, 1985), 123–128. That this may nevertheless be an inflated figure comes to mind when reading Alan B. Cobban's *The Medieval English Universities: Oxford and Cambridge to ca. 1500* (Berkeley, 1988; reprint, Berkeley, 1990), 311 ff.

32. The most important monograph on the subject is still Paul Delaunay, *La médecine et l'Eglise: Contribution à l'histoire de l'exercice médical par les clercs*, Collection Hippocrate (Paris, 1948). See, however, the more recent study of Darrel W. Amundsen, "Medieval Canon Law on Medical and Surgical Practice by the Clergy," *Bulletin of the History of Medicine* 52 (1978): 22–44.

33. Mansi, *Sacrorum conciliorum* 21:438: "Prava autem consuetudo, prout accepimus, et detestabilis inolevit, quoniam monachi et regulares canonici post susceptum habitum et professionem factam, spreta beatorum magistrorum Benedicti et Augustini regula, leges temporales et medicinam gratia lucri temporali addiscunt . . . " I follow the translation in Amundsen, "Medieval Canon Law," 28.

34. Mansi, *Sacrorum conciliorum* 21:459 (Reims) and 21:528 (Lateran II): ". . . illa etiam de quibus loqui erubescit honestas, non debet relligio pertractare. Ut ergo ordo monasticus et canonicus, Deo placens in sancto proposito inviolabiliter conservetur: ne hoc ulterius præsumatur, auctoritate apostolica interdicimus. Episcopi autem, abbates, et priores, tantæ enormitati consentientes, propriis honoribus spolientur."

35. See Mansi, *Sacrorum conciliorum* 21:1159 (Montpellier, 1162); 21:1179 (Tours, 1173); 22:670 (Montpellier, 1195); and 22:831 (Paris, 1212).

36. Amundsen, "Medieval Canon Law."

37. Mansi, *Sacrorum conciliorum* 22:225 (Lateran III, 1179), and 22:766–767 (Paris, 1208); 23:24 (Narbonne, 1227); 23:1222 (London, 1268); 23:1241–1242 (Avignon, 1279); and 22:1007 (Lateran IV, 1215).

38. See Harold J. Berman, *Law and Revolution: The Formation of the Western Legal Tradition* (Cambridge, Mass., and London, 1983), 196 and the references cited.

39. Mansi, *Sacrorum conciliorum* 22:583 (Rouen, 1189), 1152–1153 (Oxford, 1222). "Ut clerici secularibus negotiis se non inmisceant" is the title of the Oxford document.

40. Mansi, *Sacrorum conciliorum* 25:839: "Statuimus ac man-

damus, quod cura animarum habentes, et qui sunt in personalibus vel dignitatibus constituti publica officia saecularia non assumant, nec bajulas nec vicarias teneant faicorum sed in ecclesiis suis personalem et continuam residentiam faciant, sicut decet."

41. See the chapter about him in Heinrich Schipperges, *Die Assimilation der arabischen Medizin durch das lateinische Mittelalter* (Wiesbaden, 1964), 178–85. And also the more recent article by Maria Helena da Rocha Pereira, "A obra médica de Pedro Hispano," in *Memórias da academia das ciências de Lisboa: Classe de letras*, vol. 18 (Lisbon, 1977), pp. 193–208. Prof. da Rocha Pereira also published a short medical treatise (*regimen*) by Petrus in Pedro Hispano, *Livro sobre a conservação de saúde* (Porto, 1961).

42. For Theodoric and his important manual see Nancy G. Siraisi, *Taddeo Alderotti and His Pupils: Two Generations of Italian Medical Learning* (Princeton, 1981), 16–17. For Andreas Abalat, see Luis [Lluís] García-Ballester, *La medicina a la València medieval: Medicina i societat en un país medieval mediterrani* (Valencia, 1988), 71.

43. See *Histoire littéraire de la France*, vol. 34 (Paris, 1915), p. 420.

44. Jacquart, *Le milieu médical en France*, 156. For a German bishop-doctor who studied and taught in Montpellier and who spent most of his adult life around the court of Avignon, see Karl Wenck, "Johann von Göttingen: Arzt, Bischof, und Politiker zur Zeit Kaiser Ludwigs des Bayern," *Archiv für Geschichte der Medizin* 17 (1925): 141–156.

45. Jacquart, *Le milieu médical en France*, 268–269, 279.

46. Salo Wittmayer Baron, *A Social and Religious History of the Jews*, 2d ed., 18 vols. (New York and Philadelphia, 1952–1983). See esp. vol. 8 (New York, 1958), pp. 241–242.

47. For biblical and Talmudic medicine and its achievement see the still classic work of Julius Preuss, *Biblisch-talmudische Medizin: Beiträge zur Geschichte der Heilkunde und der Kultur überhaupt* (Berlin, 1911; reprint, New York, 1971), and the more recent work of Fred Rosner, *Medicine in the Bible and the Talmud: Selections from Classical Jewish Sources* (New York, 1977).

48. For the first quotation I rely on "Gaonic Responsa" published by Abraham Eliyahu Harkavi, in *Zikkaron la-Ri'shonim ve-gam la Aharonim* (in Hebrew), vol. 1, no. 4 (Berlin, 1887; reprint, Jerusalem, 1966), pp. 208–209 (no. 394). The second is according to the publication of Benjamin Menasheh Levin, *Ginze kedem* (in Hebrew), vol. 5 (Jerusalem, 1934; reprint, Bene Brak, 1986), p. 2.

49. Instead of loading this note with a lengthy bibliography, I send

the reader to Süssman Muntner's *Introduction to the Book of Asaph the Physician: The Oldest Existing Text of a Medical Book Written in Hebrew* (Jerusalem, 1957), where all previous scholarship is amply discussed.

50. Süssmann Muntner, "Concerning a New Manuscript of 'Sepher Asaph'" (in Hebrew), *Koroth* 4 (1968): 731-736. A recent defense of the antiquity of the book can be found in Aviv Melzer, "Asaph the Physician—The Man and His Book: A Historical-Philological Study of the Medical Treatise, 'The Book of Drugs,'" Ph.D. diss., University of Wisconsin, 1972, which is based on philological analysis. I tend to see the work as a tenth-century compilation and follow thus Ludwig Venetianer, "Asaf Judaeus, der Aelteste medizinische Schriftsteller in hebraeischer Sprache," *38. Jahresbericht der Landes-Rabbinerschule in Budapest für das Schuljahr 1914-1915*, 3 vols. (Budapest, 1915-1917). The most ancient copy (fragmentary) of the book seems to be of the year 1035. It used to belong to the scholar E. Carmoli and is now in Frankfurt on Main. See Ernst Róth and Leo Prijs, *Hebräische Handschriften, Teil 1B: Die Handschriften der Stadt und Universitätsbibliothek Frankfurt am Main (Fortsetzung von Teil 1A)* (Stuttgart, 1990), pp. 58-59. For a recent discussion of scholarship concerning the book, see Elinor Lieber, "Asaf's 'Book of Medicines': A Hebrew Encyclopedia of Greek and Jewish Medicine, Possibly Compiled in Byzantium on an Indian Model," *Dumbarton Oaks Papers* 38 (1984): 233-249.

51. It was published in Süssmann Muntner, *Rabbi Shabbetai Donnolo (913-985)* (in Hebrew), 2 parts in 1 vol. (Jerusalem, 1949). See also Muntner's other study, "Donnolo et la contribution des juifs aux premières oeuvres de la médecine salernitaine," *Revue d'histoire de la médecine hébraïque* 9 (1956): 155-161.

52. For this I rely on Moritz Steinschneider, *Die hebraeischen Übersetzungen des Mittelalters und die Juden als Dolmetscher* (Berlin, 1893; reprint, Graz, 1956), 672-673.

53. Joshua O. Leibowitz, "The Preface by Nathan ha-Meati to His Hebrew Translation (1279) of Ibn-Sina's 'Canon'" (in Hebrew), *Koroth* 7 (1976): 1-8, especially 7.

54. In what follows I rely principally on Max Meyerhof, "Medieval Jewish Physicians in the Near East, from Arabic Sources," *Isis* 28 (1938): 432-460, also in his *Studies in Medieval Arabic Medicine: Theory and Practice*, ed. P. Johnstone (London, 1984). For a list of Israeli works in Latin translation, see Baron, *Social and Religious History of the Jews* 8:394-395.

55. Françoise Micheau, "Hommes de sciences au prisme d'Ibn-

Qifti," in *Actes du colloque intellectuels et militants dans le monde isla-mique*, 81–106, Cahiers de la Méditerranée 37 (Nice, 1988).

56. See Moshe Perlmann, "Notes on the Position of Jewish Physicians in Medieval Muslim Countries," *Israel Oriental Studies* 2 (1972): 315–319.

57. I rely for this information on Joshua Prawer, *The History of the Jews in the Latin Kingdom of Jerusalem* (Oxford, 1988), 121.

58. Cf. Baron, *Social and Religious History of the Jews* 8:389 n. 19, and Max Meyerhof's study "Von Alexandrien nach Bagdad: Ein Beitrag zur Geschichte des philosophischen und medizinischen Unterrichts bei den Araben," which appeared in *Sitzungsberichte der Akademie der Wissenschaften* vol. 23 (Berlin, 1930), pp. 389–429, in particular pp. 424–425. Notice that the late Professor Goitein, relying on twelfth- and thirteenth-century Geniza materials from Egypt still observes Christian preponderance in the profession. See Shlomo Dov Goitein, "The Medical Profession in the Light of the Cairo Geniza Documents," *Hebrew Union College Annual* 34 (1963): 177–94, especially 179.

59. See n. 52 above. The recent publication of Geniza documents by Menaḥem Ben-Sasson, *The Jews of Sicily 825–1068: Documents and Sources* (in Hebrew) (Jerusalem, 1991), reveals the names of four Jewish doctors living in Egypt, in Alexandria, or in Fustat in the eleventh century. They are Judah ben Sa'adia, Mevorakh ben Sa'adia, Ḥanania ben Shmuel, and Ḥasan al-Bakri. For more details, see the index of Ben-Sasson's publication.

60. Felipe Martínez Pérez, "La medicina sevillana en el siglo XIII y especialmente en la época de la conquista de Sevilla," *Archivo hispalense* 12 (1950): 131–177.

61. See Goitein, "The Medical Profession in the Light of the Cairo Geniza Documents," 186.

Chapter 2

1. For this information and for what follows I rely on Harold J. Berman, *Law and Revolution: The Formation of the Western Legal Tradition* (Cambridge, Mass., and London, 1983), esp. 421; and on Antonio [Antoní] Cardoner [i] Planas, *Història de la medicina a la corona d'Aragó (1162–1479)* (Barcelona, 1973), 92–93. See also the systematic discussion of Vern L. Bullough, *The Development of Medicine as a Profession* (Basel and New York, 1966), especially his third and fifth chapters (pp. 46–73, 93–111). And more recently Nancy G. Siraisi, *Medieval and Early Renaissance Medicine: An Introduction to Knowledge and Practice* (Chicago and London, 1990), 17–23.

2. Françoise Micheau, one of the leading specialists in the field, does not believe that such examination and licensing procedures existed in the Moslem world. See her "La formation des médecins arabes au Proche-Orient (X^e–XIIIe siècle)," *Les entrées dans la vie: Initiations et apprentissages*, 105–125, Douzième congrès de la société des historiens médiévistes de l'enseignement supérieur public, Nancy 1981 (Nancy, 1982), as well as in her forthcoming "Les traités sur 'l'examen du médecin' dans le monde arabe médiéval," *Maladies, médecines et sociétés* (Paris, 1994), a history up to the present. Ghada Karmi and Juan Vernet hold a different opinion: Ghada Karmi, "State Control of the Physicians in the Middle Ages: An Islamic Model," in *Les sociétes urbaines en France méridionale et en péninsule Ibérique au moyen âge*, 63–84, Actes du colloque de Pau, 21–23 septembre 1988 (Paris, 1991); Juan Vernet, *Ce que la culture doit aux arabes d'Espagne* (Paris, 1985); note especially the evidence he brings on pp. 174–175. S. D. Goitein quotes from a Geniza letter where a doctor reprimands his assistant who was also his relative: "I heard that [a person by the name of] Menahem has already been licensed while you are still a *mu'alim*." Shlomo Dov Goitein, "The Medical Profession in the Light of the Cairo Geniza Documents," *Hebrew Union College Annual* 34 (1963): 177–94. The quote is on p. 183.

3. See, e.g., Bullough, *The Development of Medicine as a Profession*, 49–51 and the bibliography there. The text is to be found in Jean Louis Alphonse Huillard-Bréholles, *Historia diplomatica Frederici secundi*, 6 vols. (Paris, 1852–1861; reprint, Turin, 1963), vol. 4, part 1 pp. 235–237.

4. See Ch. Giraud, *Essai sur l'histoire du droit français au moyen âge*, vol. 2 (Paris, 1846), p. 49.

> Prohibemus ne quis, cuiuscumque conditionis aut status sit, in medicina aut cyrugia practicare presumat nisi prius de ipsius fide et legalitate in curia nostra testimonio sufficienti perhabito, in eadem curia, ad cuius nostro testimonio sufficienti perhabito, in eadem curia, ad cuius officium spectare censetur, de sua arte peritia idoneus approbetur. Practicantes autem contra presentis nostrae prohibitionis et determinationis edictum poenam quinquaginta librarum turonensium multandum fore sanximus nostro aerario applicandum.

5. Piero Giacosa, *Magistri Salernitani nondum editi* (Turin, 1901), 660–661, especially the paragraph entitled "Quod nullus medicus exercere artem medecine nisi fuerit examinatus."

6. For Valencia see Luis García-Ballester, *La medicina a la València medieval* (Valencia, 1988), 53–57, 63–80. See also n. 9 below, this chapter.

7. For the Cortes of Monzón see Joseph María Roca, *La medicina catalana en temps del rey Martí* (Barcelona, 1919), 114–121.

8. See Ugo Stefanutti, *Documentazioni cronologiche per la storia della medicina, chirurgia, e farmacia in Venezia dal 1258 al 1332* (Venice, 1961), 115 (doc. no. 22): "Non detur pro sufficienti peritos medicorum."

9. See Luis García-Ballester, Michael R. McVaugh, and Agustín Rubio-Vela, *Medical Licensing and Learning in Fourteenth-century Valencia*, Transactions of the American Philosophical Society, vol. 79, no. 6 (Philadelphia, 1989), pp. 22–23, 61–64. The translation to English is theirs.

10. Pilar León Tello, *Los judíos de Toledo*, 2 vols. (Madrid, 1979), 1:274.

11. See Jean Régné, *History of the Jews in Aragon* (Jerusalem, 1978), 46 (no. 525). The text was published in Alexandre Charles Germain, *Cartulaire de l'université de Montpellier*, vol. 1 (Montpellier, 1890), pp. 202–203. It reads:

> Illorum audaciam reprimamus qui presumunt ibidem sine examinatione et licentia practicare per quod non solum nomen et fama ejusdem studii denigratur, sed et multa incumbunt mortis pericula et rerum dispendia inferuntur. Et . . . prohibemus in perpetuum et districte omnibus utriusque sexus, christianis et judeis, ne quis in villa Montispessulani et tota eius dominatione audeat in facultate medicine aliquod officium practicandi exercere nisi prius ibi examinatus et licentiatus fuerit.

12. I quote the text according to the translation of Lynn Thorndike, *University Records and Life in the Middle Ages* (New York, 1944; reprint, New York, 1975), 83–85.

13. The classic study of the subject is Cecil Roth, "The Qualification of Jewish Physicians in the Middle Ages," *Speculum* 28 (1958): 834–843.

14. For Salomon Avigdor see Katharine Park, *Doctors and Medicine in Early Renaissance Florence* (Princeton, 1985), 74. See especially the study of Ladislao Münster and Mirko Malavolti, "Su alcuni documenti relativi a medici ebrei conservati nell'archivio di stato di Firenze," *Medicina nei secoli* 8 (1971): 22–53.

15. Bartolomeo and Giuseppe Lagumina, *Codice diplomatico dei giudei di Sicilia*, 3 vols. (Palermo, 1884–1895). All the information referred to below is to be found in vol. 1, pp. 69–77.

16. Ibid.

17. For reference and a somewhat different translation cf. García-Ballester, McVaugh, and Rubio-Vela, *Medical Licensing*, 28.

18. García-Ballester, McVaugh, Rubio-Vela, *Medical Licensing*, 27 and 104–105.

19. The document is preserved in the Archives départementales des Pyrénées-Orientales (Perpignan), 3E1–541, fol. 1r.

20. See García-Ballester, McVaugh, and Rubio-Vela, *Medical Licensing*, 11–18.

21. Lagumina, *Codice diplomatico dei giudei di Sicilia*, 1.

22. Leopoldo Piles Ros, "Notas sobre judíos de Aragón y Navarra," *Sefarad* 10 (1950): 176–181, especially 177.

23. Juan Torres Fontes, "Los judíos murcianos en el reinado de Juan II," in *Murgetana*, 79–107, esp. 89–91, Academia Alfonso X el Sabio (Murcia, 1965).

24. Here is the relevant part of the license as transcribed from the original in the Archivo de la Corona d'Aragón (Barcelona), reg. 894, fol. 30r:

> Et cum precipimus ratione veridica quod aliqui insutticientes et dictum artem penitus ignorantes utuntur infra terram et dominationem nostram arte ipsa, cuius rei occasione nonulli existentes sub cura eorum plerumque decedunt vel debilitati remanent propter illorum insufficientiam et ignorantiam dicti artis, concedimus tibi, prefato magistro Bonjuha quod tu, una cum aliquo cerurgico vel profisico ex sufficientioribus civitatis vel loci in quo presens fueris, per vicarium vel bajulum dicte civitatis vel loci ad hoc assignando, examinis et possis examinare dicta arte utentes et ignorantes et insufficientes denunciare dictis vicario vel bajulo qui pro penarum impositione nostro errario applicandas et aliter injungant eisdem insufficientibus ut dictam artem et scientiam exercere de cetero non presumant.

Reference to this document was made in Antonio Rubió y Lluch's article "Notes sobre la ciencia oriental a Catalunya en el XIV^en sigle," *Estudis universitaris catalans* 3 (1909): 492.

25. See the various short notes about him in Rubió y Lluch, "Notes sobre la ciencia oriental," 389–398, 489–497, esp. 493. After converting to Christianity he was known as Petrus d'Artés. See García-Ballester, *La medicina a la València medieval*, 49.

26. Ibid.

27. Raffaele Calvanico, *Fonti per la storia della medicina e della chirurgia per il regno di Napoli nel periodo angioino (1273–1410)* (Naples, 1962).

28. On this point see Jole Agrimi and Chiara Crisciani, "Medici e 'vetulae' dal duecento al quattrocento: Problemi di una ricerca," in *Cultura popolare e cultura dotta nel seicento*, 144–159, Atti del Convegno di studio di Genova, 23–25 November 1982 (Milan, 1983);

also Ronald J. Doviak, "The University of Naples and the Study and Practice of Medicine in the Thirteenth and Fourteenth Centuries," Ph.D. diss., City University of New York, 1974 (Ann Arbor, Mich.: University Microfilms, 1974).

29. Calvanico, *Fonti*, nos. 1872 and 3598.

30. Calvanico, *Fonti*, nos. 3482 and 512.

31. Calvanico, *Fonti*, no. 391: "experientiam habeat in practica cirurgie quamvis instructus non sit in theorica dicte artis." See also no. 415.

32. See Luis García-Ballester and Augustín Rubio-Vela, "L'influence de Montpellier dans le contrôle social de la profession médicale dans le royaume de Valence au XIVᵉ siècle," in *Histoire de l'école médicale de Montpellier*, pp. 19–30, esp. 25, Actes du 110ᵉ congrès national des sociétés savantes, Montpellier, 1985, Section d'histoire des sciences et des techniques, vol. 2 (Paris, 1985). The relevant statement reads in the original: "Havem a trobat en los principis de la dita sciencia de fisica introduhuit, empero ab la pratica de cuja las malatis non ha longament practicat ni usat."

33. Calvanico, *Fonti*, no. 477: "de fracturis et dislocationibus humanorum ossium"; and no. 3655: "in extratione lapidum ac in curatione vulnerum simplicium."

34. Calvanico, *Fonti*, no. 860: "curis occulorum"; and no. 2045: "peritus in curandis crepaturis seu harniis intestinalibus et in extractionibus lapidum."

35. Joseph María Roca, *L'estudi general de Lleyda* (Barcelona, n.d.), 74–75.

36. See Rubió y Lluch, "Notes sobre la ciencia oriental," 3:491.

37. García-Ballester and Rubio-Vela, "L'influence de Montpellier," 25.

38. Gustave Bayle, *Les médecins d'Avignon au moyen âge* (Avignon, 1882), 38–39.

39. García-Ballester, McVaugh, and Rubio-Vela, *Medical Licensing*, 19–20.

40. For both cases see Pearl Kibre, "The Faculty of Medicine at Paris, Charlatanism, and Unlicensed Medical Practices in the Later Middle Ages," *Bulletin of the History of Medicine* 27 (1953): 1–20. The original documents of the trials are published in Henri Denifle and Emile Chatelin, eds., *Chartularium universitatis Parisiensis*, 4 vols. (Paris, 1889–1897), 2:149–152, 255–267.

41. See Archives départementales des Bouches-du-Rhone (Marseilles), B2017, fol. 5r: "De Talardo. Mayrona judea quia contra ordinationem regiam practicavit de arte phisice in castro de Bayonis,

ne quis sine licentia curie regie et nisi aprobatur fuisset per expertos in talibus, practicavit in castro de Bayonis predicto. Condempnata fuit in solidis XL." For further information culled from Provençal archives, see Camille Arnaud, *Histoire de la viguerie de Forcalquier*, 2 vols. (Marseilles, 1874–1875), 2:273–274.

42. See Antoni Rubió y Lluch, *Documents per l'història de la cultura catalana mig-eval*, 2 vols. (Barcelona, 1908–1921), 2:67–68: "examinatus non fuerit in dicta arte ut fieri debet iuxta forum."

43. Angelina García, "Médicos judíos en la Valencia del siglo XIV," *Estudios dedicados a Juan Peset Aleixandre*, vol. 2 (Valencia, 1982), pp. 85–96, esp. p. 95, where the names of two other practitioners (Gento and Ismael), possibly Jewish, are mentioned in a similar context.

44. Cardoner [i] Planas, *Història de la medicina a la corona d'Aragó*, 116.

45. See n. 42 of this chapter.

46. Published in my *Médecine et justice en Provence médiévale: Documents de Manosque, 1262–1348* (Aix-en-Provence, 1989), 113–114 (doc. no. 26).

47. García, "Médicos judíos en la Valencia del siglo XIV," 95.

48. Cardoner [i] Planas, *Història de la medicina a la corona d'Aragó*, 110.

49. See my *Médecine et justice en Provence médiévale*, 5–7

50. See Jefim Schirmann, "Shlomo Bonfed's dispute with the Saragossa elders" (in Hebrew), *Kovets 'al-yad*, n.s., 4 (1946): 8–64, esp. 19–22.

51. For the original in Hebrew see Judah ben Samuel Ḥasid, *Sepher Ḥasidim Das Buch der Frommen* (in Hebrew), 2d ed., ed. J. Wistinetzki and J. Freimann (Frankfurt on Main, 1924), 355 (no. 1469). I have translated this *exemplum* and dealt with it in my "Doctors and Medical Practice in Germany around the Year 1200: The Evidence of 'Sefer Hasidim,'" *Journal of Jewish Studies* 33 (1982): 583–593, especially 591.

52. Isaac Alteras, "Notes généalogiques sur les médecins juifs dans le sud de la France pendant les XIIIe et XIVe siècles," *Le moyen âge* 88 (1982): 29–47, as well as his "Jewish Physicians in Southern France during the Thirteenth and Fourteenth Centuries," *The Jewish Quarterly Review* 68 (1978): 209–223.

53. Louis Barthélemy, *Les médecins à Marseille avant et pendant le moyen âge* (Marseilles, 1883), 32.

54. Noël Coulet, "Quelques aspects du milieu médical en Provence au bas moyen âge," in *Vie privée et ordre public à la fin du*

moyen âge: Etudes sur Manosque, la Provence, et le Piémont (1250–1450), ed. M. Hébert (Aix-en-Provence, 1987), 119–138, esp. 121.

55. Kalonymos ben Kalonymos, *Even Bohan* (Touchstone) (in Hebrew), ed. A. M. Habermann (Tel-Aviv, 1956), 45.

56. Pierre Pansier, "Les médecins juifs à Avignon aux XIIIe, XIVe, et XVe siècles," *Janus* 15 (1910): 421–451, esp. 443–444.

57. Pierre Pansier, "Les médecins juifs à Avignon," 442.

58. Rubió y Lluch, *Documents per l'història de la cultura catalan mig-eval* 2:246–247.

59. Louis Barthélemy, *Les médecins à Marseille*, 31.

60. See Roth, "The Qualification of Jewish Physicians," 837, and Barthélemy, *Les médecins à Marseille*, 31–32. In the past I have endorsed Barthélemy's interpretation: see the last page of my "On Becoming a Jewish Doctor in the High Middle Ages," *Sefarad* 43 (1983): 239–250. I believe my new understanding to be the correct one. The most important paragraph of the text reads: "dictus magister salomon teneatur et debeat, et ita promisit, dictos pueros et eorum quemlibet, spacio predicto unius anni, docere in scientia et lege hebraicis necessariis ipsis liberis et consuetis, et eos instruere suo posse in sua scientia, et in bonis moribus et doctrinis."

61. Lagumina, *Codice diplomatico dei giudei di Sicilia* 2:28–29 (doc. no. 491). Herewith I quote the most pertinent parts of the charter:

> liceat vobis ac possitis et valeatis vestris sumptibus et expensis, si et prout per nos vel spectabilem in dicto nostro Sicilie Viceregem, cum voluntate et assensu vestro fuerit dispositum et ordinatum, in illa civitate, villa vel loco eiusdem Regni, qua vel quo Vicerex cum dicto vestro assensu duxerit eligenda, vel eligendo, studium generale facere, doctores, legum peritos. Magistros et alios stipendiare et solvere, et in dicto studio approbatas sciencias quascumque convenientibus ad eum judicis et aliis legere et audiri facere seu permittere, et alia omnia et singula facere, que ad dictum generale studium faciendum atque tenendum pertinere quomodolibet videantur, dum illa feceritis, ut prefertur, si et prout per nos vel per dictum Viceregem fuerit dispositum et ordinatum. Nos enim doctores, legum peritos, Magistros, studentes et alios in dicto studio comorantes et ad eum, causa eiusdem, convenientes et ipsum studium sub speciali proteccione nostra de dicta nostra certa sciencia ponimus et constituimus serie cum presenti . . .

62. Note that medieval Jews labeled a Christian *studium* as *yeshivah*. Thus Benjamin of Tudela talks about the yeshivah of doctors in Salerno. Benjamin of Tudela, *The Itinerary of Benjamin of Tudela*, ed. M. N. Adler (London, 1907), 10. For other examples see the following pages.

63. Rubió y Lluch, "Notes sobre la ciencia oriental," especially 390. The relevant sentences read: "qui non adiscerent vel legerent eruditionem literarum, usque ad aetatem sexdecim . . . et qui adiscerent vel legerent, usque atingerent aetatem viginti tres annorum."

64. Lagumina, *Codice diplomatico dei giudei di Sicilia* 1:308–309: "Cum moris sit iudeorum . . . quod iudei civitatis eiusdem medicine studium sequentes gisie solucionis et ceterorum onerum collectarum mutuorum et angariarum immunes et liberi protenus conserventur."

65. Many works have been written about these alleged Jewish involvements in the establishment of Montpellier. See, e.g., Richard Kohn, "L'influence des juifs à l'origine de la faculté de médecine de Montpellier," *Revue d'histoire de la médecine hébraïque* 4 (September–December 1949): 14–34. Or the two articles by Isidore Simon, "Les médecins juifs et la fondation de l'école de médecine de Montpellier," *Revue d'histoire de la médecine hébraïque* 68 (July 1965): 79–93, and "Les médecins juifs en France, origines jusqu'à la fin du XVIIIᵉ siècle," *Revue d'histoire de la médecine hébraïque* 89 (October 1970): 89–92. See also the much more reserved tone of Joshua O. Leibowitz, "Médecins juifs à Montpellier," *Yperman* 8 (1961): 1–4. The possibility that Jacob ben Machir was a *magister regens* was raised by Jean Astruc, *Mémoires pour servir à l'histoire de la faculté de médecine de Montpellier* (Paris, 1777), 166–168.

66. The historicity of this marble plaque was demolished just a few years after it was conceived. See Ernest Wickersheimer, "La question du judéo-arabisme à Montpellier," *Janus* 21 (1927): 465–473, rev. and corrected in *Monspeliensis Hippocrates* 6 (1959): 3–7.

67. The letter is published in Alexandre Charles Germain, *Cartulaire de l'université de Montpellier*, vol. 1 (Montpellier, 1890), pp. 179–180 (doc. no. 1): "Volo . . . quod omnes homines quibus comque sint vel undecumane sint, sine aliqua interpellacione regant scolas de fisica in Montepessulano." A similar endorsement of freedom to teach is to be found in decisions of the municipality of Valencia in 1399 and in 1400. They referred to legislation (*fur*) of King Jaume I of Aragon of 1238: "allowing every master, under the last provision of the said *fur* entitled 'De metges,' that he may hold a school with or without another master in association, in whatever place that he wishes and can find within the city, without hindrance or opposition from other masters." The translation is by García-Ballester, McVaugh, and Rubio-Vela, *Medical Licensing and Learning in Fourteenth-century Valencia*, Transactions of the American Philosophical Society, vol. 79, no. 6 (Philadelphia, 1989), p. 53.

68. See my "In Search of the 'Book of Figures': Medicine and

Astrology in Montpellier at the Turn of the Fourteenth Century," *Association for Jewish Studies Review* 7–8 (1982–1983): 383–407.

69. About the 1358 list see Bernard Guillemain, "Citoyens, juifs, et courtisans dans Avignon pontificale au XIVᵉ siècle," *Bulletin philologique et historique (jusqu'à 1610)*, année 1461 (Paris, 1963), 147–160. The name of Crescas is quoted by Pierre Pansier, "Les maîtres de la faculté de médecine de Montpellier au moyen âge," *Janus* 10 (1905): 430. Cecil Roth cited this same information in "The Qualification of Jewish Physicians in the Middle Ages."

70. The treatise was published and discussed by David de Günzberg, *Be'er la-ḥai des Isak ben Todros* (in Hebrew), in *Jubelschrift zum neunzigsten Geburtstag des Dr. L. Zunz*, vol. 2 (Berlin, 1884), pp. 91–126.

71. About Jacme, Tornamira, and other members of the faculty, see Pierre Pansier, "Les maîtres de la faculté de médecine de Montpellier, *Janus* 9 (1904): 443–451, 499–511, 537–545, 593–602, and *Janus* 10 (1905): 1–11, 58–68, 113–21. See also my recent article "Etudiants juifs à la faculté de médecine de Montpellier, dernier quart du XIVᵉ siècle," *Jewish History* 6 (1992): 243–255.

72. See the article about him in Ernest Renan, "Les écrivains juifs français du XIVᵉ siècle," in *Histoire littéraire de la France*, vol. 31 (Paris, 1893), pp. 717–722. (It also appears as an independent publication, reprinted in 1969.) And see n. 73 below.

73. All quotations are according to the manuscript preserved at the Bibliothèque Nationale, Paris, ms. héb. 1054, fols. 39v, 42r, and 44r.

74. I quote the translation provided by Lynn Thorndike, *University Records and Life in the Middle Ages*, 257. Thorndike relies on Marcel Fournier, *Les statuts et privilèges des universités françaises depuis leur fondation jusqu'en 1789*, 4 vols. (Paris, 1890–1894), 2:579–580.

75. The text was published and commented on in the article concerning Leon Joseph in Ernest Renan, "*Les écrivains juifs français du XIVᵉ siècle*," 31:424–432, esp. 425–429. It has also recently been edited (Hebrew text and English translation) from a manuscript in the Bibliothèque Nationale in an article by Luis García-Ballester, Lola Ferre, and Eduard Feliu, "Jewish Appreciation of Fourteenth-century Scholastic Medicine," *Osiris*, 2d ser., 6 (1990): 85–117, esp. 107–117. In what follows I shall make reference to the pages in Renan's edition.

76. Richard W. Emery, "Documents Concerning Some Jewish Scholars in Perpignan in the Fourteenth and Early Fifteenth Centuries," in *Michael: On the History of the Jews in the Diaspora*, ed. Shlo-

mo Simonsohn and Joseph Shatzmiller, vol. 4 (Tel-Aviv, 1976), pp. 27–48, in particular pp. 40–42. In a private letter to me dated 21 December 1986 the late Professor Emery added: "I have long known . . . that his son Astruc Leo, also a physician, was still living in 1455. But I know also that Leo had two grandsons: one of them became a Cistercian monk and died around 1453; the other still living (named Bernardus Benedicti) in Barcelona in 1453 as a surgeon."

77. See n. 75 above.

78. See the Perpignan legislation in Marcel Fournier, *Les statuts et privilèges des universités françaises* 2:679–680. It reads:

> Item, fiat statutum de novo quod nullus aliene secte, sicut Judeus vel Sarracenus, vel quicunque alius, cujusque aliene secte fuerit, per aliquem doctorem, magistrum, licentiatum, baccallarium, scolarem, instruatur publice neque occulte in gramatica, logica, philosophia, medicina seu jure, aut alia scientia. Et ponatur ibi bona pena secundum quod visum fuerit, ut melius servetur.

The words "de novo" indicate that provisions for legislation on that subject existed.

79. Danielle Jacquart, *Le milieu médical en France du XIIe au XVe siècle* (Geneva and Paris, 1981), 67. See also *Histoire de Montpellier*, ed. Gérard Cholvy (Toulouse, 1984), 103–125, and in particular 117.

80. ". . . accedere voluit apud Perpinianum ubi dicebatur esse obtimi medici et bene experti." See G. Veyssière, "In Agonia," in *Pratiques du corps: Médecine, hygiène, alimentation, sexualité*, ed. J. M. Racoult and A. J. Bullier, Université de la Réunion (St.-Denis de la Réunion, 1985), 23–39. The quotation appears in n. 17 on p. 28.

81. I rely for the quote on L. Duhamel, *Inventaire-sommaire des archives municipales antérieures à 1790 de la ville d'Orange*, vol. 1: *Séries AA-CC* (Orange, 1917). It reads: "dum Montispessulani recedit seu recedere intendit a dicto loco Montispessulani et dominus noster papa fuit locutus de dicto studio cum domino nostro principe talia verba vel similia sibi dicendo: Princeps, postquam Studium recedit a Montepessulano quare non procuretis ut ipsum habeatis."

82. Adolph Neubauer, *Catalogue of the Hebrew Manuscripts in the Bodleian Library and in the College Libraries of Oxford* (Oxford, 1886), vol. 1, no. 2451.

83. See Umberto Dallari, ed., *Rotuli dei lettori e legisti e artisti dello studio bolognese dal 1384 al 1799*, vol. 1 (Bologna, 1888), pp. 9, 11–12 and 15.

84. For the information on Sassoferrato I rely on Vittore Colorni,

"Sull'ammissibilità degli ebrei alla laurea anteriormente al secolo XIX," in *La rassegna mensile di Israel: Scritti in onore di Riccardo Bachi* (1950), 16:202–216, or in *Judaica minora: Saggi sulla storia dell'ebraismo italiano dall'antichità all'età moderna* (Milan, 1983), 473–485. See esp. pp. 206–207 in *La rassegna* and pp. 477–478 in *Judaica minora.*

85. Mme. Brondy informed me of her discovery in a letter dated 26 June 1986. She is the author of an important doctoral thesis (Université de Lyon, 1986) that appeared in an abbreviated form as a book: see Réjane Brondy, *Chambéry: Histoire d'une capitale vers 1350–1560* (Lyons, 1988). For a "Mestre Ysaac juif phisicien demorant Anneysie" in 1383, see Renata Segre, "Testimonianze documentarie sugli ebrei negli stati sabaudi (1297–1398), in *Michael: On the History of the Jews in the Diaspora*, ed. Shlomo Simonsohn and Joseph Shatzmiller, vol. 4 (Tel Aviv, 1976), pp. 273–413, in particular p. 369 (no. 312).

86. Lagumina, *Codice diplomatico dei giudei di Sicilia* 1:330.

87. See Katharine Park, *Doctors and Medicine in Early Renaissance Florence*, 72–73 ff.

88. See Vittore Colorni, "Sull'ammissibilità degli ebrei alla laurea," 480, and especially Gaetano Marini, *Degli archiatri pontifici*, 2 vols. (Rome, 1784), 1:293. See also Renzo Mosti, "Medici ebrei del XIV–XV secolo a Tivoli," *Atti e memorie della società tiburtina di storia e d'arte* 27 (Tivoli, 1954): 109–156. For "doctorates" conferred on Jewish physicians in the late fifteenth century, see Anna Esposito and Micaela Procaccia, "'Iudei de Urbe': La testimonianza di un inventario," in *Un pontificato ed una città: Sisto IV (1471–1484),* 267–289, esp. 269–271, Atti del convegno, Roma, 3–7 dicembre 1984 (Rome, 1986). For a later period, see Emilia Veronese Ceseracciu, "Ebrei laureati a Padova nel cinquecento," *Quaderni per la storia dell'università di Padova* 13 (1980): 151–168.

89. Ladislao Münster, "Laurea in medicina conferita dallo studio ferrarese ad un ebreo nel 1426," *Ferrara viva: Rivista storica e di attualità* 3, no. 7–8 (1961): 63–72; and also his "Maître Guillaume feu Isaia de Urbino, docteur ès arts et en médecine à Ferrare en 1426," *Revue d'histoire de la médecine hébraïque* 11 (1958): 109–114.

90. The significance of all these symbols is explained in a similar ceremony that took place in the *studium* of Lérida [Aragon] in 1340: "cathedram magistralem in signum excellentie, librum in signum sapientie, birretam in signum glorie, osculum in signum dilectionis et amicitie, et benedictionem in signum benedictionis eterne . . ." See Michael McVaugh and Luis García-Ballester, "The Medical Faculty

in Early Fourteenth-century Lérida," *History of Universities* 8 (1989): 1–25. The quote is on p. 22.

91. See Ariel Toaff, *Il vino e la carne: Una comunità ebraica nel medioevo* (Bologna, 1989), 266–267. He was relying on Stanislao Majarelli and Ugolino Nicolini, *Il monte dei poveri di Perugia: Periodo delle origini (1462–1474)* (Perugia, 1962), 75, who states, "Il maestro Musetto di Guglielmo mantiene indisturbato la cattedra di medicina nello studio."

92. The state archives of the province of Umbria (Perugia) kindly sent me a xerox copy of the document, which carries this call number: Conservatori delle monete, vol. 36, fol. 25r.

93. Ladislao Münster, "Fu Jacob Mantino lettore effettivo dello studio di Bologna?" *Rassegna mensile di Israel* 20 (1954): 310–321.

Chapter 3

1. Aleksander Birkenmajer, "Le rôle joué par les médecins et les naturalistes dans la réception d'Aristote aux XII⁰ et XIII⁰ siècles," *Etudes d'histoire des sciences et de la philosophie du moyen âge* (Wrocław, Warsaw, and Cracow, 1970), 73–87, esp. 76–77. For a general overview of medical education in our period, see Owsei Temkin, "Medical Education in the Middle Ages," *Journal of Medical Education* 31 (1956): 383–391.

2. Vern L. Bullough, *The Development of Medicine as a Profession* (Basel and New York, 1966), 51.

3. Danielle Jacquart and Françoise Micheau, *La médecine arabe et l'occident médiéval* (Paris, 1990), 167–203. See also Luis García-Ballester, "The Diffusion of Medical Science in Thirteenth-century Castile," *Bulletin of History of Medicine* 61 (1987): 183–202; Nancy G. Siraisi, *Medieval and Early Renaissance Medicine: An Introduction to Knowledge and Practice* (Chicago and London, 1990), 70–77.

4. Luis García-Ballester and Augustín Rubio-Vela, "L'influence de Montpellier dans le contrôle social de la profession médicale dans le royaume de Valence au XIV⁰ siècle," in *Histoire de l'école médicale de Montpellier*, pp. 19–30, esp. 20–21, Actes du 110e congrès national des sociétés savantes, Montpellier, 1985, *Section d'histoire des sciences et des techniques*, vol. 2 (Paris, 1985).

5. The text and translation are to be found in Cecil Roth, "The Qualification of Jewish Physicians in the Middle Ages," *Speculum* 28 (1958): 834–843, in particular 839–840.

6. Jean Louis Alphonse Huillard-Bréholles, *Historia Diplomatica Frederici secundi*, vol. 4, part 1 (Paris, 1854), p. 235. The provision

reads: "Quia nunquam sciri potest scientia medicine nisi de logica aliquid presciatur, statuimus quod nullus studeat in medicinali scientia
nisi prius studeat ad minus triennio in scientia logicali." For the date I
count on Salvatore de Renzi, *Storia documentata della scuola medica
di Salerno* (Napoli, 1857), 77. For libraries of doctors in Sicily and for
the culture of these practitioners, see Henri Bresc, *Livre et société en
Sicile (1299-1499)* (Palermo, 1971), 34-40, 87-90, and passim.

7. I quote from Lynn Thorndike, *The Sphere of Sacrobosco and
Its Commentators* (Chicago, 1949), 344:

> Oportet medicum de necessitate scire ac considerare naturas stellarum
> et earum coniunctiones ad hoc ut diversarum egritudinum et dierum
> creticorum habeat notionem, quoniam alterabilis est equidem ipsa
> natura secundum aspectus et coniunctiones corporum superiorum, scri-
> bit Hermes *primo de speculis et de luce*, in qua verborum serie Hermes
> tria nobis innuit: primo necessitatem medici recte operantis ad istam
> scientiam capescendam, quia non potest medicus sine stellarum scientia
> perfectissime operari sed tanquam cecus ut plurimum ducitur et
> oberrat.

8. For Taddeo's treatises on astrology and logics see Nancy G.
Siraisi, *Taddeo Alderotti and His Pupils: Two Generations of Italian
Medical Learning* (Princeton, 1981), 140. For Arnold's treatise, see
Ronald J. Doviak, "The University of Naples and the Study and Practice of Medicine in the Thirteenth and Fourteenth Centuries," Ph.D.
diss., City University of New York, 1974 (Ann Arbor, Mich.: University Microfilms, 1974), 20.

9. The text was published and referred to on several occasions.
See Antonio Rubió y Lluch, "Notes sobre la ciencia oriental a Catalunya en el XIVèn sigle," *Estudis universitaris catalans* 3 (1909): 389-
398, 489-497, esp. 491-492; Fritz Baer, *Die Juden im christlichen
Spanien*, 2 vols. (Berlin, 1929-1933), 1: 578-579; and Antonio Cardoner Planas, "El médico judío Sĕlomó Caravida y algunos aspectos
de la medicina de su época," *Sefarad* 3 (1943): 377-392, especially
391. See also the data assembled recently by J. N. Hillgarth, *Readers
and Books in Majorca, 1229-1550,* 2 vols. (Paris, 1991), 1:100-101.

10. Juan Torres Fontes, "Los judíos murcianos en el reinado de
Juan II," in *Murgetana*, 79-107, esp. 106-107, Academia Alfonso X
el Sabio 24 (Murcia, 1965).

11. Torres Fontes, "Los judíos murcianos en el reinado de Juan
II," 95. A doctor who refused to operate unless the right constellation
was present was the fourteenth-century Aragonese physician Crescas
Abenrabi. See his consideration exposed in V[incente] V[ignau],

"Carta dirigida á D. Juan II de Aragón, por su médico, fijándole día para operarle los ojos," *Revista de archivos, bibliotecas, y museos* 4 (Madrid, 1874): 135–137, 230–231.

12. I rely for this on Cecil Roth, *History of the Jews of Venice* (Philadelphia, 1975), 27 n. 5.

13. See the monograph by Süssmann Muntner, *Contribution to the History of the Hebrew Language in Medical Instruction* (in Hebrew) (Jerusalem, 1940).

14. From the rich literature on the subject see the works of Manfred Ullmann, *Die Medizin im Islam* (Leyden and Cologne, 1970), 1–107; Felix Klein-Franke, *Vorlesungen über die Medizin im Islam* (Wiesbaden, 1982), 68–84; and Charles S. F. Burnett, "Some Comments on the Translating of Works from Arabic into Latin in the Mid-Twelfth Century," *Miscellanea mediaevalia* 17 (1985): 161–171.

15. David C. Lindberg, "The Transmission of Greek and Arabic Learning to the West," *Science in the Middle Ages*, ed. D. C. Lindberg (Chicago and London, 1978), 52–90, esp. 57. See also the following notes.

16. For information about Gerbert see Heinrich Schipperges, *Die Assimilation der arabischen Medizin durch das lateinische Mittelalter* (Wiesbaden, 1964), 87, and Danielle Jacquart and Françoise Micheau, *La médecine arabe et l'occident médiéval*, 87–88.

17. Aleksander Birkenmajer, "Le rôle joué par les médecins et les naturalistes dans la réception d'Aristote," 73–87; Marie-Thérèse d'Alverny, "Translations and Translators," *Renaissance and Renewal in the Twelfth Century*, ed. R. L. Benson and G. Constable (Cambridge, Mass., 1982), 421–462. For a new wave of translations from the Greek to the Latin in the second half of the thirteenth century, marked by the activity of William of Moerbeke see Agostino Paravicini Bagliani, "Guillaume de Moerbeke et la cour pontificale," *Guillaume de Moerbeke: Recueil d'études à l'occasion du 700ème anniversaire de sa mort (1286)*, ed. J. Brams and W. Vanhamed (Louvain, 1989).

18. Jacquart and Micheau, *La médecine arabe et l'occident médiéval*, 87 ff.

19. See Jose S. Gil, *La escuela de traductores de Toledo y sus collaboradores judíos* (Toledo, 1985). Jacquart and Micheau, *La médecine arabe et l'occident médiéval*, 131 ff.; and Heinrich Schipperges, *Die Assimilation der arabischen Medizin*, 85 ff. See also the magnificent articles by Charles Homer Haskins assembled in his *Studies in the History of Medieval Science* (Cambridge, Mass., 1924), 3–139, and more recently Danielle Jacquart, "Principales étapes dans la

transmission des textes de médecine (XIe–XIVe siècle)," in *Rencontres de cultures dans la philosophie médiévale* 251–271, Traductions et traducteurs de l'antiquité tardive au XIVe siècle (Louvain-la-Neuve and Cassino, 1990).

20. Antonio (Antoní) Rubió y Lluch, *Documents per l'història de la cultura catalana mig-eval*, 2 vols. (Barcelona, 1908–1921), 2:13–14.

21. See Michel Garel, *D'une main forte: Manuscrits hébreux des collections françaises* (Paris, 1991), 38 (no. 24), and 71–72 (no. 48).

22. José María Millás Vallicrosa, "The Beginning of [the Study of] Natural Sciences among Spanish Jews" (in Hebrew), *Tarbiz* 24 (Jerusalem, 1954): 48–59.

23. See José María Millás Vallicrosa, "La obra enciclopédica de R. Abraham bar Hiyya," in *Estudios sobre historia de la ciencia española*, vol. 1 (Madrid, 1987), pp. 219–262.

24. Marie-Thérèse d'Alverny, "Avendauth," in *Homenaje a Millás-Vallicrosa*, 2 vols. (Barcelona, 1954–1956), 1:19–43. Gil, *La escuela de traductores de Toledo*, 30–38.

25. Heinrich Schipperges, *Die Assimilation der arabischen Medizin*, 146–149.

26. For Anatoli (probably Antoli), see Ernest Renan, "Les rabbins français du commencement du quatorzième siècle, *in Histoire littéraire de la France*, vol. 27 (Paris, 1877), pp. 580–589.

27. See Norman Roth, "Jewish Translators of the Court of Alfonso X (1252–1284)," *Thought* 60 (1985): 439–455; as well as David Romano, "Le opere scientifiche di Alfonso X e l'intervento degli ebrei," in *Oriente e occidente nel medioevo: Filosofia e scienze*, 677–711, Convegno internazionale, 9–15 aprile 1969 (Rome, 1971), and Moisés Orfali, "Los traductores judíos de Toledo: Nexo entre oriente y occidente," *Actas del II congreso internacional, Encuentro de las tres culturas, 3–6 octubre 1983* (Toledo, 1985), 253–260. Gil, *La escuela de traductores de Toledo*, 57–87.

28. Antonio Cardoner Planas, "Nuevos datos acerca de Jafuda Bonsenyor," *Sefarad* 4 (1944): 287–293.

29. The best overview of this subject is to be found in Isadore Twersky, "Aspects of the Social and Cultural History of Provençal Jewry," *Journal of World History* 11 (1968): 185–207.

30. Henri Gross, *Gallia judaica: Dictionnaire géographique de la France d'après les sources rabbiniques* (Paris, 1897; reprint, Amsterdam, 1969), 279–281. Isadore Twersky, *Rabad of Posquières: A Twelfth-century Talmudist* (Cambridge, Mass., 1962), 12–15 and passim.

31. Twersky, "Aspects of the Social and Cultural History of Provençal Jewry." David Romano, "La transmission des sciences

arabes par les juifs en Languedoc," *Juifs et judaïsme de Languedoc XIIIᵉ siècle–début XIVᵉ siècle*, ed. Marie-Humbert Vicaire and Bernhard Blumenkranz (Paris, 1977), 363–386; Alfred L. Ivry, "Philosophical Translations from the Arabic in Hebrew during the Middle Ages," in *Rencontres de cultures dans la philosophie médiévale*, 167–186. Traductions et traducteurs de l'antiquité tardive au XIVᵉ siècle (Louvain-la-Neuve and Cassino, 1990).

32. Jacquart and Micheau, *La médecine arabe et l'occident médiéval*, 149. Danielle Jacquart, "L'école des traducteurs," in *Tolède, XIIIᵉ–XIIIᵉ: Musulmans, chrétiens, et juifs: Le savoir et la tolérance*, ed. Louis Cardaillac (Paris, 1991), 177–191. Jacquart insists in this article on the role of Archbishop Jean, which according to her was more important than that of Archbishop Raymond; see especially p. 181.

33. His letters to Samuel ibn Tibbon and to the communities of Lunel were recently published by Isaac Shilat, *Igrot ha-Rambam* (The Letters of Maimonides) (in Hebrew), 2 vols. (Jerusalem, 1987), 2:511–554 (Samuel), 2: 474–510 and 557–559 (Lunel).

34. He also had his adversaries and was at the center of the controversy over the study of philosophy, of which much has been written. See Joseph Sarachek, *Faith and Reason: The Conflict over the Rationalism of Maimonides* (New York, 1935; reprint, New York, 1970).

35. See Moritz Steinschneider, *Die hebraeischen Übersetzungen des Mittelalters und die Juden als Dolmetscher* (Berlin, 1893; reprint, Graz, 1956), 734; and Ernest Renan, "Les rabbins français," 27:573.

36. Giuliano Tamani, "Il corpus Aristotelicum nella tradizione ebraica," *Annali di Ca' Foscari* 25, no. 3 (ser. orientale 17) (1986), 5–22, esp. 16; Steinschneider, *Die hebraeischen Überersetzungen des Mittelalters und die Juden als Dolmetscher*, 132–133; and Ernest Renan, "Les rabbins français," 27: 573. And more recently, Aviezer Ravitzky, "Aristotle's 'Meteorologica' and the Maimonidean Exegesis of Creation," in *Shlomo Pines Jubilee Volume on the Occasion of His Eightieth Birthday*, 2 vols., Jerusalem Studies in Jewish Thought 9 (1990), 2:225–250.

37. For Jacob ben Machir see Ernest Renan, "Les rabbins français," 27:599–623.

38. Ernest Renan, "Les rabbins français", 27:594–599.

39. Rubió y Lluch, "Notes sobre la ciencia oriental a Catalunya en el XIVᵉⁿ sigle," 389–398, 487–496, esp. 395; Rubió y Lluch, *Documents per l'història de la cultura catalana mig-eval* 2:9.

40. See the article on Faraj in the new *Encyclopaedia Judaica* (Jerusalem, 1971), vol. 6, col. 1179–1180, and compare with Giuseppe

Sermoneta, *Un glossario filosofico ebraico-italiano del XIII secolo* (Rome, 1969), 42–55.

41. Faraj appears for the first time in our documents on 23 December 1273 and the charter describes him as "fidelem nostrum et interpretem curie nostre." See Bartolomeo and Giuseppe Lagumina, *Codice diplomatico dei giudei di Sicilia*, 3 vols. (Palermo, 1884–1895), 1:23–24 (no. 26). For more information about him, see the recent study by Colette Sirat, "Les traducteurs juifs à la cour des rois de Sicile et de Naples," in *Traduction et traducteurs au moyen âge*, 169–191, Colloque international du CNRS, IRHT, 26–28 mai 1986 (Paris, 1989). Mme. Sirat called my attention to a mistake that slipped into p. 178 of her article: Faraj did translate Razes's *Liber continens* (*al-Hawi*) and not Abu al-Kassim's *al-Zahrawi*. See also the old yet useful study of Willy Cohn indicated in n. 43 below.

42. See Jacquart and Micheau, *La médecine arabe et l'occident médiéval*, 207–208; see also the previous notes. It is unclear whether Faraj also translated the synoptic tables of Ibn Buṭlān, born in Baghdad at the beginning of the eleventh century; the tables are known in the West as *Tacuini sanitatis*. See Hosam Elkhadem, *Le Taqwīm al-Ṣiḥḥa (Tacuini sanitatis) d'Ibn Buṭlān: Un traité médical du XIᵉ siècle* (Louvain, 1990), 43.

43. Willy Cohn, "Jüdische Übersetzer am Hofe Karls I. von Anjou, Königs von Sizilien (1266–1285)," *Monatsschrift für Geschichte und Wissenschaft des Judentums*, n.s. 43 (1935): 245–260, reprinted in his *Juden und Staufer in Unteritalien und Sizilien* (Darmstadt, 1978), 50–64. In the following paragraph I rely on Cohn's information. It is not impossible that the Bibliothèque Nationale, Paris, ms. lat. 6912 in five volumes is the manuscript that Faraj proofread. Virtually every page has corrections in the margins. More information about Charles of Anjou's expenses in acquiring Arabic medical books, in translating them as well as in copying, illustrating, and binding them, was assembled by Michele Amari in his classic *La guerra del vespero siciliano*, 2d ed., ed. F. Giunta, 2 vols. in 3 (Palermo, 1969), vol. 2, pt. 1, pp. 379–383 (doc. no. 71). Most interesting is a letter of 10 June 1277 in which the king ordered a certain Master Matteo Siciliano to stay by his translator "Master Musa" and help him with the Latin: "quatenus cum eodem Magistro Musa esse debeas ad docendum et informandum eum de licteratura latina donec libri ipsi fuerint traslati." The same Musa appears in a document of 1 May 1273 as "translatorem nostrum." He could be identified with Faraj: He could also be, however, Moses ben Salomon of Salerno.

44. See Pietro Delprato, ed., *Trattati di mascalcia attribuiti ad*

Ippocrate tradotti dall'arabo in latino da maestro Moisè da Palermo (Bologna, 1865).

45. Cardoner Planas, "Nuevos datos acerca de Jafuda Bonsenyor," 287–293.

46. For more on this monumental treatise see Jacquart and Micheau, *La médecine arabe et l'occident médiéval*, 139–141 and passim, and Heinrich Schipperges, *Die Assimilation der arabischen Medizin*, 95–96.

47. Steinschneider, *Die hebraeischen Übersetzungen des Mittelalters und die Juden als Dolmetscher*, 740–746; Ernest Renan, "Les rabbins français," 27:592.

48. Published by Süssmann Muntner, "R. Shem Tov Ben Isaac of Tortosa about the Life of the European Jewish Doctor and His Ethics," in *Sinai Jubilee Volume* (Jerusalem, 1957), 321–327.

49. Steinschneider, *Die hebraeischen Übersetzungen des Mittelalters und die Juden als Dolmetscher*, 759.

50. Moritz Steinschneider, *Die europäischen Übersetzungen aus dem arabischen bis Mitte des 17. Jahrhunderts* (Graz, 1956), 76–77; and Jacquart and Micheau, *La médecine arabe et l'occident médiéval*, 210, 217–218. About Simon of Genoa as a translator, see the recent work of Agostino Paravicini Bagliani, *Medicina e scienze della natura alla corte dei papi nel duecento* (Spoleto, 1991), 191–198 and 247–251.

51. See my "Livres médicaux et éducation médicale: À propos d'un contrat de Marseille en 1316," *Medieval Studies* 38 (1980): 463–470. I follow the information in this article throughout the next paragraph.

52. Adolph Neubauer, *Catalogue of the Hebrew Manuscripts in the Bodleian Library*, vol. 1 (Oxford, 1886), nos. 2118–2119.

53. Benjamin Richler, "Another Letter from Hillel b. Samuel to Isaac the Physician?" (in Hebrew), *Kiryat Sefer* 62 (1988–1989): 450–452.

54. For Nathan, "the prince of translators," see Steinschneider, *Die hebraeischen Übersetzungen des Mittelalters und die Juden als Dolmetscher*, 753.

55. Abraham Wasserstein, ed. and trans., *Galen's Commentary on the Hippocratic Treatise Airs, Waters, Places in the Hebrew Translation of Solomon ha-Me'ati*, Proceedings of the Israel Academy of Sciences and Humanities, vol. 6, no. 3 (Jerusalem, 1982).

56. See the articles about him in Moritz Steinschneider, *Gesammelte Schriften*, vol. 1 (Berlin, 1925), pp. 196–215, and the extensive study in Ernest Renan, "Les écrivains juifs français du XIVe siècle" in *Histoire littéraire de la France*, vol. 31 (Paris, 1893), pp. 417–460.

57. See Joseph Shatzmiller, "Petite épître de l'excuse de Kalonymos ben Kalonymos," *Sefunot* 10 (Jerusalem, 1966): 9–52, and Isaia Sonne and Israel Zolli, "Iggereth ha-musar (Epistola ammonizione) di Calonimo ben Calonimo," *Qobetz al Jad*, n.s. 1 (1936): 93–110.

58. See Kalonymos ben Kalonymos, *Sendschreiben an Joseph Kaspi* (in Hebrew), ed. Joseph Perles (Munich, 1879), and Kalonymos ben Kalonymos, *Even Bohan* (Touchstone) (in Hebrew), ed. A. M. Habermann (Tel-Aviv, 1956).

59. See n. 57 above and Harry Friedenwald, *The Jews and Medicine, Essays*, 2 vols. (Baltimore, 1944; reprint, New York, 1967), 1: 178–179.

60. Immanuel of Rome, *The Cantos of Immanuel of Rome* (Mahberoth Immanuel Haromi), ed. Dov Jarden, 2 vols. (Jerusalem, 1957), 2:424–429.

61. Salomon ibn Verga, *Shevet Yehudah* (Sceptre of Judah) (in Hebrew), ed. A Shochat (Jerusalem, 1947), 60–61 and 183. See also pp. 51–52.

62. This precious piece of information reads: "Magistro Callo iudeo . . . ut circa translationem quorundam librorum in servitiis nostris vacet." See Romolo Caggese, *Roberto d'Angiò e i suoi tempi*, 2 vols. (Florence, 1930), 2:371. n. 3. We can compare this sum with the annual salaries of physicians in Sicily which run from ten ounces in 1331 to eighteen ounces in 1416 to twelve ounces in 1421. See Henri Bresc, *Un monde méditerranéen: Economie et société en Sicile 1300–1450*, 2 vols. (Rome, 1986), 2:748 n. 286. Professors at the *studium* of Naples in the 1260s and 1270s reached salaries of ten, twelve, and twenty ounces. See Ronald J. Doviak, "The University of Naples and the Study and Practice of Medicine in the Thirteenth and Fourteenth Centuries," 28–29. For the equivalency of 1 uncia = 5 floreni, I am dependent on Jacques Cambell, *Enquête pour le procès de canonisation de Dauphine de Puimichel, comtesse d'Ariano* (Turin, 1978), 324 n. 8.

63. There is ample literature about the *Canon*, some of which will be presented in the following notes. For general orientatiion, see Albert Nader, "Avicenne médecin," *Miscellanea Mediaevalia* 17 (1985): 327–343.

64. See Haim Rabin, "The Translations of the 'Canon' into the Hebrew" (in Hebrew), *Melila* 3–4 (1950): 132–147. See also Steinschneider, *Die hebraeischen Übersetzungen des Mittelalters und die Juden als Dolmetscher*, 678–686.

65. Benjamin Richler, "Manuscripts of Avicenna's 'Kanon' in Hebrew Translation: A Revised and Up-to-date List," *Koroth* 8 (1982): 145–168 (English), 137–143 (Hebrew).

66. Giuliano Tamani, "Il commento di Yeda'yah Bederši al 'Canone' di Avicenna," *Annali di Ca' Foscari* 13, no. 3 (ser. orientale 5) (1974): 1–17.

67. Steinschneider, *Die hebraeischen Übersetzungen des Mittelalters und die Juden als Dolmetscher*, 686–695. Amnon Shiloah, "'Enkol'—Commentaire hébraïque de Šem Tov Ibn Šaprūt sur le canon d'Avicenne," *Youval* 3 (1974): 267–287; J. Zvi Langermann, "Salomon ibn Ya'ish to Avicenna's canon" (in Hebrew), *Kiryat Sefer* 63 (1991): 1331–1333.

68. Heinrich Schipperges, *Die Assimilation der arabischen Medizin*, 93–95.

69. Danielle Jacquart, "La réception du 'Canon' d'Avicenne: Comparaison entre Montpellier et Paris aux XIIIe et XIVe siècles," *Histoire de l'école médicale de Montpellier*, pp. 69–77, Actes du 110e congrès national des sociétés savantes, Montpellier, 1985, vol. 2 (Paris, 1985); Nancy G. Siraisi, *Avicenna in Renaissance Italy: The 'Canon' and the Medical Teaching in Italian Universities after 1500* (Princeton, 1987), 43–53; and more recently Luis García-Ballester, "Las influencias de la medicina islámica en la obra mèdica de Arnau de Vilanova," in *Estudi general*, vol. 9 (Gerona, 1989), pp. 79–95.

70. Michael R. McVaugh, "The 'humidum radicale' in Thirteenth-century Medicine," *Traditio* 30 (1974): 259–283; Luis García-Ballester, "Arnold of Villanova (ca. 1240–1311) and the Reform of Medical Studies in Montpellier (1309): The Latin Hippocrates and the Introduction of the New Galen," *Dynamis* 2 (1982): 97–158.

71. On this subject see also Nancy G. Siraisi, *Medieval and Early Renaissance Medicine: An Introduction to Knowledge and Practice* (Chicago and London, 1990), 65–70.

72. In this paragraph I follow the lead of Tamani, "Il corpus Aristotelicum nella tradizione ebraica," 5–22.

73. Tamani, "Il corpus Aristotelicum nella tradizione ebraica," 17–18.

74. Steinschneider, *Die hebraeischen Übersetzungen des Mittelalters und die Juden als Dolmetscher*, 42–48.

75. On these scholars, see Ernest Renan, "Les écrivains juifs français du XIVe siècle," 31:359–402, 586–644, 653–655, and 717–722.

76. See n. 72 above, Tamani, "Il corpus Aristotelicum nella tradizione ebraica."

77. Steinschneider, *Die hebraeischen Übersetzungen des Mittelalters und die Juden als Dolmetscher*, 49 ff. and 276 ff.

78. Ibid., 580–582.

79. There is an English translation of this book. See F. S.

Bodenheimer, *Rabbi Gershon ben Shlomoh d'Arles: The Gates of Heaven* (Shaar ha-Shamayim) (Jerusalem, 1953).

80. Yehuda tells about this in his *Midrash ha-Khochma*. The text was published in Ben-Zion Dinur, *Israel in the Diaspora: A Documentary History of the Jewish People from Its Beginning to the Present* (in Hebrew), 2d ser., 10 vols. (Tel-Aviv and Jerusalem, 1961–1972), vol. 13, pt. 6, p. 181. It was translated into French by Colette Sirat, "Juda b. Salomon ha-Cohen philosophe, astronome, et pêut-être kabbaliste de la première moitié du XIIIᵉ siècle," *Italia* 1, no. 2 (Jerusalem, 1978): 39–61, in particular 41–42.

81. Steinschneider, *Die hebraeischen Übersetzungen des Mittelalters und die Juden als Dolmetscher*, 1–4.

82. Ibid., 5–9.

83. Ibid., 159, 294, and recently, G[ad ben Ami] Sarfati, "The Hebrew Translations of Alfarabi's 'Classification of Sciences,'" in *Memorial to H. M. Shapiro (1902–1970)*, ed. H. Z. Hirschberg, vol. 1: *Bar-Ilan*, pp. 413–422 (Hebrew), p. xlii (summary in English), Annual of Bar-Ilan University, Studies in Judaica and the Humanities 9 (Ramat-Gan, 1972).

84. J. L. Teicher, "The Latin-Hebrew School of Translators in Spain in the Twelfth Century," in *Homenaje a Millás-Vallicrosa*, 2 vols. (Barcelona, 1954–1956), 2:403–444.

85. Steinschneider, *Die hebraeischen Übersetzungen des Mittelalters und die Juden als Dolmetscher*, 284. See also Tamani, "Il corpus Aristotelicum nella tradizione ebraica," 21.

86. For Romano and his activity see Leopold Zunz, *Gesammelte Schriften*, vol. 3 (Berlin, 1876), pp. 155–161, and Steinschneider, *Gesammelte Schriften* 1:507–522. For a more recent bibliography, see Caterina Rigo, "Un passo sconosciuto di Alberto Magno nel 'Sefer 'esem ha-shamayim' di Yehudah B. Mosheh," *Henoch* 11 (1989): 295–318, and more recently Jean-Pierre Rothschild, "Un traducteur hébreu qui se cherche: R. Juda b. Moïse Romano et le De causis et processu universitatis, II, 3,2 d'Albert le Grand," *Archives d'histoire doctrinale et littéraire du moyen âge* 59 (1992): 159–173.

87. I follow here the recent study of Jean-Pierre Rothschild, "Motivations et méthodes des traductions en hébreu du milieu du XIIIᵉ à la fin du XVᵉ siècle," in *Traduction et traducteurs au moyen âge*, 277–302, Colloque international du CNRS, IRHT, 26–28 mai 1986 (Paris, 1989). See also Isak Münz, *Die jüdischen Aerzte im Mittelalter: Ein Beitrag zur Kulturgeschichte des Mittelalters* (Frankfurt on Main, 1922), 87. Hillel's *Tagmulé ha-Nefesh* has been recently published; see Hillel Ben Shemu'el of Verona, *Sefer Tagmulé ha-Nefesh*

(Book of the Rewards of the Soul) (in Hebrew), ed. Joseph Sermoneta) (Jerusalem, 1981).

88. For Jacob see the recent study by Kenneth Stow, "Jacob B[en] Eliah e l'insidiamento ebraico a Venezia nel duecento" (in Hebrew), *Italia* 5 (1985): 89–105. In the introduction to his translation of Ibn Zohr, Jacob mentions (pp. 104–105) other treatises translated by him from Latin.

89. See my "In Search of the 'Book of Figures': Medicine and Astrology in Montpellier at the Turn of the Fourteenth Century," *AJS Review* 7–8 (1982–1983): 383–407, in particular 385–391.

90. For more about this enigmatic figure see Ernest Renan, "Les écrivains juifs français du XIVe siècle," 31:655–656. It is only a guess of mine that he may have been in the circle of scholars that surrounded Jacob ben Machir.

91. For this information see my "In Search of the 'Book of Figures,'" 388 n. 19.

92. For these two translators see Ernest Renan, "Les écrivains juifs français du XIVe siècle" 31:717–722 and 732. Recently Zvi Langerman of the National Library, Jerusalem, has discovered in the library of El Escorial (Spain) (ms. G-III-a) the translation of books 1–2 of Gordon's *De conservatione vitae humanae*. As far as we know, this is a unique manuscript. I thank Dr. Langerman for sharing this information with me.

93. See Steinschneider, *Die hebraeischen Übersetzungen des Mittelalters und die Juden als Dolmetscher*, 804–805 and 833–834.

94. Cf. Ernest Renan, "Les rabbins français," 27:770–778.

95. Ron Barkaï, *Les infortunes de Dinah: Le livre de la génération: La gynécologie juive au moyen âge*, trans. J. Barnavi and M. Garel (Paris, 1991), 117–128.

96. Bibliothèque Nationale, Paris, ms. 1192, fols 6v.–7v. Cf. Ron Barkaï, *Les infortunes de Dinah*, 27, and Carolus Bernheimer, *Codices hebraici bybliothecae Ambrosianae* (Florence, 1933), 130.

97. Neubauer, *Catalogue of the Hebrew Manuscripts in the Bodleian Library*, vol. 1, nos. 2133, 2142. Sheshet Benvenisti's treatise on gynecology *Medicament for pregnancy* (or *Medicaments and confections for women*) was written originally in Arabic and translated in the first half of the thirteenth century by Judah Alharizi. See Ron Barkaï, "A Medieval Hebrew Treatise on Obstetrics," *Medical History* 33 (1988): 96–119.

98. See Joshua [O.] Leibowitz, "A[braham] Caslari's [fourteenth-century] Hebrew Manuscript 'Pestilential Fevers' Edited by H. Pinkhoff," *Koroth* 4 (1968): 69–72 (English), 517–520 (Hebrew).

99. Benjamin Richler, "Medical Treatises by Moses b. Isaac Ibn Waqar," *Koroth* 9 (1989): 253–264 (Hebrew); 700–707 (English). Prescriptions in the German language, written toward the end of the fourteenth century by the Jewish doctor Jacob of Landshut, are transcribed in Peter Assion, "Jacob von Landshut: Zur Geschichte der jüdischen Ärzte in Deutschland," *Sudhoffs Archiv* 53 (1969): 270–291.

100. See Pierre Pansier, "Inventaire de la pharmacie de Pernes en 1365," *Annales d'Avignon et du comtat Venaissin* 14 (1928): 111–123, especially 112: "Item quod judeis interdicatur quod non utantur arte medicine nisi fuerint examinati et experti et approbati et contra facientibus apponatur pena. Placet domino (Rectori) quod judei in articulo mencionato non utantur arte medicine nisi sint sufficienter approbati."

101. Francisco Cantera Burgos, *Alvar García de Santa María y su familia de conversos: Historia de la judería de Burgos y sus conversos más egregios* (Madrid, 1952), 38.

102. See Joseph María Roca, *La medicina catalana en temps del rey Martí* (Barcelona, 1919), 121–127, especially 123: "En aprés, si dels metges nostres la un tan solament serà mestre en medecina, aquell en prerogativa donor al altre serà davant anant: se emperò, amdos maestres o en altre manera de per condició seràn, lavors aquell deurà esser en la honor pus poderós qui primerament al nostre servey serà appellat." For the date I am dependent on Antonio [Antoní] Cardoner [i] Planas, *Història de la medicina a la corona d'Aragó* (1162–1479) (Barcelona, 1973), 96–97.

Chapter 4

1. The text is provided in V[ictor] Aptowitzer, *Introductio ad Sefer Rabia* (Jerusalem, 1938), 209–211. I commented on it in my "Doctors and Medical Practices in Germany around the Year 1200: The Evidence of 'Sefer Asaph,'" *Proceedings of the American Academy for Jewish Research* 50 (1983): 149–164. On R. Sheshet and his career also see H. Graetz, *Geschichte der Juden*, vol. 6 (Leipzig, 1861), pp. 392–393, and Fritz Baer, *Die Juden im christlichen Spanien*, vol. 1 (Berlin, 1929), pp. 9–10, and vol. 2 (Berlin, 1936), p. 21. Medical prescriptions made up by Sheshet are signaled by Adolph Neubauer in his *Catalogue of the Hebrew Manuscripts in the Bodleian Library and in the College Libraries of Oxford* (Oxford, 1886), entry 2135 no. 2, as well as in entry 2138 (fol. 156v).

2. See Judah's "Ethical Will" in Israel Abrahams, ed. and trans.,

Hebrew Ethical Wills, 2d ed. (Philadelphia, 1976), 51–92 and especially 59–60.

3. For Hasdai's (mostly political) career, see Elyahu Ashtor, *The Jews in Moslem Spain*, 3 vols. (Philadelphia, 1973–1984), 1:155–227; for his medical activity see especially 1:160–168. See also the antiquated yet excellent biographical dictionary by Lucien Leclerc, *Histoire de la médecine arabe*, 2 vols. (Paris, 1876; reprint, New York, 1971), 1:457–458.

4. From the many studies on "Maimonides the doctor," I single out that of Süssmann Muntner, "Aus der ärztlichen Geisteswerkstätte des Maimonides," *Miscellanea mediaevalia* 4 (1966): 128–145. Max Meyerhof, "L'oeuvre médicale de Maimonide," in his *Studies in Medieval Arabic Medicine, Theory and Practice*, ed. P. Johnstone (London, 1984), article no. 8. See also the article recently published by Fred Rosner, "Maimonides the Physician: A Bibliography," *Bulletin of the History of Medicine* 43 (1969): 221–235; and Fred Rosner, *Medicine in the Bible and the Talmud: Selections from Classical Jewish Sources* (New York, 1977). Süssman Muntner also published most of Maimonides' medical work in Hebrew translation: see Moshe ben Maimon [Maimonides], *Medical Works*, ed. Süssman Muntner, vols. 1–5 (Jerusalem, 1957–1969; reprint, Jerusalem, 1987).

5. See for this almost unknown medical author the study of Henri Paul Joseph Renaud, "Etude sur le Musta'ini d'Ibn Beklàrech, médecin juif de Saragosse au XIᵉ siècle," in *Proceedings of the Sixth International Congress of the History of Medicine* (Leyden and Amsterdam, 1927), 267–273.

6. Augustí Duran i Sanpere, *Referencies documentals del call de juhséus de Cervera*, Real academia de buenas letras de Barcelona (Barcelona, 1924), 49.

7. See Joachim Miret y Sans, "Les médecins juifs de Pierre, roi d'Aragon," *Revue des études juives* 57 (1909): 268–278, especially 273. For the composition of the court's cohort of doctors see Joseph María Roca, *La medicina catalana en temps del rey Martí* (Barcelona, 1919), 23–24; Joseph María Roca, *Mestre Guillem Colteller metge dels reys d'Aragó Pere III y Johan I* (Barcelona, 1922), 27–30. For Jewish doctors in the service of John I in Aragon, see also Joseph María Roca, *Johan I d'Aragó* (Barcelona, 1929), 235. Miret y Sans believes, however, that in the 1330s in the court of Pere, king of Aragon, Christian doctors were in a minority. He has the names of eleven Jewish doctors and only six Christian doctors. One should add that R. Nissim Gerondi (Gerundi), the most important rabbinic scholar of the mid-fourteenth century, served as a physician in the court of Pere IV of Aragon. See Leon A. Feldman, "R. Nissim ben Reuben

Gerondi—Archival Data from Barcelona," in *Exile and Diaspora: Studies in the History of the Jewish People Presented to Professor Haim Beinart*, ed. Aharon Mirsky et al. (Jerusalem, 1991), 56–97, in particular 61–62 (doc. no. 1).

8. Ramón Jordí y González, "Médicos, cirujanos, y boticarios relacionados con las Casas reales," *Boletín informativo de circular farmacéutica* 235 (Barcelona, 1969), annex 5, pp. 396–399.

9. Shlomo Dov Goitein, *A Mediterranean Society: The Jewish Communities of the Arab World as Portrayed in the Cairo Genizah*, 5 vols. (Berkeley, 1967–1988), 5:420.

10. For the Spanish *alfaquim*, see David Romano, *Los funcionarios judíos de Pedro el Grande de Aragón*, Real academia de buenas letras de Barcelona (Barcelona, 1970); David Romano, "Judíos escribanos y trujamanes de árabe en la corona de Aragón (reinados de Jaime I a Jaime II)," *Sefarad* 38 (1978): 71–105; see also the next note.

11. David Romano, "Los hermanos Abenmenassé al servicio de Pedro el Grande de Aragón," in *Homenaje a Millás-Vallicrosa*, 2 vols. (Barcelona, 1954–1956), 2:243–292.

12. See J. Vincke, "Los familiares de la Corona aragonesa alrededor del año 1300," *Anuario de estudios medievales* 1 (1964): 333–351.

13. See Baer, *Die Juden im christlichen Spanien* 1:722.

14. See Archivo de la Corona d'Aragón (Barcelona), reg. 941, fol. 51v: "te Ycach Mayr judeum ville Frage in familiarem cirurgicum domesticum admitimus et aliorum familiarium cirurgicorum et domesticorum nostrorum consortio aggregamus"; see n. 15 below.

15. Antonio Rubió y Lluch, "Notes sobre la ciencia oriental a Catalunya en el XIVèn sigle," *Estudis universitaris catalans* 3 (1909): 389–398, 489–497, esp. 490–491.

16. Camille Arnaud, *Histoire de la viguerie de Forcalquier*, 2 vols. (Marseilles, 1874–1875), 2:54–55.

17. Angelo Sacchetti Sassetti, *Maestro Salomone d'Anagni, medico del secolo* XV (Frosinone, 1964), 11–16.

18. See Shlomo Simonsohn, *The Jews in the Duchy of Milan*, 4 vols. (Jerusalem, 1982–1986), 1:438–440.

19. Shlomo Simonsohn, *The Apostolic See and the Jews*, 6 vols. (Toronto, 1988–1991), e.g., 1:511–512 (document nos. 481–482) and 1:530–531 (document no. 492).

20. See Joseph María Roca, *L'estudi general de Lleyda* (Barcelona, n.d.), 76: "sit omnibus notum quod ego magister Altazar, judeus, phisicus illustrisimi domini regis Alfonsi, confiteor et recognosco . . ."

21. Antonio Cardoner Planas and Francisca Vendrell Gallostra, "Aportaciones al estudio de la familia Abenardut, médicos reales," *Sefarad* 7 (1947): 303–348. Most of the information in this section is drawn from this rich study.

22. Michael McVaugh is still working on the subject. He kindly sent me a typewritten inventory of his findings in Aragonese archives. (In the meantime, his *Medicine before the Plague: Practitioners and Their Patients in the Crown of Aragon, 1285–1345* [Cambridge, 1993] has appeared.) For work by José Ríus Serra, see n. 24 below. See also the documents about him in Antonio Rubió y Lluch, "Notes sobre la ciencia oriental a Catalunya en el XIVèn sigle," 389–398, 487–496, esp. 489–490.

23. Cardoner Planas and Vendrell Gallostra, "Aportaciones al estudio de la familia Abenardut," 307.

24. J[osé] Ríus Serra, "Aportaciones sobre médicos judíos en Aragón en la primera mitad del siglo XIV," *Sefarad* 12 (1952): 337–350, especially 338.

25. Cardoner Planas and Vendrell Gallostra, "Aportaciones al estudio de la familia Abenardut," 319–320.

26. See n. 51 below in this chapter. On military doctors in the expeditions of the 1350s, see the recent pioneering study of Lluís Cifuentes and Luis [Lluís] García-Ballester, "Els professionals sanitaris de la corona d'Aragó en l'expedició militar a Sardenya de 1354–1355," *Arxiu de textos catalans antics* (Barcelona, 1990), 183–214.

27. Jean Régné, *History of the Jews in Aragon: Regesta and Documents 1213–1327*, ed. and annotated by Y. T. Assis in association with A. Gruzman, reprinted from *Revue des études juives* 60 [1910] to 78 [1924] (Jerusalem, 1978), 600 (doc. no. 3264).

28. Juan Torres Fontes, "Los médicos murcianos en el siglo XV," *De historia médica murciana*, vol. 1: *Los médicos* (Murcia, 1980), 13–100, especially 51.

29. Ibid., 52.

30. Cardoner Planas and Vendrell Gallostra, "Aportaciones al estudio de la familia Abenardut," 303–348, especially 326.

31. Ibid., 327.

32. Ibid., 329–330.

33. Ibid., 321.

34. Ibid., 319.

35. Miret y Sans, "Les médecins juifs de Pierre, roi d'Aragon," 268–278, esp. 276.

36. Cardoner Planas and Vendrell Gallostra, "Aportaciones al estudio de la familia Abenardut," 326.

37. Ibid., 313–314 and 333–338.

38. Ibid., 337–338.

39. Ibid., 320–321.

40. Ibid., 323.

41. Ibid., 328–339.

42. Miret y Sans, "Les médecins juifs de Pierre, roi d'Aragon," 276.

43. Cardoner Planas and Vendrell Gallostra, "Aportaciones al estudio de la familia Abenardut," 340–341 and 345–348.

44. Miret y Sans, "Les médecins juifs de Pierre, roi d'Aragon," 276–277.

45. Ríus Serra, "Aportaciones sobre médicos judíos en Aragón en la primera mitad del siglo XIV," 342.

46. Bartolomeo and Giuseppe Lagumina, *Codice diplomatico dei giudei di Sicilia*, 3 vols. (Palermo, 1884–1895), 1:457 (doc. no. 366).

47. Béatrice Leroy, "Le royaume de Navarre et les juifs aux XIVe et XVe siècles: Entre l'accueil et la tolérance," *Sefarad* 38 (1978): 263–292, especially 265 n. 6; Béatrice Leroy, *The Jews of Navarre in the Late Middle Ages* (Jerusalem, 1985), 14 n. 6, where the document is quoted more extensively.

48. Antonio Durán Gudiol, *La judería de Huesca* (Zaragoza, 1984), 76–77, and especially 177–178.

49. Rubió y Lluch, "Notes sobre la ciencia oriental a Catalunya," 494; and Durán Gudiol, *La judería de Huesca*, 77.

50. Durán Gudiol, *La judería de Huesca*, 77.

51. Miret y Sans, "Les médecins juifs de Pierre, roi d'Aragon," 275; and Régné, *History of the Jews in Aragon*, 601–602 (doc. no. 3274). A short prescription for "ailments of the legs" by a certain Moses ben Ardut is to be found in ms. 99 of the Bibliotheca Ambrosiana in Milan, fol. 167v. Cf. Carolus Bernheimer, *Codices hebraici bybliothecae Ambrosianae* (Florence, 1933), 130. It is not at all sure that he is to be identified with our royal doctor.

52. Kaspi discusses it in the introduction to his *Gelilé Kesef*. See Joseph Ibn Kaspi, *Zehn Schriften des R. Josef Ibn Kaspi* (Asarah keley kesef), ed. Isaac Last, 2 vols. (Pressburg, 1903), 2:29–40, esp. 30.

53. Joseph María Roca's *La medicina catalana en temps del rey Martí* (Barcelona, 1919), and his *Mestre Guille Colteller metge dels reys d'Aragó Pere III y Johan I* (Barcelona, 1922), and his *Johan I d'Aragó* (Barcelona, 1929).

54. Published and discussed in Baer, *Die Juden in christlichen Spanien* 1:965–966.

55. The document was first published in Claude Devic and Joseph Vaissète, *Histoire générale de Languedoc*, 15 vols. (Toulouse, 1872–1893), 8:1317–1319. It was reproduced and translated into English in

Solomon Grayzel, *The Church and the Jews in the Thirteenth Century*, rev. ed. (New York, 1966), 346–347.

56. Published by Joseph Jacobs, "Une lettre française d'un juif anglais au XIIIᵉ siècle," *Revue des études juives* 18 (1889): 256–261. Elia's appeal is translated in Franz Kobler, *Letters of Jews through the Ages*, 2 vols. (Reprint, Philadelphia, 1978), 1:246–247. See also Cecil Roth, "Jewish Physicians in Medieval England," in his *Essays and Portraits in Anglo-Jewish History* (Philadelphia, 1962), 46–51.

57. Régné, *History of the Jews in Aragon*, 214 (doc. no. 1182).

58. Antonio Pons, *Los judíos de Mallorca*, 2 vols. (Palma de Mallorca, 1984), 1:246–247 (doc. no. 56).

59. Published by Simonsohn, *The Jews in the Duchy of Milan* 1:606–607 (doc. no. 1459). See also the short reference in Emilio Ambrogio Motta, "Oculisti, dentisti, e medici ebrei nella seconda metà del secolo XV alla corte milanese," *Annali universali di medicina* 283 (1887): 326–328.

60. Renata Segre, *The Jews in Piedmont: Edited with an Introduction and Notes*, 3 vols. (Jerusalem, 1986–1990), 1:337 (doc. no. 751).

61. In depicting the career of Elia I mostly follow Ladislao Münster, "La grande figure d'Elia di Sabbato, médecin juif d'Italie du XVᵉ siècle," *Revue d'histoire de la médecine hébraïque* 9, no. 3 (1956): 125–140; 10, no. 1 (1957): 41–45; 10, no. 2: 53–65. This article appeared a year later in Italian; see "Una luminosa figura di medico ebreo del quattrocento: Maestro Elia di Sabbato da Fermo, archiatra pontificio," in *Scritti in memoria di Sally Mayer (1875–1953). Saggi sull'ebraismo italiano* (Jerusalem, 1956), 224–258. Most of my references will be to the Italian version.

62. Simonsohn, *The Jews in the Duchy of Milan* 1:27–28 (doc. no. 32).

63. Malachi Beit-Arié and Colette Sirat, *Manuscrits médiévaux en caractères hébraïques portant des indications de date jusqu'à 1540*, 2 vols. (Paris and Jerusalem, 1972–1979), 2:81. For a medal issued apparently in honor of Elia's son, see Samuel S. Kottek, "Humilitas: On a Controversial Medal of Benjamim, Son of Elijah Beer the Physician (1497?–1503?)," *Journal of Jewish Art* 11 (1985): 41–46.

64. Cf. Münster, "Una luminosa figura di medico ebreo," 236–237.

65. Ibid., 228–229. Renzo Mosti in his "Medici ebrei del XIV–XV secolo a Tivoli," *Atti e memorie della società tiburtina di storia e d'arte*, 27 (1954): 109–156, publishes (on pp. 137–143) the privilege granting Moses of Tivoli (6 July 1406) the status of *civis Romanus*. Elia's must have read the same.

66. "Propter invidiam, quia erat melior medicus quam supradictus

Helias." See Leone Luzzatto, "Medici ebrei," *Il vessillo israelitico* 50 (1902): 301–303.

67. Gaetano Marini, *Degli archiatri pontifici* (Rome, 1874), 1:134–135. For Giovanni di Anagni's opposition see Mosti, "Medici ebrei del XIV–XV secolo a Tivoli," 27:126.

68. See Münster, "Una luminosa figura di medico ebreo," 231 and 248.

69. Georg Caro, "Dr. phil. et med. Helyas Sabbati von Bologna und sein Aufenthalt in Basel 1410," *Anzeiger für schweizerische Geschichte*, n.s. 11 (1910–1913): 75–77.

70. Roger Kohn, *Les juifs de la France du nord dans la seconde moitié du XIVe siècle* (Louvain and Paris, 1988), 274.

71. Münster, "Una luminosa figura di medico ebreo," 236–237.

72. Ibid., pp. 249–250.

73. Ibid., 238.

74. See Simonsohn, *The Apostolic See and the Jews* 2:840–842. For the history of this interdiction, see Shlomo Simonsohn, "Divieto di trasportare ebrei in Palestina," in *Italia Judaica: Gli ebrei in Italia tra Rinascimento ed età barocca,* 39–53, Atti del II convegno internazionale, Genova, 10–15 giugno 1984 (Rome 1986).

75. Münster, "Una luminosa figura di medico ebreo," 255–257.

76. Ibid., 235–237.

77. Michael R. McVaugh, "Royal Surgeons and the Value of Medical Learning: The Crown of Aragon, 1300–1350," to appear in the *Actes du colloque de Barcelone sur l'histoire de la médecine* (May 1989).

78. Luis Comenge, "Formas de munificencia real para con los archiatros de Aragón," *Boletín de la real academia de buenas letras de Barcelona* 3 (1903): 1–15. Other examples are to be found in the forthcoming study of Michael R. McVaugh, "Royal Surgeons and the Value of Medical Learning: The Crown of Aragon, 1300–1350." Prof. McVaugh kindly provided me with a copy of this unpublished work.

79. Comenge, "Formas de munificencia," 3–4 and passim.

80. Salo Wittmayer Baron, *The Jewish Community: Its History and Structure to the American Revolution*, 3 vols. (Philadelphia, 1948), 1:285–286.

81. See Juan Torres Fontes, "El alcade mayor de las aljamas de moros en Castilla," *Anuario de historia del derecho español* (Madrid, 1962), 131–182. See also Eliezer Gutwirth, "Hispano-Jewish Attitudes to the Moors in the Fifteenth Century," *Sefarad* 49 (1989): 237–262, esp. 238–239 n. 4.

82. Lagumina, *Codice diplomatico dei giudei di Sicilia* 1:316–317 (doc. no. 297).

83. Ibid., 368–371 (doc. no. 301).

84. For Orabuena see Béatrice Leroy, *The Jews of Navarre in the Late Middle Ages* (Jerusalem, 1985), 123–126. For ibn Wakar and Alguades, see Fritz [Yitzhak] Baer, *A History of the Jews in Christian Spain*, 2 vols. (Philadelphia, 1971), 1:322–324, 377–378.

85. See Lagumina, *Codice diplomatico dei giudei di Sicilia*, vol. 1 passim. For favors bestowed on doctors in Sicily, see also Annamaria Precopi Lombardo, "Medici ebrei nella Sicilia medievale," *Trapani: Rassegna della provincia*, 29 (1984): 25–28, esp. 26–27.

86. Pilar León Tello, *Los judíos de Toledo*, 2 vols. (Madrid, 1979), 1:172.

87. Rubió y Lluch, "Notes sobre la ciencia oriental a Catalunya en el XIVèn sigle," 489–495.

88. Baer, *Die Juden im christlichen Spanien* 1:247–248: " . . . vos pido merced, padre ssennor . . . del quitar del ssu pecho de todo o dela meytat . . . por que el dicho maestre Salamon entienda que vale mas por mi . . ."

89. Baer, *Die Juden im christlichen Spanien*, 1:643–644 (doc. no. 400): "afirmantes pro firmo dictum Juneç pauperes et mendicos egrotantes, lesos, dolentes et macie sauciatos suis propriis sumptibus curare in domo propria et alibi animo leto . . ."

90. Lagumina, *Codice diplomatico dei giudei di Sicilia* 1:26–28 (doc. no. 30).

91. See Régné, *History of the Jews in Aragon*, 181 (doc. no. 1009, dated 24 January 1283).

92. Lagumina, *Codice diplomatico dei giudei di Sicilia* 1·40–44 (doc. no. 40).

93. Ibid., 2:180–181 (doc. no. 518).

94. Ibid., 2:203–224 (doc. no. 593); see also 1:605–606 (doc. no. 453), where in 1459 the Jewish doctors of Trapani are denied the privilege of exemption from communal taxes "comu li altri medichi et docturi cristiani."

95. See Solomon Grayzel, *The Church and the Jews in the Thirteenth Century: A Study of Their Relations during the Years 1198–1254, Based on the Papal Letters and the Conciliar Decrees of the Period*, rev. ed. (New York, 1966), 59–70.

96. Miret y Sans, "Les médecins juifs de Pierre, roi d'Aragon," 269: "te convenit per loca diversa itinera incedere de die et de nocte quod que si cum signo vel rotula quam judei portare in veste superiori tenentur incedere posses ab aliquibus christianis insipientibus agravari . . ."

97. Régné, *History of the Jews in Aragon*, 202 (doc. no. 1117).

98. All names are to be found in Miret y Sans, "Les médecins juifs

de Pierre, roi d'Aragon," 269–271.

99. Régné, *History of the Jews in Aragon*, 183 (doc. no. 1021).

100. Baer, *Die Juden im christlichen Spanien* 1:571–572 (doc. no. 374).

101. See Louis Finkelstein, *Jewish Self-Government in the Middle Ages* (Reprint, New York, 1964), 227 and 241 (for translations into English). These are the Ordinances of the Rhine communities of the first quarter of the fourteenth century: "Whoever has a *hazzan* or one to 'roll the Torah,' or any public officer appointed through Gentile influence, is excommunicated and also the *hazzan* and the one 'who rolls the Torah,' as well as he who endeavors to bring it about that a Gentile should judge a Jew is to be in excommunication, for one should try one's litigation through Jewish judges."

102. Baer, *Die Juden im christlichen Spanien*, 1:571–572:

> tu, dito Junez, al qual semblant honor que aquesta e mayor en la dita sinoga se pertenesce, havido encara esguard alos servicios por tu a nos e a nuestra cort feytos, con tenor dela present . . . atorgamos e a tu e a los de tu linatge e adaquellos, que tu querras, con tu a perpetuo dela dita solempnidat e honor de una fiesta de las vacantes o qui da [qui?] adelante vagaran por defallimiento delos ditos linatges provehimos, y es saber, daquella fiesta, que dequellas vacantes tu esleyras e querras, dando licencia e pleno poder a tu, dito Junez, e a los de tu linatge e a los, que tu querras, de puyar a la trahuna dela dita sinoga e leyr en la ley de Moysen en el rotulo o atora en e por la forma e manera, que acostumbrado yes por los otros semblantes honores havientes . . .

103. Baer, *Die Juden im christlichen Spanien*, 1:530–531 (doc. no. 350): "quia fuit et est in consiliarium et etiam aliquando in secretarium dicte aljame electus, non potest, occupatus officiis, circa eius artem medicine exercandam vaccare comode seu practicare . . ."

104. Régné, *History of the Jews in Aragon*, 518 (doc. no. 2794), 523 (doc. no. 2820), 552 and 555 (docs. no. 2985 and 3001). See also Pons, *Los judíos de Mallorca* 2:59–74 and 302.

105. Régné, *History of the Jews in Aragon*, 555 and 568 (docs. no. 3005 and 3075), and 569 (doc. no. 3083).

106. Ibid., 514 (doc. no. 2769).

107. On this aspect of Jewish private life in Spain see the study of Yom Tov Assis, "The 'Ordinance of Rabbenu Gershom' and Polygamous Marriages in Spain" (in Hebrew), *Zion* 46 (1981): 251–277.

108. For Vitàlis Almuviçuel, see Miret y Sans, "Les médecins juifs de Pierre, roi d'Aragon," 274–275. For the other two, see Rubió

y Lluch, "Notes sobre la ciencia oriental a Catalunya en el XIVèn sigle," 493–494.

109. Miret y Sans, "Les médecins juifs de Pierre, roi d'Aragon," 274–275:

> Pro parte Vitalis Almuviçuel filii Astrugi Almuviçuel fisici habitatores civitatis eiusdem, fuit coram nobis expositum reverenter quod ipse habet uxorem vocatam Ifazbuenya et quod quindecim anni sunt elapsi et prolem habere non potuit ab eadem et ut fertur de lege ebreorum est ut quicumque ebreus duxerit uxorem et infra decem annos prolem ab ea habere non poterit aliam . . . possit ducere in uxorem . . . fuit nobis humiliter supplicatum ut ducendi aliam in uxorem de benignitate solita dignaremur ei licenciam impertiri. Nos vero ipsa supplicatione suscepta vobis dicimus et mandamus quatenus si ita est ad ducendum in uxorem filiam Jacob Cerdoni . . . libere permitatis nec impedimentum ei per aliquos fieri sustineatis pro ut de lege judeorum fore inveneretis faciendum. Nos enim super hiis comitimus vices nostras.

110. The document is referred to in Rubió y Lluch, "Notes sobre la ciencia oriental a Catalunya en el XIVèn sigle." 491. I publish it from a photocopy kindly sent to me by Dr. Jaume Riera of the Archivo de la Corona d'Aragón (Barcelona) (reg. 440, fol. 288v):

> Alfonsus etc. Fideli suo Dimuto Zvalit jurisperito Cesarauguste Salutem etc. Ex parte Azarie Abenjacob phisici nostri judei Cesarauguste fuit conquerendo expositum coram nobis quod Donatus filius Sentoni Arziello judeus Cesarauguste, existens pro serviente sub certa mercede in domo dicti Azarie, fidelitatis oblitus quam famulus tenetur suo domino observare, seduxit quandam puellam nepotem dicti Azarie eamque seductam falsis inducionibus defloravit; Ex quo non solum dicto Azarie, tunc eius domino, et dicte puelle set ceteris eiusdam puelle consanguineis non modicum injuriam iregavit cum dictus Bonetus par non existat ipsi puelle, nec posset ei virum dare qualem ante dictam deflorationem dicta puella potuisset habere. Quare suplicatione propterea nobis facta admissa benigne, vobis dicimus et mandamus quatinus de persona dicti Boneti taliter vos assecuretis quod de ipso tam dictus Azarias quam alii conquerentes de eo propterea valeant habere justicie completam, quo assecuramento habito, contra ipsum ratione dicti criminis seu delicti procedatis prout de foro et ratione ac usu regni fuerit faciendum maliciis quibus libet pretermissis, sic quod penam debitam susteneat pro premissis. Nos enim vobis comitimus plenarie vires nostras. Datum Valentie v. jdus decembris anno Domini trecentesimo tricesimo.

111. See Sacchetti Sassetti, *Maestro Salomone d'Anagni*, 3–22, esp. 6–7.

112. Lagumina, *Codice diplomatico dei giudei di Sicilia* 1:397–398 (doc. no. 325) and 403–408 (doc. no. 332). I have followed Moses' career in detail in a paper presented at the fourth congress of "Italia Judaica" (Palermo, June 1992). It will appear in the conference proceedings (1994).

113. See *The Itinerary of Benjamin of Tudela*, ed. and trans. Marcus Nathan Adler (London, 1907; New York, n.d.), 16 (Hebrew), 14 (English trans.).

114. Ignaz Blumenfeld, "Letter Written by Rabbi Don Isaac Abrabanel to the Distinguished Yeḥiel of Pisa" (in Hebrew), *Ozar nechmad: Briefe und Abhandlungen jüdische Literatur betreffend* 2 (1857): 65–70, especially 70.

Chapter 5

1. John Arderne, *Treatise of "Fistula in ano": Haemorrhoids and Elysters*, ed. D'Arcy Power (London, 1910), 83–84.

2. Süssman Muntner, "R. Shem Tob Ben Isaac of Tortosa about the Life of the European Jewish Doctor and His Ethics," in *Sinai Jubilee Volume* (Jerusalem, 1957), 321–337, especially 328–329.

3. See my "Doctors' Fees and Their Medical Responsibility: Evidence from Notarial and Court Records," in *Private Acts of the Late Middle Ages*, ed. Paolo Brezzi and Egmont Lee (Toronto, 1984), 201–208.

4. See Martin Weinbaum, ed., *The London Eyre of 1276* (London, 1976), 72–73 and 131.

5. I owe this information to my colleague Thyron Sandquist of the department of history at the University of Toronto. The unpublished document, deciphered by Professor Sandquist, is to be found in Corporation of London, Miscellaneous, roll CC, membrane 17d.

6. See John Boswell, *The Royal Treasure: Muslim Communities under the Crown of Aragon in the Fourteenth Century* (New Haven and London, 1977), 158. Professor Boswell, in a letter of 12 February 1979, kindly added information about this case.

7. See Antonio (Antoní) Cardoner [i] Planas, *Història de la medicina a la corona d'Aragó (1162–1479)* (Barcelona, 1973), 223.

8. I drew this information from a file of documents (all still unpublished) deposited in the Archives départementales de l'Isère (Grenoble), série B, no. 3,804. I hope this file will be published in the near future.

9. Jean Régné, *History of the Jews in Aragon, Regesta and Documents 1213–1327*, ed. and annotated by Y. T. Assis in association

with A. Gruzman, reprinted from *Revue des études juives* 60 (1910) to 78 (1924) (Jerusalem, 1978), 587 (doc. no. 3186) and 192 (doc. no. 1065). This first document dates to 13 May 1283.

10. Joachim Miret y Sans, "Les médecins juifs de Pierre, roi d'Aragon," *Revue des études juives* 57 (1909): 268–278. The following is quoted from p. 278: "vos dictam Miram fore fisicam dedistis Sancie uxori Dominici Amargo vicini loci de Magallon et Graciete filie eorum etatis viginti mensium purgaciones aliquas ad potandum quibus mediantibus sanerentur ab infirmitatibus quibus detinebantur, quarum purgacionum occasione dicta Gracieta obiit et prefata Sancia abortavit fetum vivum quem in ventrem portaverat per sex menses."

11. The document (Archivo de la Corona d'Aragón (Barcelona), reg. 593, fol. 32v) is referred to in Antonio Rubió y Lluch, "Notes sobre la ciencia oriental a Catalunya en el XIVèn sigle," *Estudis universitaris catalans* 3 (Barcelona, 1909): 389–398, 489–497, especially 495. Here is my deciphering of its first part:

Petrus etc. Fideli suo justicie Alagonis vel eius locum tenenti, salutem. Ad tantum seu quotiensquam Maria Egidii uxor Egidii Eximini quondam vicina loci de Bagnena Aldea Daroce, movit aut movere intendit adversus Mahyl judeus cirurgicum Alagonis super eo quia ipsa Maria asserit Romenam filiam suam deffunctam existendo sub cura dicti judei pretextu cujusdam infirmitatis quam patiebatur in altero pedum, fuisse mortua ob culpam judei eiusdem   , XVI Kalendas Februarii anno domini millesimo CCCXXXVII.

12. Carmen Martínez Loscos, "Orígenes de la medicina en Aragón: Los médicos árabes y judíos," *Jerónimo Zurita: Cuadernos de historia* 6–7 (Zaragoza, 1954): 7–55, esp. 48.

13. Elena Lourie, "Jewish Moneylenders in the Local Catalan Community, ca. 1300: Vilafranca del Penedés, Besalú, and Montblanc," in *Michael: On the History of the Jews in the Diaspora*, ed. Eliezer Gutwirth and Shlomo Simonsohn, vol. 11 (Tel-Aviv, 1989), 33–98, esp. 50–52.

14. David Jacobi, "Jewish Doctors and Surgeons in Crete under Venetian Rule" (in Hebrew), in *Culture and Society in Medieval Jewry: Studies Dedicated to the Memory of Haim Hillel Ben-Sasson*, ed. M. Ben-Sasson et al. (Jerusalem, 1989), 431–444, in particular 439–442.

15. The text is still unpublished; it is described in much detail in Félix Portal, *Un procès en responsabilité médicale à Marseille en 1390* (Marseilles, 1902). I have tried unsuccessfully to track down the original in the archives of Marseilles.

16. Süssmann Muntner, "R. Shem Tob Ben Isaac of Tortosa

about the Life of the European Jewish Doctor and His Ethics," esp. 328.

17. Published in my *Médecine et justice en Provence médiévale: Documents de Manosque, 1262–1348* (Aix-en-Provence, 1989), 80–85 (docs. no. 10 and 11).

18. Adolph Neubauer, *Catalogue of the Hebrew Manuscripts in the Bodleian Library and in the College Libraries of Oxford*, vol. 1 (Oxford, 1886), 733–734 (ms. no. 2134).

19. Quoted by Moritz Güdemann, *Geschichte des Erziehungswesens und der Cultur der abendländischen Juden während des Mittelalters und der neueren Zeit*, 3 vols. (Vienna, 1884–1888; reprint, Amsterdam, 1966), 3:196:

> Die Juden, so sich für artzte auszgeben, bringen die Christen, welche ihre artzney brauchen, umb leib und gut, denn sie halten es gewisz dar für, lehren es auch ihre Kinder und discipul, wenn sien nur die Christen weidlich plagen, heimlich umbringen, oder inen ja vorliegen, sie thun gott einen dienst daran. Und wir Christen seind gleichwol solche unbesunnen narren, dasz wir zuflucht in gefahr unsers leben und umb errettung desselbigen bey unsern ertzfeinden und widerwertigen haben, damit wir gott, mit verschmehung rechtschaffener christlicher medicorum medicamentis, versuchen.

20. Jean Marx, *L'inquisition en Dauphiné: Etude sur le développement et la répression de l'hérésie et de la sorcellerie du XIVe siècle au début du règne de François Ier* (Paris, 1914; reprint, Geneva and Paris, 1978), 218–228. The quote is on p. 221:

> Item plus, dixit et fuit confessus quod Judei multum inimicantur Christianis, et in constitucionibus suis habent, ut eciam medici nullos liberent, sed quotquot poterunt interficiant, et in diebus Jovis et Vencris sanctis faciunt ymaginem Virginis Marie et ejus Filii, quam in contemptum ipsorum comburunt, et agnum unum cruciffigunt, et carnes inde canibus tradunt, et plura alia turpia, exsecrabilia contra Dominum nostrum Jesum Christum et Christianos continue faciunt, licet in partu judee Virginem Mariam invocent, quam incontinenti post renegant et possethinus expellunt.

21. [Charles-Albert] Costa de Beauregard, "Notes et documents sur la condition des juifs en Savoie [dans le moyen âge]," *Mémoires de l'académie des sciences, belles-lettres et arts de Savoie*, 2d ser., 2 (1854): 81–126; I refer to the independent publication of this study published in Chambéry, 1851, pp. 35–36.

22. Joseph ben Meir Iben Zabara, *Sepher Sha'ashu'im le R[abbi] Joseph ben Meir Iben Zabara* (in Hebrew), ed. I. Davidson (Berlin, 1924–1925), 65. The therapeutic potential of ground bones and the

teeth of the dead, of the genitalia of dead animals, of dogs' milk and the like intrigued the mind of no less than Petrus Hispanus, the famous pope-doctor John XXI. See Heath Dillard, *Daughters of the Reconquest: Women in Castilian Town Society 1100–1300* (Cambridge, 1984; reprint, Cambridge, 1989), 210–211.

23. See Pierrette Paravy, "A propos de la genèse médiévale des chasses aux sorcières: Le traité de Claude Tholosan, juge dauphinois (vers 1436)," *Mélanges de l'Ecole française de Rome: Moyen âge, temps modernes* 91 (1979): 333–379; Pierrette Paravy "Faire croire: Quelques hypothèses de recherche basées sur l'étude des procès de sorcellerie du Dauphiné au XVᵉ siècle," in *Faire croire: Modalités de la diffusion et de la réception des messages religieux du XIIᵉ au XVᵉ siècle*, 119–130, Table ronde organisée par l'Ecole française de Rome, en collaboration avec l'Institut d'histoire médiévale de l'université de Padoue, Rome, 22–23 juin 1979 (Rome, 1981).

24. The Hebrew lamentation was published several times: first by Moritz Steinschneider in *He-Halutz*, vol. 4 (Breslau, 1858), pp. 66–70, and then as an independent booklet by Mosheh Rimos, *Kinah le-Mosheh Rimos* (Lamentation by Mosheh Rimos) (in Hebrew), ed. David Kahana (Odessa, 1893). A third publication, accompanied by a translation of the English, is Israel Abrahams, ed. and trans., *Hebrew Ethical Wills*, vol. 2 (Philadelphia, 1926; reprinted in 1 vol., 1976), pp. 235–248. For the above quotation I have used Abrahams' translation, p. 247. In dating the document I have followed David Kaufmann, "Das Sendschreiben des Mose Rimos aus Majorca an Benjamin b. Mordechai in Rom," in *Festschrift zum achtzigsten Geburtstage Moritz Steinschneider's* (Leipzig, 1896; reprint, Jerusalem, 1970), 227–232. Nahum Slousch, who also published the document, suggests it is from the 1530s or even the 1540s. See his "Élégie de Moïse Rimos, martyr juif à Palerme au XVIᵉ siècle," in *Centenario della nascita di Michele Amari*, vol. 2 (Palermo, 1910), pp. 186–204; there were no Jews on the island at that date.

25. See Katharine Park, *Doctors and Medicine in Early Renaissance Florence* (Princeton, 1985), 74.

26. I follow here the calendar of Edgard Boutaric, *Actes du parlement de Paris: Première série, de l'an 1254 à l'an 1328*, 2 vols. (Paris, 1863–1867; reprint, Hildesheim, 1975), 2:210. For a Jewish doctor charged in 1490 with poisoning some of his coreligionists, members of the family of Vitalis Isaac of Pisa, see Michele Luzzati, "Lucca e gli ebrei fra quattro e cinquecento," in *La casa dell'ebreo: Saggi sugli ebrei a Pisa e in Toscana nel medioevo e nel Rinascimento* (Pisa, 1985), 171–172.

27. For the text and its translation and for discussion see Dwayne

E. Carpenter, *Alfonso X and the Jews: An Edition of and Commentary on* Siete Partidas *7.24, "De los judíos"* (Berkeley, Los Angeles, London, 1986), 34–35.

28. See Fritz Baer, *Die Juden im christlichen Spanien*, 2 vols. (Berlin, 1929–1933), 1:732–734:

> Ulterius, quia dicti judei perfidi velut inimici sitiunt christianorum sanguinem et ipsis christianis periculosum est a judeis medicis in eorum infirmitatibus benefficium assumere medicine, ordinamus et statuimus, quod aliquis judeus utens arte medicine in aliqua christiani infirmitate suum medicine non audeat officium exercere, nisi in ipsa cura intervenerit alius medicus christianus, sub pena privacionis dicti officii et decem librarum barchinonensium, quodque nullus apothecarius ab eis recipiat receptam aliquam nec ex ea letovarium, collirium audeant facere vel xiropum sub pena consimili dictarum X librarum.

29. Giovanni Domenico Mansi, ed., *Sacrorum conciliorum nova et amplissima collectio*, 58 vols. (Florence and Venice, 1759–1798), 25:720 (Valladolid), 25:1055–1056 (Salamanca).

30. I owe this information to my friend Noël Coulet, who discovered (and dated) the manuscript in the Bibliothèque Nationale, Paris, N. acq. lat. 1358, fol. 6r. The Latin reads: "quod judeus cirurgicus debeat gustare de vino dando egrotibus ne pro vini assumptione intemperata langor arrestat, non obstante consuetudine vestra de non bibendo inter christicolas ad quam vestra lex scripta judayca non astringit." We notice that in 1348 Jews were accused of poisoning Christians and causing the plague.

31. See Antonio Pons, *Los judíos de Mallorca*, 2 vols. (Palma de Mallorca, 1984), 2:248–249. For the Barcelona pharmacist, see Régné, *History of the Jews in Aragon*, 611 (doc. no. 3336).

32. Mansi, *Sacrorum conciliorum* 25:1105, quoted in n. 46 below of this chapter.

33. Shlomo Simonsohn, *The Jews in the Duchy of Milan*, 4 vols. (Jerusalem, 1982–1986), 1:528–529 (doc. no. 1252) and 1:531 (doc. no. 1258).

34. Ibid., 1:379 (doc. no. 869); see also 1:286 (doc. no. 836).

35. The document was published in full and discussed in his article: Rodrigue Lavoie, "La délinquance sexuelle à Manosque: Schéma général et singularités juives," *Provence historique* 37 (1987): 571–587, in particular 583–587. A partial publication appears in my *Médecine et justice en Provence médiévale*, 229–230.

36. Oldradus de Ponte, the fourteenth-century canonist (d. 1337?), reported on a similar situation he witnessed where "a Jew whose name was Pandonus was condemned to castration" for having had carnal relations with a Christian woman. "I saw the physical evi-

dence of the excision before the palace," he wrote. See Norman Zacour, *Jews and Saracens in the Consilia of Oldradus de Ponte* (Toronto, 1990), 70. In Castile, *Las Siete Partidas* decreed the death sentence on a Jew who lies with a Christian woman.

> Forbidden Unions 7.24.9: Law 9: "What punishment a Jew deserves who lies with a Christian woman": Jews who lie with Christian women are guilty of great insolence and presumption. As such, we order that henceforth all Jews guilty of having committed such an act shall die. Since Christians who commit adultery with married women deserve death, how much more so do Jews who lie with Christian women, for these are spiritually espoused to Our Lord Jesus Christ by virtue of the faith and baptism they received in His name. And the Christian woman who commits such a transgression should not remain unpunished. We decree, therefore, that if she be a virgin, married woman, widow, or profligate whore, she shall receive the same punishment as the Christian woman who lies with a Muslim, as we indicated in the last law of the title dealing with Muslims.

I quote the translation of Dwayne E. Carpenter in his *Alfonso X and the Jews*, 35.

37. Published in my *Médecine et justice en Provence médiévale*, 106–107 (doc. no. 22).

38. For the legislation of the Fourth Lateran Council see Mansi, *Sacrorum conciliorum* 22:1054–1058, as well as Solomon Grayzel, *The Church and the Jews in the Thirteenth Century: A Study of Their Relations during the Years 1198–1254, Based on the Papal Letters and the Conciliar Decrees of the Period*, rev. ed. (New York, 1966), 307–312, for the texts and the English translations.

39. See Mansi, *Sacrorum conciliorum* 23:33. "Item precipimus quod sacerdotes . . . praecipiant omnibus subditis suis ne aliquam potationem vel medicinam ab eis sumant." A similar exemption is awarded to the Jew Joseph di Montalto on 28 April 1400. He will be examined by Master Nicolà Pagano di Cosenza and has not to appear personally in court. The reason: the way from his place to the court is long and dangerous. See Cesare Colafemmina, "Presenza ebraica nel marchesato di Crotone," *Studi storici meridionali* 9 (1989): 287–308, in particular 288–289.

40. Mansi, *Sacrorum conciliorum* 23:850. "Excommunicentur preterea christiani qui causa medicine cure se commiserint judeorum."

41. Archives départementales des Bouches-du-Rhône (Marseilles), B1372, fol. 54r, 10 October 1306.

> Eidem Magistri David presenti et postulanti in arte phisice licentiam contulimus libere practicandi in civitate Arelate usque ad beneplacitum domini nostri regis, sub hac forma ut infirmum aliquem seu infirmam

adhire vel ei super cura prebere consilium non audat, nisi prius infirmus
vel infirma confessus seu confessa fuerit et receperit corpus Christi, sub
pena contenta in statuto illustris domini ducis Calabrie primoginiti dicti
domini nostri regis.

See also below, p. 93 and n. 48.

42. For the Avignon synod of 1341 see below, n. 46 of this chapter; for Barcelona see J. N. Hillgarth and Giulio Silano, "A Compilation of the Diocesan Synods of Barcelona (1354): Critical Edition
and Analysis," *Mediaeval Studies* 46 (1984): 78–157, in particular
136–137. According to the 1354 synod decree, Jewish doctors should
approach a Christian patient only in the presence of a Christian colleague "lest a fraud be committed in their soul or body."

43. Juan Torres Fontes, "Los médicos murcianos en el siglo XV,"
De historia médica murciana, vol. 1: *Los médicos* (Murcia, 1980), 13–
100, in particular 61; and Shlomo Simonsohn, *The Apostolic See and
the Jews*, 6 vols. (Toronto, 1988–1991), 2:808 (doc. no. 685).

44. Mansi, *Sacrorum conciliorum* 25:720:

Adversus Judaeorum and Sarracenorum induratam malitiam, (qui sub
velamine medicinae, chirurgiae, & apothecariae, callide insidianter &
nocent populo Christiano; dum eis medicamenta proponant, ex quibus
nonnunquam pericula mortis incurrunt) sanctorum patrum canones
salubriter providerunt, prohibentes, ne Christiani eos in infirmitatibus
suis vocent, aut ab eis recipiant medicinam. Quia vero praedicti
canones propter praelatorum negligentiam non servantur, in virtute
sanctae obedientiae praecipiendo mandamus, ut praelati ipsi praecepta
canonum tam circa praedicta, quam circa eorumdem evitanda cibaria,
per censuram ecclesiasticam faciant inviolabiliter observari.

45. Mansi, *Sacrorum conciliorum* 25:1055–1056:

Quia impraevisus jaculis homo saepe percutitur, quae si fuissent
praevisa, vel potuissent vitari vel levius sustineri; quibus expedit in pro-
cessibus initiis opportunis remediis subveniri, ne amplius cum multorum
scandalo in suarum animarum periculum damnosius invalescant: ea
propter detestabilem quorumdam Christianorum abusum, qui Hebraeos
et Sarracenos in infirmitatibus suis, et nonnumquam in convalescentia,
pro suorum corporum cura advocant, et ab eisdem medicinas recipiunt;
non attendentes ipsorum malitiam, quae sub velamine chirurgiae et
medicinae callide insidiantur, et nocent populo Christiano volentes pro
viribus exstirpare; statuimus, ut nullus Christianus, clericus vel laicus,
in infirmitatibus, vel etiam convalescentia, aliquando Sarracenum seu
Hebraeum vocet, ut ab eis medicinam recipiat.

Qui vero contra praemissa, seu praemissorum aliquid attentare
praesumpserit, per dioecesanum, vel ejus vicarium, ab introitu ecclesiae
et communione fidelium arceatur: et si infidelis fidelis filium nutriverit,

seu lactaverit, vel fidelis infideli ut mancipium famuletur, seu familiariter scripserit, in excommunicationis sententiam ipso facto incidant.

46. For the Avignon council in 1337 see Mansi, *Sacrorum conciliorum* 25:1105. I have reproduced here the statute as published in Charles Giraud, *Essai sur l'histoire du droit français au moyen âge*, 2 vols. (Paris and Leipzig, 1846), 2:126:

> De Judeis pro medicina exhibenda non requirendis, nec, si se ingesserint, admittendis. Item quia inter christianos non sine catholicae fidei opprobrio adeo invaluit perniciosus abusus, ut hii qui Judeorum, utpote nostrae inimicorum fidei, foetidos actus et opera spernere et abhorrere deberent, ad ipsos Judeos qui se physicos vel cyrurgicos asserunt, pro medicamentis, imo, verius nocumentis, indifferenter recurrant: propter quod eorumdem Judeorum servilis status ultra methas erigitur, inflatur et superbit cecitas, et ipsi fidem catholicam parvipendunt et ex inde familiaritates et conversationes multiplices, multorum, utique incentiva malorum, inter ipsos Christianos et Judeos prodeuntes, pluribus nefandis sceleribus quae reperiuntur perpetrata, causam credunt verisimilcter prebuisse; et darent in posterum aliis sceleribus, hiis forsitan pejoribus, occasionem sive causam, nisi salubris provisio talibus obviaret. Idcirco nos quibus est cura diligens per omnia superni numinis religionem tueri, subditosque nostros a noxiis quantium cum Deo possumus preservare; statuimus et etiam ordinamus ut a modo nullus christianus nostrarum provinciarum, civitatum et dyocesum, cujusvis sexus, status, conditionis aut dignitatis existat, in infirmitate sua vel alias, Judeum quemquam physicum vel cyrurgicum pro aliqua cujuscunque conditionis medicina vel medicamine sive cura recipientis ab eodem, adeat, requirat, aut re quiri faciat: nec etiam ipsius Judei ad eum sponte vel venientis aut mittentis recipere audeat per se vel per alium, quovis exquisito colore, medicinam, consilium alias quam facturus fuerat sive curam, nisi facienti immineret periculum et christiani periti, medici physici ve cyrurgici haberi commode in prefato periculo copia non valeret. Interdicentes pari modo Judeis utriusque sexus ut in curandis infirmitatibus christianorum nullatenus se audeant immiscere. Qui autem hujus statuti extiterit violator, si Judeus fuerit, eidem communi fidelium substrahatur; christianus vero superioris sui arbitrio puniatur.

47. The constitution of Frederick III was issued at Messina on 15 October 1310. For the text see Bartolomeo and Giuseppe Lagumina, *Codice diplomatico dei giudei di Sicilia*, 3 vols. (Palermo, 1884–1895), 1:31–35; for the paragraph concerning doctors, see 1:34–35:

> "Ut nullus Iudeus audeat medendi artem exercere in christianum vel medicinam ei dare vel conficere. In his confidere non possumus qui fidem non habent nec alijs poterunt esse fideles qui eorum dominum prodiderunt et propterea providimus et iubemus ut nullus Iudeorum qui

cum de illius spectaremur consilio sive cura forte nobis cum nos odio habeant et procurent imperpendibiliter dispendia vel nociva medendi artem in christianos audeat exercere vel medicinas pro christianis conficere aut medicinas eisdem christianis vendere vel eciam ministrare quod si contra fecerint iubemus quod Iudeus ipse per annum unum carceri detineatur inclusus ducens per tempus predictum in pane tribulactionis et aqua miserie vitam suam christianus vero qui ad curam ipsum vocaverit vel a Iudeo medicinam sibi aut suis propinari vel confici fecerit vel medicinam aut medicinali scienter emerit carceri per tres menses detineatur in penam et totum quod dederat aut daturus esset ipsi Iudeo salarii aut precii nomine ad curie manus perveniat per eam postmodum pauperius erogandum.

48. For the legislation see Archives départementales des Bouches-du-Rhône (Marseilles), B1372, fol. 35r, reproduced by Camille Arnaud, *Essai sur la condition des juifs en Provence au moyen âge* (Forcalquier, 1879), 37:

Nullus in infirmitate vocare debeat medicum judeum, vel aliter infidelem, vel ab eo, seu ejeo consilio recepere medicinam; nec per senescallum, vel officialem alium, judeo . . . inter fideles licencia in posterum concedatur. Et si forte alicui ante hoc tempus sit concessa, eam decernimus non tenere, revocantes eamdem . . . Judeus vero qui contra presentem ordinationem vocatus accesserit in librarum reforciatarum penam incidat, nostre curie applicamdam; quam si solvere nequiverit, corpore eum castigari jubemus Vocans vero fidelis arbitrio judicis cujus jurisdictionis est puniatur.

49. For the revocation of the legislation of 1306 in Provence see Emile Camau, *Les juifs en Provence* (Paris, 1928), 308. For the revocation in Avignon of the previous statute in 1341, see Pierre Pansier, "Les médecins juifs à Avignon aux XIIIe, XIVe, et XVe siècles," *Janus* 15 (1910): 421–451, esp. 427. I herewith reproduce the text of the revocation as copied by Pansier on 427–428 (n. 1) of his study:

Item cum non sit novum nec irreprehensibile, si secundum varietatem temporum, maxime necessitate urgente, aut utilitate publica evidente, humana statua in melius mutentur, seu verius reformentur, a nostrisque predecessoribus synodaliter et per aliquos officiales judicialiter fuerit constitutum, quod nullus Christianus vel Christiana, cujuscumque status existat, sub gravi pena quam facientes ipso facto incurrere decernebant, auderet pro ipsius cura aliquem judeum medicum evocare, nec pro infirmitate sua consilium curationis recipere; ab eodem quoque nullus hipotecarius vel speciator receptas ordinatas per talem judeum medicum auderet seu attentaret sub eadem pena conficere, nec ministrare alicui Christiano.

Et propterea nos attendentes quod tempore constitutionis hujusmo-

di erat major medicorum Christianorum copia, qui sic ad Christianorum curandas egritudines poterant evocari, quamquam quamplurimi Christiani metu dicte sentente excommunicationis licet graviter egrotantes non auderent judeos medicos evocare, quodque Christianorum medicorum penuriam paterentur, et ideo forsitan citius decedebant.

Nos volentes, ut expedit super his apponere remedium opportunum, dictum statutum sive constitutiones ac penas aut excommunicationis sententias in eis, premissorum occasione appositas, duximus synodaliter suspendendas, donec consultius ordinaverimus super hiis.

50. See Isak Münz, *Die jüdischen Aerzte im Mittelalter: Ein Beitrag zur Kulturgeschichte des Mittelalters* (Frankfurt on Main, 1922), 101–102.

51. Fausto Garofalo, "I papi ed i medici ebrei in Roma," *Pagine di scienza e tecnica* (Rome, 1948), 1–25. See also the less important study by Vincenzo Rocchi, "Gli ebrei e l'esercizio della medicina di fronte alle leggi della Chiesa e del governo di Roma papale,"*Rivista di storia critica delle scienze mediche e naturali* 1 (1910): 32–39. See also Jacques Pinès, "Des médecins juifs au service de la papauté du XIIe au XVIIe siècle," *Revue d'histoire de la médecine hébraïque* 18 (1965): 123–132.

52. Simonsohn, *The Apostolic See and the Jews* 1:511–513 (docs. no. 481–482).

53. Ibid., 1:628 (doc. no. 564) and 662–663 (doc. no. 585).

54. See Pilar León Tello, *Los judíos de Toledo*, 2 vols. (Madrid, 1979), 1:172, and Noël Coulet, "Autour d'un quinzain des métiers de la communauté juive d'Aix en 1437," *Minorités, techniques et métiers*, 79–104, in particular 99 n. 2, Actes de la table ronde du groupement d'intérêt scientifique: Sciences humaines sur l'aire méditerranéenne, Abbaye de Sénanque, octobre 1978 (Aix-en-Provence, 1980).

55. Coulet, "Autour d'un quinzain des métiers," 82.

56. Louis Stouff, *Arles à la fin du moyen âge*, 2 vols. (Aix-en-Provence and Lille, 1986), 2:707.

57. See Isak Münz, *Die jüdischen Aerzte im Mittelalter*, 47 (for Trèves) and Ernest Wickersheimer, *Dictionnaire biographique des médecins en France au moyen âge*, 2 vols. (Paris, 1936; reprint, Geneva and Paris, 1979–1981), 2:775.

58. Pilar León Tello, *Los judíos de Toledo* 1:172.

59. Françoise Gasparri, *La principauté d'Orange au moyen âge (fin XIIIe–XVe siècle)* (Paris, 1985), 52.

60. Pierre Pansier, "Les médecins juifs à Avignon," 421–451, in particular 430–431, 433, and 446.

61. Noël Coulet, "Autour d'un quinzain des métiers," 99.

62. Augustin Fabre, *Histoire des hôpitaux et des institutions de bienfaisance de Marseille*, 2 vols. (Marseilles, 1854–1855; reprint, Marseilles, 1973), 1:186 and 191–194.

63. V. Lieutaud, *Un séminaire à Manosque il y a cinq siècles* (4 juin 1365) (Aix-en-Provence, 1901), 11. For the *studium* see also Abbé Chaillan, *Documents nouveaux sur le studium du pape Urbain V à Trets-Manosque 1364–1367* (Aix-en-Provence, 1904).

64. See Louis Israel Newman, *Jewish Influence on Christian Reform Movements* (New York, 1925), 189. I was unable to verify this information at its source.

65. Juan Torres Fontes, "Los médicos murcianos en el siglo XV," 47, 55, and 124 (see n. 43 above).

66. Francisco Cantera Burgos, *Alvar García de Santa María y su familia de conversos: Historia de la judería de Burgos y de sus conversos más egregios* (Madrid, 1952), 38–39.

67. Isak Münz, *Die jüdischen Aerzte im Mittelalter*, 318.

68. See Michele Luzzati, "Lucca e gli ebrei fra quattro e cinquecento," in his *La casa dell'ebreo: Saggi sugli ebrei a Pisa e in Toscana nel medioevo e nel Rinascimento* (Pisa, 1985), 149–175, in particular 171–172.

69. Simonsohn, *The Apostolic See and the Jews*, docs. no. 797 (2:972), 845 (2:1037–1038), 848 (2:1040–1041), 884 (2:1093–1094), and the documents referred to in the following four notes.

70. Ibid., docs. no. 638 (2:742–743), 644 (2:750), and for the year 1464, doc. no. 911 (2:1130).

71. The reference to preachers' propaganda is in doc. no. 911 (2:1130) mentioned above. It reads: "contingat nonnullos predicatores verbi Dei in suis predicationibus eosdem fideles retrahere, ne se curari a te permittant, asserentes id sine peccato fieri non posse, nec fieri quoquomodo debere . . ." The hope for eventual conversion of the Jewish doctor is formulated in doc. no. 851 (2:1043–1044) in the following words: "ea spe ut per fidelium conversationem, cecitate deposita, possint veritatis lumen agnoscere et timere." See also in the same vein doc. no. 852 (2:1045).

72. Doc. no. 851 (2:1044): "Ita tamen, quod eos qui fideles fuerint ab ecclesiasticis sacramentis . . . nullatenus retrahas." See also doc. no. 852 (2:1045). The third, doc. no. 896 (2:1106–1107), in which the doctor is expected to enjoin the patient to receive sacraments, reads: "a sacramentis ecclesiasticis suscipiendis nullatenus retrahas, quin ymmo . . . ipsis iuxta ritum vere fidei christianis, dicta sacramenta recipiant suadeas."

73. Doc. no. 852 (2:1044–1045): "Iudeos . . . ad honorem gradus inter fideles provehi, canonica prohibent instituta," and "non obstan-

tibus constitutionibus et ordinationibus apostolicis ac statutis et constitutionibus provinciarum etc. . . ."

74. See R. Sassi, "Un famoso medico ebreo a Fabrino nel secolo
XV," *Studia picena* 6 (1930): 113–123. "Ut sit providendum de altero
medico Christiano cum multi sunt qui nolunt a medico hebraico nuper
conducto." (p. 119)

75. Ariel Toaff, *Il vino e la carne: Una comunità ebraica nel
medioevo* (Bologna, 1989), 279–280.

76. Ariel Toaff, *The Jews in Medieval Assisi, 1305–1487: A Social
and Economic History of a Small Jewish Community in Italy* (Florence, 1979), 187–194, in particular 193–194: "neque per ipsam de
futuro tempore aliquod salarium petere aut petere posse quomodo
etc., quia intelligit non placere populo quod ipse serviat ex quo est
Judeus etc. . . . "

77. See, for example, Leah Lydia Otis, "Prostitution and Repen-
tance in Late Medieval Perpignan," in *Women in the Medieval World:
Essays in Honor of John H. Mundy*, ed. Julius Kirshner and Suzanne
F. Wemple (Oxford, 1985; reprint, Oxford, 1987), 137–160, in particular 153 where Sister Catherine, wounded, found herself under the
"power" of a physician: "la dita Caterina . . . stet en poder de metge
be un mcs." For what Henri de Mondeville, the famous Parisian
surgeon of the first half of the fourteenth century, thought about
obedience and disobedience in doctor-patient relations, see Mary
Catherine Welborn, "The Long Tradition. A Study in Fourteenth-
century Medical Deontology," in *Medieval and Historiographical
Essays in Honor of James Westfall Thompson*, ed. J. L. Cate and E.
N. Anderson (Chicago, 1959), 344–359.

78. See n. 46 of this chapter.

Chapter 6

1. See Huling E. Ussery, *Chaucer's Physician: Medicine and Literature in Fourteenth-century England*, Toulane Studies in English 19
(New Orleans, 1971). For Boccacio, see *Decameron*, day three, ninth
tale; day eight, ninth tale; day nine, third tale; and the introduction.

2. Judah (ben Salomon) al-Ḥarizi, *Taḥkemoni* (in Hebrew), ed.
Y. Toporowsky (Tel-Aviv, 1952), 254–257, chap. 30; see also the English translation by Victor Emanuel Reichert, *The Taḥkemoni of
Judah Al-Harisi*, 2 vols. (Jerusalem, 1965–1973), 2:156–162. For an
inventory of an Avignon surgeon in 1392, see Pierre Pansier, "La
médecine juive à Avignon au moyen âge," *Cahiers de pratique
médico-chirurgicale* 8 (1934): 123–135, in particular 129. It contained a
scalpel with a handle of ivory shaped in the image of a man with a sil-

ver helmet; another scalpel with a gilded handle; a small scalpel; a case and a chest both full of instruments for surgery; a wooden vice with its screw for doctors; a basin made of copper and one of the same kind for shaving the beard; two small basins of brass and one small flask of Damascus glass for rosewater.

3. Ad. Jellinek, ed., *Dialog zwischen einem Orthodoxen und einem Philosophen von Schem-Tob b. Josef Palquera* (Iggeret ha-Vikuah) (in Hebrew) (Vienna, 1875), 31–32. My translation is inspired by that of M. Herschel Levine, *The Book of the Seeker* (Sefer Ha-Mebaqqesh) *by Shem Tob ben Joseph ibn Falaquera* (New York, 1976), 40–41; however, my translation differs in many instances.

4. Kalonymos ben Kalonymos, *Even Bohan* (Touchstone) (in Hebrew), ed. A. M. Habermann (Tel-Aviv, 1956), 44–48. See also J. Chotzner, "Kalonymos ben Kalonymos, Thirteenth-century Satirist," *Jewish Quarterly Review* 13 (1901): 128–146, and Judith Dishon, *The Book of Delight Composed by Joseph ben Meir Zabara* (in Hebrew) (Jerusalem, 1985), 185–196. Dishon also provides an overview of the topos of villain doctors in medieval Hebrew literature. Another useful overview is that of Harry Friedenwald, "Wit and Satire about the Physician in Hebrew Literature," *The Jews and Medicine: Essays*, vol. 1 (Baltimore, 1944; reprint, New York, 1967), pp. 69–83.

5. For similar parodies in German literature in the Middle Ages see Melitta Weiss-Amer, "*Von stichellinges magin vnd mucken fuezzen*: Mittelalterliche Rezeptliteratur in der Parodie," *Seminar: Journal of Germanic Studies* 28 (Toronto, 1992): 1–16, particularly 9–10, 14–16. A list of medications administered by master Samuel Cavaller of Corvera to a family of a local notary in June and July of 1489 was published by Augustí Duran i Sanpere. We have there digestive syrups, laxatives, and even narcotic materials to induce sleep. The list gives the exact date for each and every treatment and, of course, the cost of the medicine. See Augustí Duran i Sanpere, *Referencies documentals del call de juhséus de Cervera*, Discursos llegits en la real academia de buenas letres de Barcelona en la solemne recepció pública de D. Lluis Via y Pegès el dia 9 de desembre de 1924 (Barcelona, 1924), 50 and, for the list, 60–62.

6. Another scene of a uroscopy performed in front of an audience is depicted in a miniature of the thirteenth century in the "Cantigas de Santa Maria" of King Alfonso X of Castille. But there we have also a scene of a uroscopy done in private. Both miniatures are reproduced in Ramón Jordí González's study "Consideraciones sobre la legislación sanitaria peninsular," *Boletín informativo de circular farmacéutica* 224 (Barcelona, 1969), (no pagination).

7. Ms. 2197, University Library, Bologna. See Giuliano Tamani,

Il "Canon medicinae" di Avicenna nella tradizione ebraica (Padua, 1988); for the present discussion, see in particular 26–27 and 66–67. See also the publication by Samuel S. Kottek, Mendel Metzger, and Thérèse Metzger, "Manuscrits hébraïques décorés ou illustrés du Canon d'Avicenne," *Twenty-seventh International Congress of the History of Medicine, Acta*, vol. 2 (Barcelona, 1981), pp. 739–745.

8. Luis García-Ballester, Michael R. McVaugh, and Agustín Rubio-Vela, *Medical Licensing and Learning in Fourteenth-century Valencia*, Transactions of the American Philosophical Society, vol. 79, no. 6 (Philadelphia, 1989), p. 33.

9. See my *Médecine et justice en Provence médiévale: Documents de Manosque, 1262–1348* (Aix-en-Provence, 1989), 8–21, 46–47.

10. Manuel Grau i Monserrat, "Medicina a Besalú (s. XIV) (Metges, apotecaris, i manescals)," in *Patronat d'estudis històrics d'Olot i Comarca*, 103–133, Annals 1982–1983 (1984).

11. Christian Guilleré, "Le milieu médical géronais au XIVᵉ siècle," *Santé, médecine, et assistance au moyen âge*, pp. 263–281, Actes du 110ème congrès national des sociétés savantes, Montpellier, 1985, vol. 1 (Paris, 1987).

12. Richard W. Emery, "Documents Concerning Some Jewish Scholars in Perpignan in the Fourteenth and Fifteenth Centuries," in *Michael: On the History of the Jews in the Diaspora*, ed. Shlomo Simon-sohn and Joseph Shatzmiller, vol. 4 (Tel-Aviv, 1976), pp. 27–48.

13. José Cabezudo Astrain, "Médicos y curanderos zaragozanos en el siglo XV," *Archivo iberoamericano de historia de la medicina* 7 (1955): 119–126, in particular 125–126.

14. See Danielle Jacquart, *Le milieu médical en France du XIIᵉ au XVᵉ siècle* (Geneva and Paris, 1981), 254.

15. Ibid., 252–253.

16. See Louis Stouff, "Activités et professions dans une communauté juive de Provence au bas moyen âge: La juiverie d'Arles, 1400–1450," in *Minorités, techniques et métiers*, 57–77, esp. 70, Actes de la table ronde du groupement d'intérêt scientifique: Sciences humaines sur l'aire méditerranéenne, Abbaye de Sénanque, octobre 1978 (Aix-en-Provence, 1980).

17. Françoise Gasparri, "Juifs et Italiens à Orange au XIVᵉ siècle: Métiers comparés," in *Minorités, techniques, et métiers*, 47–56, esp. 52–53, Actes de la table ronde du groupement d'intérêt scientifique: Sciences humaines sur l'aire méditerranéenne, Abbaye de Sénanque, octobre 1978 (Aix-en-Provence, 1980).

18. García-Ballester, McVaugh, and Rubio-Vela, *Medical Licensing and Learning in Fourteenth-century Valencia*, 31–37.

19. See my *Médecine et justice en Provence médiévale*, 13–18.

20. Ibid., see references to particular studies, 18–19 and 46–47.

21. Franz Rosenthal, "The Physician in Medieval Muslim Society," *Bulletin of the History of Medicine* 52 (1978): 475–491, in particular 478–480.

22. Shatzmiller, *Médecine et justice en Provence médiévale*, 8–29.

23. See n. 13 above and also Salo Wittmayer Baron, *A Social and Religious History of the Jews*, 18 vols., 2d ed. (New York and Philadelphia, 1952–1983), 12:84.

24. Elisabeth Santschi, "Médecine et justice en Crète vénitienne au XIVe siècle," *Thèsaurismata* 8 (1971): 17–48, especially 25–27.

25. See Danielle Jacquart, *Le milieu médical en France du XIIe au XVe siècle*, 252–253. Jacquart relies on the findings of Louis Barthélemy in his *Les médecins à Marseille avant et pendant le moyen âge* (Marseilles, 1883).

26. Pierre Pansier, "Les médecins juifs à Avignon aux XIIIe, XIVe, et XVe siècles," *Janus* 15 (1910): 421–451. We may add that in the Castilian city Victoria in the early 1490s all doctors are reported to have been Jewish. When they left, following the decree of expulsion in 1492, the municipality had to face a crisis because no one "practiced this profession" in the city. See Enrique Cantera Montenegro, *Las juderías de la diócesis de Calahorra en la baja edad media* (Logroño, 1987), 206.

27. For the size of the Manosque community see my *Recherches sur la communauté juive de Manosque au moyen âge 1241–1329* (Paris and The Hague, 1973), 27–31.

28. See Édouard Baratier, *La démographie provençale du XIIIe au XVIe siècle* (Paris, 1961), 69–72.

29. For Venosa see Alfonso Silvestri, "Gli ebrei nel regno di Napoli durante la dominazione aragonese," *Campania sacra* 18 (1987): 21–77, especially 33. For Rome see Anna Esposito, "Gli ebrei a Roma nella seconda metà del '400 attraverso i protocolli del notaio Giovanni Angelo Amati," in *Aspetti e problemi della presenza ebraica nell'Italia centrosettentrionale (secoli XIV e XV)*, 29–125, esp. 71–73, Quaderni dell'istituto di scienze storiche dell'università di Roma 2 (Rome, 1983).

30. For a recent bibliographic study see Monica Green, "Women's Medical Practice and Health Care in Medieval Europe," *Signs: Journal of Women in Culture and Society* 14 (1989): 434–473. One has to add now the very interesting chapter about the marginalization of women in obstetrics and in medicine in general by Renate Blumenfeld-Kosinski, *Not of Woman Born: Representations of Caesarean Birth in Medieval and Renaissance Culture* (Ithaca, N.Y., and London, 1990), 91–119. In this section I rely also on my "Femmes

médecins au moyen âge: Témoignages sur leurs pratiques (1250–1350)," in *Histoire et société: Mélanges offerts à Georges Duby*, vol. 1: *Le couple, l'ami et le prochain* (Aix-en-Provence, 1992), pp. 167–175. I must mention here the pioneering article of Harry Friedenwald, "Jewish Doctoresses in the Middle Ages," in his *The Jews and Medicine: Essays*, 2 vols. (Baltimore, 1944; reprint, New York, 1967), 1:217–220.

31. See my *Médecine et justice en Provence médiévale*, 74–76 (doc. no. 7).

32. Ibid., 150–151 (doc. no. 47).

33. Ibid., 5–6.

34. See n. 32 above for Hava; see also Annamaria Precopi Lombardo, "Viridimura, dottoressa ebrea del medio evo siciliano," *La Fardelliana* 3 (1984): 361–364; Annamaria Precopi Lombardo, "Medici ebrei nella Sicilia medievale," *Trapani* 29 (1984): 25–28. Viridimura's license was published in Bartolomeo and Giuseppe Lagumina, *Codice diplomatico dei giudei di Sicilia*, 3 vols. (Palermo, 1884–1895), 1:99. It states: "per Viridimuram Iudeam uxorem Pascalis de Medico de Cathania Judei . . ."

35. Antonio Cardoner Planas, "Seis mujeres hebreas practicando la medicina en el reino de Aragón," *Sefarad* 9 (1949): 441–445, in particular 444.

36. See Louis Barthélemy, *Les médecins à Marseille avant et pendant le moyen âge*, 31.

Notum sit . . . & . . . quod Salvetus de Burgonovo, filius Davini de Burgonovo de Sallono, judei quondam, bona fide, se posuit et collocavit pro discipulo, seu scolari et nuncio, cum Sara de Sancto Egidio, uxore Abrahe de Sancto Egidio, presenti et recipienti, ad standum cum eadem, et ejus servitium et mandatum faciendum, tam in civitate Massilie quam extra, et ad addiscendum artem medicine et phisice, hinc ad festum Paschatis proxime venturum, promittens dicte Sare presenti se esse bonum et sufficientem et obedientem per totum tempus supradictum, et omnia servitia facere.
Et versa vice dicta Sara promisit dicto Salveto presenti eum instruere bonis moribus, et eum docere artem predictam, et eum non expelere ad se per totum tempus supradictum, nisi culpa dicti Salveti, et sibi providere in vestitu, victu et cibo, sic itque quod totum lucrum quod faciet dictus Salvetus de arte predicta det et consignet dicte Sare per totum tempus predictum; quod facere promisit dictus Salvetus dicte Sare presenti et recipient. Actum Massilie in botiga mei notarii, testes . . . etc. . . . .

37. See Raffaele Calvanico, *Fonti per la storia della medicina e della chirurgia per il regno di Napoli nel periodo angioino (1273–1410)*

(Naples, 1962), 141 (doc. no. 1165): "in crepaturis et in apostematibus matricis et in aliis accidentibus matricis"; 256 (doc. no. 3534): "in curandis vulneribus et apostematibus periculosis in mamallis et matrice"; 159 (doc. no. 1451): "ad mulieres curandas egrotas"; see also 219 (doc. no. 3071) and 224 (doc. no. 3127).

38. Ibid., 119 (doc. no. 916). See other licenses for women "without limitations" on 262 (doc. no. 3572) and 271 (doc. no. 3621).

39. N. Barone, "Notizie raccolte dai registri di cancelleria del re Ladislao di Durazzo," *Archivio storico per le province napoletane* 13 (1888): 22–25. I owe this reference to Professor Cesare Colafemmina of the University of Bari.

40. The paragraph is copied in four of the licenses published by Calvanico. There are some minor differences between them and what I offer is a "composite" text. See p. 194 (doc. no. 1872), p. 261 (doc. no. 3571), p. 262 (doc. no. 3572), and pp. 277–278 (doc. no. 3643): "Licet alienum sit feminis conventibus intresse virorum, ut in matronalis pudoris contumeliam metuant, propter quod culpam vetite transgressionis incurrant: quo quia inde jure edicto medicine officium mulieribus est concessum expediter, actento quod ad mulieres curandas egrotas precipue in morbis eisdem de honestate morum virorum sunt femine aptiores."

41. See Pearl Kibre, "The Faculty of Medicine at Paris, Charlatanism, and Unlicensed Medical Practices in the Later Middle Ages," *Bulletin of the History of Medicine* 17 (1953): 1–20; Henri Denifle and Emile Chatelain, eds., *Chartularium universitatis Parisiensis*, 4 vols. (Paris, 1889–1897), 1:258–262.

42. Klaus Wagner, *Regesto de documentos del archivo de protocolos de Sevilla referentes a judíos y moros* (Seville, 1978), 36–37 (docs. no. 116, 120, 122, 124). These sums can be compared to yearly honoraria awarded to municipal doctors in Castile (see the next section in this chapter) which could be as low as five hundred maravedi.

43. See for southern Italy Ronald J. Doviak, "The University of Naples and the Study and Practice of Medicine in the Thirteenth and Fourteenth Centuries," Ph.D. diss., City University of New York, 1974 (Ann Arbor, Mich.: University Microfilms 1974), 43–46.

44. I quote here the translation of Israel Abrahams, ed. and trans., *Hebrew Ethical Wills*, 2d ed. (Philadelphia, 1976), 165–166.

45. See my *Médecine et justice en Provence médiévale*, 150–151 (doc. no. 47): "Interrogata si palpavit eum dixit quod non, set ipsum in lecto invenit."

46. In this section I rely principally on my study "Médecins municipaux en Provence, Catalogne, et autres régions de l'Europe méridionale (1350–1400)," in *Les sociétés urbaines en France méridionale*

et en péninsule ibérique au moyen âge, 329–336, Actes du colloque franco-espagnol, Pau, 21–23 septembre 1988 (Paris, 1991). See also Andrew W. Russel, ed., *The Town and State Physician in Europe from the Middle Ages to Enlightenment* (Wolfenbüttel, 1981). For other professionals (smiths, bakers, butchers) hired by Provençal municipalities, see F. Sauve, "Les services publics communaux et les abonnements en nature au moyen âge dans la région aptésienne," *Annales de la société d'études provençales* 5 (1908): 89–110.

47. Ugo Stefanutti, *Documentazioni cronologiche per la storia della medicina, chirurgia, e farmacia in Venezia dal 1258 al 1332* (Venice, 1961), 62 and 107–108. For a contract done there four years later with a certain "magister Anselmus medicus," see p. 109.

48. For expenditures on municipal doctors in Marseilles see Alain Droguet, "Une ville au miroir de ses comptes: Les dépenses de Marseille à la fin du XIVe siècle," *Provence historique* 30 (1980): 171–213, especially 175.

49. See Duran i Sanpere, *Referencies documentals del call de juhséus de Cervera*, 62–63.

50. Shlomo Simonsohn, *The Jews in the Duchy of Milan*, 4 vols. (Jerusalem, 1982–1986), 1:379 (doc. no. 869).

51. For Digne see Noël Coulet, "Autour d'un quinzain des métiers de la communauté juive d'Aix en 1437," in *Minorités, techniques, et métiers*, 79–104, esp. 81–82, Actes de la table ronde du groupement d'intérêt scientifique: Sciences humaines sur l'aire méditerranéenne (Aix-en-Provence, 1980). For Murcia see Juan Torres Fontes, "Los médicos murcianos en el siglo XV," in Juan Torres Fontes et al., *De historia médica murciana*, vol. 1: *Los Médicos* (Murcia, 1980), 13–110, esp. 43.

52. Justiniano Rodríguez Fernández, *La judería de la ciudad de León* (Leon, 1969), 133.

53. Manuel Grau i Monserrat, "Meteges Jueus de Besalú (s. XIV et XV), Sa Sala, Des Portal i Coret," *Tercer congres d'historia de la medicina catalana* (Lleida, 1981), 165–81, esp. 181. For the agreement in Castolló d'Empúries, see Michael McVaugh, "Bernat de Berriacho (fl. 1301–1343) and the "Ordinacio" of Bishop Ponç de Gualba," *Arxiu de textos catalans antics* 9 (1990): 240–254. Bernat, by the way, obtained permission to be absent temporarily from the city, mostly to pursue his studies in Montpellier in three consecutive terms "causa recipiendi suum magisterium." For the above mentioned quotation see p. 251. It reads:

Et e converso dictus magister Bernardus promisit et obligavit se dictis consulibus et proceribus ville Castilionis quod ipse quamdiu vivet faciet

continuam residenciam in villa Castilionis et quod bene et legaliter pro
posse suo videbit et iudicabit omnes orinas que apportabuntur sibi per
omnes habitatores dicte ville et dabit eis consilia tam super flebotomiis
quam etiam dietis et generaliter regimina et consilia, excepto quod non
teneatur eosdem infirmos visitare, et quod de hoc nichil accipiet ab eis
nec ab alio ipsorum, immo libere et gratis predicta exhibebit pro posse
suo.

54. Pierre Vidal, "Les juifs des anciens comtés de Roussillon et de
Cerdagne," *Revue des études juives* 15 (1887): 19–55 and 16 (1888):
1–23, 170–203, esp. 171–174 of number 16 of the series.

55. Réjane Brondy, "Chambéry 1350 environ–1560 environ:
Etude d'histoire urbaine," 2 vols., Ph.D. diss., Université de Lyon
III, 1986, 2:542.

56. Pierre Pansier, "Inventaire de la pharmacie de Pernes en
1365,"*Annales d'Avignon et du comtat Venaissin* 14 (1928): 111–123,
esp. 114 n. 1. This arrangement was concluded on 31 August 1450.

57. R. Sassi, "Un famoso medico ebreo a Fabriano nel secolo
XV," *Studia picena* 6 (1930): 113–123, esp. 120–121. A similar contract, which also included the *contado*, was agreed on in 1474 between the city council of Assisi and the Jewish doctor Elia di Manu-
ele. See Ariel Toaff, *Il vino e la carne: Una comunità ebraica nel
medioevo* (Bologna, 1989), 270–271.

58. José Ramón Magdalena, "Estructura socio-económica de las
aljamas castellonenses a finales del siglo XV," *Sefarad* 32 (1972):
341–370, esp. 350.

59. See Pierre Pansier, "Inventaire de la pharmacie de Pernes en
1365," 114 n. 1.

60. Manuel Grau i Monserrat, "Meteges jueus de Besalú," 165–
181, esp. 181.

61. Pierre Pansier, "Inventaire de la pharmacie de Pernes en
1365," 111–112.

62. Ibid., 112 nn. 3 and 4: "Fuit conclusum quod Monetus Caroli
junior accedat Carpentoracte pro loquendo et concludendo cum
magistro Vitali medico de veniendo et serviendo in presentem locum
pro exercendo suum officium medicine, prout alias fuit sepe ordinatum."

63. Ibid.: "Fuit ordinatum quod syndici factant ventre magistrum
Vitalem, medicum, pro conveniendo cum eo de serviendo et veniendo bis seu tribus diebus in septimana quando mandabitur."

64. Ibid., 111–112. The process of bargaining in other parts of
Europe is described by Vivian Nutton, "Continuity or Rediscovery?
The City Physician in Classical Antiquity and Mediaeval Italy," in

The Town and State Physician in Europe from the Middle Ages to the Enlightenment, ed. Andrew W. Russell, 9–61, esp. 30–31, Wolfenbütteler Forschungen 17 (Wolfenbüttel, 1981).

65. Ibid.

66. Toaff, *Il vino e la carne*, 266–268.

67. Adolphe Crémieux, "Les juifs de Marseille au moyen âge," *Revue des études juives* 47 (1903): 243–261, especially 244; and Brondy, "Chambéry 1350 environ–1560 environ," 2:542.

68. Crémieux, "Les juifs de Marseille au moyen âge," 243–261, esp. 244.

69. See Noël Coulet, "Autour d'un quinzain des métiers," 81–82. See also Camille Arnaud, *Histoire de la viguerie de Forcalquier*, 2 vols. (Marseilles, 1874–1875), 2:272.

70. Crémieux, "Les juifs de Marseille au moyen âge," 244.

71. Toaff, *Il vino e la carne*, 266–267.

72. Droguet, "Une ville au miroir de ses comptes: Les dépenses de Marseille à la fin du XIVᵉ siècle," 175.

73. Brondy, "Chambéry 1350 environ–1560 environ," 2:542.

74. Juan Torres Fontes, "Tres epidemias de peste en Murcia en el siglo XIV: 1348–1349, 1379–1380, 1395–1396," in Juan Torres Fontes et al., *De historia médica murciana*, vol. 2: *Las epidemias* (Murcia, 1981), 9–66, esp. 51, 44–45, 46–47.

75. Jesús Oesada Sanz, "Algunos aspectos de la medicina en Murcia durante la época de los reyes católicos," in Juan Torres Fontes et al., *De historia médica murciana*, vol. 1: *Los médicos* (Murcia, 1980), 101–167, esp. 134.

76. Francisco Cantera Burgos, *Alvar García de Santa María y su familia de conversos: Historia de la judería de Burgos y de sus conversos más egregios* (Madrid, 1952), 37–39.

Chapter 7

1. See Emeric Deutsch, "Les Français sont-ils antisémites?" *L'arche: Le mensuel du judaïsme français* 270–271 (1979): 60–66. I would like to express my thanks to my friend Dr. Simon Elbaum of Aix-en-Provence who brought this article to my attention.

2. I have already mentioned this syncretism concerning miraculous medicine, in which even Jews turn to Christian sanctuaries for help, in my study "Doctors and Medical Practice in Germany around the Year 1200: The Evidence of 'Sefer Ḥasidim,'" *Journal of Jewish Studies* 33 (1982): 583–593. I return to this issue later in this section. It went both ways, however: for the description of a Christian nobleman

who asked for a Jewish amulet (*mezuza*) to be fixed at the gate of his castle and for the use of Jewish amulets by Christians in other instances, see Yedidiah Alter Dinari, *The Sages of Germany and Austria in the Later Middle Ages* (in Hebrew) (Jerusalem, 1984), 53 and n. 192.

3. Published (from the manuscript in the Bibliothèque Nationale, Paris, ms. héb. 1130) by Ben-Zion Dinur, *Israel in the Diaspora: A Documentary History of the Jewish People from Its Beginning to the Present* (in Hebrew), 2d ser., 10 vols. (Tel-Aviv and Jerusalem, 1961–1972), vol. B(6) (=10), p. 214.

4. Süssmann Muntner, "R. Shem Tob Ben Isaac of Tortosa about the Life of the European Jewish Doctor and His Ethics," in *Sinai Jubilee Volume* (Jerusalem, 1957), 321–337, esp. 324–325.

5. Published according to manuscript of the Jewish Theological Seminary (New York), Rabb. no. 577, fol. 79r–86r, by Joseph Buxenboim, "Responsa of Askenazic Sages, R. Zalman of St. Goar with R. Loewe Landau and Maharam Mintz" (in Hebrew), *Moria* 12 (1983): 139–141. I owe the reference to this manuscript to Arye Maimon, ed., *Germania judaica*, vol. 3(1) (Tübingen, 1987), pp. 703–711. Zalman of Sankt Goar is known as a devoted student of the great scholar Jacob Moelin ("Maharil") (ca. 1360–1427) who collected and then published his teacher's *minhagim* (particular customs in daily religious life). Landau was also Maharil's student. See Yedidiah Alter Dinari, *The Sages of Germany and Austria*, 272–296. And more recently Israel Jacob Yuval, *Scholars in Their Time: The Religious Leadership of German Jewry in the Late Middle Ages* (in Hebrew) (Jerusalem, 1988), 97–114 (about Zalman of Sankt Goar) and 256–264 (about Liwa Landau). See also the more recent summary by Israel Jacob Yuval, "Juden, Hussiten, und Deutsche nach einer hebräischen Chronik," in *Juden in der christlichen Umwelt während des späten Mittelalters*, ed. A. Haverkamp and F.-J. Ziwes (Berlin, 1992), 59–102, in particular 61–62.

6. See Shalom Albeck, "Rabbenu Tam's Attitude to the Problems of His Time" (in Hebrew), *Zion* 19 (1954): 104–141, especially 125. See also Ephraim Elimelech Urbach, *The Tosaphists: Their History, Writings, and Methods* (in Hebrew), 2 vols. (Jerusalem, 1980), 1:262.

7. Published in my *Médecine et justice en Provence médiévale: Documents de Manosque, 1262–1348* (Aix-en-Provence, 1989), 57–60 (doc. no. 1).

8. See Moritz Güdemann, *Geschichte des Erziehungswesens und der Cultur der abendländischen Juden während des Mittelalters und der neueren Zeit*, 3 vols. (Vienna, 1884–1888; reprint, Amsterdam, 1966), 1:197–198.

9. The document was published by Haim Beinart, "A Fifteenth-century Hebrew Formulary from Spain," *Sefunot* 5 (1961): 75-134, especially 117-119.

10. See Elena Lourie, "Jewish Moneylenders in the Local Catalan Community, ca. 1300: Vilafranca del Penedés, Besalú, and Montblanc," in *Michael: On the History of the Jews in the Diaspora*, ed. Eliezer Gutwirth and Shlomo Simonsohn, vol. 11 (Tel-Aviv, 1989), pp. 33-98, in particular p. 52 n. 43.

11. Judah ben Samuel Ḥasid, *Sepher Ḥasidim (Das Buch der Frommen)* (in Hebrew), 2d ed., ed. J. Wistinetzki and J. Freimann (Frankfurt on Main, 1924), 332-333 (doc. no. 1352). Translated in my "Doctors and Medical Practice in Germany around the Year 1200: The Evidence of 'Sefer Ḥasidim,'" 593. For Blanche of Castile's saying she would rather see her sick son dead than visiting (as the doctor recommended) a whore (and committing a mortal sin), see "Chronique de Primat traduite par Jean du Vignay," in Bouquet, *Recueil des historiens des Gaules et de France*, vol. 23 (Paris, 1840), p. 16. I thank Dr. Margaret Wade Labarge of Ottawa (Canada) for indicating this document to me.

12. Originally published in J. C. Robertson, *Materials for the History of Thomas Becket* (London, 1876), 2:71. Here the text is quoted as published by Joseph Jacobs, *The Jews in Angevin England: Documents and Records* (London, 1893; reprint, Westmead, Farnborough, 1969), 153.

13. Jacques Cambell, ed., *Enquête pour le Procès de canonisation de Dauphine de Puimichel, comtesse d'Ariano* (Turin, 1978), 412, 421, 433, where Asher's name is transcribed "Ausseres" and "Aitos."

14. Manuel Grau i Monserrat, "Medicina a Besalú (s. XIV) (Metges, apotecaris, i manescals)," in *Patronat d'estudis històrics d'Olot i Comarca*, 101-133, esp. 104, Annals 1982-1983 (1984).

15. See my *Médecine et justice en Provence médiévale*, 229-230 (doc. no. 76).

16. Henri Bresc, *Un monde méditerranéen: Economie et société en Sicile 1300-1450*, 2 vols. (Rome 1986), 2:748.

17. Michael McVaugh, "Bernat de Berriacho (fl. 1301-1343) and the "Ordinacio" of Bishop Ponç de Gualba," *Arxiu de textos catalans antics* 9 (1990): 240-254.

18. The document is published in my *Médecine et justice en Provence médiévale*, 47-48 n. 11.

19. See, for example, the documents published by Ariel Toaff, *The Jews in Medieval Assisi 1305-1487: A Social and Economic History of a Small Jewish Community in Italy* (Florence, 1979), 174-185.

20. *Le corps souffrant: maladies et médications*, vol. 4 of *Razo:*

Cahiers du centre d'études médiévales de Nice (1984).

21. Michele Luzzati, "Il medico ebreo e il contadino: Un documento pisano del 1462," in his *La casa dell'ebreo: Saggi sugli ebrei a Pisa e in Toscana nel medioevo e nel Rinascimento* (Pisa, 1985), 49–57.

22. See the series of articles published by Jérôme de Duranti La Calade, "Notes sur les rues d'Aix au XIVᵉ et au XVᵉ siècle," *Annales de Provence* 7 (1910): 207–220 to 23 (1926): 22–41. The present document is published and commented on in 9 (1912): 122–125.

23. Louis Stouff, "Documents arlésiens," *Razo: Cahiers du centre d'études médiévales de Nice* 4 (1984): 126.

24. Noël Coulet, "Documents aixois (première moitié du XVᵉ siècle)," *Razo: Cahiers du centre d'études médiévales de Nice* 4 (1984): 115–125, in particular 122.

25. Pierre Pansier, "Les médecins juifs à Avignon aux XIIIᵉ, XIVᵉ, et XVᵉ siècles," *Janus* 15 (1910): 421–451, csp. 445.

26. Roger Kohn, "Les juifs de la France du nord à travers les archives du parlement de Paris (1359?–1394)," *Revue des études juives* 141 (1982): 5–138, in particular 79.

27. Salomon Kahn, "Les juifs de la sénéchaussée de Beaucaire," *Revue des études juives* 65 (1913): 181–195; 66 (1913): 75–97; see in particular 66:81: "debet sibi x libras melgoriensium pro salario suo seu mercede quas solvere contradicit."

28. For the document relating to Maria Comtessa (Comptessa), see n. 73 of this chapter. It is unclear in the document whether the child is female or male. The second document concerning Tolosa is published in my *Médecine et justice en Provence médiévale*, 48 n. 12.

29. The document, dated Feb. 8, 1431, is published by Toaff, *The Jews in Medieval Assisi*, 180–181 (doc. no. 84).

30. For the case in Valencia see Luis [Lluís] García-Ballester, *La medicina a la València medieval: Medicina i societat en un país medieval mediterrani* (Valencia, 1988), 48–49. For Majorca see Antonio Pons, *Los judíos de Mallorca*, 2 vols. (Palma de Mallorca, 1984), 1:212.

31. Kalonymos ben Kalonymos, *Even Bohan* (Touchstone) (in Hebrew), ed. A. M. Habermann (Tel-Aviv, 1956), 47.

32. Published in my *Médecine et justice en Provence médiévale*, 104–105 (doc. no. 21).

33. See Richard W. Emery, "Documents Concerning Some Jewish Scholars in Perpignan in the Fourteenth and Early Fifteenth Centuries," in *Michael: On the History of the Jews in the Diaspora*, ed. Shlomo Simonsohn and Joseph Shatzmiller, vol. 4 (Tel-Aviv, 1976), pp. 27–48, esp. p. 37.

34. Manuel Grau i Monserrat, "Meteges jueus de Besalú (s. XIV et XV), Sa Sala, Des Portal i Coret," *Tercer congres d'historia de la medicina catalana* (Lleida, 1981), 165–181, esp. 170: "pro diversis visitationibus per me factis infirmitate dicti defuncti."

35. Augustí Duran i Sanpere, *Referencies documentals del call de juhséus de Cervera*, Discursos llegit en la real academia de buenas letras de Barcelona (Barcelona, 1924), 49.

36. See my article, "Doctors' Fees and Their Medical Responsibility: Evidence from Notarial and Court Records," in *Private Acts of the Late Middle Ages*, ed. Paolo Brezzi and Egmont Lee (Toronto, 1984), 201–208.

37. See Ariel Toaff, *Il vino e la carne: Una comunità ebraica nel medioevo* (Bologna, 1989), 272.

38. Ibid.

39. Noël Coulet, "Documents aixois," 123–124. A fourth document was pointed out to me by Noël Coulet: Bibliothèque Nationale, Paris, N. acq. lat. 1340, no. 22; it was written in Marseilles on 7 February 1404 and reads:

> Anno Domini millesimo CCCC tertio, die Jovis septima mensis februarii post vesperos. Noverint universi etc. quod, cum domina Johanneta Arnaude de Massilia patiatur et a longo tempore citra passa fuit in ore suo sive maxilla quendam morbum vocatum vulgariter "lo crant," requirit ideo magistrum Mosse Salves judeum surgicum dicte civitatis ut de dicto morbo sive infirmitate sanare vellit et ipsam recipere in curam pro sanando ipsam a predicto morbo suo posse satisfacto ei de suo labore condecenti. Et vice versa dictus magister Mosse Salves respondit et dicit quod dictus morbus est incurabilis et est quidam morbus vocatus vulgariter "lo crant" et non acciperet ipsam ad suum periculum pro sanando eam, neque ipsam teneret in curam.
>
> Sed, postquam ipsa eumdem magistrum Mosse requisivit et adhuc requirat quod ipsam accipiat in curam, dicit et exponit coram dicta domina Johanneta ac testibus infrascriptis quod ipsam non acciperet ad suum periculum quia morbus ille incurabilis est, sed faciet et dabit ei remedium quod poterit prout asseruit.
>
> Protestans idem Mosse quod, casu quo dicta domina Johanneta pro dicto morbo decederet, quod ipse dampnum aliquod pati non possit neque debeat, cum ipsam non accipiat ad suum periculum sed pro dando ei remedium quo poterat.
>
> "De quibus etc. Actum Massilia in butiga etc. Johannes Audeberti filius Johanne; Petrus de Fossis; Petrus Gamenlli. Hugo Plante de Areis de Massilia.

40. José Cabezudo Astrain, "Médicos y curanderos zaragosanos en el siglo XV," *Archivo ibéroamericano de historia de la medicina* 7 (1955): 119–126, esp. 120–123.

41. Published in my *Médecine et justice en Provence médiévale*, 128 (doc. no. 32). I have discussed the case in more detail in "Notes sur les médecins juifs en Provence au moyen âge," *Revue des études juives* 128 (1969): 259–266, especially 266.

42. See the numerous publications of Alessandro Simili: "Bartolomeo da Varignana e una sua perizia giudiziaria," *La riforma medica* 36 (1941): 1101–1105; "Considerazioni su una perizia medico-legale inedita del '300," *Giornale di clinica medica* 17 (1941): 921–927; "Appunti su quattro referti medico-legali inediti del '300," *Minerva medica* 33 (1942): 3–15; "Un consiglio inedito di Bartolomeo da Varignana e Giovanni da Parma," *Minerva medica* 33 (1942): 1–12; "Sui primordi e sulla procedura della medicina legale in Bologna," *Atti e memorie dell'Accademia di storia dell'arte sanitaria*, 2d ser., 9 (1943): 41–56; "Un referto medico-legale inedito e autografo di Bartolomeo da Varignana," *Il policlinico: Periodico di medicina, chirurgia, e igiene* 58 (1951): 150–156.

43. See my "Médecins et expertise médicale dans la ville médiévale: Manosque 1280–1348," in *Vie privée et ordre public à la fin du moyen âge: Etudes sur Manosque, la Provence, et le Piémont (1250–1450)*, ed. M. Hébert (Aix-en-Provence, 1987), 105–117.

44. Shatzmiller, *Médecine et justice en Provence médiévale*, 145–146 (doc. no. 44).

45. Ibid., 140 (doc. no. 41).

46. "Astrugus surgicus" appears in six documents published in my *Médecine et justice en Provence médiévale*. The first (no. 5 on pp. 70–71) is dated 1 December 1290; he is referred to as "Astrugus judeus aurificerius" but is also part of a group of "sirurgici." In the last, doc. no. 18 on p. 95, dated 17 May 1306, just a few months before his death, he appears with Fossonus, diminutive of Bonafos, who is expressly referred to as his son. In doc. no. 17 (pp. 93–94) he is referred to once more as "magister Astrugus Aurificerius sirurgicus." See also pp. 74–77 and 93–94 (docs. no. 7, 8, 16) where Hana (or Hava) appears as his wife in the list of the Jews of the year 1296 as, according to my deciphering, "Fana uxor Astrugi Aurificerii"; see my *Recherches sur le communauté juive de Manosque au moyen âge 1241–1329* (Paris and The Hague, 1973), 158. "Jocepus judeus filius magistri Bonafosii" appears as *sirurgicus* on 29 January 1338 (see pp. 205–206, doc. no. 68) and with his father in an agreement with a patient to end their medical relationship in February 1341 (p. 224, doc. no. 76). Less than two months later they both provided medical expertise concerning the murder of a Jew of Manosque named Leon Frances (pp. 225–226, doc. no. 77).

47. Published in my *Médecine et justice en Provence médiévale*, 194 (doc. no. 63), 235 (doc. no. 82), and 193 (doc. no. 62).

48. Ibid., 184 (doc. no. 57).

49. Ibid., 185–186 (doc. no. 58).

50. Ibid., 215–217 (doc. no. 73).

51. Ibid., 152–153 (doc. no. 48).

52. Ibid., 147–148 (doc. no. 45): "tunc non erat locus neque hora inspiciendi ipsum vulneratum."

53. Ibid., 156–158 (doc. no. 49).

54. Ibid., 171–172 (doc. no. 54). See also, for example, 199–200, 205–206, 233–234, 236–237 (docs. no. 66, 68, 81, and 83).

55. Ibid., 132–133 (doc. no. 35).

56. Ibid., 233–234 (doc. no. 81).

57. Ibid., 150–151 (doc. no. 47).

58. See Pierre Pansier, "Les médecins juifs à Avignon," 431.

59. Jacques Cambell, ed., *Enquête pour le procès de canonisation de Dauphine de Puimichel, comtesse d'Ariano* (Turin, 1978), 412–413.

60. See Coulet, "Document aixois," 122–123, and Danièle Iancu-Agou, "Documents sur les juifs aixois et la médecine au XVᵉ siècle: Médications et ouvrages," *Santé, médecine, et assistance au moyen âge*, pp. 251–262 Actes du 110ᵉ congrès national des sociétés savantes, Montpellier, 1985, vol. 1 (Paris, 1987). In 1479 in the small city of Randezzo, western Sicily, such a collaboration is sanctioned through a notarial agreement. The Jewish practitioner Manuel Servideu, "medicus" and "surgicus," establishes an association for the duration of two years with two local surgeons, the Christians Bernardus de Oriolo and Antonius Marrota. The Jewish doctor is described in the document as "old," in contradiction to his two associates. For this reason he will deal only with difficult cases. The Latin reads at this point:

> Item primo et ante omnia prefati magistri Antonius et magister Bernaldus eo quo sunt juniores dicti magistri Manueli ipsos se obligaverunt in omnes curas sollicite eos gerere, licet quod si non in omnibus prefatus magister Manuel non intervenerit maxime in minimis, non sit ei aliquod per alios dictum, quia est senes et non potest ita prout ipsi caminare. Set in omnibus curis arduis et periculosis casis semper intervenire se obligavit et promisit. See Archivio di stato di Catania, Prot. Randano, notaio G. Marrota, reg. 10 car. 32r. I am indebted for this information to Professor R. Rizzo-Pavone, director of the Catania state archive.

61. See my *Médecine et justice en Provence médiévale*, 115–118 (doc. no. 27).

62. Ibid., 153–155 (doc. no. 48).

63. Ibid., 126–127 (doc. no. 31) for Bertrandus Arduini; 170 (doc. no. 53) for Raymundus Gaudii; and 195–196 (doc. no. 64) for Michael Tartona.

64. Ibid., 152–155 (doc. no. 48), 159–164 (doc. no. 50), 173–175 (doc. no. 55), 191–192 (doc. no. 61), 224–226 (docs. no. 76, 77).

65. Archives départementales des Bouches-du-Rhône (Marseilles), 56H960, fol. 39v: "denuntiavit Fossonus Levi judeus quod Fossonus filius Astrugi judei Aurielerii dum verbis cum ei contendebat dixit ei malitiose et iniuriose 'Tu habes unum fratrum messema' quod verbum ebraicum interpretatur renegat de la ley . . .

"Eodem die dictus Fossonus accusatus . . . negavit omnia 'exepto quod ipse dixit' si tu mihi facias aliquam iniuriam ego faciam tibi."

66. I discussed this case and the possible meaning of the word *mehares* in my *Recherches sur la communauté juive de Manosque*, 54–55. The Latin reads: "Mihares quod verbum ebraycum interpretatur rebellis de lege."

67. I discussed the case in *Recherches sur la communauté juive de Manosque*, 46–49. Part of the documentation was also published in *Médecine et justice en Provence médiévale*, 115–118 (doc. no. 27).

68. Archives départementales des Bouches-du-Rhônes (Marseilles) 56H1093, fol. 115r, 117v, 121r. Bonafos' mother, designated as "Fava judea uxor quodam Astrugi Aurificerii," is purchasing on credit 7 sestarii of wheat on 25 March 1313 (ibid., fol. 130r).

69. See my *Médecine et justice en Provence médiévale*, 6–7.

70. In this section I shall provide evidence about extramedical activity from Provençal documentation only. But similar evidence was found elsewhere. See, for example, Robert S. Gottfried, *Doctors and Medicine in Medieval England 1340–1530* (Princeton, 1986), 57–58.

71. See n. 28 above in this chapter. The court injunction is preserved in the Archives départementales des Bouches-du-Rhône (Marseilles), 381E372, fol. 84v, and reads:

Eodem die (kalendas Octobris), dictus dominus judex injunxit etc. Marie comptesse, uxori Bernardi Compte quondam, presenti et confitenti, obligant res et jura, etc. quatinus, ad voluntatem et requisitionem creditoris suprascripti, det et solvat Magistro Guillelmo Brocho, fisico, presenti et petenti, sexaginta solidos reforciatos, quorum XL solidos confessa sibi debere pro salario cure dicte Marie et fili[e] su[e] et XX solidos ex causa mutui, et quos XX solidos ex causa predicta confessit habuisse et recepisse dicta Maria a dicto Magistro Guillelmo.

A similar situation is revealed in a notarial contract in Arles in 1440: Peyre Gulard owes eight florins to Master Bendich de Canet,

part of it as a loan, part of it as a medical fee. See Louis Stouff, *Arles à la fin du moyen âge*, 2 vols. (Aix-en-Provence et Lille, 1986), 1:309 and 2:574 n. 16. For doctors lending money in the region of Béarn, southwestern France, in the fifteenth century, see Muriel Laharie, "Le milieu médical en Béarn à la fin du moyen âge," *Annales du Midi* 102 (1990): 349-357, in particular 355.

72. Louis Barthélemy, *Les médecins à Marseille avant et pendant le moyen âge* (Marseilles, 1883), 13-14.

73. Ibid., 27-28.

74. The document is preserved at the Archives municipales de la ville de Marseille, ms. 9 ii 187. A typewritten transcription and translation can be found in Pierre Paul, *Transcription et traduction du "livre de raison" de Jean Blaise: Un manuscrit en ancien provençal des archives communales de Marseille*, Mémoire pour le diplôme de langue et culture régionales de l'université de Provence, 2 vols. (Aix-en-Provence, 1980). Another translation exists by D. Hauck, *Das Kaufmannsbuch des Johan Blasi, 1329-1337: Ausgabe mit sprachlichen und wirtschaftsgeschichtlichen Kommentar*, 2 vols. (Saarbruck, 1965).

75. The will was published by Miguel Batllori, "La documentación de Marsella sobre Arnau de Vilanova y Joan Blasi," *Analecta sacra tarraconensia* 21 (1948): 75-119, especially 91-98. Parts of the aforementioned account book are also published on pp. 98-105.

76. See Maurice de Dainville et al., *Inventaire analytique, série BB (notaire et greffiers du consulat 1293-1387)*, Archives de la ville de Montpellier (Montpellier, 1984), 18, no. 188.

77. The documents, still in manuscript, are preserved in the Archives départementales des Bouches-du-Rhône (Marseilles), 381E9, fols. 31r-50r.

78. Both are summarized, but not published, in my *Médecine et justice en Provence médiévale*, 242 (docs. no. 8, 9).

79. Published by Shlomo Simonsohn, *The Jews in the Duchy of Milan*, 4 vols. (Jerusalem, 1982-1986), 1: 24-27 (doc. no. 31).

80. See Toaff, *Il vino e la carne*, 268. I depend here on Toaff's translation to modern Italian.

81. Ibid., 268-269.

82. Antonio Durán Gudiol, *La judería de Huesca* (Zaragoza, 1984), 35; Duran i Sanpere, *Referencies documentals del call de juhséus de Cervera*, 49.

83. Richard W. Emery, "Jewish Physicians in Medieval Perpignan," in *Michael: On the History of the Jews in the Diaspora*, ed. Shlomo Simonsohn and Joseph Shatzmiller, vol. 12 (Tel-Aviv, 1991), pp. 113-134.

84. Jean Régné, *History of the Jews in Aragon: Regesta and Docu-*

ments 1213–1327, ed. and annotated by Y. T. Assis in association with A. Gruzman, reprinted from *Revue des études juives* 60 (1910) to 78 (1924) (Jerusalem, 1978), 555 (docs. no. 3001, 3005).

85. Shlomo Simonsohn, *The Jews of the Duchy of Milan*, 1:557 (doc. no. 1327).

86. Bartolomeo and Giuseppe Lagumina, *Codice diplomatico dei giudei di Sicilia*, 3 vols. (Palermo, 1884–1895), 1:168 (doc. no. 124). "Supplicavit quod cum ipse vacet in studio sue artis medicine ut plurimum die noctuaque ob quod in Sinagoga seu misquita publica iudeorum suas cerimonias et oraciones minime facere potest." See also chapter 2 n. 16.

Select Bibliography

Abraham Ibn Ezra. *Sefer Hanisyonot: The Book of Medical Experiences*. Ed. and trans. J. O. Leibowitz and S. Marcus. Jerusalem, 1984.

Agrimi, Jole, and Chiara Crisciani. *Malato, medico, e medicina nel medioevo*. Turin, 1980.

———. "Medici e 'vetulae' dal duecento al quattrocento: Problemi di una ricerca." In *Cultura popolare e cultura dotta nel seicento*, 144–159. Atti del convegno di studio di Genova, 23–25 novembre 1982. Milan, 1983.

Albucasis, *On Surgery and Instruments*. Ed. and trans. M. S. Spink and G. L. Lewis. Berkeley and Los Angeles, 1973.

Alteras, Isaac. "Jewish Physicians in Southern France during the Thirteenth and Fourteenth Centuries." *The Jewish Quarterly Review* 68 (1978): 209–223.

———. "Notes généalogiques sur les médecins juifs dans le sud de la France pendant les XIIIe et XIVe siècles." *Le moyen âge* 88 (1982): 29–47.

D'Alverny, Marie-Thérèse. "Translations and Translators." In *Renaissance and Renewal in the Twelfth Century*, ed. R. L. Benson and G. Constable, 421–462. Cambridge, Mass., 1982.

Amundsen, Darrel W. "Medieval Canon Law on Medical and Surgical Practice by the Clergy." *Bulletin of the History of Medicine* 52 (1978): 22–44.

Arderne, John. *Treatise of Fistula in Ano: Haemorrhoids and Elysters*. Ed. D'Arcy Power. London, 1910.

Ascheri, Mario. "'Consilium sapientis,' perizia medica, e 'res iudicata': Diritto dei 'dottori' e istituzioni comunali." In *Proceedings of the Fifth International Congress of Medieval Canon Law*, 533–579. *Monumenta iuris canonici*, series C: subsidia, vol. 6. Ed. S. Kuttner and K. Pennington. Vatican City, 1980.

Assion, Peter. "Jacob von Landshut: Zur Geschichte der jüdischen Aerzte in Deutschland." *Sudhoffs Archiv* 53 (1969): 270–291.

Astruc, Jean. *Mémoire pour servir à l'histoire de la faculté de médecine de Montpellier.* Paris, 1777.

Barkaï, Ron. *Les infortunes de Dinah: Le Livre de la génération: La gynécologie juive au moyen âge.* Trans. J. Barnavi and M. Garel. Paris, 1991.

———. "A Medieval Hebrew Treatise on Obstetrics." *Medical History* 33 (1988): 96–119.

Barthélemy, Louis. *Les médecins à Marseille avant et pendant le moyen âge.* Marseilles, 1883.

Batllori, Miguel. "La documentación de Marsella sobre Arnau de Vilanova y Joan Blasi." *Analecta sacra tarraconensia* 21 (1948): 75–119.

Bayle, Gustav. *Les médecins d'Avignon au moyen âge.* Avignon, 1882.

Bériac, Françoise. *Histoire des lépreux au moyen âge.* Paris, 1988.

Birkenmajer, Aleksander. "Le rôle joué par les médecins et les naturalistes dans la réception d'Aristote aux XIIe et XIIIe siècles." In *Etudes d'histoire des sciences et de la philosophie du moyen âge,* 73–87. Wrocław, Warsaw, and Cracow, 1970.

Blumenfeld-Kosinski, Renate. *Not of Woman Born: Representations of Caesarean Birth in Medieval and Renaissance Culture.* Ithaca, N. Y., and London, 1990.

Bodenheimer, F. S. *Rabbi Gershon ben Shlomoh d'Arles: The Gates of Heaven.* Jerusalem, 1953.

Bullough, Vern L. *The Development of Medicine as a Profession.* Basel and New York, 1966.

Burnett, Charles S. F. "Some Comments on the Translating of Works from Arabic into Latin in the Mid-Twelfth Century." *Miscellanea mediaevalia* 17 (1985): 161–171.

Cabezudo Astrain, José. "Médicos y curanderos zaragosanos en el siglo XV." *Archivo iberoamericano de historia de la medicina* 7 (1955): 119–126.

Calvanico, Raffaele. *Fonti per la storia della medicina e della chirurgia per il regno di Napoli nel periodo angioino (1273–1410).* Naples, 1962.

Della Campana, G. P. *Archiatri pontifici ebrei nel Rinascimento.* Montecatini, 1968.

Campbell Hurdmead, Kate. *A History of Women in Medicine from Earliest Times to the Beginning of the Nineteenth Century.* Haddam, Conn., 1938.

Cantera Burgos, Francisco. *Alvar García de Santa María y su familia*

de conversos: Historia de la judería de Burgos y de sus conversos más egregios. Madrid, 1952.

Capparoni, Pietro. *Magistri Salernitani nondum cogniti: A Contribution to the History of the Medical School of Salerno*. London, 1923.

Cardoner [i] Planas, Antonio [Antoní]. *Història de la medicina a la corona d'Aragó (1162–1479)*. Barcelona, 1973.

————. "El 'Hospital para judíos pobres' de Barcelona." *Sefarad* 22 (1962): 373–375.

————. "El linaje de los Cabrit en relación con la medicina del siglo XIV." *Sefarad* 16 (1956): 357–368.

————. "El médico judío Benvenist Samuel y su parentesco con Samuel Benvenist de Barcelona." *Sefarad* 1 (1941): 327–345.

————. "El médico judío Sělomó Caravida y algunos aspectos de la medicina de su época." *Sefarad* 3 (1943): 377–392.

————. "Muestra de protección real a físicos judíos españoles conversos." *Sefarad* 12 (1952): 378–380.

————. "Nuevos datos acerca de Jafuda Bonsenyor." *Sefarad* 4 (1944): 287–293.

————. "Seis mujeres hebreas practicando la medicina en el reino de Aragón." *Sefarad* 9 (1949): 441–445.

Cardoner Planas, Antonio, and Francisca Vendrell Gallostra. "Aportaciones al estudio de la familia Abenardut, médicos reales." *Sefarad* 7 (1947): 303–348.

Carmoly, Eliakim. *Histoire des médecins juifs, anciens et modernes*. Brussels, 1844.

Carnevali, Luigi. *Il ghetto di Mantova: Con appendice sui medici ebrei*. Mantua, 1884.

Caro, Georg. "Dr. phil. et med. Helyas Sabbati von Bologna und sein Aufenthalt in Basel 1410." *Anzeiger für schweizerische Geschichte*, n.s. 11 (1910–1913): 75–77.

Carpi, Daniel. "Note su alcuni ebrei laureati a Padova nel cinquecento e all'inizio del seicento." *Quaderni per la storia dell'università di Padova* 19 (1986): 145–156.

————. "R. Judah Messer Leon and His Activity as a Physician" (in Hebrew). *Koroth* 6 (1974): 277–301.

Cifuentes Lluís, and Luis (Lluís) García-Ballester. "Els professionals sanitaris de la corona d'Aragó en l'expedició militar a Sardenya de 1354–1355." *Arxiu de textos catalans antics* 9 (1990): 183–214.

Cipolla, Carlo M. *Public Health and the Medical Profession in the Renaissance*. Cambridge, 1976.

Cobban, Alan B. *The Medieval English Universities: Oxford and Cambridge to ca. 1500*. Berkeley, 1988. Reprint. Berkeley, 1990.

Cohn, Willy. "Jüdische Übersetzer am Hofe Karls I. von Anjou,

Königs von Sizilien (1266–1285)." *Monatsschrift für Geschichte und Wissenschaft des Judentums*, n.s. 43 (1935): 245–260. Reprinted in his *Juden und Staufer in Unteritalien und Sizilien*, 50–64. Darmstadt, 1978.

Colorni, Vittore. "Sull'ammissibilità degli ebrei alla laurea anteriormente al secolo XIX." In *La rassegna mensile di Israel: Scritti in onore di Riccardo Bachi* vol. 16, pp. 202–216. 1950. Or *Judaica minora: Saggi sulla storia dell'ebraismo italiano dall'antichità all'età moderna*, 473–485. Milan, 1983.

Comenge [y Ferrer], Luis. "Formas de munificencia real para con los archiatros de Aragón." *Bolétin de la real academia de buenas letras de Barcelona* 3 (1903): 1–15.

Comenge [y Ferrer], Luis. *La medicina en Cataluña (bosquejo histórico)*. Barcelona, 1908.

———."La medicina en el reino de Aragón." *El siglo médico* 44 (1897): 449–566. Reprint: *La medicina en el reino de Aragón (siglo XIV)*. Valladolid, 1974.

Le Corps souffrant: Maladies et médications. *Razo: Cahiers du centre d'études médiévales de Nice* 4 (1984).

Cotturi, Enrico. "Medici e medicina a Pistoia nel medioevo." *Incontri pistoiesi di storia arte cultura* 13 (1982):1–14.

Coulet, Noël. "Autour d'un quinzain des métiers de la communauté juive d'Aix en 1437." In *Minorités, techniques et métiers*, 79–104. Actes de la table ronde du groupement d'intérêt scientifique: Sciences humaines sur l'aire méditerranéenne, Abbaye de Sénanque, octobre 1978. Aix-en-Provence, 1980.

———."Documents aixois (première moitié du XVe siècle)." *Razo: Cahiers du centre d'études médiévales de Nice* 4 (1984): 115–125.

———."Quelques aspects du milieu médical en Provence au bas moyen âge." In *Vie privée et ordre public à la fin du moyen âge: Etudes sur Manosque, la Provence, et le Piémont (1250–1450)*, ed. M. Hébert, 119–138. Aix-en-Provence, 1987.

Dallari, Umberto, ed. *Rotuli dei lettori e legisti e artisti dello studio bolognese dal 1384 al 1799*. Bologna, 1888.

Daumet, Georges. "Une femme médecin au XIIIe siècle." *Revue des études historiques* 44 (1918):69–71.

Delaunay, Paul. *La médecine et l'Eglise: Contribution à l'histoire de l'exercice médical par les clercs*. Collection Hippocrate. Paris, 1948.

Delprato, Pietro, ed. *Trattati di mascalcia attribuiti ad Ippocrate tradotti dall'arabo in latino da maestro Moisè da Palermo*. Bologna, 1865.

Demaitre, Luke E. *Doctor Bernard de Gordon: Professor and Practitioner*. Toronto, 1980.

Denifle, Henri, and Emile Chatelain, eds. *Chartularium universitatis Parisiensis*. 4 vols. Paris, 1889–1897.

Donnolo, Shabbetai. *Medical Writings* (in Hebrew). Ed. Süssmann Muntner. 2 vols. Jerusalem, 1949.

Doviak, Ronald J. "The University of Naples and the Study and Practice of Medicine in the Thirteenth and Fourteenth Centuries". Ph.D. diss., City University of New York, 1974. University Microfilms, Ann Arbor, Michigan, 1974.

Dulieu, Louis. *La médecine à Montpellier*. Vol. 1: *Le moyen âge*. Avignon, 1975.

Elkhadem, Hosam. *Le Taqwīm al-Ṣiḥḥa (Tacuini sanitatis) d'Ibn Buṭlān: Un traité médical du XIᵉ siècle*. Louvain, 1990.

Emery, Richard W. "Documents Concerning Some Jewish Scholars in Perpignan in the Fourteenth and Early Fifteenth Centuries." In *Michael: On the History of the Jews in the Diaspora*, ed. Shlomo Simonsohn and Joseph Shatzmiller, vol. 4, pp. 27–48. Tel-Aviv, 1976.

———. "Jewish Physicians in Medieval Perpignan." In *Michael: On the History of the Jews in the Diaspora*, ed. Shlomo Simonsohn and Joseph Shatzmiller, vol. 12, pp. 113–134. Tel-Aviv, 1991.

Esposito, Anna. "Notai, medici, convertiti: Figure di intermediari nella società romana del tardo quattrocento," In *Atti del VI congresso internazionale dell'associazione italiana per lo studio del giudaismo*, 113–121. Rome, 1988.

Fabre, Augustin. *Histoire des hôpitaux et des institutions de bienfaisance de Marseille*. 2 vols. Marseilles, 1854–1855. Reprint. Marseilles, 1973.

Faur, Joseph. "Doctor's Right for Remuneration according to the Jewish Sources" (in Hebrew). *Diney Israel* 7 (1976): 79–98.

Fernandez, F. *La medicina árabe en España*. Barcelona, 1936.

Fort, George F. *Medical Economy during the Middle Ages*. London and New York, 1883. Reprint. New York, 1970.

Fournier, Marcel. *Les statuts et privilèges des universités françaises depuis leur fondation jusqu'en 1789*. 4 vols. Paris, 1890–1894. Reprint. Bologna, 1969, and Aalen, 1970.

Friedenwald, Harry. *The Jews and Medicine: Essays*. 2 vols. Baltimore, 1944. Reprint. New York, 1967.

———. "Wit and Satire about the Physician in Hebrew Literature." In his *The Jews and Medicine: Essays*, vol. 1, pp. 69–83. Baltimore, 1944. Reprint. New York, 1967.

Fürst, Livius. "Beiträge zur Geschichte der jüdischen Aerzte in Italien." In *Jahrbuch für die Geschichte der Juden und des Judentums*, vol. 5. Leipzig, 1861.

García, Angelina. "Médicos judíos en la Valencia del siglo XIV." In *Estudios dedicados a Juan Peset Aleixandre*, vol. 2, pp. 85–96. Valencia, 1982.

García-Ballester, Luis [Lluís]. "Arnold of Vilanova (ca. 1240–1311) and the Reform of Medical Studies in Montpellier (1309): The Latin Hippocrates and the Introduction of the New Galen." *Dynamis: Acta Hispanica ad medicinae scientiarumque historiam illustrandam* 2 (1982): 97–158.

————."Dietetic and Pharmacological Therapy: A Dilemma among Fourteenth-century Jewish Practitioners in the Montpellier Area." *Clio Medica: Essays in the History of Therapeutics* 22 (1991): 23–37.

————. "Las influencias de la medicina islámica en la obra mèdica de Arnau de Vilanova." *Estudi general* 9 (1989): 79–95.

————. "Medical Science in Thirteenth-century Castile: Problems and Prospects." *Bulletin of the History of Medicine* 61 (1987): 183–202.

————. *La medicina a la València medieval: Medicina i societat en un país medieval mediterrani*. Valencia, 1988.

————. "Los orígenes de la profesión médica en Cataluña: El 'collegium' de médicos de Barcelona (1342)." In *Estudios dedicados a Juan Peset Aleixandre*, vol. 1, pp. 129–149. Valencia, 1982.

————. "El papel de las instituciones de consumo y difusión de ciencia médica en la Castilla del siglo XIII: El monasterio, la catedral, y la universidad." *Dynamis: Acta Hispanica ad medicinae sicentiarumque historiam illustrandam* 4 (1984): 33–63.

García-Ballester, Luis, and Agustín Rubio-Vela. "L'influence de Montpellier dans le contrôle social de la profession médicale dans le royaume de Valence au XIVe siècle." In *Histoire de l'école médicale de Montpellier*. Actes du 110ème congrès national des sociétés savantes (Montpellier, 1985), Section d'histoire des sciences et des techniques, vol. 2, pp. 19–30. Paris, 1985.

García-Ballester, Luis, Lola Ferre, and Eduard Feliu. "Jewish Appreciation of Fourteenth-century Scholastic Medicine." *Osiris*, 2d ser., 6 (1990): 85–117.

García-Ballester, Luis, Michael R. McVaugh, and Agustín Rubio-Vela. *Medical Licensing and Learning in Fourteenth-century Valencia*. Transactions of the American Philosophical Society, vol. 79, no. 6. Philadelphia, 1989.

Garofalo, Fausto. "I papi ed i medici ebrei in Roma." In *Pagine di scienza e tecnica*, 1–25. Rome, 1948.

Germain, Alexandre Charles. *Cartulaire de l'université de Montpellier.* vol. 1. Montpellier, 1890.

Gershon ben Shlomoh d'Arles. *The Gate of Heaven* (Shaar ha-Shamayim). Ed. and trans. F. S. Bodenheimer. Jerusalem, 1953.

Giacosa, Piero. *Magistri Salernitani nondum editi.* Turin, 1901.

Gil, José S. *La escuela de traductores de Toledo y los colaboradores judíos.* Toledo, 1985.

Goitein, Shlomo Dov. "The Medical Profession in the Light of the Cairo Geniza Documents." *Hebrew Union College Annual* 34 (1963): 177–194.

Gottfried, Robert S. *Doctors and Medicine in Medieval England 1340–1530.* Princeton, 1986.

Grau i Monserrat, Manuel. "Medicina a Besalú (s. XIV) (Metges, apotecaris, i manescals)." *Patronat d'estudis històrics d'Olot i Comarca,* 101–133. Annals 1982–1983. Olot, 1984.

———. "Meteges jueus a Besalú (s. XIV)." *Amics de Besalú.* I Assemblea d'estudis del seu comtat, 29–33. Olot, 1968.

———. "Meteges jueus de Besalú (s. XIV et XV), Sa Sala, Des Portal i Coret." *Tercer congres d'historia de la medicina catalana,* 165–181. Lleida, 1981.

Grava, Yves. "Pratique médicale en milieu rural: Istres au XVᵉ siècle." *Razo: Cahiers du centre d'études médiévales de Nice* 4 (1984): 95–99.

Green, Monica. "Women's Medical Practice and Health Care in Medieval Europe." *Signs: Journal of Women in Culture and Society* 14 (1989): 434–473.

Güdemann, Moritz. *Geschichte des Erziehungswesens und der Cultur der abendländischen Juden während des Mittelalters und der neueren Zeit.* 3 vols. Vienna, 1884–1888. Reprint. Amsterdam. 1966.

Guilleré, Christian. "Le milieu médical géronais au XIVᵉ siècle." In *Santé, médecine, et assistance au moyen âge.* Actes du 110ᵉᵐᵉ congrès national des sociétés savantes (Montpellier, 1985), vol. 1, pp. 263–281. Paris, 1987.

de Günzberg, David. "Be'er la-hai des Isak ben Todros." In *Jubelschrift zum neunzigsten Geburtstag des Dr. L. Zunz,* vol 2. Berlin, 1884.

Haskins, Charles Homer. *Studies in the History of Mediaeval Science.* Cambridge, Mass., 1924.

Hauck, Dietrich. *Das Kaufmannsbuch des Johan Blasi, 1329–1337:*

Ausgabe mit sprachlichen und wirtschaftsgeschichtlichen Kommentar. Saarbruck, 1965.

Hillel ben Shemu'el of Verona. *Sefer Tagmulé ha-Nefesh* (Book of the Rewards of the Soul). Ed. Joseph Sermoneta. Jerusalem, 1981.

Hillgarth, J. N. *Readers and Books in Majorca, 1229–1550.* 2 vols. Paris, 1991.

Hillgarth, J. N. and Giulio Silano. "A Compilation of the Diocesan Synods of Barcelona (1354): Critical Edition and Analysis." *Mediaeval Studies* 46 (1984): 78–157.

Hinojosa Montalvo, José. "El préstamo judío en la ciudad de Valencia en la segunda mitad del siglo XIV." *Sefarad* 45 (1985): 315–339.

Hugues, Muriel Joy. *Women Healers in Medieval Life and Literature.* New York, 1943. Reprint. Freeport, 1968.

Huillard-Bréholles, Jean Louis Alphonse. *Historia diplomatica Frederici secundi.* 6 vols. Paris, 1852–1861. Reprint. Turin, 1963.

Iancu-Agou, Danièle. "Documents sur les juifs aixois et la médecine au XVᵉ siècle: Médications et ouvrages." In *Santé, médecine, et assistance au moyen âge.* Actes du 110ᵉᵐᵉ congrès national des sociétés savantes (Montpellier, 1985), vol. 1, pp. 251–262. Paris, 1987.

———. "L'inventaire de la bibliothèque et du mobilier d'un médecin juif d'Aix-en-Provence au milieu du XVᵉ siècle." *Revue des études juives* 134 (1975): 47–80.

———. "Les médecins juifs en Provence au XVᵉ siècle: Praticiens, notables, et lettrés." *Yod: Judaïsme et médecine* 26 (1987): 33–43.

———. "Préoccupations intellectuelles des médecins juifs au moyen âge." *Provence historique* 103 (1976): 21–44

———. "Une strate mince et influente: Les médecins juifs aixois à la fin du XVᵉ siècle (1480–1500): Activités économiques et état social." In *Minorités, techniques, et métiers*, 105–126. Actes de la table ronde du groupement d'intérêt scientifique: Sciences humaines sur l'aire méditerranéenne, Abbaye de Sénanque, octobre 1978. Aix-en-Provence, 1980.

———. "Une vente de livres hébreux à Arles en 1434: Tableau de l'élite juive arlésienne." *Revue des études juives* 146 (1987): 5–62.

Imbault-Huart, Maire-José. *La médecine au moyen âge à travers les manuscrits de la Bibliothèque nationale.* Paris, 1983.

[Isak ben Todros]. "Beer la-hai des Isak ben Todros" (in Hebrew). Ed. D. de Günzburg. In *Jubelschrift zum neunzigsten Geburtstag des Dr. L. Zunz*, part 2, pp. 91–126. Berlin, 1884.

Ivry, Alfred L. "Philosophical Translations from the Arabic in Hebrew during the Middle Ages." *Rencontres de cultures dans la philo-*

sophie médiévale, 167–186. Traductions et traducteurs de l'anti-quité tardive au XIVe siècle. Louvain-la-Neuve and Cassino, 1990.

Jacobi, David. "Jewish Doctors and Surgeons in Crete under Vene-tian Rule" (in Hebrew). In *Culture and Society in Medieval Jewry: Studies Dedicated to the Memory of Haim Hillel Ben-Sasson*, ed. M. Ben-Sasson et al., 431–444. Jerusalem, 1989.

Jacobs, Joseph. "Une lettre française d'un juif anglais au XIIIe siè-cle." *Revue des études juives* 18 (1889): 256–261.

Jacquart, Danielle. "L'école des traducteurs." In *Tolède, XIIe–XIIIe: Musulmans, chrétiens, et juifs: Le savoir et la tolérance*. Ed. Louis Cardaillac, 177–191. Paris, 1991.

———. *Le milieu médical en France du XIIe au XVe siècle*. Geneva and Paris, 1981.

———."Un 'physicien' des ducs de Bourgogne: Hacquin de Vesoul." *Archives juives* 8 (1971–1972): 30.

———. "Principales étapes dans la transmission des textes de méde cine (XIe–XIVe siècle)." In *Rencontres de cultures dans la philo-sophie médiévale*, 251–271. Traductions et traducteurs de l'anti-quité tardive au XIVe siècle. Louvain-la-Neuve and Cassino, 1990.

———. "La réception du 'Canon' d'Avicenne: Comparaison entre Montpellier et Paris aux XIIIe et XIVe siècles." *Histoire de l'école médicale de Montpellier*, Actes du 100ème congrès national des so-ciétés savantes (Montpellier, 1985), vol. 2, pp. 69–77. Paris, 1985.

———. *Supplément* to Ernest Wickersheimer, *Dictionnaire bio-graphique des médecins en France au moyen âge*. Geneva and Paris, 1979.

Jacquart, Danielle, and Françoise Micheau. *La médecine arabe et l'occident médiéval*. Paris, 1990.

Jordí [y] González, Ramón. "Consideraciones sobre la legislación sanitaria peninsular." *Boletín informativo de circular farmacéutica* 224 (separata, no pagination). Barcelona, 1969.

———. "Médicos, cirujanos, y boticarios relacionados con las Casas reales." *Boletín informativo de circular farmacéutica* 235, annex 5, pp. 396–399. Barcelona, 1969.

Judaïsme et médecine. Yod 26. Paris, 1987.

Kantorowicz, Hermann. "Cino da Pistoia ed il primo trattato di medi-cina legale." In *Rechtshistorische Schriften*. Ed. H. Coing and G. Immel. Karlsruhe, 1970.

Karmi, Ghada. "State Control of the Physicians in the Middle Ages: An Islamic Model." In *Les sociétés urbaines en France méridionale et en péninsule ibérique au moyen âge*, 63–84. Actes du colloque de Pau, 21–23 septembre 1988. Paris, 1991.

Kaufmann, David. "Trois docteurs de Padoue." *Revue des études*

juives 18 (1889): 293–298.

———. "Das Sendschreiben des Mose Rimos aus Majorca an Benjamin b. Mordechai in Rom." In *Festschrift zum achtzigsten Geburtstage Moritz Steinschneiders*, 227–232. Leipzig, 1896. Reprint. Jerusalem, 1970.

Kayserling, Moritz. "Zur Geschichte der jüdischen Aerzte." *Monatsschrift für Geschichte und Wissenschaft des Judentums* 7 (1858): 393–395; 8 (1859): 161–170, 330–339; 9 (1860): 92–98, 478; 10 (1861): 38–40; 11 (1862): 350–353; 12 (1863): 182–183; 17 (1868): 151–152, 185–188.

Kibre, Pearl. "The Faculty of Medicine at Paris, Charlatanism, and Unlicensed Medical Practices in the Later Middle Ages." *Bulletin of the History of Medicine* 27 (1953): 1–20.

Klein-Franke, Felix. *Vorlesungen über die Medizin im Islam.* Wiesbaden, 1982.

Kohlberg, Etan, and B. Z. Kedar. "A Melkite Physician in Frankish Jerusalem and Ayyubid Damascus: Muwaffaq al-Dīn Ya'qūb b. Siqlāb." *Asian and African Studies* 22 (1988): 113–126.

Kohn, Richard. "L'influence des juifs à l'origine de la faculté de médecine de Montpellier." *Revue d'histoire de la médecine hébraïque* (4 September–December 1949): 14–34.

Kottek, Samuel S. "Humilitas: On a Controversial Medal of Benjamin Son of Elijah Beer the Physician (1497?–1503?)." *Journal of Jewish Art* 11 (1985): 41–46.

Kottek, Samuel S., Mendel Metzger, and Thérèse Metzger. "Manuscrits hébraïques décorés ou illustrés du canon d'Avicenne." *Acta of the Twenty-seventh International Congress of the History of Medicine*, vol. 2, pp. 739–745. Barcelona, 1981.

Krauss, Samuel. *Geschichte der jüdischen Aerzte vom frühesten Mittelalter bis zur Gleichberechtigung.* Vienna, 1930.

Lahaire, Muriel. "Le milieu médical en Béarn à la fin du moyen âge." *Annales du Midi* 102 (1990): 349–357.

Landau, Richard. *Geschichte der jüdischen Aerzte.* Berlin, 1895.

Langermann, Zvi J. "Salomon ibn Ya'ish to Avicenna's canon" (in Hebrew). *Kiryat sefer* 63 (1991): 133–1333.

Lavoie, Rodrigue. "La délinquance sexuelle à Manosque: Schéma général et singularités juives." *Provence historique* 37 (1987): 571–587.

Lavoie, Rodrigue, and Joseph Shatzmiller. "Médecine et gynécologie au moyen âge: Un exemple provençal." *Razo: Cahiers du centre d'études médiévales de Nice* 4 (1984): 133–143.

Leclerc, Lucien. *Histoire de la médecine arabe.* 2 vols. Paris, 1876. Reprint. New York, 1971.

Leibowitz, Joshua [O.]. "A [braham] Caslari's [Fourteenth-century] Hebrew Manuscript 'Pestilential Fevers' Edited by H. Pinkhoff." *Koroth* 4 (1968): lxix–lxxii (English); 517–520 (Hebrew).

———. "Historical Aspects of the Persecution of Jewish Physicians [in the Middle Ages]" (in Hebrew). *Dapim refuiim* (Medical Journal) 12 (1953): 3–7.

———. "Médecins juifs à Montpellier." *Yperman* 8 (1961): 1–4.

———. "The Preface by Nathan ha-Meati to His Hebrew Translation (1279) of Ibn-Sina's Canon." *Koroth* 7 (1976): i–viii.

Lieber, Elinor. "Asaf's 'Book of Medicines': A Hebrew Encyclopedia of Greek and Jewish Medicine, Possibly Compiled in Byzantium on an Indian Model." *Dumbarton Oaks Papers* 38 (1984): 233–249.

Lieutaud, V. *Un séminaire à Manosque il y a cinq siècles (4 juin 1365)*. Aix-en-Provence, 1901.

Lindberg, David C. "The Transmission of Greek and Arabic Learning to the West." In *Science in the Middle Ages*, ed. D. C. Lindberg, 52–90. Chicago and London, 1978.

Lipinska, Mélanie *Histoire des femmes médecins depuis l'antiquité jusqu'à nos jours*. Paris, 1900.

López de Meneses, Amada. "Crescas de Viviers, astrólogo de Juan I el Cazador." *Sefarad* 14 (1954): 99–115, 265–293.

———."Seis mujeres hebreas practicando la medicina en el reino de Aragón." *Sefarad* 9 (1949): 441–445.

Luzzati, Michele. "Il medico ebreo e il contadino: Un documento pisano del 1462." *La casa dell'ebreo: Saggi sugli ebrei a Pisa e in Toscana nel Mediœvo e nel Rinascimento*, 49–57. Pisa, 1985.

Luzzatto, Leone. "Ricordi storici": "Medici ebrei nei secoli XV–XVI." *Il vessillo israelitico* 33 (1885): 316–317.

———. "Medici ebrei," *Il ressillo israelitico* 50 (1902): 301–303.

Mac Kinney, Loren. *Medical Illustrations in Medieval Manuscripts*. Wellcome Historical Library. London, 1965.

McVaugh, Michae R. "Bernat de Berriacho (fl. 1301–1343) and the 'Ordinacio' of Bishop Ponç de Gualba." *Arxiu de textos catalans antics* 9 (1990): 240–254.

———. "The humidum radicale' in Thirteenth-century Medicine." *Traditio* 30 (1974): 259–283.

———. *Medicine before the Plague: Practitioners and Their Patients in the Crown of Aragon, 1285–1345*. Cambridge, 1993.

———."Professional Rivalries Among Medical Practitioners." Paper read at conference Dissent and Repression in the Middle Ages, January 1991, University of California, Los Angeles.

———. "Royal Surgeons and the Value of Medical Learning: The

Crown of Aragon, 1300–1350." *Actes du colloque de Barcelone sur l'histoire de la médecine*, May 1989. Forthcoming.

McVaugh, Michael, and Luis García-Ballester. "The Medical Faculty at Early Fourteenth-century Lérida." *History of Universities* 8 (1989): 1–25.

[Maimonides] Moshe ben Maimon. *Medical Works*. Ed. Süssmann Muntner, 5 vols. Jerusalem, 1957–1969. Reprint. Jerusalem, 1987.

Margalith, David. "The Ideal Doctor as Depicted in Ancient Hebrew Writings." *Journal of the History of Medicine* 12 (1957): 37–41.

———. *The Scholars of the Jews* (in Hebrew). Jerusalem, 1962.

Marini, Gaetano. *Degli archiatri pontifici*. 2 vols. Rome, 1784.

Martínez Loscos, Carmen. "Orígenes de la medicina en Aragón: Los médicos árabes y judíos." *Jerónimo Zurita: Cuadernos de historia* 6–7 (1954): 7–61.

Martínez Pérez, Felipe. "La medicina sevillana en el siglo XIII y especialmente en la época de la conquista de Sevilla." *Archivo hispalense* 12 (1950): 131–177.

Melzer, Aviv. "Asaph the Physician—The Man and His Book: A Historical-Philological Study of the Medical Treatise, 'The Book of Drugs.'" Ph.D. diss., University of Wisconsin, 1972.

Meyerhof, Max. "Von Alexandrien nach Bagdad: Ein Beitrag zur Geschichte des philosophen und medizinischen Unterrichts bei den Arabern." *Sitzungsberichte der preussischen Akademie der Wissenschaften* 23 (1930): 389–429.

———. "Medieval Jewish Physicians in the Near East, from Arabic Sources." *Isis* 28 (1938): 432–460. Also in his *Studies in Medieval Arabic Medicine: Theory and Practice*, ed. P. Johnstone. London, 1984.

———. "L'œuvre médicale de Maïmonide." In his *Studies in Medieval Arabic Medicine: Theory and Practice*, ed. P. Johnstone. London, 1984.

———. *Studies in Medieval Arabic Medicine: Theory and Practice*. Ed. P. Johnstone. London, 1984.

———. "La surveillance des professions médicales et paramédicales chez les arabes." *Bulletin de l'institut d'Egypte* 26 (1944): 119–134. Also in his *Studies in Medieval Arabic Medicine: Theory and Practice*, ed. P. Johnstone. London, 1984.

Micheau, Françoise. "La formation des médecins arabes au Proche-Orient (Xe–XIIIe siècle)." *Les entrées dans la vie: Initiations et apprentissages*. Douzième congrès de la société des historiens médiévistes de l'enseignement supérieur public, Nancy, 1981, 105–125. Nancy, 1982.

———. "Hommes de sciences au prisme d'Ibn-Qifti." In *Actes du*

colloque intellectuels et militants dans le monde islamique. Cahiers de la Méditerranée, vol. 37, pp. 81–106. Nice, 1988.

―――. "Les traités sur 'l'examen du médecin' dans le monde arabe médiéval." In *Maladies, médecines, et sociétés,* vol. 2, *Histoire au présent.* Paris. Forthcoming.

Millás Vallicrosa, José María. "The Beginning of [the Study of] Natural Sciences among Spanish Jews" (in Hebrew). *Tarbiz* 24 (1954): 48–59.

―――. *Estudios sobre historia de la ciencia española.* 2 vols. Madrid, 1987.

―――. "La obra enciclopédica de R. Abraham bar Ḥiyya." In *Estudios sobre historia de la ciencia española,* vol. 1, pp. 219–262. Madrid, 1987.

Miret y Sans, Joachim. "Les médecins juifs de Pierre, roi d'Aragon." *Revue des études juives* 57 (1909): 268–278.

Mondeville, Henri de. *Chirurgie de maître Henri de Mondeville, chirurgien de Philippe le Bel.* Ed. E. Nicaise. Paris, 1893.

Moshe ben Maimon [Maimonides]. *Medical Works.* Ed. Süssmann Muntner. 5 vols. Jerusalem, 1957–1969. Reprint. Jerusalem, 1987.

Mosheh Rimos. *Lamentation by Mosheh Rimos* (Kinah le-Mosheh Rimos) (in Hebrew). Ed. David Kahana. Odessa, 1893.

Mosti, Renzo. "Medici ebrei del XIV–XV secolo a Tivoli." *Atti e memorie della società tiburtina di storia e d'arte* 27 (1954): 109–156.

Motta, Emilio Ambrogio. "Oculisti, dentisti, e medici ebrei nella seconda metà del secolo XV alla corte milanese." *Annali universali di medicina* 283 (1887): 326–328.

Münster, Ladislao. "Alcuni episodi sconosciuti o poco noti sulla vita e sull'attività di Bartolomeo da Varignana." *Castalia: Rivista di storia della medicina* 5–6 (1954): 207–215.

―――. "L'enarratio brevis de senum affectibus' de David de Pomis, le plus grand médecin israélite en Italie au XVIe siècle." *Revue d'histoire de la médecine hébraïque* 7 (1954): 7–16, 125–136.

―――. "Fu Jacob Mantino lettore effettivo dello Studio di Bologna?" *Rassegna mensile di Israel* 20 (1954): 310–321.

―――. "La grande figure d'Elia di Sabbato, médecin juif d'Italie du XVe siècle." *Revue d'histoire de la médecine hébraïque* 32 (July 1956): 125–140; 35 (March 1957): 41–45; 36 (July 1957): 53–65.

―――. "Laurea in medicina conferita ad un ebreo spagnolo a Napoli nel 1488: Contributo alla questione dell'ammissione degli ebrei al grado dottorale in Italia nell'ultimo secolo del medioevo." *Atti del XV congresso internazionale di storia della medicina,* vol. 1, pp. 291–297. Madrid, 1956.

————. "Laurea in medicina conferita dallo studio ferrarese ad un ebreo nel 1426." *Ferrara viva: Rivista storica e di attualità* 3, nos. 7–8 (1961): 63–72.

————. "Una luminosa figura di medico ebreo del quattrocento, maestro Elia di Sabbato da Fermo, archiatra pontificio." In *Scritti in memoria di Sally Mayer (1875–1953): Saggi sull'ebraismo italiano*, 224–258. Jerusalem, 1956.

————. "Maître Guillaume feu Isaia de Urbino, docteur ès arts et en médecine à Ferrare en 1426." *Revue d'histoire de la médecine hébraïque* 11 (1958): 109–114.

————. "Medichesse italiane dal XIII al XV secolo." *Lo smeraldo* 6 (1952): 1–11.

————. "La medicina legale in Bologna dai suoi albori alla fine del secolo XIV." *Bollettino dell'accademia medica pistoiese Filippo Pacini* 26 (1955): 257–271.

————. "Notizie di alcune medichesse veneziane nelle prima metà del trecento." In *Scritti in onore di Adalberto Pazzini*, 180–187. Milan, 1954.

Münster, Ladislao, and Mirko Malavolti. "Su alcuni documenti relativi a medici ebrei conservati nell'archivio di stato di Firenze." *Medicina nei secoli* 8 (1971): 22–53.

Muntner, Süssmann. *Accusations against Jewish Physicians in the Light of Medical History* (in Hebrew). Jerusalem, 1953.

————. "Aus der ärztlichen Geisteswerkstätte des Maimonides," *Miscellanea mediaevalia* 4 (1966): 128–145.

————. "Concerning a New Manuscript of 'Sepher Asaph'" (in Hebrew). *Koroth* 4 (1968): 731–736.

————. *Contribution to the History of the Hebrew Language in Medical Instruction* (in Hebrew). Jerusalem, 1940.

————. "Donnolo et la contribution des juifs aux premières œuvres de la médecine salernitaine." *Revue d'histoire de la médecine hébraïque* 9 (1956): 155–161.

————. *Introduction to the Book of Asaph the Physician: The Oldest Existing Text of a Medical Book Written in Hebrew.* Jerusalem, 1957.

————. *Rabbi Shabbetai Donnolo (913–985)* (in Hebrew). 2 parts in 1 vol. Jerusalem, 1949.

————. "R. Shem Tob Ben Isaac of Tortosa about the Life of the European Jewish Doctor and His Ethics." In *Sinai Jubilee Volume*, 321–337. Jerusalem, 1957.

Münz, Isak. *Die jüdischen Aerzte in Mittelalter: Ein Beitrag zur Kulturgeschichte des Mittelalters.* Frankfurt on Main, 1922.

Nader, Albert. "Avicenne médecin." *Miscellanea mediaevalia* 17 (1985): 327–343.

Naso, Irma. *Medici e strutture sanitarie nella società tardo medioevale.* Milan, 1982.

Nutton, Vivian. "Continuity or Rediscovery? The City Physician in Classical Antiquity and Mediaeval Italy." In *The Town and State Physician in Europe from the Middle Ages to the Enlightenment,* ed. Andrew W. Russell, 9–61. Wolfenbütteler Forschungen 17. Wolfenbüttel, 1981.

Orfali, Moisés. "Los traductores judíos de Toledo: Nexo entre oriente y occidente." *Actas del II congreso internacional, Encuentro de las tres culturas, 3–6 octubre 1983,* 253–260. Toledo, 1985.

Ortalli, Edgardo. "La perizia medica a Bologna nei secoli XXIIe XIV: Normativa e pratica di un istituto giudiziario." *Deputazione di storia patria per le province di Romagna, Atti e memorie,* n.s. 17–19 (1969): 223–259.

Dall'Osso, Eugenio. *L'organizzazione medico-legale a Bologna e a Venezia nei secoli XII–XIV.* Cesena, 1954.

Pansier, Pierre. "Jean de Tournemire: Etude bio-bibliographique." *Les mémoires de l'académie de Vaucluse,* 2d ser., 4 (1904): 89–102, and *Monspeliensis Hippocrates* 42 (1968): 5–12.

———. "Inventaire de la pharmacie de Pernes en 1365." *Annales d'Avignon et du comtat Venaissin* 14 (1928): 111–123.

———. "Les maîtres de la faculté de médecine de Montpellier au moyen âge." *Janus* 9 (1904): 443–451, 499–511, 537–545, 593–602; 10 (1905): 1–11, 58–68, 113–121.

———. "La médecine juive à Avignon au moyen âge." *Cahiers de pratique médico-chirurgicale* 8 (1934): 123–135.

———. "Les médecins juifs à Avignon aux XIIIᵉ, XIVᶜ et XVᶜ siècles." *Janus* 15 (1910): 421–451.

Paravicini Bagliani, Agostino. "L'Eglise médiévale et la renaissance de l'anatomie." *Revue médicale de la Suisse romande* 109 (1989): 987–991.

———. "Guillaume de Moerbeke et la cour pontificale." In *Guillaume de Moerbeke: Recueil d'études à l'occasion du 700ᵉᵐᵉ anniversaire de sa mort (1286),* ed. J. Brams and W. Vanhamed. Louvain, 1989.

———. *Medicina e scienze della nature alla corte dei papi nel duecento.* Spoleto, 1991.

Park, Katharine. *Doctors and Medicine in Early Renaissance Florence.* Princeton, 1985.

Paul, Pierre. *Transcription et traduction du livre de raison de Jean*

Blaise: Un manuscrit en ancien provençal des archives communales de Marseille. 2 vols. Mémoire pour le diplôme de langue et culture régionales de l'université de Provence. Aix-en-Provence, 1980.

Pedro Hispano. *Livro sobre a conservação da saúde.* Ed. M. H. da Rocha Pereira. Porto, 1961.

Perlmann, Moshe. "Notes on the Position of Jewish Physicians in Medieval Muslim Countries." *Israel Oriental Studies* 2 (1972): 315–319.

Pesaro, Abramo. "Notizie intorno al medico ferrarese Mosè Coen." *Il vessillo israelitico* 25 (1877): 285–286.

Pesenti Marangon, Tiziana. "'Professores chirurgie,' 'medici ciroici,' e 'barbitonsores' a Padova nell'età di Leonardo Buffi da Bertipaglia (†dopo il 1448)." *Quaderni per la storia dell'università di Padova* 11 (1978): 1–38.

Pierro, Francesco. "Nuovi contributi alla conoscenza delle medichesse nel regno di Napoli negli ultimi tre secoli del medioevo." *Archivio storico pugliese* 27 (1964): 231–241.

Piles Ros, Leopoldo. "Notas sobre judíos de Aragón y Navarra (Ejercicio de la medicina. Fiscalización de recaudaciones)." *Sefarad* 10 (1950): 176–181.

Pinès, Jacques. "Des médecins juifs au service de la papauté du XIIe au XVIIe siècle." *Revue d'histoire de la médecine hébraïque* 18 (1965): 123–132.

Portal, Félix. *Un procès en responsabilité médicale à Marseille en 1390.* Marseilles, 1902.

Power, Eileen. "Some Women Practitioners of Medicine in the Middle Ages." *Proceedings of the Royal Society of Medicine* 15 (1922): 20–22.

Precopi Lombardo, Annamaria. "Medici ebrei nella Sicilia medievale." *Trapani* 29 (1984): 25–28.

———. "Viridimura, dottoressa ebrea del medio evo siciliano." *La Fardelliana* 3 (1984): 361–364.

Preuss, Julius. *Biblisch-talmudische Medizin: Beiträge zur Geschichte der Heilkunde und der Kultur überhaupt.* Berlin, 1911. Reprint. New York, 1971.

Qesada Sanz, Jesús. "Algunos aspectos de la medicina en Murcia durante la época de los reyes católicos." In Juan Torres Fontes et al., *De historia médica murciana,* vol. 1, *Los médicos,* pp. 101–167. Murcia, 1980.

Rabin, Haim. "The Translations of the 'Canon' into the Hebrew." *Melila* 3–4 (1950): 132–147.

Ravitzky, Aviezer. "Aristotle's '*Meteorologica*' and the Maimonidean

Exegesis of Creation." In *Shlomo Pines Jubilee Volume on the Occasion of His Eightieth Birthday*, vol. 2, pp. 225–250. Jerusalem studies in Jewish Thought 9. Jerusalem, 1990.

Renan, Ernest. "Les écrivains juifs français du XIVᵉ siècle." In *Histoire littéraire de la France* 31. Paris, 1893.

———. "Les rabbins français du commencement du quatorzième siècle." In *Histoire littéraire de la France* 27. Paris, 1877.

Renaud, Henri Paul Joseph. "Etude sur le Mustaʿini d'Ibn Beklàrech, médecin juif de Saragosse au XIᵉ siècle." In *Proceedings of the Sixth International Congress of the History of Medicine*, 267–273. Leyden and Amsterdam, 1927.

De Renzi, Salvatore. *Storia documentata della scuola medica di Salerno*. Naples, 1857.

Reynaud, Félix. *La commanderie de l'hôpital de Saint-Jean de Jérusalem, de Rhodes, et de Malte à Manosque*. Gap, 1981.

Richler, Benjamin. "Another Letter from Hillel b. Samuel to Isaac the Physician?" (in Hebrew). *Kiryat sefer* 62 (1988–1989): 450–452.

———. "Manuscripts of Avicenna's Kanon in Hebrew Translation: A Revised and Up-to-date List." *Koroth* 8 (1982): 145–168 (English); 137–143 (Hebrew).

———. "Medical Treatises by Moses b. Isaac Ibn Waqar." *Koroth* 9 (1989): 253–264 (Hebrew); 700–707 (English).

Rigo, Caterina. "Un passo sconosciuto di Alberto Magno nel ʿSefer ʿeṣem ha-shamayim' di Yehudah b. Mosheh." *Henoch* 11 (1989): 295–318.

Rimos, Mosheh. *Kinah le-Mosheh Rimos* (Lamentation by Mosheh Rimos) (in Hebrew). Ed. David Kahana. Odessa, 1893.

Ríus Serra, J[osé]. "Aportaciones sobre médicos judíos en Aragón en la primera mitad del siglo XIV." *Sefarad* 12 (1952): 337–350.

Roca, Joseph María. *L'Estudi general de Lleyda*. Barcelona, n.d.

———. *La medicina catalana en temps del rey Martí*. Barcelona, 1919.

———. *Mestre Guillem Colteller metge dels reys d'Aragó Pere III y Johan I*. Barcelona, 1922.

Rocchi, Vincenzo. "Gli ebrei e l'esercizio della medicina di fronte alle leggi della Chiesa e del governo di Roma papale." *Rivista di storia critica delle scienze mediche e naturali* 1 (1910): 32–39.

Da Rocha Pereira, Maria Helena. "A obra médica de Pedro Hispano." In *Memórias da academia das ciências de Lisboa: Classe de letras*, vol. 18, pp. 193–208. Lisbon, 1977.

Romano, David. "Judíos escribanos y trujamanes de árabe en la

corona de Aragón (reinados de Jaime I a Jaime II)." *Sefarad* 38 (1978): 71–105.

———. "Le opere scientifiche di Alfonso X e l'intervento degli ebrei." In *Oriente e occidente nel medioevo: filosofia e scienze,* 677–711. Convegno internazionale, 9–15 aprile 1969. Rome, 1971.

———. "La transmission des sciences arabes par les juifs en Languedoc." In *Juifs et judaïsme de Languedoc: XIIIᵉ siècle–début XIVᵉ siècle,* ed. Marie-Humbert Vicaire and Bernhard Blumenkranz, 363–386. Paris, 1977.

Rosenthal, Franz. "The Physician in Medieval Muslim Society." *Bulletin of the History of Medicine* 52 (1978): 475–491.

Rosner, Fred. "Maimonides the Physician: A Bibliography." *Bulletin of the History of Medicine* 43 (1969): 221–235.

———. *Medicine in the Bible and the Talmud: Selections from Classical Jewish Sources.* New York, 1977.

———. *Medicine in the "Mishneh Torah" of Maimonides.* New York, 1984.

Roth, Cecil. "Jewish Physicians in Medieval England." *Medical Leaves* 5 (1943): 42–45. Reprinted in Cecil Roth, *Essays and Portraits in Anglo-Jewish History,* 46–51. Philadelphia, 1962.

———. "The Qualification of Jewish Physicians in the Middle Ages." *Speculum* 28 (1958): 834–843.

Roth, Norman. "Jewish Translators of the Court of Alfonso X." *Thought* 60 (1985): 439–455.

Rothschild, Jean-Pierre. "Motivations et méthodes des traductions en hébreu du milieu du XIIᵉ à la fin du XVᵉ siècle." In *Traduction et traducteurs au moyen âge,* 277–302. Colloque international du CNRS, IRHT, 26–28 mai 1986. Paris, 1989.

———. "Un traducteur hébreu qui se cherche: R. Juda b. Moïse Romano et le 'De causis et processu universitatis' II, 3,2 d'Albert le Grand." *Archives d'histoire doctrinale et littéraire du moyen âge* 59 (1992): 159–173.

Rowland, Beryl, ed. and trans. *Medieval Woman's Guide to Health: The First Gynecological Handbook.* Kent, Ohio, 1981.

Rovinski, Jacques. Introduction to "Dossier: Guérir au moyen âge: Médecine et société au XIVᵉ et au XVᵉ siècle." *Razo: Cahiers du centre d'études médiévales de Nice* 4 (1984): 107–108.

Rubió y Lluch, Antonio [Antoní]. *Documents per l'història de la cultura catalana mig-eval.* 2 vols. Barcelona, 1908–1921.

———. "Notes sobre la ciencia oriental a Catalunya en el XIVᵉⁿ sigle." *Estudis universitaris catalans* 3 (1909): 389–398, 489–497.

Russel, Andrew W., ed. *The Town and State Physician in Europe from the Middle Ages to Enlightenment.* Wolfenbüttel, 1981.

H. S. "The Jewish Doctor 600 Years Ago." *Moment* (November 1988): 36–40.

Sacchetti Sassetti, Angelo. *Maestro Salomone d'Anagni, medico del secolo XV*, 3–22. Frosinone, 1964.

Santschi, Elisabeth. "Médecine et justice en Crète vénitienne au XIVᵉ siècle." *Thèsaurismata* 8 (1971): 17–48.

Sarachek, Joseph. *Faith and Reason: The Conflict over the Rationalism of Maimonides*. New York, 1935. Reprint. New York, 1970.

Sarfati, G[ad ben Ami]. "The Hebrew Translations of Alfarabi's 'Classification of Sciences.'" In *Memorial to H. M. Shapiro (1902–1970)*, ed. H. Z. Hirschberg, vol. 1, *Bar-Ilan*, pp. 413–422 (Hebrew), xlii (summary in English). Annual of Bar-Ilan University, Studies in Judaica and the Humanities 9. Ramat-Gan, 1972.

Sarton, George. *Introduction to the History of Science*. Vol. 2, part, 1. New York, 1975.

Sassi, R. "Un famoso medico ebreo a Fabriano nel secolo XV." *Studia picena* 6 (1930): 113–123.

Scalvanti, Oscar. "Lauree in medicina di studenti israeliti a Perugia nel secolo XVI." *Annali della facoltà di giurisprudenza* 8 (1910): 91–129.

Schipperges, Heinrich. *Die Assimilation der arabischen Medizin durch das lateinische Mittelalter*. Wiesbaden, 1964.

———. *Die Kranken im Mittelalter*. Munich, 1990.

Segre, Marcello. "Dottoresse ebree nel medioevo." *Pagine di storia della medicina* 15 (1970): 98–106.

Shatzmiller, Joseph. "On Becoming a Jewish Doctor in the High Middle Ages." *Sefarad* 43 (1983): 239–250.

———. "Contacts et échanges entre savants juifs et chrétiens à Montpellier vers 1300." *Cahiers de Fanjeaux* 12 (1977): 337–344.

———. "Doctors and Medical Practices in Germany around the Year 1200: The Evidence of 'Sefer Asaph.'" *Proceedings of the American Academy for Jewish Research* 50 (1983): 149–164.

———. "Doctors and Medical Practice in Germany around the Year 1200: The Evidence of 'Sefer Hasidim.'" *Journal of Jewish Studies* 33 (1982): 583–593.

———. "Doctors' Fees and Their Medical Responsibility: Evidence from Notarial and Court Records." In *Private Acts of the Late Middle Ages*, ed. Paolo Brezzi and Egmont Lee, 201–208. Toronto, 1984.

———. "Etudiants juifs à la faculté de médecine de Montpellier, dernier quart du XIVᵉ siècle." In *The Frank Talmage Memorial Volume*, vol. 2, pp. 243–255. Jewish History 6. Haifa and Hanover, N.H., 1992.

————. "Femmes médecins au moyen âge: Témoignages sur leurs, pratiques (1250–1350)." In *Histoire et société: Mélanges offerts à Georges Duby*, vol. 1, *Le couple, l'ami, et le prochain*, pp. 167–175. Aix-en-Provence, 1992.

————. "Legal Records and Medical Practices." In *La typologie des sources du moyen âge: Médecine*, ed. D. Jacquart. Forthcoming.

————. "Livres médicaux et éducation médicale: À propos d'un contrat de Marseille en 1316." *Medieval Studies* 38 (1980): 463–470.

————. *Médecine et justice en Provence médiévale: Documents de Manosque, 1262–1348*. Aix-en-Provence, 1989.

————. "Médecins et expertise médicale dans la ville médiévale: Manosque 1280–1348." In *Vie privée et ordre public à la fin du moyen âge: Etudes sur Manosque, la Provence, et le Piémont (1250–1450)*, ed. M. Hébert, 105–117. Aix-en-Provence, 1987.

————. "Médecins municipaux en Provence, Catalogne, et autres régions de l'Europe méridionale (1350–1400)." *Les sociétés urbaines en France méridionale et en péninsule Ibérique au moyen âge*, 329–336. Actes du colloque de Pau, 21–23 septembre 1988. Paris, 1991.

————. "Notes sur les médecins juifs en Provence au moyen âge." *Revue des études juives* 128 (1969): 259–266.

————. "In Search of the 'Book of Figures': Medicine and Astrology in Montpellier at the Turn of the Fourteenth Century." *Association for Jewish Studies Review* 78 (1982–1983): 383–407.

————. "Soigner le corps souffrant: Pratiques médicales au tournant du XIVe siècle." In *Mélanges offerts à Georges Duby par le Collège de France*, ed. C. Amado and G. Lobrichon. Forthcoming.

Shiloah, Amnon. "'En-Kol'—Commentaire hébraïque de Šem Tov ibn Šaprūt sur le canon d'Avicenne." *Youval* 3 (1974): 267–287.

Sigerist, Henry E. *On the History of Medicine*. Ed. Felix Marti-Ibañez. New York, 1960.

Simili, Alessandro. "Appunti su quattro referti medico-legali inediti del '300." *Minerva medica* 33 (1942): 3–15.

————. "Bartolomeo da Varignana e una sua perizia giudiziaria." *La riforma medica* 36 (1941): 1101–1105.

————. "Considerazioni su una perizia medico-legale inedita del '300." *Giornale di clinica medica* 17 (1941): 921–927.

————. "Un consiglio inedito di Bartolomeo da Varignana e Giovanni da Parma." *Minerva medica* 33 (1942): 1–12.

————. "Sui primordi e sulla procedura della medicina legale in Bologna." *Atti e memorie dell'accademia di storia dell'arte sanitaria*, 2d ser., 9 (1943): 41–56.

————. "Un referto medico-legale inedito e autografo di Bartolomeo

da Varignana." *Il policlinico, periodico di medicina, chirurgia, e igiene* 58 (1951): 150–156.

Simon, Isidore. "Les médecins juifs en France, origines jusqu'à la fin du XVIIIe siècle." *Revue d'histoire de la médecine hébraïque* 89 (October 1970): 89–92.

———. "Les médecins juifs et la fondation de l'école de médecine de Montpellier" (in English). *Revue d'histoire de la médecine hébraïque* 68 (July 1965): 79–93.

———. "La vie et l'œuvre des médecins juifs d'origine espagnole et portugaise du moyen âge à la fin du XVIIIe siècle." *Revue d'histoire de la médecine hébraïque* 130 (October 1979): 55–58; 131 (December 1979): 73–76; 132 (March–April 1980): 17–20; 133 (July 1980): 39–42; 134 (October 1980): 47–52; 135 (December 1980): 69–72; 136 (March–April 1981): 9–12; 137 (July 1981): 25–28.

Simón de Gilleuma, José María. "Crescas Abnarrabí, médico oculista de la aljama leridana." *Sefarad* 18 (1958): 83–97.

Singer, Charles, and E. Ashworth Underwood. *A Short History of Medicine.* 2d ed. Oxford, 1962.

Siraisi, Nancy G. *Avicenna in Renaissance Italy: The 'Canon' and Medical Teaching in Italian Universities after 1500.* Princeton, 1987.

———. *Medieval and Early Renaissance Medicine: An Introduction to Knowledge and Practice.* Chicago and London, 1990.

———. *Taddeo Alderotti and His Pupils: Two Generations of Italian Medical Learning.* Princeton, 1981.

Sirat, Colette. "Juda b. Salomon ha-Cohen, philosophe, astronome et peut-être kabbaliste de la première moitié du XIIIe siècle." *Italia* 1 (1978): 39–61.

———. "Les traducteurs juifs à la cour des rois de Sicile et de Naples." *Traduction et traducteurs au moyen âge*, 169–191. Colloque international du CNRS, IRHT, 26–28 mai 1986. Paris, 1989.

Stefanutti, Ugo. *Documentazioni cronologiche per la storia della medicina, chirurgia, e farmacia in Venezia dal 1258 al 1332.* Venice, 1961.

Steinschneider, Moritz. *Die europäischen Übersetzungen aus dem Arabischen bis Mitte des 17. Jahrhunderts.* Graz, 1956.

———. *Die hebraeischen Übersetzungen des Mittelalters und die Juden als Dolmetscher.* Berlin, 1893. Reprint. Graz, 1956.

———. "Jüdische Aerzte." *Zeitschrift für hebräische Bibliographie* 17 (1914): 63–96, 121–167; 18 (1915): 25–57.

Tamani, Giuliano. *Il 'Canon medicinae' di Avicenna nella tradizione ebraica.* Padua, 1988.

————. "Il commento di Yeda'yah Bederši al 'Canone' di Avicenna."
Annali di Ca' Foscari 13, no. 3 (ser. orientale 5) (1974): 1–17.
————. "Il 'Corpus Aristotelicum' nella tradizione ebraica." *Annali di Ca' Foscari* 25, no. 3 (ser. orientale 17) (1986): 5–22.

Tani, Tommaso. "Archiatri israeliti tiburtini." *Bollettino di studi storici ed archeologici di Tivoli* 10 (1932): 2065–2067.

Teicher, J. L. "The Latin-Hebrew School of Translators in Spain in the Twelfth Century." In *Homenaje a Millás-Vallicrosa*, vol. 2, pp. 403–444. Barcelona, 1956.

Temkin, Owsei. "Medical Education in the Middle Ages." *Journal of Medical Education* 31 (1956): 383–391.

Terracina, Sergio. "Medici ebrei minori, in Spagna, dal IX al XV secolo." *Rivista di storia della medicina* 4 (1960): 129–151.

Thorndike, Lynn. *The 'Sphere' of Sacrobosco and Its Commentators*. Chicago, 1949.

————. *University Records and Life in the Middle Ages*. New York, 1944. Reprint. New York, 1975.

Torres Fontes, Juan. "Los médicos murcianos en el siglo XV." In Juan Torres Fuentes et al., *De historia médica murciana*, vol. 1, *Los médicos*, pp. 13–100. Murcia, 1980.

————. "Tres epidemias de peste en Murcia en el siglo XIV: 1348–1349, 1379–1380, 1395–1396." In Juan Torres Fuentes et al., *De historia médica murciana*, vol. 2, *Las epidemias*, pp. 9–66. Murcia, 1981.

Torres Fontes, Juan et al. *De historia médica murciana*. 3 vols. Murcia, 1980, 1981, 1982. Or: Academia Alfonso X el Sabio, *Biblioteca Murciana de Bolsillo*, vols. 11, 21, 31.

Twersky, Isadore. "Aspects of the Social and Cultural History of Provençal Jewry." *Journal of World History* 11 (1968): 185–207.

Ullmann, Manfred. *Die Medizin im Islam*. Leyden and Cologne, 1970.

Ussery, Huling E. *Chaucer's Physician: Medicine and Literature in Fourteenth-century England*. Toulane Studies in English 19. New Orleans, 1971.

Vajda, Georges. "Brèves notes sur quatre manuscrits médicaux." *Revue des études juives* 123 (1964): 125–130.

————. "Contribution à l'histoire de la controverse entre la philosophie et la religion." *Tarbiz* 24 (1955): 307–322.

Venetianer, Ludwig. "Asaf Judaeus, der Aelteste medizinische Schriftsteller in hebraeischer Sprache." In *38. Jahresbericht der Landes-Rabbinerschule in Budapest für das Schuljahr 1914–1915*. 3 vols. Budapest, 1915–1917.

Vernet, Juan. *Ce que la culture doit aux arabes d'Espagne.* Paris, 1985.

Veronese Ceseracciu, Emilia. "Ebrei laureati a Padova nel cinquecento." *Quaderni per la storia dell'università di Padova* 13 (1980): 151–168.

Veyssière, G. "In Agonia." In *Pratiques du corps, médecine, hygiène, alimentation, sexualité,* ed. J.-M. Racoult and A. J. Bullier, 23–39. St-Denis de la Réunion, 1985.

V[ignau], V[icente]. "Carta dirigida á D. Juan II de Aragón, por su médico, fijándole día para operarle los ojos." *Revista de archivos, bibliotecas, y museos* 4 (1874): 135–137, 230–231.

Arnaud de Villeneuve. *Medicationis parabole in Arnaldi de Villanova opera medica omnia,* VI.1. Ed. J. A. Paniagua. Barcelona, 1990.

Wasserstein, Abraham, ed. and trans. *Galen's Commentary on the Hippocratic Treatise Airs, Waters, Places in the Hebrew Translation of Solomon ha-Me'ati.* Proceedings of the Israel Academy of Sciences and Humanities 6, no. 3. Jerusalem, 1982.

Weiss-Amer, Melitta. "Von stichellinges magin vnd mucken fuezzen: Mittelalterliche Rezeptliteratur in der Parodie." *Seminar: Journal of Germanic Studies* 28 (1992): 1–16.

Welborn, Mary Catherine. "The Long Tradition: A Study in Fourteenth-century Medical Deontology." In *Medieval and Historiographical Essays in Honor of James Westfall Thompson,* ed. J. L. Cate and E. N. Anderson, 344–359. Chicago, 1959.

White, Lynn. *Medieval Religion and Technology.* Berkeley, 1978.

Wickersheimer, Ernest. *Dictionnaire biographique des médecins en France au moyen âge.* 2 vols. Paris, 1936. Reprint. Geneva and Paris, 1979–1981.

———. "La question du judéo-arabisme à Montpellier." *Janus* 21 (1927): 465–473, and, revised and corrected, *Monspeliensis Hippocrates* 6 (1959): 3–7.

Wolff, Philippe. "Recherches sur les médecins de Toulouse aux XIVᵉ et XVᵉ siècles." In *Regards sur le Midi médiéval,* 125–147. Toulouse, 1978.

Yuval, Israel Jacob. *Scholars in Their Time: The Religious Leadership of German Jewry in the Late Middle Ages* (in Hebrew). Jerusalem, 1988.

Zimmels, Hirsch Jacob. *Magicians, Theologians, and Doctors.* New York, 1952.

Index

Abalat, Andreas, 9
Abdalhac of Majorca, 75
Abenafia, Joseph, 17, 139
Abenardut dynasty, 23, 60–64
Abenardut, El'azar, 17, 60–65, 70, 72
Abenardut, Joseph, 20, 63
Abenardut, Moses, 64
Abenardut, Salomon, 63
Abencrespi, Isma'el, 128
Abenjacob, Azariah, 61–62
Abenjacob, Salomon, 75
Abenmenasse, Samuel, 59
Abenvives, Jaffudà, 17
Abin Ardut, El'azar, 64. See also Abenardut dynasty
Abin Ardut, Hayyim, 64. See also Abenardut dynasty
Abin Ardut, Joseph (Juce), 64. See also Abenardut dynasty
Abortion, 84
Abu 'Ali ibn Ghazāla, 43
Abu-Qasim Khalaf ibn 'Abbas al-Zahrāwī (Abulcasis), 44
Abrabanel, Don Isaac, 77
Abraham al-Faquim (Ibn Wakar), 41
Abraham bar Hiya of Barcelona, 40
Abraham Boniac of Carcassonne, 116
Abraham Chalom, 113
Abraham ibn David (Avendaut), 40
Abraham di Sabatuccio, Master, 129
Abraham of Carcassonne, 95
Abraham of Tortosa, 45
Addaran, Joseph, 76
Adhud, 12
Albi, synod of, 91

Alderotti, Taddeo, 112
Alfaquim, 58–59, 64
Alfarābi, 51
Alguades, Meir, 72
'Ali Ibn Ridwan, 42, 47, 52
Almelich, Baron, 75
Almuviçuel, Vitalis, 76
Alonso de Spina, 96
Alphonso, King of Aragon, 61
d'Alverny, Marie-Thérèse, 39
Aminorise, Isma'el, 76
Amundsen, Darrel W., 8
Anatoli, Jacob, 40, 42, 50
Angelo of Cesena, 89, 113
Antonius, Master, 137
Apprenticeship, 19
Arabic, as language of medicine, 39–40, 41, 43, 52, 57
Aragon: examination and licensing in, 17, 18; Jewish doctors in, 60–65; malpractice trials in, 81; medical texts in, 39–40
Arderne, John, 79
Aristotelian commentaries, 47, 50, 69
Arnold of Villanova, 28, 29, 37, 50, 136–137; on doctors to clergy, 95; as translator, 52, 53
Aron, Vidal, 20
Astrology, in study of medicine, 37–38
Astruc of Sestiers, Master, 133
Astruc Vidal Levi of Besalú, Master, 124
Astrugii, Abraham, 25
Astrugus de Marnovilla of Arles, Master, 115

Astrugus of Manosque, 131
Aucemont, Michael, 21
Avenarduç Joseph (Jucef), 64. *See also* Abenardut dynasty
Avenardusi, Salomon, 64
Avendita, Joseph, 24
Aventuriel, Samuel, 38
Averroës, 13, 42; Aristotelian commentaries of, 47, 50, 69
Avicenna, 13, 36, 42, 52; *Canon of Medicine* of, 47, 48–50, 103–104
Avigdor, Abraham, 29–30, 50, 53
Avigdor, Salomon ben Abraham, 16, 37
Avignon: anti-Jewish legislation in, 92; Jewish doctors in, 1; private medical education in, 24; synod of (1337), 89
Axaques, Joseph, 62
Aycardi, Petrus, 134, 137
Azariah ibn Jacob, Rabbi of Saragossa, 75, 76, 138

Baer, Fritz, 74
Bahya ibn Pakuda, 41
Barkaï, Ron, 53–54
Baron, Salo W., 10–11, 12, 71
Barthélemy, Louis, 25, 135
Bartholet Johannis, Master of Aix, 126
Benedict XII, Pope, 7
Benjamin di Sabbato, 69
Benjamin of Tudela, 77
Benvenist de Porta, Vitalis, 43
Benveniste Samuel of Barcelona, 59
Benvenisti Isamel, 7
St. Bernard, 9
Bernat de Berriacho, Master, 113–114, 125
Birkenmajer, Aleksander, 39
Black Death, 2–3, 54
Blaise, Armengaud, 27
Blaise, Jean, 136–137
Boccaccio, Giovanni, 101
Bologna, medical education in, 7, 32
Bonafilia, Joseph, 17
Bonafos of Manosque, Master, 124–125, 130, 131–135, 138
Bonastruch Baço, Master, 81, 83
Bonavita de Tivoli, 138
Bondavin, Abraham, 82
Bonfed, Shlomo, 23
Boniaquet Durand, 24

Boniface IX, Pope, 94
Bonjuda Carbit, Master, 18
Bonjuda Durant, 23
Bonomo of Pisa, 126
Bresc, Henri, 125
Breuer, Mordechai, 22–23
Broche, Guillelmus, 127
Brondy, Réjane, 33
Bruno di Lungoburgo, 52
Busach family of Salerno, 73

Cabrit, Master Isaac, 128
Calvanico, Raffaele, 19
Çaravida, Bendit, 37–38
Carbo, Abraham, 81, 83
Caslari, Abraham, 54
Caslari, Israel, 52
Catalonia, 4, 105, 107
Catholic Church, 141; acts against Jewish doctors, 88–89, 91–92; on clerics in professions, 8–10. *See also* Christian-Jewish relations
Cavalaire (Cavaller), Joseph (Juceff), 128–129, 138
Cavaller, Samuel, 138
Caveti, Petrus, 19
Cecho de Ascoli, 37
Certification (medical excuses for illness), 3–5
Charles, Count of Anjou and Provence, 15, 44, 93
Chaucer, Geoffrey, 101, 108
Christian-Jewish relations, 89, 96, 99, 119, 141; in accusing Jewish doctors of denying last rites, 91, 92; in accusing Jewish doctors of killing Christian patients, 85–88, 92; in collaboration of Jewish and Christian doctors, 133–134; in Jewish doctors' salary differences, 116–117; in Jews treating Christian patients, 16, 20, 96–98; in Jews using Christian doctors and medicines, 121–123
Cirurgicus, ix
Clarissa of Rouen, 20
Clergy: in medicine, 8–10; treated by Jewish doctors, 70, 94–95. *See also* Popes
Cohen, Aaron, of Jajora, 59
Cohen, Boniac, 5
Cohen, Joseph, 25
Cohen, Judah, 32, 50

Cohen, Vitalis, 4, 5, 25
Cohen de Talardo, Isaac, 134
Cohn, Willy, 44
Comenge, Luis, 71
Commentaries, 50–51
Community/civic role of doctors, 75, 138, 140
Constantine Africanus, 39
Contier, Pierre, 4, 5
Contracts, doctor-patient, 2, 124–131; disagreements in, 127–130; remuneration in, 124, 125, 126
Correto, Pierre, 136
Coulet, Noël, 125, 129, 133
Council of Clermont (1130), 8, 9
Council of Reims (1139), 8
Crescas Creyssent (Creysse), Master, 23–24, 94
Crescas de Caylar, 133
Crescas of Nimes (Crescas of Mirabeau), 89–90
Crescas Vidon, Master, 127
Cresconus de Sancto Paulo, 28
Cusina di Filippo, 110

Daniel da Castro, 98
David of Arles, 91
David of Marseilles, Master, 71–72
David "the Young," 87
Davinus Bonet Bourjorn, 17–18
Diego Rodrigues, 18
Dieulosal, Master, 95
Domingo Polo, 18
Donolo, Shabetai, 11
Dünash ben Tamim, 12
Duran de Cortali, 76
Durandus Tamani, Master, 95
Duranti La Calade, Jérôme de, 126

Education, medical, 15, 22–35; in academies, 22–23; by apprenticeship, 19; auxiliary sciences in, 37–38, 50; cost of, 7, 24; language of, 38–42; length of, 24; license dependent on, 19–20; marriage contracts provide for, 23–24; private, 23, 24, 25; tax exemption for, 26; universities ban Jews from, 27, 32–33, 35; university-based, 7, 25–26, 27–31, 32–35; for women, 27, 109–110
Elia di Sabbato of Fermo, 33, 35, 68–70, 72

Elia of Assisi, Master, 98
Elia of London, Master (Eliahu ben Menahem), 66, 67
Elia (Helias) of Narbonne, 116
Emery, Richard W., 105, 138
Empiricists, 21, 22
Espeçero, Vidal, 67
Eugenius IV, Pope, 70, 91–92
Examination process: auxiliary disciplines in, 37; bibliography required in, 36–38; Jewish proto-medici in, 17, 18–19; license based on, 14, 15–16; monopoly controlled by, 16; of practicing physicians, 18; technical reading as part of, 37
Exemption: from community or civic duties, 75, 138; Jewish community on, 73–74; for medical students, 26; from sumptuary laws, 74; from taxes, 63, 71, 72–73

Falaquera, Nathan, 53–54
Falaquera, Shem Tov, 51, 101–103
Familiaris, 59–60, 69, 94
Faraj (Mose) of Agrigento, 40, 43–44
Farrusol, Joseph, 24
Farussol, Crescas, 128
Ferdinand, King of Sicily, 26
Ferrarius Saladi, 17
Ferrerius Marvani, 25
Forensic medicine, 130
France: doctors' remuneration in, 116, 117; public health doctors in, 113–114. See also Manosque; Marseilles; Montpellier
Francisca of Viesti, 110
Frederick II, 15, 37
Frederick III, 92–93

Gaio di Sabatuccio, 129
Gaio the Jew (Isaac ben Mordecai), Master, 46, 94
Galen, 13, 36; translated, 42, 46, 47, 52
Gamel, Pierre, 135
García, Angelina, 22
Garofalo, Fausto, 94
Gaucelin, Robert, 66
Ge'onim, 11
Gerard de Solo, 29, 30, 53
Gerbert of Aurillac (Pope Sylvester II), 39

Gerhard of Cremona, 39, 40, 49, 50
Gershon ben Salomon of Arles, 51
Gersonides (Levi ben Gershon), 50
Giovanni di Anagni, 69
Goitein, S. D., 58
Goldsmith, physician as, 131, 135
Gordon, Bernard, 27, 29, 50, 53
Graçian, 49
Grau i Monserrat, Manuel, 105
Greek, medical texts in, 39
Gui de Chauliac, 24, 53
Guild, doctors', 16
Guillelmo, Benjamin, of Urbino, 33–34
Guillem, Count of Montpellier, 27
Guilleré, Christian, 105

ha-Levi, Hayyim, 72, 94
ha-Levi, Judah, 41
ha-Levi, Samuel, 41
ha-Me'ati, Nathan ben Eli'ezer, 46–47, 49
Hamet of Valencia, 21
ha-Penini, Jeda'iah, 49, 50
al-Harizi, Judah, 41, 101
Hasdai, Bonsenior (Azday), 59
Hasdai ben Shaprut, 12, 58
Hava of Manosque, 109, 112, 131
Hebrew, medical texts in, 38–42, 49, 51, 53
Hillel ben Samuel of Verona, 46, 52
Hippocrates, 13, 42, 46
Hunayn ibn Ishāq, 36, 39

Ibn-al-Qifti, 12
Ibn al-Shaffar, 51
Ibn Zohr, 52
Immanuel of Rome, 47
Innocent VII, Pope, 94
Inquisition, 86
Insurance, medical. See Contracts, doctor-patient
Isaac, Master, 33
Isaac ben Abraham of Montpellier, 27
Isaac ha-Hazan ben Sid, 41
Isaac (Icach) Gabriel, 19
Isaac Judeus (Isaac ibn Sulaiman al Israili), 11–12, 36, 45, 58
Isaac of Annecy, Master, 114
Isaac of Carcassonne, 114–115

Isaac of Cremona, 68, 137
Isaac of Manosque, Master, 84
Isnard, Gaufré, 9–10
Italy, xi, 6; Jews in universities in, 32–35; licensing in, 19–20, 110; public health doctors in, 112, 114; remuneration in, 116–117
Itinerant doctors, 114–115

Jacme, Jean, 28–29, 53
Jacob ben Elia, 52
Jacob ben Joseph ha-Levi (Jacob of Alesto), 52
Jacob ben Machir, 11, 27–28, 42, 51, 52
Jacob de Villanova, 28
Jacobi, David, 82
Jacob Leon, 24
Jacob of Cremona, 138
Jacob of Milan, Master, 67–68
Jacquart, Danielle, 10
Jacqueline Felicie de Alamania, 20, 21, 111
Jāhiz, 12
Jaime de Limiaña 117, 118
James I, King of Aragon, 16
Jean, Archbishop of Toledo, 41–42
Jean of Saint Nicholas (Abraham of Bari), 86
Jekuthiel ben Salmon, 53
Johanna, Queen of Naples, 60
Johanna, Queen of Navarre, 65
John of Damascus, 121
John XXI, Pope (Petrus Hispanus), 9
John XXIII, Pope (Baldassare Cossa), 94
Jordí y González, Ramón, 58
Joseph ben Isaac ibn Bilkirish, 58
Joseph ben Joshua ha-Lorki, 49
Joseph (Josse) de Novis, 127, 136
Joseph ibn Zabara, 41, 86
Joseph Leon of Cavaillon, Master, 24
Joseph Moses de Çeret, 128
Joseph of Manosque, 131
Juan de Leon, Don, 3
Judah ben Moses, 40
Judah ben Salomon ha-Cohen ibn Matka, 51
Judah ben Saul Ibn Tibbon, 13, 41, 57
Judah Bonseniyor dez Cortal, 76

Judah ibn Wakar, 72
Judah (Jafuda) Bonsenior, of Catalonia, 41, 44
Judah Mosconi, Master, 67
Judah of Damascus, Master, 82
Judeus, ix
Judges, Jewish doctors as, 71–72
Judicial role of physicians, 3, 130, 132–133
Junec (Junez) Trigo of Saragossa, Master, 73, 74–75

Kalonymos ben Kalonymos of Arles, 24, 41, 47–48, 51, 101, 103, 128
Kaspi, Joseph ibn, 65
Kimhi, Joseph and David, 41
Kirchhoff, Hans Wilhelm, 85
Knighthood, for doctors, 69

Lagumina, Bartolomeo and Giuseppe, 16–17, 18, 26, 33
Landau, Rabbi Liwa, 121–122
Lanfranc, 24
Lateran Council: Fourth, 91; Second, 8
Latin, medical texts in, 39, 40, 43, 49, 52, 53
Laura de Digna, 109
Laurea, 32–33
Leal, Doña, 111
Legislation, against Jewish doctors, 91, 92–94
Lentilosus, Rufus, 86
Leon Joseph of Carcassonne, 30–31, 53
Leprosy, 4–5
Libraries, 10–11, 46, 36–55. See also Translations
Licensing, 14–22; as anti-Semitic, 93; apprenticeship-based, 19; in Aragon, 18; as control, 5, 20–22; education-based, 19–20; exam-based, 14, 15–16; experience-based, 19, 21, 110; limited/restricted, 20, 110; in Naples, 19–20, 110; via protomedicus, 18–19; in Sicily, 14–15, 16–17, 18; in Valencia, 20; of women, 110
Literature, doctors depicted in, 101–104
Luzzati, Michele, 126

McVaugh, Michael, 61
Magister, 5
Maimonides (Moshe ben Maimon), vii, 13, 41, 42, 46, 58
Malavolti, Mirko, 16
Malpractice, 79–85; in Aragon, 81; Jews discriminated against in, 83–85; penalties for, 80, 81, 82, 83, 84; verdicts of, appealed, 82–83; waivers, 129–130
Manosque: contracts in, 2; medical certificates in, 3–4; number of doctors in, x, 6, 105, 106–107, 108
Mantino, Jacob, 34
Manuelis, Angelo, 94
Maria, Queen of Aragon, 87–88
María Roca, Joseph, 65
Marseilles: medical certificates in, 4; number of doctors in, x, 6, 106, 107–108; private medical school in, 25; remuneration in, 116, 117
Martin V, Pope, 69, 70
Matheus Saducinus Judeus, 17
Matthias of Cremona, 137
Mayrona of Bayons, 20 21, 22
Mayrona of Manosque, 22, 109, 135
Medicus, ix, 5, 64, 69
Meir, Master Isaac, 59
Meir, Moses, 62
Mercadel, Isaac, 81
Meschulam ben Isaac, 27
Meshullam ben Jacob of Lunel, 41
Meyer, Etienne, 135
Meyerhof, Max, 12–13
Micheau, Françoise, 12
Miles, 69
Military duties, of physicians, 61–62
Millás Vallicrosa, José María, 40
Mira, 81, 83
Miret y Sans, Joachim, 58
Moneylending, 1, 141; by physicians, 135, 137–138
Monsoniego, Mordecai, 117
Montpellier: bibliography studied at, 36–37, 50; Jewish students allowed at, 27–31; Jewish students expelled from, 35; translations done at, 52, 53
Morcas, Isma'el, 20
Mordecai Astruc Abraham, 24
Moses of Palermo, 40
Moses ben Isaac ibn Waqar, 54

Moses ben Salomon of Salerno, 43
Moses Boaç, Master, 115
Moses Bonavogla, 26, 33, 64, 71, 76–
    77
Moses Bonsegnor, 23
Moses de Portal, 21
Moses de Roquemart, 94
Moses Gasendi, 73
Moses ibn Ardut of Huesca, 40
Moses ibn Tibbon, 42, 50
Moses of Rieti, 114
Moses of Spain, 33
Moses of Tivoli, 33, 35, 69
Münster, Ladislao, 16, 34
al-Muquaddasi, 12

Na Bellaire, 109
Na Pla, 109
Naples, licensing in, 19–20, 110
Na Regina, 81, 83
Nicholas IV, Pope, 94
Nicolo di Fava, 32
Nissim Gerondi (Gerundi), Rabbi,
    173–174 n.7
Notary, physician as, 135
Numbers of doctors, 1, 6–8, 100–
    118; in Aragon, 60–65, 105; in
    Manosque, x, 6, 105, 106–107,
    108; in Marseilles, x, 6, 106, 107–
    108; scarcity of, 6–8

Omār Tawil of Valencia, 18–19, 75, 138
Ophthalmology, 111
Orabuena, Joseph, 72

Padua, medical education at, 7, 35
Paris, medical examination at, 16
Patarinus, 52
Paul de Viterbo, 133
Pedro, King of Aragon, 61, 62, 63
Pedro Tenorio, Archbishop of
    Toledo, 94
Peter the Ceremonious, 55
Petrus Alphonsi (Moses), 40
Pharmacy, 88
Physician: -patient relationship, 119–
    139 (see also Contracts); vs.
    surgeon, ix
Pietro d'Alessandro, Master, 18
Plato of Tivoli, 40
Poisoning, alleged, 87–88
Political role, of physicians, 62–63,
    67–68, 69–70, 76–77, 140

Popes: give dispensation for Jews
    to treat Christians, 96–98; have
    Jewish physicians, 60, 70, 94
Portaleone, Guillelmo, 60
Privileges, granted to physicians, 70–
    77
Protomedicus, 18–19
Provence. See Manosque; Marseilles
Public health doctors, 2–3, 112–118;
    in France, 113–114; in Italy, 112,
    114; remuneration for, 113, 114–
    118; in Spain, 113

Rabbis, physicians as, 140
Rav major, 71–72
Raymond de la Sauvetat, 41
al-Razi (Razes), 13, 42, 43, 44, 50
Remuneration, 2, 5, 70–71, 131; in
    contract, 124, 125, 126; discrimina-
    tion in, 116–117; in Italy, 116–117;
    in Marseilles, 116, 117; from non-
    medical sources, 63–64; not paid,
    127–129; for public health doctors,
    113, 114–118; in Spain, 117–118;
    for translators, 42, 43–48
Richler, Benjamin, 49
Rimoch, Astruch, 24
Rimos, Moses, 86–87
Ríus Serra, José, 61
Robert the Wise, King of Naples,
    47
Roger II, King of Sicily, 14–15
Romano, David, 58, 59
Romano, Judah ben Moses ben
    Daniel, 52
Rosenthal, Franz, 107
Roth, Cecil, 25
Royalty, doctors for, 56–64
Rubió y Lluch, Antoni, 72

Sa'adiah, 41
Safe conduct, for physicians, 65–67
Sahon, Vital, 88
Salamonis, Benjamin (Guillelmo), 97
Salera, Ramon, 20
Salamon of Calatayud, 73
Salomen ben Moses of Melgueil, 52
Salomon ben Abraham ibn David, 11
Salomon de Matasia de Sabauducio,
    94
Salomone de Benaventura, 117, 138
Salomon Gerundini, 25
Salomon ibn Verga, 47

Salomon of Anagni, Master, 60, 76
Salomon of Castellón, Master, 114
Salomon of Cremona, 137
Salomon of Languedoc, Master, 127
Salomon of Salerno, 95
Salomon of Tudela, 65
Salvetus de Burgenovo, 24–25
Samuel de Valencia, 74
Samuel ibn Tibbon, 41, 42
Sandei, Felino, 96
Sara of Saint-Gilles, 24–25, 109–110
Sargusia, Abram, 125
Sassoferrato, Bartolo, 32–33
Sefer Asaph, 11
Sepher Hasidim, 123
Sefer-ha Yakar, 11
Sefer ha-Yosher, 84–85
Sexual misconduct, alleged, 88–90
Shem Tov ben Isaac of Tortosa, 27,
    44–45, 46, 79, 83–84, 121
Shem Tov of Leon, Master, 113
Sherira Ga'on, Rabbi, 11
Sheshet of Barcelona, 57
Sicily: anti-Semitic legislation in, 92–
    93; Jewish doctors in, 16–17; Jew-
    ish university in, 25–26; licensing
    in, 14–15, 16–17, 18; medical
    certificates in, 3–4
Las Siete Partidas, 87, 88
Signs, Jews had to wear, 71, 73–74,
    91
Simon of Genua, 45
Simonsohn, Shlomo, 89, 96
Slave trade, 4
Soranos of Ephesus, 53
Spain, xi, 57–58; medical certificates
    in, 3–4; public health doctors in,
    113; remuneration in, 117–118;
    scarcity of doctors in, 6–7
Steinschneider, Moritz, 43, 49, 52
Stouff, Louis, 106, 126

Taddeo of Parma, 37
Talmud, 11
Tam, Rabbi Jacob, 122
Taurosii, Master Joseph, 115
Teicher, J. L., 52
Theodoric, Bishop of Bari and
    Ravenna, 9
Tibbon dynasty. See Anatoli, Jacob;
    Jacobben Machir; Judah ibn
    Tibbon; Moses ibn Tibbon;
    Samuel ibn Tibbon

Titles, given to physicians, ix, 5, 55,
    59–60, 64, 69, 94, 109
Todrosi, Isaac, 28–29
Tornamira, Jean de, 28–29, 30, 31,
    53
Translations (of medical texts): in
    Arabic, 39–40, 41, 43, 52, 57; by
    Arnold of Villanova, 52, 53; of
    auxiliary sciences, 50; of Averroës,
    42, 47; of Avicenna, 47, 48–50; of
    Galen, 42, 46, 47, 52; generations
    required for, 45, 46–47; in Greek,
    39; into Hebrew, 38–42, 49, 51,
    53; Jewish doctors denied access
    to, 53; in Latin, 39, 40, 43, 49, 52,
    53; at Montpellier, 52, 53; remun-
    eration for, 42, 43–48; of al-
    Zahrawi, 44–47
Treves, synod of, 91

Valencia: examination in, 18–19;
    licensing in, 20
Vidal, Abulbaça, 138
Vincent, Pierre, 135
Viridimura, 109
Vitale de Salomone, 117
Vitalis, 6
Vitalis, Bonsenior, 94, 95
Vitalis Amelhuti, 25
Vitalis Habib, 20
Vitalis of Carpentras, Master, 115
Vitalis of Marseilles, Master, 127
Vitalis Salves, 80–81

Wickersheimer, Ernst, 10, 27
Witch-hunts, 86
Women physicians, 100, 109–112,
    131, 135; discriminated against,
    20, 21–22, 27; education for, 27,
    109–110; restricted licenses for,
    110; specialties of, 111; titles for,
    109; treat women patients, 110–
    111

Yehuda ben Salomon (Ibn Mosca),
    41
Yeshiva, 22–23
Yeshu'ah, Joseph Gallouf, 23

al-Zahrawi, 44–47, 79
Zalman, Rabbi of Sankt Goar, 121–
    122
Zerahiah ben Shealtiel Hen, 49

Designer: U.C. Press Staff
Compositor: Asco Trade Typesetting, Ltd.
Text: 10/12 Times Roman
Display: Goudy Bold
Printer: Braun-Brumfield, Inc.
Binder: Braun-Brumfield, Inc.

Reinventing Anarchy

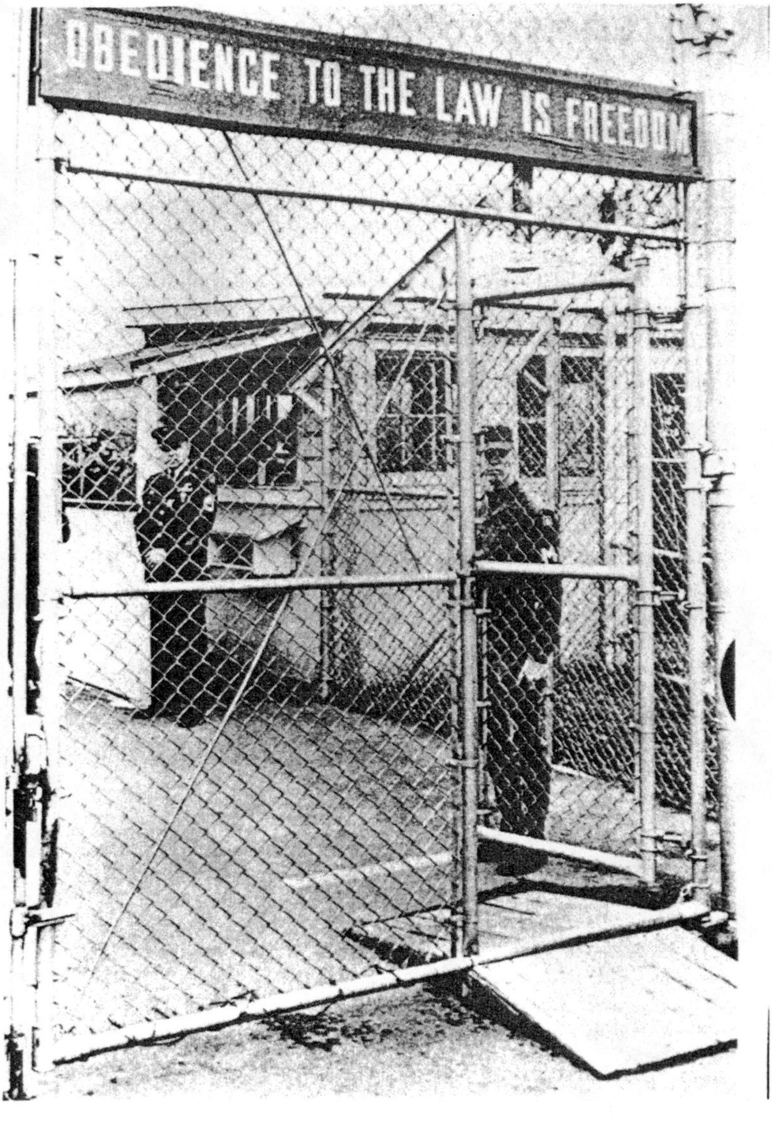
OBEDIENCE TO THE LAW IS FREEDOM

Reinventing Anarchy

What are anarchists thinking
these days?

Edited by

Howard J. Ehrlich
Carol Ehrlich
David DeLeon
Glenda Morris

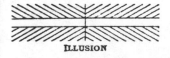

ILLUSION

Routledge & Kegan Paul
London, Boston and Henley

First published in 1979
by Routledge & Kegan Paul Ltd
39 Store Street, London WC1E 7DD,
Broadway House, Newtown Road,
Henley-on-Thames, Oxon RG9 1EN and
9 Park Street, Boston, Mass. 02108, USA
Set in Press Roman by
Hope Services, Abingdon
and printed in Great Britain by
Lowe & Brydone Ltd
Thetford, Norfolk

British Library Cataloguing in Publication Data

Reinventing anarchy.

1. Anarchism and anarchists – Addresses, essays, lectures
I. Ehrlich, Howard J
335'.83'08   HX833   78-41022

ISBN 0 7100 0128 2

Contents

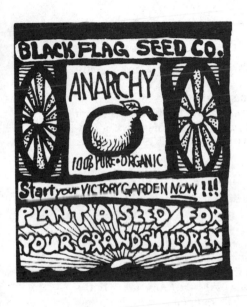

Introduction   1

The Editors   7

Part One What is anarchism?   11

1   *The editors*: Questions and answers about anarchism   13
2   *Fred Woodworth*: Anarchism   29
3   *Nicolas Walter*: About anarchism   42

Contents

Part Two The state and social organization   65

Introduction   67
4   *David DeLeon*: Anarchism on the origins and functions of the state: some basic notes   70
5   *Gar Alperovitz*: Towards a decentralist commonwealth   84
6   *Howard J. Ehrlich*: Anarchism and formal organizations – some notes on the sociological study of organizations from an anarchist perspective   96

Part Three Criticisms of the left: old and new   113

Introduction   115
7   *Radical Decentralist Project*: Toward a post-scarcity society: the American perspective and SDS   120
8   *Point-Blank!*:The storms of youth   127
9   *David Thoreau Wieck*: The negativity of anarchism   138
10   *C. George Benello*: Anarchism and Marxism: a confrontation of traditions   156
11   Why the black flag?   172

Part Four The liberation of self   175

Introduction   177
12   *Kingsley Widmer*: Three times around the track: how American workouts helped me become an anarchist   182
13   *Diane di Prima*: Revolutionary letter no. 1   193
14   *Situationist students at Strasbourg University*: On the poverty of student life (Once upon a time the universities were respected)   194
15   *Robert Cooperstein*: The production and consumption of humans   206
16   *Jay Amrod and Lev Chernyi*: Beyond character and morality: toward transparent communications and coherent organization   209
17   *David Porter*: Revolutionary realization: the motivational energy   214
18   *Peggy Kornegger*: red emma   229

Part Five Anarcha-feminism   231

   Introduction   233
19 *Peggy Kornegger*: Anarchism: the feminist connection   237
20 *Champaign-Urbana SRAF*: For a general contestation!   250
21 *Siren*: Who we are: the anarcho-feminist manifesto 251
22 *Marian Leighton*: Anarcho-feminism   253
23 *Carol Ehrlich*: Socialism, anarchism, and feminism 259
24 *Tuli Kupferberg*: Newspoem   278

Part Six The liberation of labor   281

   Introduction   283
25 *John Zerzan*: Organized labor versus 'the revolt against
   work': the critical contest   285
26 *Diane di Prima*: Revolutionary letter no. 19   302
27 *David DeLeon*: For democracy where we work: a
   rationale for social self-management   304

Part Seven Reinventing anarchist tactics   325

   Introduction   327
28 *David Wieck*: The habit of direct action   331
29 *Dick Lourie*: Civics I: Nothing Fancy   334
30 *Judith Malina*: Anarchists and the pro-hierarchical left 335
31 *Anti-Mass*: Anti-mass – methods of organization for
   collectives   342
32 *Howard J. Ehrlich*: The logic of alternative institutions 346
33 *Murray Rosenblith*: Surrounded by acres of clams   347
34 *Anon*: Paris 1968   360
35 *HJE*: Notes and queries of an anarchist critic   361
36 Fear and powerlessness   365
37 Letter from the mayor   368

TUMBLER

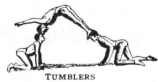

TUMBLERS

Introduction

Reinventing anarchy

In this book we offer a new synthesis of anarchist ideas. We have inter-twined statements of theory and action, and we have tried to present statements that are models of anarchist and intellectual inquiry. We think we have come closer than anyone, or any collection, to articulating a theory of social anarchism. The elements are almost all here. Through our synthesis we have generated a new paradigm – a new way of looking at anarchism and the world.

Anarchism is a theory of society that embodies both a moral philos-ophy and a guide to everyday behavior. How do we know we are right? We don't. Is there, after all, any theory of human behavior that one can declare to be true in an absolutist sense? The call for certainty is for the immature or the insecure.

As theorists, however, we are ruthlessly instrumental. Our paradigm 'works' if it helps you, and us, better comprehend the world we live in. It works if it extends the range of our comprehension and the precision of our knowledge. It works, too, if it can lead us to know what is false about other claims to knowledge. Finally, our theory works if it leads us to revolutionary projects that work. If a theory cannot be imple-mented in practice, it is not a good theory.

Our commitment as anarchists has its fundamental basis in two beliefs. We believe that true social justice is possible, but possible only in an anarchist society. (The outlines of that society are the subject of the selections by Woodworth, Walter and ourselves that follow.) We also believe that our engagement in the revolutionary struggle to bring about anarchism is inescapable. It is not only that we perceive that being engaged in that struggle brings us more dignity, but we cannot be anarchists unless we are so engaged. Anarchism is not just a political philosophy or social theory; it is a matter of living.

Revolution as process

Since the Russian Revolution of October 1917, Marxism–Leninism has dominated revolutionary theory. The primary concern of Marxism has been the criticism of social–economic relations. The theory points to what is wrong or false, to what you can *not* do. It is a crucial defect of that theory, however, that it provides little direction for what you should do.

Marxist–Leninist arguments are based on the premise that political systems have purely economic foundations. By that profound misunderstanding of society, the Marxist Left has confused the seizure of state power with genuine revolutionary change. Richard Gombin writes in his book, *The Origins of Modern Leftism* (that which he calls 'leftism' we would call social anarchism):

> In the last analysis, Marx emerges as the theoretician of the bourgeois revolution pushed to the limits of its potentialities. The whole of the Leninist theory of organization, its very conception of revolution as the seizure of political power at the summit, bears all the marks of bourgeois thought. To a leftist, it is therefore not surprising that the Russian Revolution should have resulted in a State-capitalist régime reproducing a more refined and more concentrated version of the system of class domination.
>
> The leftist critique therefore repudiates all the revolutions of the twentieth century, or rather denies them the label 'socialist'; it sees in them the last of the bourgeois revolutions.

For the social anarchist, revolution is a process, not an event. It is not an historical inevitability, nor is it a political moment of history. The state is not destroyed by a revolutionary upheaval. As Gustav Landauer, a German anarchist, wrote in 1910,

> The State is a condition, a certain relationship among human beings . . . we destroy it by contracting other relationships, by behaving differently toward one another . . . . We are the State, and we shall continue to be the State until we have created the institutions that form a real community and society.

The critique of everyday lives

The critique of the capitalist state must also be transformed into a critique of ourselves. Capitalism and the state are genuine social structures, but like most matters of social structure they have also been

internalized. In that sense, we are the state. It exists in our minds, and we reproduce it in our day-to-day existence. The banalities of everyday life, the meaninglessness of most work, our profound isolation from others, and our being treated (and treating others) as objects – these are not byproducts of capitalism: they are key mechanisms of social control.

Social anarchism begins with the transformation of our everyday lives. In Parts Four and Six, on the 'liberation of self' and the 'liberation of work,' we will talk concretely about this transformation. In Part Seven, on anarchist tactics, we will present very specific proposals for building anarchist institutions.

We are all products of a particular society, and are bound by it – perhaps more than we like to admit. Nevertheless, we must live its negation. We must refuse to become prisoners of its standards of reality and practicality. Our task, as the old anarchist slogan goes, is to 'build the new society in the vacant lots of the old.' Or, as Marge Piercy puts it in her poem, *Rough Times*, 'We are trying to live as if we were an experiment conducted by the future.'

The habits of freedom

You can set people loose from the constraints of oppressive institutions, but even unlocking prison doors does not automatically free them. A free individual is competent, self-confident, autonomous. Freedom is a habit, in the old-fashioned sense of habits. It takes years of practice.

People are not born free; the human child has a long period of helplessness and dependency. The totality of institutional arrangements of modern societies operates to socialize children and young adults to submissiveness to, and even fear of, authority. Independence training and the teaching of critical thought are more often slogans than commonplace occurrences. Nonconformity is risky, and it often wrenches people from comfortable circles of family and friends. Deviants are often treated as enemies of the state – and in a sense, they are.

None of us was born free, and almost all of us need to unlearn the lethal thoughtways that were seared into our heads. Anarchy takes practice: most people fear freedom and cannot cope with it. The need for leadership is not human nature, but human learning. The incapacity of many people to cope with the world they live in is not a problem of basic inabilities, but a problem of trained incompetence.

Central to anarchist behaviour is the principle of consistency between means and ends. To build a nonviolent society, people must learn how to act today in nonviolent relation to others. To build a non-hierarchical

3

society, people must learn how to work collectively. To build a society free of racism and sexism, people must practice equalitarian relations. To build a free society, it is necessary that people learn the habits of freedom in the process of building.

The limiting conditions

We do not know the limiting conditions of anarchy. As social anarchists we do know that, any time people come together to live or work, their social organization sets some limits on their behavior. All social organization entails some conflict between individual autonomy and social control. We believe that such conflict is inescapable, but that there may be some ascertainable level of 'creative conflict.' At that level we can build organizations that maximize the nurturance of people, their creativity and autonomy.

A realistic anarchist manifesto will be drafted as a network of contingencies. There are no lists of contradictions or ordering of these as primary and secondary; crises are not automatic outcomes of political economy; and there is no historical inevitability. Anarchist collectives will create their own forms of struggle as anarchy and the conflicts with agents of the state grow.

The anarchist movement will be its own laboratory. Ken Knabb, an American 'Situationist' writing in a 1974 pamphlet in his, *Bureau of Public Secrets* series, puts the issue cogently.

> Its own failures are the lodes which contain the richest ore. Its first task is always to expose its own poverties, which will be continually present, whether in the form of simple lapses into the dominant poverties of the world it combats or the new poverties which its very successes create for itself . . . . What we must aim at is to fail clearly, each time, over and over . . . . Be cruel with your past and those who would keep you there.

This anthology

We began talking about the need for a good collection of anarchist materials in early 1973. Not only did we feel that we personally weren't ready for the undertaking; we also felt that there simply weren't enough good contemporary materials. We were not satisfied with earlier anthologies that excerpted long-dead anarchist writers or mixed together liberals and libertarians, socialists and capitalists. And we certainly did not want detached discourses on the nature of authority or political

events that the writer studied at a safe distance. We wanted to bring together the works of living, working anarchists.

By the spring of 1976, we not only felt more secure in our own knowledge, but we had now accumulated an extraordinary collection of anarchist materials. We also came to the realization that some topics we would have to write about ourselves, and that some other important topics would have to go uncovered since anarchists today weren't writing about them, or weren't writing very carefully about them.

In selecting articles we had several explicit criteria. First of all, the articles had to be in English. This is simply because it is the only language that the four of us, as editors, are fully comfortable with. Second, the materials had to be current. Third, we included only articles that were reasonably well written and that offered new ideas or a new synthesis of old ideas. Fourth, fifth, sixth and seventh: we wanted mainly new materials, by practicing anarchists, by anarchists whose orientation was social (as opposed to individualist), and by anarchists who addressed themselves to the political and social questions that people are asking today. We had no interest, for example, in a new discussion of the Paris Commune or the Kronstadt uprising.

We think that we were quite successful in satisfying those criteria. We worked hard with some writers, abridged or excerpted the lengthy essays of others, and collected a diversity of materials which are stimulating and new. Ten of our selections have not been published before and perhaps all but three could not be found in the average public or even college library. All but one of the articles are less than ten years old. Finally, we also included examples of anarchist leaflets as well as the kinds of graphic art that decorates anarchist publications.

In the course of collecting materials, we discovered a number of interesting things about contemporary anarchism. We were surprised to see how much sexist language forms still pervade anarchist writings. We should no longer overlook that coercive component of our language. It is certainly not good anarchist practice. To talk about 'mankind' when one means women and men or to use 'he' to mean he or she perpetuates an insidious form of male domination. Sexism in language can be easily avoided.

We were disturbed also by the almost total absence of women contributors outside the section on feminism. Anarchism has not escaped the cultural ravages of sexism. But while our section on anarcha-feminism is quite strong, we found nothing to offer on racism. Now, neither racism nor sexism nor any other artificial division of humankind has any place in an anarchist society. Doubtless, all social anarchists would agree. Although very little racism or ethnic prejudice can be found in anarchist writings, just the same there have been very few analyses of this problem from an anarchist perspective.

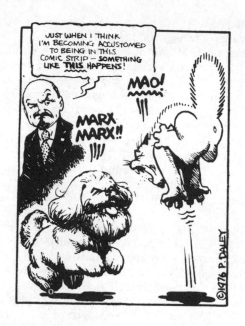

There are also a number of other critical issues that are not represented by a single essay in this collection. There is nothing here on the role of popular culture; there is nothing on ecology and technology; there is nothing on economics; and there is nothing on anarchist education. We mention these in particular because we looked hard to fill those vacancies. Our search reminded us of Francisco Ferrer's attempt to stock his Modern School's library with books appropriate to his view of libertarian education. He opened the school with an empty library. While our book is full, and all of these issues are in fact touched on in various essays, we should be aware that these are important gaps in the development of anarchism. Also missing are selections from two major anarchist writers, Colin Ward and Murray Bookchin. Ward's book, *Anarchy in Action*, and Bookchin's collected essays in his *Post-Scarcity Anarchism* are important anarchist works of this decade.

The Editors

We solicited from all of our contributors a brief statement about themselves. Personally we were interested and assumed you would be too. Having collected these capsule biographies (they appear at the end of each selection), we realized that we could do no less for ourselves.

Howard J. Ehrlich: I don't know what to write about myself briefly. There'd be no problem if I could take a page or five or six. I enjoy producing political radio programs; I like to write and to teach. I like to explore cities, eating, cooking, wine.

I started out as a bright, wiseguy, New York Jewish kid. I was a difficult angry adolescent iconoclast. I matriculated from the New Deal to the New Left – dodging the draft during the Korean War and fighting the government during the Vietnam War. I began to explore Left alternatives partly by accident and partly through my growing dissatisfaction with the elitism, authoritarianism, and anti-intellectualism of American Left groups. The process of discovering I was a 'radical' was very painful. My discovery of anarchism several years later was very gratifying.

I made my way through two graduate schools selling parakeets and ladies' shoes. In the course of schooling I was certified as a social psychologist and sociologist. I eventually became a professor; I soon became a professor drop-out. I like that better.

Carol Ehrlich was born in Missouri and until moving to Baltimore spent most of her life in assorted Midwestern cities in the United States. She came of age politically in Iowa City, Iowa, in the late 1960s, and became active in various radical feminist and non-sectarian Left groups. Since 1971 she has been on the faculty of the American Studies Department at the University of Maryland Baltimore County, where she teaches courses on feminism and social change. She continues to explore the connections between anarchism and radical feminism.

David DeLeon: I was born and 'raised' in a peasant village on the

Siberian plains of North Dakota, semi-civilized within the sylvan confines of the University of Iowa, and corrupted by living in the exotic
East. Over the years, I have traversed the ideological spectrum, being a
Young Republican, a militant member of a right-wing youth group (the
Young Americans for Freedom), a campaign worker for Nelson Rockefeller and Eugene McCarthy, an enthusiastic communard in several
collectives, a counselor for RESIST and the American Friends Service
Committee, and a member of SDS, the Peace and Freedom Party and
the New University Conference. Much of that, of course, was in the
past, when I was a firebreathing young fanatic. Now I am an older and
cooler fanatic . . . an aging delinquent. Part of my work has been devoted
to making sense of this history, and its cultural context, in my book on
The American as Anarchist; Reflections on Indigenous Radicalism
(Baltimore and London, Johns Hopkins University Press, 1978).

Glenda Morris has served time in a family, several colleges and a civilian-
military bureaucracy. She has waitressed, been a union organizer, and a
maker of neurophysiological microelectrodes. She has worked in five
collectively managed enterprises in Baltimore – a feminist newsletter, a
food co-op, a research group, a radio collective, and an alternative
school for adults. At the school she has taught 'anarchism for beginners'
and 'simplified breadbaking.' Out of that course, she wrote and published *The Different Bread Book*. She is particularly interested in the
problems of economic survival in and of alternative organizations, as
well as in the connections between anarchism and feminism.

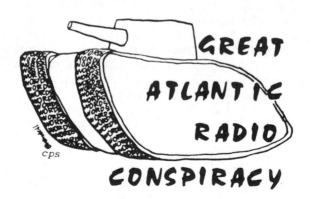

The four editors are members of the Great Atlantic Radio Conspiracy.
Since 1972 the Conspiracy has been producing audio-programs for
radio broadcast, libraries, teachers and studygroups. We are organized

as an anti-profit work collective. Each week Conspiracy regulars and irregulars produce a thirty-minute program – a combination of script, interviews and music. Some programs are in-depth analyses of particular topics, such as our program on abortion or our program on Patuxent (an especially grim and savage prison). Other programs, like 'The Politics of Psychosurgery,' combine dramatization with a documentary format. Still others, such as 'The Poetry of Work' and 'Recording the Music of Struggle,' present the poetry and music of radical artists. We have produced programs de-mystifying holidays such as Christmas and Mother's Day, and we have commemorated Wounded Knee and the centennial of Bakunin.

We sell our taped programs on reel or cassette as close to cost as we can. We have available an annotated catalog.

9

Part One

What is anarchism?

1 Questions and answers about anarchism

The editors

1 How would an anarchist revolution come about?

For social anarchists revolution is a process, a process leading to the total deflation of state authority. That process entails self- and collective education and the building of alternative institutions as mechanisms of survival, of training and as models of a new society. Continuing parts of that process are repeated symbolic protests and direct assaults on ruling-class institutions.

As more and more people regard the anarchist alternatives as preferable to the status quo, state power begins to be deflated. When the state can no longer maintain the confidence of substantial segments of the population, its agents will have to rely increasingly on the mobilization of the police and the military. Of course, that increase in force has multiple possible outcomes, ranging from the total repression of the Left to the further leftward mobilization of the population that regards this increased use of force illegitimate.

Our scenario does not rule out guerrilla warfare and armed struggle. But in the United States, for example, with its mammoth police apparatus, extensive files and surveillance of radicals, and its over 3,600 underground 'emergency operating centers' for ruling-class and military retreats, the idea of a *primarily* military revolution is an atavistic Marxist fantasy.

So where do we go from here? The next act in the revolutionary drama remains to be written. Drawing a battle plan today seems pointless. The overthrow of the state – the building of anarchist societies – will be an overwhelming majoritarian act. It cannot be otherwise. When, say, 5-10 per cent of the population identify themselves as anarchists, it is our guess that there would be a range of contingencies available that we could not possibly anticipate today.

2 Who will make the anarchist revolution?

Everyone. Every day in their daily lives.

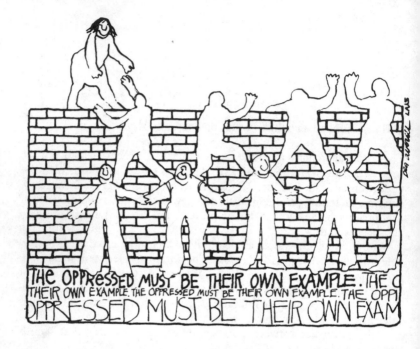

3 How can an anarchist society prevent the development of informal elites, new bureaucracies and a reconcentration of power?

There is nothing integral to the nature of human social organization that makes hierarchy, centralization and elitism inescapable. These organizational forms persist, in part because they serve the interests of those at the top. They persist, too, because we have learned to accept roles of leadership and followership; we have come to define hierarchy as necessary, and centralization as efficient. All of this is to say that we learned the ideological justifications for elite organizational forms quite well.

We could dismiss the question by pointing out that social motivations to power, elites and elitism and bureaucracy would not exist in an anarchist society. The question should not be dismissed, however, when we talk about building an anarchist society in the shell of another. In

such a context we will inevitably be struggling against the life-denying values of our socialization. Hierarchy, dominance and submission, repression and power – these are facts of everyday life. Revolution is a process, and even the eradication of coercive institutions will not automatically create a liberatory society. We create that society by building new institutions, by changing the character of our social relationships, by changing ourselves – and throughout that process by changing the distribution of power in society. It is by the constant building of new forms of organization, by the continual critical evaluation of our successes and failures, that we prevent old ideas and old forms of organization from re-emerging.

If we cannot begin this revolutionary project here and now, then we cannot make a revolution.

4 How will decisions be made? by consensus? by majority?

Groups will make decisions by consensus because majority rule is unacceptable for people who think that everyone should run his or her own life. Decision-making by majority rule means that the minority voluntarily gives up control over the policies that affect them.

To operate by consensus, groups will discuss an issue until it is resolved to the satisfaction of everyone. This doesn't mean that there's only one way of doing things. People must accept that many ways can coexist. They also must realize that there can be multiple policies on most issues with people free to choose which policy they want.

The principle of consensus can be effective because membership in a community is voluntary and because that membership entails agreements on its basic goals and values.

The workings of consensual decisions have many advantages. It is the only way to prevent a permanent minority from developing. It takes into consideration the strength of feelings. It is more efficient for group action because people are genuinely involved in achieving consensus and are therefore more likely to act on their decisions.

One of the things people have difficulty understanding about group consensus is that it does take into account the strength of feelings and differences in perspectives of all of the people involved. In a social anarchist meeting the process of decision-making is as important as the outcome itself.

Of course, people will have to learn to recognize what they want and to express their desires in a constructive way. If they do not know what they want a false consensus develops because people are just trying to go along with the group so as not to make trouble. If decisions are reached this way people remain unhappy about the outcome; their

participation may drop to a low level and they may ultimately feel that they have to leave the group.

5 How can people be motivated to participate in decisions that affect them if they don't want to participate?

In the kinds of societies in which we live now, this is a pseudo-question. People are managed; they are rarely asked to participate. The unmotivated citizen of the capitalist/socialist state has sized up the situation correctly, and has concluded that non-participation is the only realistic choice.

What about an anarchist community, where everyone would have genuine control over his or her life? We would assume that non-participants would be few – but if they existed, we would have to ask why. This is no idle question: if it wished to survive, an anarchist community would have to solve this problem. If it failed to do so, the community would be on the road back to social inequality. And it would no longer be anarchist.

There are two reasons why a person might not participate in making decisions. The first would be lack of time. But if a person is too busy, then either s/he has voluntarily taken on too much work, or the others are shirking. In neither case is the community functioning on genuine social anarchist principles.

The second reason is quite different. Non-participation would be due not to working too much out of a misplaced sense of priorities, but to failure to see the linkage between personal autonomy and community functioning. Some people may feel that community decision-making is beneath them; this 'star' mentality needs to be effectively challenged every time it occurs. Others may genuinely believe that the community affords them everything they need for their physical and psychological wellbeing, so they are perfectly happy letting others make the decisions. Still others may feel alienated, or lack confidence in their ability to make competent decisions.

All of these people are handicapped by 'old ideas.' These are well suited to a stratified society in which a few run the lives of everyone, but they are severely damaging to an anarchist community. People who think in these ways need loving support from others, a feeling of being an essential part of the community, and gentle (but firm) pressure to participate. This may take time, but it can be done.

6 When does a community become too large to operate with direct participation by everyone? Is a system of representation ever justified?

We do not really know the maximum or optimum size of a community that would still allow effective participation, but there are numerous examples of communities, some as large as 8,000 people, where all the people actively participated in self-government. For example, during the Spanish Revolution self-governed villages all over Spain formed into federations to co-ordinate decisions affecting all of them. In Denmark in 1971 about 600 people occupied an army camp and set up a viable functioning community that not only lasted for years but was able to defend itself nonviolently from attacks by the government.

In these examples everyone made decisions about the goals of the community and how to achieve them. Then the people who were actually doing the particular tasks were able to work in their own way.

In a decentralized society that is composed of many communities the lines of communication go in multiple directions. Two-way television and other technological improvements make direct democracy possible in larger groups, but there will probably still be times when representatives will be necessary. Selection procedures for these representatives would no doubt vary. Sometimes representatives could be drawn by lot and other times on the basis of task-specific skills or abilities.

The system of representation, however, must meet certain criteria. Representatives must come from the group of people whom they represent and they must be accountable to that group. To make them accountable, representatives should be assigned for a brief period of time or to do a specific task. In an anarchist society nobody could make a career of 'politics.' The role of representative could be rotated among members of the community. All important decisions would be made by the group as a whole; the representatives would just communicate the decisions of their group to the larger group. Representatives must also be subject to immediate recall.

The decisions about what functions best for one community or one group will have to be made by that group at the time depending upon the circumstances. But there is every reason to believe that people can effectively participate in managing their own lives.

7 Will there still be experts and specialization? If so, how will experts be trained? How will we know they are competent? Can we have experts in a non-hierarchical society?

Differences in skill and knowledge will continue to exist. Such differences are compatible with a free and egalitarian society. People may also want to develop their abilities in their own way. And this too is compatible with social anarchism.

Much of the work that is now done by specialists can be learned in

a relatively short time so that it could be done by nearly everyone. One problem with specialists in our society is that they restrain the number of people who are trained. Obviously there is some work, such as surgery or architecture, that requires a high degree of skill acquired through lengthy training. No one wants to be operated on by someone who has only two weeks of training, and few people would feel comfortable in a five-story building assembled without blueprints. The real problem becomes training specialists who will be accountable to the people they serve. We want co-operation between specialist and 'client,' not solidarity among specialists. To ensure this there could be no positions of privilege for specialists, and they must be committed to sharing their knowledge with everyone.

In a decentralized or small society, judging the competence of someone whose labor is highly visible, such as a carpenter, is not difficult. In somewhat more complex cases, say in judging the competence of a surgeon, one possibility is to have the people who work with the surgeon along with those from the community be the judge of the quality of work.

Expertise and non-hierarchy can co-exist only if specialization does not convey special privileges; only if people who are experts do not monopolize or control resources or information; and only if people are committed to co-operative and collective work rather than destructive competition.

8 Who will do the dirty work?

We all will. In an anarchist community, people wouldn't categorize work as 'dirty' or 'clean,' as 'white-collar' or 'blue-collar.' That way of thinking can exist only in a class-stratified society – one that teaches its members that maintenance tasks are undignified, demeaning, and to be avoided if possible. For anarchists, all socially useful work has dignity, and everyone would co-operate to sustain the community at a mutually agreed-upon level of health, comfort and beauty. Those who refuse to collect the garbage, clean streets and buildings, trim the grass, provide a clean water supply and so on would be acting in a most irresponsible fashion. It they continued to refuse, they would be asked to leave.

Does this seem coercive? A successfully self-governed community must be comprised of people who voluntarily live and work together, who agree on the necessary tasks, and who have the self-discipline to carry out their share of these tasks (no more and no less). Those who refuse are coercing others; they are implicitly saying that *their* time is to be spent doing more important things; that *they* are above such menial tasks. In an anarchist community no one is 'above' anyone else;

no one is more important than anyone else. To think so will destroy both equality and freedom.

One of the things that makes 'dirty' work so onerous is that only some people do it, and they work at it full-time. Very few maintenance tasks would seem totally awful if they were rotated, and each person knew s/he would be doing it for a short period of time. Short work periods on the garbage truck, or cleaning public bathrooms, or fertilizing fields would seem – well, not *fun* of course (anarchists aren't stupid) – but would be tolerable if each person knew they would end soon.

9 Will any people have more money and property than others? Who will control the means of production and how will profits be distributed?

In an anarchist society everyone will have an equal right to the basic liberties and material goods, which is consistent with a similar right for others. People would, of course, maintain personal possessions, but we would expect that the matter of the accumulation of property and property rights would be very different. Certainly the meaning of money and property would be quite different in an egalitarian and non-hierarchical society.

It is hard to conceive of a serious alternative to a market economy. However, unlike the capitalist market place, the anarchist economy would not be based on the maximization of control and profit. Therefore, there would be no need to monopolize resources, expand markets or create useless products and/or consumer demands. Worker and community control of the workplace would be the organizational form for regulating productivity and profits in keeping with the needs of the community.

While an anarchist economic theory remains to be written, its theorems will all have to be derived from principles of social justice, from principles that claim the maximum values of freedom and equality for all people.

10 Aren't anarchists ignoring the complexity of urban life? Aren't they rejecting technology and industrial development? Don't they really want to go back to a simpler society?

Any anarchists who ignore the complexities of modern urban–industrial societies are wrong. A return to a 'simpler' society' is a fantasy of escapists, not of persons seriously committed to building a new society.

The underlying issue for us as social anarchists is the determination of the optimum size for urban settlements. The equation for an optimum

size would doubtless have to balance factors of self-sufficiency, self-governance and the minimizing of damage to the ecosystem.

The related technological problems must be taken seriously by all anarchists. Can we satisfy our energy requirements with technologies that do minimal environmental damage? Can we develop a technology that can be comprehended by most people? Can we develop a technology that is a genuine substitute for human labor? The answer to these questions is yes. The technology and knowledge are already here: the issue is their implementation.

The result of implementing such technological changes and building self-governing and relatively self-sufficient communities would probably bring about substantial differences in urban settlements. We suspect that these differences would yield even more 'complex' urban arrangements than we now have. We suspect, too, that they would result in more genuinely humane cities.

11 How will an anarchist society meet the threat of foreign invasion?

Paradoxically, the more successfully it meets the threat of armed force, the more likely it is to move away from anarchist principles. War always seems to turn relatively free and open societies into repressive ones. Why? Because war is irrational: it fosters fear and hopelessness in the gentle; it brings out aggression, hatred and brutality in the truculent; it destroys the balance between people and nature; it shrinks the sense of community down to one's immediately endangered group; and under conditions of starvation and deprivation it pits neighbor against neighbor in the fight for survival. If a besieged anarchist community did successfully resist foreign invasion, then it should immediately work to reestablish the interrelationships of trust, mutual aid, equality and freedom that have probably been damaged. 'War is the health of the state;' but it can be a fatal disease for an anarchist community.

If war came, however, how would the society organize to defend itself? Let us assume that the anarchist federation of North America is invaded by troops of the Chinese, Swedish, Saudi Arabian or Brazilian government. What would happen? There would be no state apparatus to seize; instead, the invaders would have to conquer a network of small communities, one by one. There would be no single army to defeat, but an entire, armed population. The people would challenge the invasion with resistance – strikes, psychological warfare, and non-co-operation – as well as with guerrilla tactics and larger armed actions. Under these circumstances, it is unlikely that the invaders would conquer the federation.

12 What about crime?

Much of what is now defined as crime would no longer exist. The communalization of property and an ethic of mutual aid would reduce both the necessity and the motivation for property crimes. Crimes against people seem more complex, but we reject the idea that they are rooted in 'original sin' or 'human nature.' To the degree that such crimes stem from societally based disorders of personality, we can only anticipate that their incidence – as well as their actual form – would be radically altered.

In a social anarchist society, crime would be defined solely as an act harmful to the liberties of others. It would not be a crime to be different from other people, but it would be a crime to harm someone. Such hostile acts against the community could be prevented, above all, by inculcating a respect for the dignity of each person. Anarchist values would be reinforced with the strongest of human bonds, those of affection and self-respect.

Remaining crimes would not be administered by masses of lawyers, police and judges; and criminals would not be tossed into prisons, which Kropotkin once labeled 'universities of crime.' Common law and regularly rotated juries could decide whether a particular act was a crime, and could criticize, censure, ostracize or even banish the criminal. However, in most cases we anticipate that criminals would be placed in the care and guidance of members of the community.

13 How shall public health issues be handled?

Public health issues would be handled like all other issues. This means that decisions about inoculations and other health issues would be made at the local level by the people who would be affected by the decision. This would result in a very different type of health care. Health care workers would be members of the community where they worked. Their function would be to provide day-to-day care and advice to people on how to remain healthy. People would have a chance to talk frequently with these workers and would know that they were really concerned about health and not about making money or gaining status in the community.

If there were a threatened epidemic of some deadly flu and a vaccine were developed the people in the community would be able to get together to discuss the risks and benefits of the inoculations. Once the group decided that inoculations would benefit the community they would try to persuade everyone to be inoculated because the more people who were protected the less likelihood there would be of an

epidemic. If there were a clear case of people being a danger to the health of the entire community then they would be asked to make a choice between being vaccinated and remaining in the community, or leaving to find another group that was more compatible.

14 There are times when the state takes care of the sick and elderly, or protects individuals against coercion (for example, children brutalized by parents; blacks attacked by whites). If the state disappears, who will take over these functions?

People who look at the world this way believe that there are only two possibilities: either there is state regulation and an orderly society, or there is a stateless chaos in which life is nasty, brutish and short. In fact, even when the state functions in a benevolent or protective manner, it is capricious: sometimes it helps the helpless; other times it doesn't. Sometimes social welfare workers remove a child from a vicious environment – and other times the child is left at home, perhaps to be further brutalized, even killed. Sometimes the state protects the civil rights of oppressed minorities; other times it ignores these rights, or even joins in the persecution. We cannot count on the state to do anything to protect us. It is, after all, the major task of the agents of the state to protect the distribution of power. Social justice is a secondary concern.

In fact, we can only count on ourselves, or on those with whom we are freely associated in community. This means that helping functions will be performed by those groups that have always done them, with or without the state: voluntary associations. However, in an anarchist community, the need for such services will be less frequent. For example, if there is no longer systematic poisoning of the environment, diseases caused by this pollution (pesticide poisoning, asbestosis, Minimata disease) won't happen; if there are no longer extremes of wealth and poverty, diseases caused by lack of adequate food, shelter, and medical care will not exist; if children and adults can freely choose whether or not to live together, much violence against 'loved ones' will disappear; if racism is systematically attacked, then the majority ethnic group won't harass minorities. There will, of course, still be a need for mutual aid and protection – but this will be provided by the community, for *all* its members.

15 Would an anarchist society be less likely to be sexist? racist?

Anarchists usually talk about the illegitimacy of authority, basing their

arguments on the premise that no person should have power over another. A logical extension of this argument is to attack the power relationships in which men dominate women and some racial and ethnic groups dominate others. Thus anarchism creates the preconditions for abolishing sexism and racism.

Anarchism is philosophically opposed to all manifestations of racism and sexism. Equally important as its philosophical commitments is the fact that with anarchism there would be no economic basis to support racist or sexist ideas or practices. Work and income would be divided equitably, so there would be no need to subordinate a class of people to do the dirty work or to work at low pay to support the dominant class.

Sexism and racism would not automatically disappear in the process of building an anarchist society. A conscious effort would have to be made to change old behavior and attitudes.

16 What do anarchists think about sex, monogamy, and family?

Anarchists believe that how you live your daily life is an important political statement. Most people in industrialized societies spend a significant portion of their lives in what may be the last bulwark of capitalism and state socialism – the monogamous nuclear family. The family serves as the primary agent for reproducing the dominant values of the society, both through the socialization of children and the social control of its members. Within the family all of the pathologies of the larger society are reproduced: privatized social relations, escapism patriarchal dominance, economic dependency (in capitalist society), consumerism, and the treatment of people as property.

In an anarchist society, social relations will be based on trust, mutual aid, friendship and love. These may occur in the context of the family (if people choose to live in a family setting), but they certainly do not have to. Indeed, these conditions may be more easily achieved outside the family.

Will there be monogamous relations in an anarchist society? Clearly, people will have the option to choose how they want to live, with whom, and how long they want to live in these relationships. This will of course include the option of monogamy. However, without a system based on patriarchy, economic insecurity and religious or state authority, we doubt that monogamy would be anything more than an anachronism. If and when people did elect to live monogamously, it presumably would be seen as a choice made by both persons. Today, of course, monogamy is considered far more important for women than for men. This is called the double standard; and it has no place in a society of free and equal women and men.

The family? The nuclear family is not universal, but social systems for the rearing of the young, the care of the elderly, and companionate relations are. We think that whole new forms of communal and collective living arrangements will grow to replace the traditional family system.

Sex? Of course. But this does not mean that all kinds of sexual behavior would be condoned. We cannot imagine a truly anarchist society condoning rape, sexual exploitation of children, or sex that inflicts pain or humiliation, or involves dominance and submission. In sexual behavior, as in all other forms of behavior, social anarchism is based on freedom, trust and respect for the dignity of others. In fact, in an anarchist society sexuality would lose all the inegalitarian and oppressive meanings it now has.

17 Is it coercive to require education for children? What should its content and structure be?

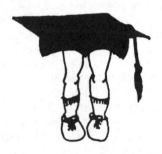

When people today worry about the coercive character of mandatory public education, we think that their concern really stems from the authoritarian character of schooling. Schools are an extension of the state; they reproduce the class, sex, race and other divisions on which the state is built. In an anarchist society, the social function of schools and the potential of education would be quite different.

Even today, we think that the implications of withholding basic education from young children are far more coercive than the requirement that they be educated. Without at least a minimal level of literacy, people would be much worse off than they already are. In an anarchist society education would, of course, provide far more. Education would be fundamentally liberating because it would help people learn how to learn; and it would teach them much more than they could ever acquire on their own about the physical world and the world of ideas. It would

also help them learn to be free and self-directed.

Such education is so important for young children that neither they nor their parents should be able to decide that the child doesn't need it. Bakunin stated the reason well:

> Children do not constitute anyone's property . . . they belong only to their own future freedom. But in children this freedom is not yet real; it is only potential. For real freedom - . . . based upon a feeling of one's dignity and upon the genuine respect for someone else's freedom and dignity, i.e., upon justice - such freedom can develop in children only through the rational development of their minds, character, and will.

What would anarchist education teach the young? Intellectual and physical skills that help to develop literate, healthy and competent people should be taught. Essential intellectual materials would include some that children now learn, and some that they don't: reading and writing, self-care (emotional and physical), farming and carpentry, cooking, and physical education. Children in the upper elementary grades would be introduced to literature and the other arts, cross-cultural materials, and the principles of anarchist community organization and economics. However, the content of these materials should reflect anarchist values: it would be senseless to teach the principles of capitalist politics and economics (except perhaps as a horrible example), an acceptance of stratification, or materials that advocate racist, sexist or other inegalitarian ideas.

Not only the content, but also the structure of anarchist education is vitally important. It is difficult to develop liberatory modes of thought and action in an atmosphere of intimidation, regimentation, boredom and respect for authority. We do not mean to imply that children should devalue teachers; but genuine respect must be based upon what someone knows and how effectively s/he teaches it, not upon position, age or credentials. It will be difficult to create an atmosphere of mutual respect and orderly process without imposing discipline. But liberatory education cannot take place in an authoritarian setting.

What else? Well, schools should be small, so that each child can get the attention and stimulation s/he needs. Activities should be varied, and distinctions between work and play narrowed as far as possible. Grading and competition with each other would be eliminated. Students would learn to set standards for themselves, and to try to meet them. (If they did not, the child should not evaluate him/herself negatively. Guilt and self-deprecation are enemies of autonomy and healthy functioning.) Teachers would be selected on the basis of knowledge and interpersonal competence, not upon the possession of formal

credentials. Probably few people would make a career of teaching, but many members of the community (including some older children) would spend time doing it. Schools would be integrated into the community, and everyone would participate in the direction of the schools.

When would education end? Ideally, never. Instead of being a prison, which inmates flee as soon as the guard's back is turned (which is what many public schools are like today), the anarchist school would encourage people to see education as a lifelong process. As the child becomes an adult, education would increasingly become an informal, self-directed activity which would take place outside the school. But people would return for further formal study as often, and as long, as they wish.

18 What is the relation of children to authority?

The line between nurturance and the authoritarian control of children is difficult to draw. Perhaps in an anarchist society that boundary line will be more clearly sketched.

Infants and young children are unquestionably dependent on others for their survival. Perhaps the difference between nurturance and authoritarianism arises when a child has acquired the skills for her or his own survival. If we accept that boundary, then we will have to work at determining what those skills minimally are. The skills themselves – once we go beyond the acquisition of language – are not absolute. They are relative to the social conditions under which people live. For example, under capitalism, where income and work are tied together and where both are prerequisites for food, housing, medical care and the like, survival training must last longer. Partly because of this long period of dependency, there has been a strong tradition in such settings to view the child (and young adult) as property, hence at the disposal of the family or state. Certainly, the political economy is one condition that fosters dependence on authority.

Fostering authoritarian dependence is, in fact, a major mechanism of social control in capitalist and state socialist societies. Today it is easier to catalog examples of dependence and authoritarian social conditions than it is to provide examples of social conditions that encourage self-management and autonomous behavior.

The quintessence of nurturant child-rearing in an anarchist community would be the teaching of children to like themselves, to learn how to learn, and how to set standards for self-evaluation.

19 Has there ever been a successful anarchist organization? If so, why don't they last longer?

Yes, there has been. In fact, there have been many groups that have been organized without centralized government, hierarchy, privilege and formal authority. Some have been explicitly anarchist: perhaps the best-known examples are the Spanish industrial and agricultural collectives, which functioned quite successfully for several years until destroyed by the combined forces of the authoritarian Left and the Right.

Most anarchist organizations are not called that – even by their members. Anthropological literature is full of descriptions of human societies that have existed without centralized government or institutionalized authority. (However, as contemporary feminist anthropologists point out, many so-called 'egalitarian' cultures are sexist.)

Industrialized societies also contain many groups that are anarchist in practice. As the British anarchist, Colin Ward, says, 'an anarchist society, a society which organizes itself without authority, is always in existence, like a seed beneath the snow.' Examples include the leaderless small groups developed by radical feminists, co-ops, clinics, learning networks, media collectives, direct action organizations such as the Clamshell Alliance; the spontaneous groupings that occur in response to disasters, strikes, revolutions and emergencies; community-controlled day-care centers; neighborhood groups; tenant and workplace organizing; and so on. Not all such groups are anarchist, of course, but a surprising number function without leadership and authority to provide mutual aid, resist the government, and develop better ways of doing things.

Why don't they last longer? People who ask this question expect anarchist organizations to meet standards of permanence that most anarchists, who value flexibility and change, do not hold; and that most non-anarchist groups cannot meet. There is, of course, another reason why many anarchist organizations do not last longer than they do. Anarchists are enemies of the state – and the state managers do not react kindly to enemies. Anarchist organizations are blocked, harassed, and sometimes (as in the case of Spain, and more recently Portugal) deliberately smashed. Under such circumstances, it is a tribute to the persistence and capabilities of many anarchists that their organizations last as long as they often do.

1,000 REWARDS

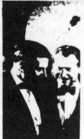

David Rockefeller (*l.*)
President of the Chase
Manhattan Bank and
an unknown accômplice

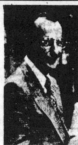

Roy E. Weber–Pres-
ident of the Michigan
Savings & Loan
League

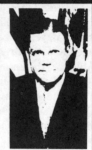

Robert McNamara–
President of the
World Bank

1,000 REWARDS FOR INFORMATION
LEADING TO THE   SUPPRESSION
AND ELIMINATION OF BANKERS

You can help eliminate the number of BANKS and BANKERS who hold up and rob people everyday, and win a new and creative life for yourself and others. If you have information that you believe will lead to the suppression and consequent elimination of any BANKERS responsible for the daylight robbery of you and your fellow workers, call your neighbor or friend for assistance.

With the money we're *given* for surrendering 40-60 hours of our life each week, BANKS like Chase Manhattan not only finance the functioning of capitalism by giving loans to the factories, shops and offices to which we are wage-slaves, they also *invest* our dead labor in the stocks of international conglomerates like General Motors and IT&T, becoming the major stockholders and controllers of such corporations.

As their financial control becomes global, BANKS become involved in wars and revolutions in other countries as the main money backers of counter-revolution everywhere, giving loans to puppet governments and CIA fronts in places such as Chile, Canada, Spain, Angola, Vietnam, Korea and the U.S.

Thus they are the representatives and manipulators of a social system, the every action and mere existence of which is the absolute negation of freedom.

Help make the world a better and safer place to live by preventing BANKERS and everything they represent.

DETROIT AREA BANKS

Bank of the Commonwealth · Dearborn Bank & Trust Company · Liberty State Bank & Trust · City National Bank of Detroit · Detroit Bank & Trust · Manufacturers National Bank of Detroit · Michigan National Bank of Detroit · Peoples Bank, Trenton · Wyandotte Savings Bank · National Bank of Detroit · Security Bank & Trust National Bank of Dearborn · Michigan National Bank of Dearborn · Detroit Bank, Livonia · Detroit Bank, Southfield · Detroit Bank, Troy · Detroit Bank, Warren · First Federal Savings & Loan

FIFTH ESTATE

2 Anarchism*

Fred Woodworth

What is anarchism?

As defined by anarchists themselves, it is 'the philosophy of a new social order based on liberty unrestricted by man-made law; the theory that all forms of government rest on violence, and are therefore wrong and harmful, as well as unnecessary.' An anarchist named Emma Goldman wrote this definition about fifty years ago, but the idea of human society being better off not having governments did not originate with Emma Goldman or any other one person whom we are aware of today. There have been people of a more or less anarchistic leaning in every era and place, although the actual word 'anarchy,' compounded out of Greek root-words meaning 'without rule' was coined comparatively recently.

You say 'more or less.' Aren't all anarchists in complete agreement?

No. Among those who have accepted the label of anarchist to describe themselves, various differences exist. There are individualists and collectivists, holding varied opinions about economics, organization, and other matters; and there are numerous combinations of these views. But all anarchists have found common cause in opposing the existence of government.

Anarchists believe that no possible reforms can halt the maltreatment of a subject populace – short of the outright abolishment of government – because the state is an institution that has in its nature a predisposition to always increase its power and authority. This unavoidable shift toward growing interference in people's affairs and lives makes governments all tend to approach the same authoritarian end, no matter what initial 'liberal' goals. Governments of the past and present have behaved this way, and it is an inescapable conclusion that future ones will do the same.

* This essay first appeared in the *Match!*, a monthly anarchist journal, vol. 4, nos. 9, 10 and 11, September, October, November 1973.

What is anarchism?

But according to the widest traditions of humanity, government is, in fact, absolutely necessary. Do anarchists suppose they are right while the vast majority of people, who do believe we need governments, are wrong? It would seem that to compare the relative numbers of each philosophy's adherents, anarchists are so badly outnumbered as to be virtually discredited.

This argument that the majority is against us is not really so profound. It would be trite to point out specific instances where majorities were completely wrong. History is filled with them. But more importantly, anarchists do not even believe that the majority of the people have in reality consciously chosen to have any government. Rather, we feel, they were simply conditioned to believe the rationales for governments; and in any event these governments usually existed even before the birth of any person who is ruled by them, making the question so moot that most people have failed to consider it at all. The acceptance of government is acculturated. Who questions the germ theory of disease? This is not to imply that that theory is necessarily wrong, but considering the way everyone accepts it virtually on faith, for all we know it might be wrong. This is the same way in which people used to be certain that demons and spirits existed and caused misfortune and so on. The current age may indeed be one of enlightenment, or at least enlightenment of a type pertaining to scientific theory; but let's not pretend that people today are any less gullible than they ever have been.

If people have 'accepted' government, it is no wonder. But whether this kind of acceptance has anything in common with a true conscious choice by a person who fairly considers alternatives and is not forced into some mental set by schooling or early training, ought to be obvious – it is not any kind of conscious decision at all. The truth of the matter is that the people are believers in the necessity of the State only because of the engineering of – the deliberate creation of – this belief by governments themselves. They accomplish this feat through the indoctrinations of their schools, churches, and the rest of the means of propaganda which permeate the entire culture of nations. But whatever the truth may happen to be with respect to any particular question, we repeat that this truth is in no way affected by what the majority may believe.

 +35

Supposing that this is true – that governments further the very attitudes required to ensure their own survival; how is it that anyone ever comes to be an anarchist within such a milieu?

There can be no one answer to this question. Some anarchists become so after discovering some item of literature by or about anarchists, or else they meet and talk with anarchists and are swayed by their arguments. Still others (but this is the exception) reason out governmentless philosophies of their own by themselves, and only later discover what

correct label to affix to their logic. But aside from just a few tendencies, very little is known about the psychology of getting to be an anarchist.

What do anarchists do?
Like anyone who is concerned with changing society, they try to convince other people that government is unnecessarily intruding in this or that area, and also provide a consistent analysis showing from this that there is no necessity for it in other areas. To change people's minds is the task of anarchists, since this is literally the only way to topple the state. The nature of government is such that if people did not, as we say, *legitimize* it by permitting it to make decisions binding them, it could not exist.

Our re-educational efforts can be expressed through the word, in writing, public speaking or personal conversations; or, in certain instances, through demonstrations specifically against government (as contrasted to demonstrations which call upon the government to perform some action). But in no sense do we attempt to force our analysis on anyone, as governments do. We want to convince people in a rational way, not create another reflection of the unthinking acceptance which people now possess and apply toward government. To try to create an anarchist society by making people blindly believe our ideas would be disastrous, since blind acceptance of anything is antithetical to our concept of freedom. This concept is of the freedom that exists when people can think and act for themselves.

Your answers make no mention of assassinations or the use of bombs, activities with which anarchists are inevitably associated in the public's mind. What about this association with violence which anarchism has; is there any basis for it?
We feel there is not. The philosophy of anarchism is not intrinsically related to any use of violence. It may happen, once in a great while, that some anarchist individual may (as all kinds of people do) commit an act of violence. But the same could be said of the adherents to any political philosophy, or, indeed, of any class of people. Anarchists are unfairly linked with violence. When some Democrat kills another in a

bar, no newspaper ever reports that 'A self-avowed Democrat killed one man and injured two in a brawl at the . . .' etc. But let an anarchist do something like this and see the condemnation which is heaped upon the whole movement. In reality, we have heard of clean-cut Republicans who have climbed with rifles up into high towers from where they insanely kill innocent passers-by below. Are Republicans universally stigmatized because of this?

Violence is, at least at the present stage of human development, something of a universal activity. At times it may even be necessary, when one must defend oneself, resist a dictator, or something similar. But violence is in no way integral to anarchism.

In fact, violence *is* integral to the philosophy and actions of statists. The state rests upon violence; its threat is used to maintain artificial order amidst the social unrest and inequality-bred anger that governments themselves create. The brandishment of a club should be the universal symbol of the state. Behind every law, every facet of 'international diplomacy,' every decree or court order, is the implicit promise of violence to those who do not comply. Governments, not anarchists, have been responsible for the vicious bombing of unoffending people, for the kidnapping and imprisonment of hundreds of thousands, for the robbery of untold wealth from the human race. Who deserves the label of 'Violent' – anarchists, or the minions of the state?

This is unfortunate if anarchism is precluded from an intelligent appraisal because of its bad name. Why don't anarchists call themselves by some other name and get around the problem?
Because that doesn't work. The only reason anarchism has such a bad name is that people with a vested interest in government have deliberately slandered us. The syllables of the word did not just magically acquire all this connotation of evil, and the fact is that we anarchists are not the monsters that we are made out to be – so somebody had to see to it that we were systematically denigrated. Thus we feel that if we called ourselves 'sans-governists' or 'anticrats,' or some other name we could invent, *it* would eventually suffer also the same predictable libel in newspaper articles and children's textbooks, and so what's the use? Anyhow, as anarchism has no leaders to impose usage, there is no way of ensuring uniformity even if we desired it, which, at least here, we don't. Governments can change whole nations from one system of terminology to another merely by imposing it as law. Anarchists think that that itself is an evil.

How would public services be organized under anarchy?
First of all, I should remark that it is a mistake to talk about life 'under' anarchy. There is no 'under' about it. The implication of 'under' is that

a uniform system is to be imposed upon everyone, and that standard solutions to societal problems will be accepted and take precedence over the ones of today, so that instead of living under the present system, we live under a new one. In reality, the nature of the projected pluralistic anarchy is such that a whole diversity is not only tolerated, but encouraged. Many kinds of non-coercive social modes, not merely a single one, would find acceptance among varying groups of people who had different ideas about what they wanted to accomplish, and different criteria to determine if they were succeeding at it.

'Public services' would be organized by whatever persons wanted to see them exist and expected to benefit from them. So-called public services which are actually coercive governmentalist functions, of course, would not exist at all. Today many of these supposed 'services' are forcibly imposed upon persons who openly detest them and all but rebel under their yoke. The police, for example, are often claimed to be 'servants of the people,' or to be providing a 'service,' whereas actually they are dictatorial autocrats forcibly maintaining a rigid, fear-inspired control over the people, while using as a justification for their existence the pretext of the very crime which the state itself fosters by its policies of tax robbery, imposed morality, inequality, etc.

People's opinions about what services are necessary are often greatly unlike each other, and this is as it should be. But today, under the governmental system, even people who oppose the public schools and never make use of them are still compelled to pay for them – and this is to name only a single one of the many forms of this same injustice. The essence of the current system is standardization and uniformity. Under government, everyone in the entire country can be forced to aid in the realization of some one person's or some tiny minority's pet project. In an anarchistic society of free and voluntary relationships, 'public services' would be organized anywhere that people were interested in seeing them made reality, and would be made possible by the help of like-minded persons who would support the projects if they wanted them. Similarly, people would be under no compulsion to support projects which they felt were undeserving, and if *nobody* thought some 'service' was necessary, perhaps it wasn't a service at all; very likely it would disappear until such time, if ever, that interest rekindled and people were willing to extend support.

This is the reply to every question about roads, schools, hospitals, post offices, and the like. As for the objection that people might, for example, travel on a road that they had not helped to pay for, my answer is: so what? Is that an argument against the free society? If so, it is an argument against the coercive, governmentalist society, too, because even with compulsory funding and taxation, some people never do contribute to the maintenance of services which they use. If one-

third of the whole population saw the necessity for establishing medical centers, and did so, and if then deadbeats from the other two-thirds of the people began to 'steal' use of the service, such a service could probably not continue to function, and would cease. In the event that this happened, and if there was still a need for medical services, personal responsibility would of necessity reappear among the irresponsible portion of the people.

But more likely than this is that changes in attitudes resulting from the abandonment of the present governmental system of institutionalized irresponsibility would already have precluded any such desire arising to evade payment for services rendered. In any case, within a short time, free interaction would tend to establish a high level of personal responsibility. Importantly, as long as government exists, self-reliance and responsibility are constantly eroded, making more laws 'necessary' to force compliance; and of course, this has the effect of eroding self-reliance even further.

Admittedly there are many wrongs and abuses. We all recognize that government has become too large and that its bureaucracy has intruded into areas where it is completely unneeded. But wouldn't you agree that it is somewhat unrealistic to demand an end to government altogether? Wouldn't it be better to try to simply reduce government to an acceptable level?

For us, no level is acceptable. We refuse to pay for 'services' which we hate and reject, and, needless to say, government cannot function at all without taxation. 'Liberal' governments only reshuffle priorities. And so-called limited governments somehow never stay limited at all. The government of the United States is a fine example of a government which once operated on a much lower scale but which, in a process greatly resembling biological maturation, grew up from its 'limited' infancy into an unlimited, monstrous adulthood. What good were its limits?

The reason there can be no acceptable level, even if a lower level of government could be attained and kept, is that, as the basis of all governments is robbery, or compulsory taxation, any talk of 'good governments' is at best only pretense that there is such a thing as good robbery. As with murder, the principle itself is wrong. There are no good governments.

The only meaningful change that can be made in government is to change its gathering of income from a demanded requirement to a request which can be ignored, and to remove the authoritarian nature from it so that no one *must* listen to it, abide by its decisions, support it, be bound by it. But since to remove these authoritarian attributes from government is to remove the very qualities that make it itself, we

say that there can be no meaningful change in it except that kind, just described, which actually abolishes it.

As for the objection that we are 'unrealistic,' government itself is, in our view, the more unrealistic: it promises peace but delivers war. It institutionalizes robbery as its means of 'protection' against the criminals who might commit robbery. Its conscription enslaves us so as to force us to 'defend' ourselves against enslavement by foreign countries' governments. Its police surveillance, its continually augmenting pile of laws to which no one can be safe from accidental disobedience or selective prosecution, show that in 'protecting' us, government actually invades farther than the alleged anti-freedom elements from which government 'protects' us. Government is an unrealistic, unworkable, utopian dream. It has been so *demonstrated* and *proved* countless times.

People feel that without a system of laws and police, there would be chaos in human society. Don't you think there is some real basis for this fear?

If there is such a basis in reality, it is only a product of the present authoritarian order. Suppose a heroin addict claims he cannot live without his drug; does that mean that heroin is a basic human need? That would be getting things backward – mistaking effects for causes. In other words, I mean that the supposed 'need' for government is an artificial dependency, manufactured by those in control who naturally want to stay in control. We anarchists think that people can live in peace with a really low incidence of true crime, once the responsibility-destroying cause of today's crimes – namely, the authoritarian system of laws and enforced morality – is finally removed.

You mean you are saying that the anarchist society might still have some crime? Isn't this a justification for retaining government?

Not unless government itself could reduce crime to nothing. The fact of the matter is, government increases all the time, but *so does crime*. If the governmentalists were right, as government increased, crime would decrease. Yet this does not happen; in fact, the opposite happens. It is possible that random, arbitrary crimes will always take place. However, we do know that all of the so-called victimless crimes are not really crimes in any sense, and with the abolition of government this whole category of crimes occasioned by the existence of government now, including tax evasion, draft resistance, sedition, etc., simply would no longer exist. As for the true crimes such as murder, rape, robbery, and so on, these appear to be symptoms of the present cultural disorder perpetuated by government, rather than the justification for government as some people erroneously imagine.

What is anarchism?

In a social situation wherein a cancerously expanding series of laws renders more and more possible varieties of behavior illegal and 'criminal,' the number of so-called criminals is bound to increase. This is an obvious reason to stop before everyone is turned into a criminal, and it is equally a reason to reverse the process so that the laws diminish. The end of the diminishment of laws, the condition of no laws, is our ideal.

So you do admit that some random violence against persons might occur as a result of unpredictable factors and unbalanced individuals. Wouldn't we need protection from these acts of violence?
By 'protection', I presume you mean police.

Yes.
Then what if the 'unbalanced individual' whom you are so worried about happened to be a policeman?

I suppose I would have to protect myself.
Indeed you would, provided that you had not already delegated so much responsibility and power to your protector–attacker that you had no defenses left. But this is an argument against the state again, not against anarchy, for in the free society the ultimate protector is yourself – you who are in this incorruptible.

But as for the original objection, I answer that life is a series of risks which everybody has to take. Intelligence or stupidity will maximize or minimize our chances for survival, but there is never any guarantee that a person is absolutely safe. As you amble along the city sidewalk, you risk having a flowerpot plunge into your skull from a point seventeen stories above. You may burden yourself with a steel umbrella, or drive an armored car everyplace you go, from neurotic fear of falling objects, but you have really solved nothing. Such 'solutions' only substitute a more onerous burden for that posed by the original risk, and lower life's quality farther than the previous danger did. Exactly the same is true in the case of the state and in the case of police, armies, and other such stultifying and ruinous remedies for the unknown problems of our existences.

Regardless of their several faults which you have pointed out – that they are ordered in compulsion, based on a technical theft which is taxation, and maintained solely by popular prejudice excited through propaganda – haven't the world's governments still done the best that could be done to make civilization progress?
And isn't it true that for all their lackings, governments are familiar and predictable, while anarchy, which has never been tried, is complete-

ly unpredictable?

What about revolutionary governments, such as those of the Soviet Union or the People's Republic of China – aren't those at least closer to your position, and therefore less to be condemned?

I will answer these questions in order, with a short preface.

Government is essentially a hysterical reaction to existing conditions. Whereas ordinary people will normally rank interpersonal violence as a last resort of social breakdown or crisis, governments operate with violence as their immediate priority all the time. Determined courses of action are *decreed*, not voluntarily decided upon; *ordered*, not freely accepted. If the principle of government were extended consistently and uniformly throughout society, true chaos would result. Every civilized relationship would give way to the gun or knife, to force instead of persuasion. We have only the principle of anarchy operating – the principle of no compulsion – to thank for the fact that the present social condition is not as faulty as it might be. Numerous social interactions even today still take place with an absence of compulsion, although governmentally ordained procedures are of course increasing all the time. In these spontaneous relationships between persons there is no ubiquitous policeman interceding (yet); none the less, most transactions, conversations, even quarrels, are accomplished without resort to coercion. Government's standard operating procedure is to use coercion first and to discuss matters afterward: 'Under penalty of three years in the federal penitentiary or $10,000 fine, or both, you are herewith required to . . .' etc. This reversal of normal order is, we anarchists contend, completely typical of governments. The tendency to place social compulsion uppermost is certainly not natural to correctly functioning human beings. None the less, most individuals of our species seem to have the remarkable ability to overlook the insanity of the premises upon which governments operate, even while they reject these premises in their own private lives, and base their behavior on different ones.

To the extent that people have been able to ignore their various governments, then civilization has progressed. If we were to have a method to calculate what the world would be like today had the thousands of wars of recorded history not occurred; if we could determine what negative effect of retrogression was exercised by the numberless benighted laws, arrogances and interferences of government, we would doubtless see that the actual advance of mankind has been retarded rather than aided by governments.

True, governments are familiar and predictable. But notice how so: in all the literature of the subject there is not one recorded instance of a government following any other course than that of compulsion and arbitrary authority, growing constantly in power, until the principle of the government is forcibly intruded into the whole of the interactions

of society, at which point society ceases to function and a revolution is made necessary to throw off the chains of bureaucracy and repression which the people discover binding themselves. Then, promptly – tragicomically – they institute a new government which itself travels full circle and is overthrown in a few years more. Yes, all this is as familiar and predictable as the movement of the bodies in the solar system.

But the social principle of anarchy is familiar and predictable also. Whenever one person helps another, whenever people solve their problems and no policeman or law instructs or compels – in short, at the taking place of any human development which is not mandated, ordained, decreed, controlled or interfered in by a legislature or by someone acting so as to force a result, we have the principle of anarchy at work. It is ordinarily claimed that this social anarchy, which is thought to be evil, needs to be overcome and regulated by governments, which are thought to be necessary so that society can 'work.' I assert that this explanation is false and is the exact opposite of the correct description of affairs, which is that the social principle of government, itself evil (in the sense that it does harm), is only overcome so that society can work, by the principle of anarchy, or freedom, spontaneously asserting itself in the uncontrolled interstices of the social matrix.

An industrial analogy is the 'work to rule,' a type of collective action for the same purposes as a strike, only that this involves not a stoppage of work but a strict obedience to all the regulations of the job-place. Since no business or factory can operate under such conditions – i.e., since the rules have to be disregarded somewhat so that the place can function – this is often an effective alternative to a strike. In the larger society, only selective enforcement of the laws and widespread disobedience of them prevents the chaos of unworkable regimentation. If the laws are 'made to be broken,' why make them at all?

Whoever has had an idea which would have increased the leisure and pleasure of all people (this is the purpose and definition of progress) has labored to defy the massed force of social compulsion – government – and, when succeeding, has achieved a true victory for anarchy. Perhaps we will never know what contributions could have been made by those who were long on invention or science or literature or art, but who were short on political cunning, strength, craftiness or wealth, and who could not, therefore, fight and win. This has been the double hindrance to true progress: governments' actual augmentation of ignorance or wrongness, and continual persecutions of any who would rectify these.

The self-styled revolutionary nature of some governments deserves little more than contemptuous disdain from anarchists. Revolutionary

government is the purest form of reactionary politics, and as the reactionaries are possessed of a fanaticism and zeal not to be found among the minions of so-called bourgeois governments, and since fanaticism and zeal among rulers are properties which are especially dangerous to freedom, the fact of the matter is that the revolutionary – that is, reactionary – governments tend to be *worse* than the bourgeois ones. Some perpetual crisis of 'the heroic party,' or some alleged danger to 'the People's State' inevitably provides a justification for the suspension of civil liberties, crackdowns on artists, stoppage of critical commentary, etc., while science is subjugated to the demands of the new regime. That these crises multiply and never end until reasons of political expedience may replace them with other repressive factors decades later, is well known.

Meanwhile, a generation of dissidents, unapproved artists, etc., is deported, confined in prison till death, or, in some cases, shot. This has the effect of 'removing the anarchists' from the society – i.e., the uncontrollable elements – and if the society then 'works' for a while until some sort of spontaneity can reassert itself, it only 'works' to the extent that everybody is told what to do, and is watched and checked, and everyone salutes, robotlike, or parrots slogans upon command. Every ideological 'revolutionary government' of modern times has imposed the same systematic mechanization of human life. These are not 'closer' to the anarchist position, but rather are more remote from it than are most.

Find the country where the people have the most liberty to criticize, where the press has the fewest regulations on it, where the least repression exists, where there are the fewest police and prisoners, where people have maximum self-determination; and there, for purposes of comparison only, you will find the closest counterpart of the anarchist society that exists among government-ruled orders. Even so, the anarchist still finds much there to oppose and disagree with, for, although it tends toward anarchy, it is not enough. Importantly, however, anarchists make whatever judgments they make about the condition of freedom anywhere, not upon what names or slogans are used to describe a particular regime, but upon the extent to which actions of the regime meddle in the anarchy of the people. It is not inconceivable that an authoritarian structure could someday attempt to conceal its true nature by terming itself an 'anarchist government' or a 'libertarian government.' We would oppose it all the same. Names mean nothing to us; what counts is what *is*.

But wouldn't an anarchist society be just as repressive as the statist ones, only to a different class of people? For instance, wouldn't the occasional governmentalist be in the same position then that the

anarchist is now, that is, as a detested radical?

Today there is a legal–judicial system in existence, responsive to the whims of a ruling class, which carries out sanctions against people who are 'different.' In the contemplated anarchist order, there is neither a judicial system nor a ruling class. Nor are we anarchists worried about 'subversion' of our society's principles because the very same forces that grew powerful enough to force the demise of the state through refusal to support it any longer, would presumably act to assure that it did not reappear. Provided that there was anybody who felt masochistically displeased at the scarcity of bosses or tyrants or ruling cliques to order their lives for them, perhaps such pathetic individuals would cater to each other's peculiar deviance. If there were any such frustrated authoritarians, they would naturally be quite free to denounce the anarchist society through their own press and through speeches, and so on. Undoubtedly they would provoke lively discussions and disagreements – perhaps even serve a necessary function by way of contrasting as 'horrible examples,' and so illustrate the advantages of the free society.

Here it would be worthwhile to remark that the word 'revolution' is actually a good one to describe all previous political turmoils, which were meaningless, because it suggests the image of a wheel, the turning of which exchanges the upper for the lower. Most 'revolutions' are just like this; they change nothing except the relative positions of the rulers and the ruled, and leave the dominating relationship itself untouched. But the anarchist 'revolution' is not intended to substitute any new ruling group for the old. This 'revolution' might perhaps be better termed 'insurrection,' which shatters the hierarchical structure itself, rather than merely plugging new rulers into vacant slots in a replacement government. Unlike other revolutionaries, anarchists have no ulterior motives for carrying on their work: no promised positions in any 'provisional government' or assured berths as prominent officials 'after the revolution.' There's nothing in it for anarchists except the satisfaction of working for their own freedom and that of others.

Can the goal of anarchism be achieved, and if so, how?

A tremendous amount of re-education will have to be accomplished before people will come to see the desirability and the necessity of ending domination by governments. Unless people agree that government is not necessary, simple destruction of the existing structure can accomplish nothing; popular demand would immediately put a new one in its place. When people do agree that government is unneeded, total withdrawal of support will render the government impotent without resources and will signal its imminent collapse. As there is no anarchist society without anarchists, and as these are only created by rational

discourse and understanding, these processes ought to be encouraged and actively helped along by those who oppose government already.

It is both easy and difficult to be a 'member' of the anarchist movement. There are no entrance fees or membership cards, but everyone who has a sincere wish to participate in this quest for freedom is welcome.

Seek out other anarchists and add your efforts to theirs: add their efforts to yours. Improve your understanding of all subjects which can be useful in this work. Constantly question every aspect of authoritarian society, launch an unremitting assault on all ignorance and superstition, and on every common, unthinkingly accepted notion which helps to justify the continuing delay of total emancipation. Read and listen to what other anarchists have had to say, and disagree with them unhesitatingly at those points where they seem to be wrong. Publish, speak, write, or assist these activities; organize like-minded people so that collective as well as individual effort can be put to use to achieve our common goal.

Even so doing, success is not guaranteed. Can anarchy be achieved? Even among anarchists the spectrum of opinion ranges from that of the extreme pessimists, who believe that anarchy is a beautiful ideal, but one which we will never reach, to those cheerful optimists who think that government is all but dead already. And usually today's pessimists are the optimists of two years ago.

Somewhere in between these positions of great certainty, the remainder of anarchists goes on, sometimes doubtfully, but always hopefully.

Fred Woodworth is the editor of the *Match!*, an anarchist monthly newspaper published in Tucson, Arizona.

3 About anarchism*

Nicolas Walter

What anarchists believe

The first anarchists were people in the English and French revolutions
of the seventeenth and eighteenth centuries who were given the name
as an insult to suggest that they wanted anarchy in the sense of chaos or
confusion. But from the 1840s anarchists were people who accepted
the name as a sign to show that they wanted anarchy in the sense of
absence of government. The Greek word *anarkhia*, like the English
word 'anarchy', has both meanings; people who are not anarchists take
them to come to the same thing, but anarchists insist on keeping them
apart. For more than a century, anarchists have been people who
believe not only that absence of government need not mean chaos and
confusion, but that a society without government will actually be
better than the society we live in now.

Anarchism is the political elaboration of the psychological reaction
against authority which appears in all human groups. Everyone knows
the natural anarchists who will not believe or do something just because
someone tells them to. Throughout history the practical tendency towards anarchy is seen among individuals and groups rebelling against
those who rule them. The theoretical idea of anarchy is also very old;
thus the description of a past golden age without government may be
found in the thought of ancient China and India, Egypt and Mesopo-
tamia, and Greece and Rome, and in the same way the wish for a future
utopia without government may be found in the thought of countless

---

* These two sections are from an essay, 'About Anarchism', which was
  first published as the hundredth issue of the British magazine *Anarchy*
  in June 1969, and was immediately republished as a separate pamphlet; it was translated into several languages, and a slightly revised
  edition was published in June 1977. The pamphlet is available from
  the publishers, Freedom Press, 84B Whitechapel High Street, London
  E 1, England.

religious and political writers and communities. But the application of anarchy to the present situation is more recent, and it is only in the anarchist movement of the past century that we find the demand for a society without government here and now.

Other groups on both left and right want to get rid of government in theory, either when the market is so free that it needs no more supervision, or when the people are so equal that they need no more restraint; but the measures they take seem to make government stronger and stronger. It is the anarchists, and the anarchists alone who want to get rid of government in practice. This does not mean that anarchists think all men are naturally good, or identical, or perfectible, or any romantic nonsense of that kind. It means that anarchists think almost all men are sociable, and similar, and capable of living their own lives. Many people say that government is necessary because some men cannot be trusted to look after themselves, but anarchists say that government is harmful because no men can be trusted to look after anyone else. If all men are so bad that they need to be ruled by others, anarchists ask, how can any men be good enough to rule others? Power tends to corrupt, and absolute power corrupts absolutely. At the same time, the wealth of the earth is the product of the labour of mankind as a whole, and all men have an equal right to take part in continuing the labour and enjoying the product. Anarchism is an ideal type which demands at the same time total freedom and total equality.

Liberalism and socialism

Anarchism may be seen as a development from either liberalism or socialism, or from both liberalism and socialism. Like liberals, anarchists want freedom; like socialists, anarchists want equality. But we are not satisfied by liberalism alone or by socialism alone. Freedom without equality means that the poor and weak are less free than the rich and strong, and equality without freedom means that we are all slaves together. Freedom and equality are not contradictory, but complementary; in place of the old polarisation of freedom versus equality – according to which we are told that more freedom equals less equality, and more equality equals less freedom – anarchists point out that in practice you cannot have one without the other. Freedom is not genuine if some people are too poor or too weak to enjoy it, and equality is not genuine if some people are ruled by others. The crucial contribution to political theory made by anarchists is this realisation that freedom and equality are in the end the same thing.

Anarchism also departs from both liberalism and socialism in taking a different view of progress. Liberals see history as a linear development

from savagery, superstition, intolerance and tyranny to civilisation, enlightenment, tolerance and emancipation. There are advances and retreats, but the true progress of mankind is from a bad past to a good future. Socialists see history as a dialectical development from savagery, through despotism, feudalism and capitalism, to the triumph of the proletariat and the abolition of the class system. There are revolutions and reactions, but the true progress of mankind is again from a bad past to a good future.

Anarchists see progress quite differently; in fact they often do not see progress at all. We see history not as a linear or a dialectical development in one direction, but as a dualistic process. The history of all human society is the story of a struggle between the rulers and the ruled, between the haves and the have-nots, between the people who want to govern and be governed and the people who want to free themselves and their fellows; the principles of authority and liberty, of government and rebellion, of state and society, are in perpetual opposition. This tension is never resolved; the movement of mankind is now in one direction, now in another. The rise of a new regime or the fall of an old one is not a mysterious break in development or an even more mysterious part of development, but is exactly what it seems to be. Historical events are welcome only to the extent that they increase freedom and equality for the whole people; there is no hidden reason for calling a bad thing good because it is inevitable. We cannot make any useful predictions of the future, and we cannot be sure that the world is going to get better. Our only hope is that, as knowledge and consciousness increase, people will become more aware that they can look after themselves without any need for authority.

Nevertheless, anarchism does derive from liberalism and socialism both historically and ideologically. Liberalism and socialism came before anarchism, and anarchism arose from the contradiction between them; most anarchists still begin as either liberals or socialists, or both. The spirit of revolt is seldom born fully grown, and it generally grows into rather than within anarchism. In a sense, anarchists always remain liberals and socialists, and whenever they reject what is good in either they betray anarchism itself. On one hand we depend on freedom of speech, assembly, movement, behaviour, and especially on the freedom to differ; on the other hand we depend on equality of possessions, on human solidarity, and especially on the sharing of power. We are liberals but more so, and socialists but more so.

Yet anarchism is not just a mixture of liberalism and socialism; that is social democracy, or welfare capitalism, the system which prevails in this country. Whatever we owe to and however close we are to liberals and socialists, we differ fundamentally from them – and from social democrats – in rejecting the institution of government. Both liberals

and socialists depend on government – liberals ostensibly to preserve freedom but actually to prevent equality, socialists ostensibly to preserve equality but actually to prevent freedom. Even the most extreme liberals and socialists cannot do without government, the exercise of authority by some people over other people. The essence of anarchism, the one thing without which it is not anarchism, is the negation of authority over anyone by anyone.

Democracy and representation

Many people oppose undemocratic government, but anarchists differ from them in also opposing democratic government. Some people oppose democratic government as well, but anarchists differ from them in doing so not because they fear or hate the rule of the people but because they believe that democracy is not the rule of the people – that democracy is in fact a logical contradiction, a physical impossibility. Genuine democracy is possible only in a small community where everyone can take part in every decision; and then it is not necessary. What is called democracy and is alleged to be the government of the people by themselves is in fact the government of the people by elected rulers and would be better called 'consenting oligarchy'.

Government by rulers whom we have chosen is different from and generally better than government by rulers who have chosen themselves, but it is still government of some people by other people. Even the most democratic government still depends on someone making someone else do something or stopping someone else doing something. Even when we are governed by our representatives we are still governed, and as soon as they begin to govern us against our will they cease to be our representatives. Most people now agree that we have no obligation to a government in which we have no voice; anarchists go further and insist that we have no obligation to a government we have chosen. We may obey it because we agree with it or because we are too weak to disobey it, but we have no obligation to obey it when we disagree with it and are strong enough not to do so. Most people now agree that those who are involved in any change should be consulted about it before any decision is made; anarchists go further and insist that they should themselves make the decision and go on to put it into effect.

So anarchists reject the idea of a social contract and the idea of representation. In practice, no doubt, most things will always be done by a few people – by those who are interested in a problem and are capable of solving it – but there is no need for them to be selected or elected. They will always emerge anyway, and it is better for them to do so naturally. The point is that leaders and experts do not have to be

rulers, that leadership and expertise are not necessarily connected with authority. And when representation is convenient, that is all it is; the only true representative is the delegate or deputy who is mandated by those who send him and who is subject to instant recall by them. In some ways the ruler who claims to be a representative is worse than the ruler who is obviously a usurper, because it is more difficult to grapple with authority when it is wrapped up in fine words and abstract arguments. The fact that we are able to vote for our rulers once every few years does not mean that we have to obey them for the rest of the time. If we do, it is for practical reasons, not on moral grounds. Anarchists are against government, however it is built up.

State and class

Anarchists have traditionally concentrated their opposition to authority on the state – that is, the institution which claims the monopoly of power within a certain area. This is because the state is the supreme example of authority in a society and also the source of confirmation of the use of authority throughout it. Moreover, anarchists have traditionally opposed all kinds of state – not just the obvious tyranny of a king, dictator or conqueror, but also such variations as enlightened despotism, progressive monarchy, feudal or commercial oligarchy, parliamentary democracy, soviet communism, and so on. Anarchists have even tended to say that all states are the same, and that there is nothing to choose between them.

This is an oversimplification. All states are certainly authoritarian, but some states are just as certainly more authoritarian than others, and every normal person would prefer to live under a less authoritarian rather than a more authoritarian one. To give a simple example, this statement of anarchism could not have been published under most states of the past, and it still could not be published under most states of both left and right, in both East and West; I would rather live where it can be published, and so would most of my readers.

Few anarchists still have such a simplistic attitude to an abstract thing called 'the state', and anarchists concentrate on attacking the central government and the institutions which derive from it not just because they are part of the state but because they are the extreme examples of the use of authority in society. We contrast the state with society, but we no longer see it as alien to society, as an artificial growth; instead we see it as part of society, as a natural growth. Authority is a normal form of behaviour, just as aggression is; but it is a form of behaviour which must be controlled and grown out of. This will not be done by trying to find ways of institutionalising it, but only by find-

ing ways of doing without it.

Anarchists object to the obviously repressive institutions of government – officials, laws, police, courts, prisons, armies, and so on – and also to those which are apparently benevolent – subsidised bodies and local councils, nationalised industries and public corporations, banks and insurance companies, schools and universities, press and broadcasting, and all the rest. Anyone can see that the former depend not on consent but on compulsion and ultimately on force; anarchists insist that the latter have the same iron hand, even if it does wear a velvet glove.

Nevertheless, the institutions which derive directly or indirectly from the state cannot be understood if they are thought of as being purely bad. They can have a good side, in two ways. They have a useful negative function when they challenge the use of authority by other institutions, such as cruel parents, greedy landlords, brutal bosses, violent criminals; and they have a useful positive function when they promote desirable social activities, such as public works, disaster operations, communication and transport systems, art and culture, medical services, pension schemes, poor relief, education, broadcasting. Thus we have the liberatory state and the welfare state, the state working for freedom and the state working for equality.

The first anarchist answer to this is that we also have the oppressive state – that the main function of the state is in fact to hold down the people, to limit freedom – and that all the benevolent functions of the state can be exercised and often have been exercised by voluntary associations. Here the state resembles the medieval church. In the Middle Ages the church was involved in all essential social activities, and it was difficult to believe that the activities were possible without it. Only the church could baptise, marry and bury people, and they had to learn that it did not actually control birth, love and death. Every public act needed an official religious blessing – many still have one – and people had to learn that the act was just as effective without the blessing. The church interfered in and often controlled those aspects of communal life which are now dominated by the state. People have learnt to realise that the participation of the church is unnecessary and even harmful; what they now have to learn is that the domination of the state is equally pernicious and superfluous. We need the state just as long as we think we do, and everything it does can be done just as well or even better without the sanction of authority.

The second anarchist answer is that the essential function of the state is to maintain the existing inequality. Anarchists do not agree with Marxists that the basic unit of society is the class, but most agree that the state is the political expression of the economic structure, that it is the representative of the people who own or control the wealth of the

community and the oppressor of the people who do the work which creates that wealth. The state cannot redistribute wealth fairly because it is the main agency of the unfair distribution. Anarchists agree with Marxists that the present system must be destroyed, but they do not agree that the future system can be established by a state in different hands; the state is a cause as well as a result of the class system, and a classless society which is established by a state will soon become a class society again. The state will not wither away – it must be deliberately abolished by people taking power away from the rulers and wealth away from the rich; these two actions are linked, and one without the other will always be futile. Anarchy in its truest sense means a society without either rulers or rich men.

Organization and bureaucracy

This does not mean that anarchists reject organisation, though here is one of the strongest prejudices about anarchism. People can accept that anarchy may not mean just chaos or confusion, and that anarchists want not disorder but order without government, but they are sure that anarchy means order which arises spontaneously and that anarchists do not want organisation. This is the reverse of the truth. Anarchists actually want much more organisation, though organisation without authority. The prejudice about anarchism derives from a prejudice about organisation; people cannot see that organisation does not depend on authority, that it actually works best without authority.

A moment's thought will show that when compulsion is replaced by consent there will have to be more discussion and planning, not less. Everyone who is involved in a decision will be able to take part in making it, and no one will be able to leave the work to paid officials or elected representatives. Without rules to observe or precedents to follow, every decision will have to be made afresh. Without rulers to obey or leaders to follow, everyone will be able to make up his or her own mind. To keep all this going, the multiplicity and complexity of links between individuals will be increased, not reduced. Such organisation may be untidy and inefficient, but it will be much closer to the needs and feelings of the people concerned. If something cannot be done without the old kind of organisation, without authority and compulsion, it probably isn't worth doing and would be better left undone.

What anarchists do reject is the institutionalisation of organisation, the establishment of a special group of people whose function is to organise other people. Anarchist organisation would be fluid and open; as soon as organisation becomes hardened and closed, it falls into the hands of a bureaucracy, becomes the instrument of a particular class, and reverts to

the expression of authority instead of the co-ordination of society. Every group tends towards oligarchy, the rule of the few, and every organisation tends towards bureaucracy, the rule of the professionals, anarchists must always struggle against these tendencies, in the future as well as the present, and among themselves as well as among others.

Property

Nor do anarchists reject property, though we have a peculiar view of it. In one sense property is theft – that is, the exclusive appropriation of anything by anyone is a deprivation of everyone else. This does not mean that we are all communists; what it means is that any particular person's right to any particular thing depends not on whether he made it or found it or bought it or was given it or is using it or wants it or has a legal right to it, but on whether he *needs* it – and, more to the point, whether he needs it more than someone else. This is a matter not of abstract justice or natural law, but of human solidarity and obvious commonsense. If I have a loaf of bread and you are hungry, it is yours, not mine. If I have a coat and you are cold, it belongs to you. If I have a house and you have none, you have the right to use at least one of my rooms. But in another sense property is liberty – that is, the private enjoyment of goods and chattels in a sufficient quantity is an essential condition of the good life for the individual.

Anarchists are in favour of the private property which cannot be used by one person to exploit another – those personal possessions which we accumulate from childhood and which become part of our lives. What we are against is the public property which is no use in itself and can be used only to exploit people – land and buildings, instruments of production and distribution, raw materials and manufactured articles, money and capital. The principle at issue is that a man may be said to have a right to what he produces by his own labour, but not to what he gets from the labour of others; he has a right to what he needs and uses, but not to what he does not need and cannot use. As soon as a man has more than enough, it either goes to waste or it stops another man having enough.

This means that rich men have no right to their property, for they are rich not because they work a lot but because a lot of people work for them; and poor men have a right to rich men's property, for they are poor not because they work little but because they work for others. Indeed, poor people almost always work longer hours at duller jobs in worse conditions than rich people. No one ever became rich or remained rich through his own labour, only by exploiting the labour of others. A man may have a house and a piece of land, the tools of his trade and

good health all his life, and he may work as hard as he can as long as he can – he will produce enough for his family, but little more; and even then he will not be really self-sufficient, for he will depend on others to provide some of his materials and to take some of his produce in exchange.

Public property is not only a matter of ownership, but also one of control. It is not necessary to possess property to be able to exploit others. Rich men have always used other people to manage their property, and, now that anonymous corporations and state enterprises are replacing individual property owners, managers are becoming the leading exploiters of other people's labour. In both advanced and backward countries, both capitalist and communist states, a tiny minority of the population still owns or otherwise controls the overwhelming proportion of public property.

Despite appearances, this is not an economic or legal problem. What matters is not the distribution of money or the system of land tenure or the organisation of taxation or the method of taxation or the law of inheritance, but the basic fact that some people will work for other people, just as some people will obey other people. If we refused to work for the rich and powerful, property would disappear – in the same way that, if we refused to obey rulers, authority would disappear. For anarchists, property is based on authority, and not the other way round. The point is not how peasants put food into the landlord's mouths or how workers put money into the bosses' pockets, but *why* they do so, and this is a political point.

Some people try to solve the problem of property by changing the law or the government, whether by reform or by revolution. Anarchists have no faith in such solutions, but they do not all agree on the right solution. Some anarchists want the division of everything among everyone, so that we all have an equal share in the world's wealth, and a *laissez-faire* commercial system with free credit to prevent excessive accumulation. But most anarchists have no faith in this solution either, and want the expropriation of all public property from those who have more than they need, so that we all have equal access to the world's wealth, and the control is in the hands of the whole community. But at least it is agreed that the present system of property must be destroyed together with the present system of authority.

God and church

Anarchists have traditionally been anti-clerical, and also atheist. The early anarchists were opposed to the church as much as to the state, and most of them have been opposed to religion itself. The slogan,

'Neither God nor master', has often been used to sum u
message. Many people still take the first step towards
abandoning their faith and becoming rationalists or
rejection of divine authority encourages the rejection of
ity. Nearly all anarchists today are probably atheists, or at

But there have been religious anarchists, though they a̶̶̶̶ ̶̶̶̶̶̶̶̶̶̶̶ ̶̶̶ out
side the mainstream of the anarchist movement. Obvious examples are
the heretical sects which anticipated some anarchist ideas before the
nineteenth century, and groups of religious pacifists in Europe and North
America during the nineteenth and twentieth centuries, especially
Tolstoy and his followers at the beginning of the twentieth century and
the Catholic Worker movement in the United States since the 1930s.

The general anarchist hatred of religion has declined as the power of
the church has declined, and most anarchists now think of it as a personal matter. They would oppose the discouragement of religion by
force, but they would also oppose the revival of religion by force. They
would let anyone believe and do what he wants, so long as it affects
only himself; but they would not let the church have any more power.

In the meantime, the history of religion is a model for the history of
government. Once it was thought impossible to have a society without
God; now God is dead. It is still thought impossible to have a society
without the state; now we must destroy the state.

War and violence

Anarchists have always opposed war, but not all have opposed violence.
They are anti-militarists, but not necessarily pacifists. For anarchists,
war is the supreme example of authority outside a society, and at the
same time a powerful reinforcement of authority within society. The
organised violence and destruction of war are an enormously magnified
version of the organised violence and destruction of the state, and war
is the health of the state. The anarchist movement has a strong tradition
of resistance to war and to preparations for war. A few anarchists have
supported some wars, but they have always been recognised as renegades
by their comrades, and this total opposition to national wars is one of
the great unifying factors among anarchists.

But anarchists have distinguished between national wars between
states and civil wars between classes. The revolutionary anarchist movement since the late nineteenth century has called for a violent insurrection to destroy the state, and anarchists have taken an active part in
many armed risings and civil wars, especially those in Russia and Spain.
Though they were involved in such fighting, however, they were under
no illusions that it would itself bring about the revolution. Violence

.t be necessary for the work of destroying the old system, but it is useless and indeed dangerous for the work of building a new system. A people's army can defeat a ruling class and destroy a government, but it cannot help the people to create a free society, and it is no good winning a war if you cannot win the peace.

Many anarchists have in fact doubted whether violence plays any useful part at all. Like the state, it is not a neutral force whose effects depend on who uses it, and it will not do the right things just because it is in the right hands. Of course the violence of the oppressed is not the same as the violence of the oppressor, but even when it is the best way out of an intolerable situation it is only a second best. It is one of the most unpleasant features of present society, and it remains unpleasant however good its purpose; moreover, it tends to destroy its purpose, even in situations where it seems appropriate – such as revolution. The experience of history suggests that revolutions are not guaranteed by violence; on the contrary, the more violence, the less revolution.

All this may seem absurd to people who are not anarchists. One of the oldest and most persistent prejudices about anarchism is that anarchists are above all men of violence. The stereotype of the anarchist with a bomb under his cloak is eighty years old, but it is still going strong. Many anarchists have indeed favoured violence, some have favoured the assassination of public figures, and a few have even favoured terrorism of the population, to help destroy the present system. There is a dark side to anarchism, and there is no point denying it. But it is only one side of anarchism, and a small one. Most anarchists have always opposed any violence which is not really necessary – the inevitable violence occurs when the people shake off their rulers and exploiters.

The main perpetrators of violence have been those who maintain authority, not those who attack it. The great bomb-throwers have not been the tragic individuals driven to desperation in southern Europe more than half a century ago, but the military machines of every state in the world throughout history. No anarchist can rival the Blitz and the Bomb, no Ravachol or Bonnot can stand beside Hitler or Stalin. We would encourage workers to seize their factory or peasants to seize their land, and we might break windows or build barricades; but we have no soldiers, no aeroplanes, no police, no prisons, no camps, no firing squads, no gas chambers, no hangmen. For anarchists, violence is the extreme example of the use of power by one person against another, the culmination of everything we are against.

Some anarchists have even been pacifists, though this is not usual. Many pacifists have been (or become) anarchists, and anarchists have tended to move towards pacifism as the world has moved towards destruction. Some have been especially attracted by the militant type of pacifism advocated by Tolstoy and Gandhi and by the use of non-

violence as a technique of direct action, and many anarchists h.
part in anti-war movements and have sometimes had a significan
ence on them. But most anarchists – even those who are closely invoi.
– find pacifism too wide in its rejection of all violence by all people in
all circumstances, and too narrow in its belief that the elimination of
violence alone will make a fundamental difference to society. Where
pacifists see authority as a weaker version of violence, anarchists see
violence as a stronger version of authority. They are also repelled by the
moralistic side of pacifism, the asceticism and self-righteousness, and by
its tender-minded view of the world. To repeat, they are anti-militarists,
but not necessarily pacifists.

The individual and society

The basic unit of mankind is man, the individual human being. Nearly
all individuals live in society, but society is nothing more than a collection of individuals, and its only purpose is to give them a full life. Anarchists do not believe that people have natural rights, but this applies
to everyone; an individual has no right to do anything, but no other
individual has a right to stop him doing anything. There is no general
will, no social norm to which we should conform. We are equal, but not
identical. Competition and mutual aid, aggression and tenderness, intolerance and tolerance, violence and gentleness, authority and rebellion –
all these are natural forms of social behaviour, but some help and others
hinder the full life of the individuals. Anarchists believe that the best
way to guarantee it is to secure equal freedom for every member of
society.

We therefore have no time for morality in the traditional sense, and
we are not interested in what people do in their own lives. Let every
individual do exactly what he wants, within the limits of his natural
capacity, provided he lets every other individual do exactly what *he*
wants. Such things as dress, appearance, speech, manners, acquaintance,
and so on, are matters of personal preference. So is sex. We are in favour
of free love, but this does not mean that we advocate universal promis-
cuity; it means that all love is free, except prostitution and rape, and
that people should be able to choose (or reject) forms of sexual behavior
and sexual partners for themselves. Extreme indulgence may suit one
person, extreme chastity another – though most anarchists feel that the
world would be a better place if there had been a lot less fussing and a
lot more fucking. The same principle applies to such things as drugs.
People can intoxicate themselves with alcohol or caffeine, cannabis or
amphetamine, tobacco or opiates, and we have no right to prevent them,
let alone punish them, though we may try to help them. Similarly, let

orship in his own way, so long as he lets other
in their own way, or not worship at all. It doesn't
e offended; what does matter is if people are injured.
o worry about differences in personal behaviour; the
out is the gross injustice of authoritarian society.
e always opposed every form of national, social, racial
sion, and have always supported every movement for
natio.., racial or sexual emancipation. But they tend to differ
from their allies in seeing all forms of oppression as being political in
nature, and in seeing all victims of oppression as individual human beings
rather than as members of a nationality, class, race, or sex.

The main enemy of the free individual is the overwhelming power of
the state, but anarchists are also opposed to every other form of authority which limits freedom – in the family, in the school, at work, in the
neighbourhood – and to every attempt to make the individual conform.
However, before considering how society may be organised to give the
greatest freedom to its members, it is necessary to describe the various
forms anarchism has taken according to the various views of the relationship between the individual and society.

What anarchists want

It is difficult to say what anarchists want, not just because they differ
so much, but because they hesitate to make detailed proposals about a
future which they are neither able nor willing to control. After all,
anarchists want a society without government, and such a society
would obviously vary widely from time to time and from place to place.
The whole point of the society anarchists want is that it would be what
its members themselves want. Nevertheless, it is possible to say what
most anarchists would like to see in a free society, though it must always
be remembered that there is no official line, and also no way of recon-
ciling the extremes of individualism and communism.

The free individual

Most anarchists begin with a libertarian attitude towards private life,
and want a much wider choice for personal behaviour and for social
relationships between individuals. But if the individual is the atom of
society, the family is the molecule, and family life would continue even
if all the coercion enforcing it were removed. Nevertheless, though the
family may be natural, it is no longer necessary; efficient contraception
and intelligent division of labour have released mankind from the narrow

choice to have children, and children could be brought up by more or less than two parents. People could live alone and still have sexual partners and children, or live in communes with no permanent partnerships or official parenthood at all.

No doubt most people will go on practising some form of marriage and most children will be brought up in a family environment, whatever happens to society, but there could be a great variety of personal arrangements within a single community. The fundamental requirement is that women should be freed from the oppression of men and that children should be freed from that of parents. The exercise of authority is no better in the microcosm of the family than in the macrocosm of society.

Personal relationships outside the family would be regulated not by arbitrary laws or economic competition but by the natural solidarity of the human species. Almost all of us know how to treat our fellow-men – as we would like them to treat us – and self-respect and public opinion are far better guides to action than fear or guilt. Some opponents of anarchism have suggested that the moral oppression of society would be worse than the physical oppression of the state, but a greater danger is surely the unregulated authority of the vigilante group, the lynch mob, the robber band, or the criminal gang – the rudimentary forms of the state which come to the surface when the regulated authority of the real state is for some reason absent.

But anarchists disagree little about private life, and there is not much of a problem here. After all, a great many people have already made their own new arrangements, without waiting for a revolution or anything else. All that is needed for the liberation of the individual is the emancipation from old prejudices and the achievement of a certain standard of living. The real problem is the liberation of society.

The free society

The first priority of a free society would be the abolition of authority and the expropriation of property. In place of government by permanent representatives who are subject to occasional election and by career bureaucrats who are virtually unmovable, anarchists want co-ordination by temporary delegates who are subject to instant recall and by professional experts who are genuinely accountable. In such a system, all those social activities which involve organisation would probably be managed by free associations. These might be called councils or cooperatives or collectives or communes or committees or unions or syndicates or soviets, or anything else – their title would be irrelevant, the important thing would be their function.

There would be work associations from the workshop or smallholding up to the largest industrial or agricultural complex, to handle the production and transport of goods, decide conditions of work, and run the economy. There would be area associations from the neighbourhood or village up to the largest residential unit, to handle the life of the community – housing, streets, refuse, amenities. There would be associations to handle the social aspects of such activities as communications, culture, recreation, research, health and education.

One result of co-ordination by free association rather than administration by established hierarchies would be extreme decentralisation on federalist lines. This may seem an argument against anarchism, but we would say that it is an argument for it. One of the oddest things about modern political thought is that wars are often blamed on the existence of many small nations when the worst wars in history have been caused by a few large ones. In the same way, governments are always trying to create larger and larger administrative units when observation suggests that the best ones are small. The breakdown of big political systems would be one of the greatest benefits of anarchism, and countries could become cultural entities once more, while nations would disappear.

The association concerned with any kind of wealth or property would have the crucial responsibility of either making sure that it was fairly divided among the people involved or else of holding it in common and making sure that the use of it was fairly shared among the people involved. Anarchists differ about which system is best, and no doubt the members of a free society would also differ; it would be up to the people in each association to adopt whichever method they preferred. There might be equal pay for all, or pay according to need, or no pay at all. Some associations might use money for all exchange, some just for large or complex transactions, and some might not use it at all. Goods might be bought, or hired, or rationed, or free. If this sort of speculation seems absurdly unrealistic or utopian, it may be worth remembering just how much we already hold in common, and how many things may be used without payment.

In Britain, the community owns some heavy industries, air and rail transport, ferries and buses, broadcasting systems, water, gas and electricity, though we pay to use them; but roads, bridges, rivers, beaches, parks, libraries, playgrounds, lavatories, schools, universities, hospitals and emergency services are not only owned by the community but may be used without payment. The distinction between what is owned privately and what is owned communally, and between what may be used for payment and what may be used freely, is quite arbitrary. It may seem obvious that we should be able to use roads and beaches without payment, but this was not always the case, and the free use of

hospitals and universities has come only during this century. In the same way, it may seem obvious that we should pay for transport and fuel, but this may not always be the case, and there is no reason why they should not be free.

One result of the equal division or free distribution of wealth rather than the accumulation of property would be the end of the class system based on ownership. But anarchists also want to end the class system based on control. This would mean constant vigilance to prevent the growth of bureaucracy in every association, and above all it would mean the reorganisation of work without a managerial class.

Work

The first need of man is for food, shelter and clothing which make life livable; the second is for the further comforts which make live worth living. The prime economic activity of any human group is the production and distribution of the things which satisfy these needs; and the most important aspect of a society - after the personal relations on which it is based - is the organisation of the necessary work. Anarchists have two characteristic ideas about work: the first is that most work is unpleasant but could be organised to be more bearable and even pleasurable; and the second is that all work should be organised by the people who actually do it.

Anarchists agree with Marxists that work in present society alienates the worker. It is not his life, but what he does to be able to live; his life is what he does outside work, and when he does something he enjoys he does not call it work. This is true of most work for most people in all places, and it is bound to be true of a lot of work for a lot of people at all times. The tiring and repetitive labour which has to be done to make plants grow and animals thrive, to run production lines and transport systems, to get to people what they want and to take from them what they do not want, could not be abolished without a drastic decline in the material standard of living; and automation, which can make it less tiring, makes it even more repetitive. But anarchists insist that the solution is not to condition people into believing that the situation is inevitable, but to reorganise essential labour so that, in the first place, it is normal for everyone who is capable of it to take a share in doing it, and for no one to spend more than a few hours a day on it; and so that, in the second place, it is possible for everyone to alternate between different kinds of boring labour, which would become less boring through greater variety. It is a matter not just of fair shares for all, but also of fair work for all.

Anarchists also agree with syndicalists that work should be run by

the workers. This does not mean that the working class – or the trade unions or a working-class party (that is, a party claiming to represent the working class) – runs the economy and has ultimate control of work. Nor does it mean the same thing on a smaller scale, that the staff of a factory can elect managers or see the accounts. It means quite simply that the people doing a particular job are in direct and total control of what they do, without any bosses or managers or inspectors at all. Some people may be good co-ordinators, and they can concentrate on co-ordination, but there is no need for them to have power over the people who do the actual work. Some people may be lazy or inefficient, but they are already. The point is to have the greatest possible control over one's own work, as well as one's own life.

This principle applies to all kinds of work – in fields as well as factories, in large cóncerns as well as small, in unskilled as well as skilled occupations, and in dirty jobs as well as liberal professions – and it is not just a useful gesture to make workers happy but a fundamental principle of any kind of free economy. An obvious objection is that complete workers' control would lead to wasteful competition between different workplaces and to production of unwanted things; an obvious answer is that complete lack of workers' control leads to exactly the same things. What is needed is intelligent planning, and despite what most people seem to think, this depends not on more control from above but on more information below.

Most economists have been concerned with production rather than consumption – with the manufacture of things rather than their use. Right-wingers and left-wingers both want workers to produce more, whether to make the rich richer or to make the state stronger, and the result is 'overproduction' alongside poverty, growing productivity together with growing unemployment, higher blocks of offices at the same time as increasing homelessness, greater yields of crops per acre when more acres are left uncultivated. Anarchists are concerned with consumption rather than production – with the use of things to satisfy the needs of the whole people instead of to increase the profits and power of the rich and strong.

Necessities and luxuries

A society with any pretension to decency cannot allow the exploitation of basic needs. It may be acceptable for luxuries to be bought and sold, since we have a choice whether we use them or not; but necessities are not mere commodities, since we have no choice about using them. If anything should be taken off the commercial market and out of the hands of exclusive groups, it is surely the land we live on, the food

which grows on it, the homes which are built on it, and those essential things which make up the material basis of human life – clothes, tools, amenities, fuel, and so on. It is also surely obvious that when there is plenty of any necessity everyone should be able to take what he needs; but that when there is a scarcity, there should be a freely agreed system of rationing so that everyone gets a fair share. It is clear that there is something wrong with any system in which waste and want exist side by side, in which some people have more than they need, while other people go without.

Above all it is clear that the first task of a healthy society is to eliminate the scarcity of necessities – such as the lack of food in undeveloped countries and the lack of housing in advanced countries – by the proper use of technical knowledge and of social resources. If the available skill and labour in Britain were used properly, for instance, there is no reason why enough food could not be grown and enough homes could not be built to feed and house the whole population. It does not happen now because present society has other priorities, not because it cannot happen. At one time it was assumed that it was impossible for everyone to be clothed properly, and poor people always wore rags; now there are plenty of clothes, and there could be plenty of everything else too.

Luxuries, by a strange paradox, are also necessities, though not basic necessities. The second task of a healthy society is to make luxuries freely available as well, though this may be a place where money would still have a useful function – provided it were not distributed according to the ludicrous lack of system in capitalist countries, or the even more ludicrous system in communist ones. The essential point is that everyone should have free and equal access to luxury.

But man does not live by bread alone, or even by cake. Anarchists would not like to see recreational, intellectual, cultural, and other such activities in the hands of society – even the most libertarian society. But there are other activities which cannot be left to individuals in free associations but must be handled by society as a whole. These are what may be called welfare activities – mutual aid beyond the reach of family and friends and outside the place of residence or work. Let us consider three of these.

The welfare society

Education is very important in human society, because we take so long to grow and take so long learning facts and skills necessary for social life, and anarchists have always been much concerned about the problems of education. Many anarchist leaders have made valuable contributions to

educational theory and practice, and many educational reformers have had libertarian tendencies – from Rousseau and Pestalozzi to Montessori and Neill. Ideas about education which were once thought of as utopian are now a normal part of the curriculum both inside and outside the state educational system in Britain, and education is perhaps the most stimulating area of society for practical anarchists. When people say that anarchy sounds nice but cannot work, we can point to a good primary or comprehensive school, or a good adventure playground or youth club. But even the best educational system is still under the control of people in authority – teachers, administrators, governors, officials, inspectors, and so on. The adults concerned in any educational process are bound to dominate it to some extent, but there is no need for them – let alone people not directly concerned in it at all – to control it.

Anarchists want the current educational reforms to go much further. Not only should strict discipline and corporal punishment be abolished – so should all imposed discipline and all penal methods. Not only should educational institutions be freed from the power of outside authorities, but students should be freed from the power of teachers or administrators. In a healthy education relationship the fact that one person knows more than another is no reason for the teacher having authority over the learner. The status of teachers in present society is based on age, strength, experience, and law; the only status teachers should have would be based on their knowledge of a subject and their ability to teach it, and ultimately on their capacity to inspire admiration and respect. What is needed is not so much student power – though that is a useful corrective to teachers' power and bureaucrats' power – as workers' control by all the people involved in an educational institution. The essential point is to break the link between teaching and governing and to make education free.

This break is actually nearer in health than in education. Doctors are no longer magicians and nurses are no longer saints, and in many countries – including Britain – the right of free medical treatment is accepted. What is needed is the extension of the principle of freedom from the economic to the political side of the health system. People should be able to go to hospital without any payment, and people should also be able to work in hospitals without any hierarchy. Once again, what is needed is workers' control by all the people involved in a medical institution. And just as education is for students, so health is for patients.

The treatment of delinquency has also progressed a long way, but it is still far from satisfactory. Anarchists have two characteristic ideas about delinquency: the first is that most so-called criminals are much the same as other people, just poorer, weaker, sillier or unluckier; the

second is that people who persistently hurt other people should not be hurt in turn but should be looked after. The biggest criminals are not burglars but bosses, not gangsters but rulers, not murderers but mass-murderers. A few minor injustices are exposed and punished by the state, while the many major injustices of present society are disguised and actually perpetrated by the state. In general punishment does more damage to society than crime does; it is more extensive, better organised, and much more effective. Nevertheless, even the most libertarian society would have to protect itself against some people, and this would inevitably involve some compulsion. But proper treatment of delinquency would be part of the education and health system, and would not become an institutionalised system of punishment. The last resort would not be imprisonment or death, but boycott or expulsion.

Pluralism

This might work the other way. An individual or a group might refuse to join or insist on leaving the best possible society; there would be nothing to stop him. In theory it is possible for a man to support himself by his own efforts, though in practice he would depend on the community to provide some materials and to take some products in exchange, so it is difficult to be literally self-sufficient. A collectivist or communist society should tolerate and even encourage such pockets of individualism. What would be unacceptable would be an independent person trying to exploit other people's labour by employing them at unfair wages or exchanging goods at unfair prices. This should not happen, because people would not normally work or buy for someone else's benefit rather than their own; and while no law would prevent appropriation, no law would prevent expropriation either – you could take something from someone, but he could take it back again. Authority and property could hardly be restored by isolated individuals.

A greater danger would come from independent groups. A separate community could easily exist within society, and this might cause severe strains; if such a community reverted to authority and property, which might raise the standard of living of the few, there would be a temptation for people to join the secession, especially if society at large were going through a bad time.

But a free society would have to be pluralist and put up with not only differences of opinion about how freedom and equality should be put into practice but also deviations from the theory of freedom and equality altogether. The only condition would be that no one is forced to join such tendencies against his will, and here some kind of authoritarian pressure would have to be available to protect even the most

libertarian society. But anarchists want to replace mass society by a mass of societies, all living together as freely as the individuals within them. The greatest danger to the free societies that have been established has been not internal regression but external aggression, and the real problem is not so much how to keep a free society going as how to get it going in the first place.

Revolution or reform

Anarchists have traditionally advocated a violent revolution to establish a free society, but some have rejected violence or revolution or both – violence is so often followed by counter-violence and revolution by counter-revolution. On the other hand, few anarchists have advocated mere reform, realising that while the system of authority and property exists superficial changes will never threaten the basic structure of society. The difficulty is that what anarchists want is revolutionary, but a revolution will not necessarily – or even probably – lead to what anarchists want. This is why anarchists have tended to resort to desperate actions or to relapse into hopeless inactivity.

In practice most disputes between reformist and revolutionary anarchists are meaningless, for only the wildest revolutionary refuses to welcome reforms and only the mildest reformist refuses to welcome revolutions, and all revolutionaries know that their work will generally lead to no more than reform and all reformists know that their work is generally leading to some kind of revolution. What most anarchists want is a constant pressure of all kinds, bringing about the conversion of individuals, the formation of groups, the reform of institutions, the rising of the people, and the destruction of authority and property. If this happened without trouble, we would be delighted; but it never has, and it probably never will. In the end it is necessary to go out and confront the forces of the state in the neighbourhood, at work, and in the streets – and if the state is defeated it is even more necessary to go on working to prevent the establishment of a new state and to begin the construction of a free society instead. There is a place for everyone in this process, and all anarchists find something to do in the struggle for what they want.

Nicolas Walter is an English journalist and editor of the *New Humanist*. He edited Kropotkin's *Memoirs of a Revolutionist* and Bakunin's *Paris Commune and the Idea of the State*. He has written in the libertarian press on both sides of the Atlantic, and has contributed to numerous anthologies of anarchism. During the 1960s he was a member of the

Committee of 100, the London Committee of 100, the Spies for Peace, and the Vietnam Action Group. He has several convictions for taking part in political demonstrations.

Part Two

The state and social organization

Introduction

The state and organization

Marxist theorists of the state have usually asked two basic questions: 'How does the state serve the ruling class?' and 'How does the state actually operate so as to maintain capitalism?' (They have seldom asked questions about the functioning of the socialist state.) Marxists have not given any unified answer. Members of the Kapitalistate Collective writing in the *Monthly Review* (1975) indicate that there have been at least three different *categories* of answers to these questions. And they go on to call for a new synthesis.

Marxists have come to reject the simplistic notion that the state is purely an instrument of the ruling class. While they have shifted more closely to the anarchist emphasis on ideology and consciousness, the question of how the state or its agents actually do operate is still open.

There has been an obvious revival of interest in the state among Marxist social scientists. There has been no such revival among anarchist theorists. For them, the very character of socialist states has made such theory to be of little concern, and they have steadfastly pointed to 'bureaucratic position and privilege' as the post-revolutionary, socialist state equivalent of class. While Maoists and some other Marxists may call for a 'continuing revolution' through which the state is to be continually remade, anarchists have always maintained that the state can not change itself. Perhaps the present-day interest in the state by Marxists reflects unstated fears of the resiliency of the capitalist state and of the authoritarianism of the socialist state (which is a tragic contradiction of socialist philosophy).

DeLeon reviews the traditional Marxist and anarchist theories on the origins and functions of the state. 'The capitalist state,' he writes, 'is virtually a gyroscope centered in capital, balancing the system.'

The pivot of Gar Alperovitz's scheme is that of preventing the centralization of power that characterizes the nation-state. He proposes to do this in the context of building a framework of localities linked by

67

co-ordinating institutions on a regional and continental scale. In his proposal for a 'pluralist commonwealth,' Alperovitz's focus on the problems of resolving inequities between communities is an important complement to those anarchist writings that are solely concerned with problems of individual equality and freedom.

While DeLeon's essay alludes to the centrality of organizational forms, and Alperovitz presents a sketch for decentralization, Ehrlich directly tackles the problems of developing a theory of anarchist organization. He selected the strategy of attacking sociological theories of organization as his means of approach. His rationale was twofold. First, he believes that we need to develop a social science based on anarchist philosophy. Second, he argues that the major societal consequence of sociology and the other social sciences is that they create ways of looking at the world that typically provide a scientific justification for the existing distribution of power. Today's justifications for organizational models are generally stated in the rhetoric of social science, and make their way from college texts to matters of common knowledge and popular culture.

The central task of the revolutionary project is to build liberatory organizational forms. And that task will require a comprehension of what is true and what is false in the handbook of sociological principles.

WANTED

THE STATE

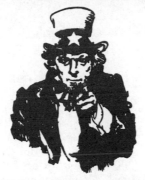

FOR CRIMES AGAINST INDIVIDUALS

THEFT — Taxation, eminent domain, confiscation of drugs, books, weapons, etc.

REPRESSION — censorship, liquor laws, sex laws, anti-trust laws, etc.

SLAVERY — Selective Slavery System (conscription)

KIDNAPPING — compulsory indoctrination of children in statist schools

NUISANCE — licensing, drug raids, vice raids, "blue" laws, etc.

FRAUD — Social Security, public education, foreign aid, and various other social experiments

ALIASES:	Uncle Sam, Public Servant, Welfare State, Big Brother, World Peacemaker, et al.
DESCRIPTION:	height — piled higher and deeper weight — as much as he can throw around eyes — his "EYE" is everywhere
OCCUPATION:	professional thug of the "silent majority"
CAUTION:	subject is heavily armed and dangerous and is frequently found lurking in and around world councils, in the company of other states.

ISSUED BY: THE NEW BANNER   **PLEASE POST**
BOX 1972
COLUMBIA, SOUTH CAROLINA 29202

4 Anarchism on the origins and functions of the state: some basic notes*

David DeLeon

We live in a world divided into more than 180 states. While this seems natural to us, these organizations were absent from most of human history. The oldest states were formed in Egypt, Iraq and elsewhere about 5,500 years ago, whereas a speaking and tool-making humanity has been present for approximately 1 million years. Although both figures can be disputed, that would not alter the fact that states have existed for as little as 1/200th of our history.[1] Early societies did not have police, courts, political administrations and armies. They were 'governed' by customs, the sexual division of labor (with the women doing certain tasks and the men others), and the collective struggle for survival.

With the evolution of societies that produced a surplus, whether it was more food, more cattle or more goods than could be immediately consumed, economic inequality was likely to occur. In some cultures this surplus came to be redistributed by various mechanisms, but in others it persisted and grew. Then, primitive communism was replaced by property and society was split into classes, based upon ownership of the means of production and the social division of labor. In these cultures it often became necessary for the economically advantaged to have some means to protect their property. The organization, control and direction of a property society fostered a separate police force (instead of the armed people), formal laws and types of governance, all needing taxes to maintain. This process was accelerated in some areas by regimenting the population to build and preserve irrigation systems. More generally, wealth and territorial expansion provoked wars which, in turn, were justifications for the enlargement of institutional powers.[2]

Most anarchists and Marxists agree that the state was founded in conflict, not consensus. It was built upon the ruins of early community. A sovereign power, having a monopoly on interior force (police and law) and exterior violence (war-making capacity), ruling over a definite

---

* This article is printed here for the first time.

territory, was vital for the preservation of a society of inequality. Bakunin remarked that 'the State is the organized authority, domination and power of the possessing classes over the masses,' and Daniel DeLeon, a Marxist, made a similar argument:[3]

> The 'political state' is that social structure which marks the epoch since which society was ruptured into classes, and class-rule began. This fact determines the foundation of the political State. The foundation of the political State is not, as it was with previous society, man; the foundation of the political State is property.

Why had people accepted this inequality? Marxists and anarchists concurred, in the nineteenth century, that it was a slow process that had not triumphed everywhere, although the spread of capitalism would intrude forms of state organization into the most remote corners of the planet. Marxists regarded this tendency, however brutal, as a progressive stage from primitive communism toward the full utilization of resources and realization of humanity within a higher form of communism. Anarchists, even when they agreed that the division of labor and the state had laid the foundations for possible utopia, were more likely to emphasize the crimes of the state than to emphasize its historical necessity. Neither group, however, believed that the state was eternal, or that it was rooted in 'human nature,' such as a desire for domination, some sense of territoriality, or aggressive instincts.

Beyond these generalities, however, neither the Marxists nor the anarchists of the nineteenth century wrote extensively on the state. Marx had planned to devote the fourth book of a six-volume study called *Economics* to the role of the state, but this was never done. Both his comments and those of the anarchists were brief. A century ago, this neglect was understandable. Most states had small bureaucracies, restricted taxing powers, few social welfare programs, no nationalized industries, and relatively limited military forces. Today, Marxists have become vitally concerned with the activities of the state.[4]

What are the essential functions of the state today, and some of the means that it can use to achieve its purposes? Above all, the state remains an institution for the continuance of dominant socioeconomic relations, whether through such agencies as the military, courts, politics or police. Because it has a monopoly on 'legitimate' force, the anarchists have always claimed that the state is the greatest terrorist, at home and abroad. While Josiah Warren could comment, in the 1870s, on the 'civilized cannibalism' of elite power, modern examples of systematic terror are more obvious: colonialism, Stalinist dictatorship, Nazism, the Second World War, and Vietnam. Although anarchists may concede that the Western liberal democracies are (in Herbert Marcuse's words)

71

non-terroristic totalitarianisms, they insist that all states are fundamentally unjust, if not equally unjust.

Contemporary states have acquired, for example, less primitive means
to reinforce their property systems. States can regulate, moderate or
resolve tensions in the economy by preventing the bankruptcies of key
corporations, manipulating the economy through interest rates, supporting hierarchical ideology through tax benefits for churches and schools,
and other tactics. In essence, it is not a neutral institution; it is powerfully for the status quo. The capitalist state, for example, is virtually a
gyroscope centered in capital, balancing the system. If one sector of the
economy earns a level of profit, let us say, that harms the rest of the
system – such as oil producers' causing public resentment and increased
manufacturing costs – the state may redistribute some of that profit
through taxation, or offer encouragement to competitors.

But these institutional mechanisms, by themselves, are not the only
reasons for public control. No state can survive without at least the
passive support of the populace. While the size of the government and
the majesty of its buildings, rituals and elaborate regulations partly
explain the resignation or awe of the majority ('What can I do? You
can't fight City Hall'), there are other reasons. The modern state benefits
from various psychological and social appeals, fostering an ideological
hegemony where a basic critique of the state becomes almost unthink-
able.

First, there are appeals to patriotism, to 'our nation.' The highest
values of the culture are said to be embodied in the agencies of authority, hierarchy and domination: the Supreme Court, the people's legislature, the President of the Republic. Ceremonies, awards, medals, titles
and pomp add to the aura of solemn importance. Marx once commented
that, just as the image of God derived from human desires for perfection
that were thwarted, the mythology of the good state represented the
yearning for community, but through a false community that was
really dominated by elites and the demands of capital. One commenta-
tor has claimed that Marx perceived the state as 'the most characteristic
institution of man's alienated condition.'[5]

Patriotism can be used, like religion and socialist ideology, to justify
repressing critics of the established order. 'Reasons of state' have been
excuses for monstrous crimes, and even the basis for praising destruction
and murder as acts of virtue. Emma Goldman captured the typical
anarchist sentiment when she entitled one of her essays 'Patriotism: A
Menace of Liberty.'

Second, modern governments tend to emphasize their justice, or their
defense of human rights. By one estimate, the United States has over
65 million laws. The labyrinthine complexity of this appals, mystifies
or impresses the majority of the population. Yet the anarchists are

convinced that behind noble rhetoric is usually the aggrandizing re
of politics: 'The Congressmen have gone home. Of course the treasury
is empty and there is a big deficit for us to make good. Long live "law
and order"!'[6]

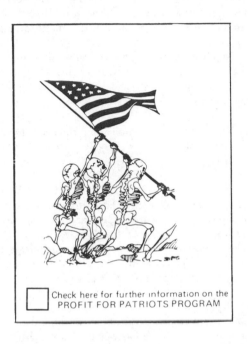

Check here for further information on the
PROFIT FOR PATRIOTS PROGRAM

Third, states are now generally cloaked in the fiction or the reality
of popular validation. Even dictatorships are 'democratic people's
republics' or 'free world governments.' Myths like this can be powerful
narcotics, if believed.[7] 'Democracies' that actually allow participation
have the most convincing case, even if participation is not necessarily
power. For a citizen to cast a slip of paper for a representative who
cannot be removed easily, and is likely to be controlled by corporate
interests, is shallow democracy. The democratic state is often an elaborate maze of 'proper channels' into which the public's demands may
enter only to be trapped.

Fourth, all states appeal to stability. Most people will suffer known
evils rather than trying a potential good. They feel helpless before
historical continuity, the enormity of society, the unintelligible language
of 'experts,' and the implications that they are unimportant. The
citizen becomes a passive being, waiting for the central authority to act,

...ne phrase 'I only obeyed orders.'[8]

...are modern equivalents to bread and circuses in welfare ...trionic foreign policies and other activities.

...these economic, social and symbolic justifications of the ...been acceptable to the anarchists. While liberals and social ...s may argue that the state can be reformed, both anarchists and Marxists reply that it must be abolished.[9] As Engels stated:[10]

> The society which reorganizes production on the basis of free and equal association of the producers will put the whole state machinery where it will then belong – into the museum of antiquities, next to the spinning wheel and the bronze axe.

Marx spoke of 'transcending' or 'abolishing' the state; Engels coined the phrase that the state must 'wither away.' The revolution would make a clean sweep:[11]

> Along with the state disappear its representatives; ministers, parliaments, regular armies, police and gendarms, courts, lawyers and public prosecutors, prison wardens, tax and custom authorities, in a word – the whole political apparatus. Barracks and other military buildings, court and administrative premises, prisons, etc. will be turned to better use. Tens of thousands of laws, decrees and regulations will have become waste paper, and will possess only historical value.

As an alternative to centralized coercion, the early Marxists envisioned the free commune, 'an association in which the free development of each is the condition of the free development of all' (*Communist Manifesto*). Neither the anarchists nor the Marxists disagreed with Saint-Simon that the government of people should be replaced by the administration of things.

They differed radically, however, on the means. The Marxists ridiculed the anarchists as impatient utopians who often refused to differentiate between authoritarian and democratic governments, scorned reforms as trivial, failed to create effective groups, and denied the necessity for rigid centralization (such as the dictatorship of the proletariat) in order to defend the revolution from internal and external enemies. Discipline, the Marxists said, was imperative during the transitional period.[12]

Anarchists and Marxists were already divided in the 1840s by this question, which influenced all of their other views. Marxists, for example, commonly welcomed the growing centralizations of power, the triumphs of colonialism, and concentrations of capital as precursors

of socialism. These trends would presumably culminate in a final monopoly, the popularly controlled state, which was, perhaps, a transitional stage. Anarchists, of all types, were horrified. The Marxists said little about ultimate decentralization or human rights for all. The anarchists favored regions and cities, rather than nations; individuals and communes, not 'the masses.' They believed that the Marxist reliance on large units would inevitably poison their libertarian goals, producing 'the indivisibility of public power, all-consuming centralization, systematic destruction of all individual, co-operative and regional thought [regarded as disruptive], and inquisitorial police.'[13] When such criticism was raised in the First International, Marx had termed it nonsense, while purging the critics.[14]

The twentieth century has witnessed the validation of much of the anarchist critique of any Marxist provisional state. As Marxist parties came to power, their anti-statist goals were retained only verbally, in a process 'analogous to the transformation of revolutionary, anti-statist Christianity into the official religion of the Roman state.'[15] Bakunin's prediction of a new class, 'the red bourgeoisie,' was realized in the party elite, with special benefits in housing, food and cars, and their comfortable isolation in an ever-expanding bureaucracy. Proudhon's specter of 'barracks socialism' was also achieved in all of the people's democracies, where socialism means more and more state power, often exploiting the people in the name of the people. Workers in nationalized factories are denied independent unions, and often discover that the management is remote, centralized and authoritarian. Political life is discouraged, other than obediently voting in elections with no choices. Lenin began these policies in the USSR with the plea that they constituted 'a thoroughgoing material preparation for socialism, the entrance gate to it.'[16]

History has mocked this dream; the USSR has become a model of state monopoly capital. One critic has jokingly compared the modern reality with Lenin's vision in *State and Revolution*, 'the greatest pre-election pamphlet ever written: "Elect us and we will wither away".'[17] Trotskyists may argue that Stalin 'betrayed' the Revolution, but anarchists say that Trotskyism is merely Stalinism out of power. At any rate, Stalin is now dead, but neo-Stalinism lives on. Others plead that the USSR was born in difficult circumstances; but so were other socialist governments, like Yugoslavia and China, whose resulting states have not been so cruelly repressive.

The market socialism of Yugoslavia and the genuine elements of mass participation in China have been exceptions to the command society, directed from the top, that is typical of the Marxist world. Even these exceptions may be defeated by capitalism and/or nationalism. To date, it is not obvious that the political state, by protecting and encouraging property relations, is creating the potential for the abolition of the

state. Rather, the merging of political and civil societies has produced all-invading governments. One century after Bakunin's prophecy, it sounds truer than ever:[18]

> In the People's State of Marx, there will be, we are told, no privileged class at all. . . . But there will be a government and, note this well, an extremely complex government, which will not be content with governing and administering the masses politically, as all governments do today, but will also administer them economically, concentrating in its own hands the production and just division of wealth. . . . It will be the reign of *scientific intelligence*, the most aristocratic, despotic, arrogant, and contemptuous of all regimes. There will be a new class, a new hierarchy of real and pretended scientists and scholars, and the world will be divided into a minority ruling in the name of knowledge and an immense majority.

The greatest victories of Marxism during this century must also be numbered among its most stunning defeats. Statist communists could learn much from the anarcho-communists.

It is also true, however, that the theories of the anarchists have often been impressionistic (however insightful), their constituencies disorganized, and their goals obscure. Some anarchists have even engaged in political activity to promote anti-statism – such as many in the Spanish Civil War – but most have shunned this activity as incompatible with their ideals. The problem of building a stateless society remains.

It is difficult even to present an outline of such a society because the anarchists have resisted any description of life after a revolution, just as Marx refused to predict the future. Both assumed that needs would be met by popular ingenuity. When people asked 'what will replace the state?' the anarchists said[19]

> this is akin to such questions as: – If you abolish slavery, what do you propose to do with four million ignorant 'niggers'? If you abolish popes, priests and organized religion, what do you propose to do with the rude and vicious masses? If you abolish marriage, what do you propose to do with the children? etc., etc.

For anarchists like Goldman, these were 'trifling details.' When society was freed from the bonds of the state, natural patterns of organization would spontaneously develop. Until then, it was absurd to predict 'A Complete Representation of Universal Progress for the Balance of Eternity.'[20]

One myth about the anarchists must be dispelled, however. They have seldom envisioned anarchy as the abolition of all organizations.

Instead, it would mean new forms of organization. Kropotkin urged the creation of voluntary 'communities of interest,' and S. P. Andrews pointed to such models as common nurseries, infant schools and co-operative cafeterias. These would be more economical, efficient and varied than tiny separate facilities. They would also assist in the abolition of 'the unmitigated drudgery and undevelopment of the female sex.'[21] Josiah Warren agreed that something like a common kitchen would be cheaper, more convenient and would 'relieve the female of the family from the full, mill-horse drudgery to which they otherwise are irretrievably doomed.'[22] Forms of economic production could also be enormously diverse. Andrews could imagine vast 'combined houses' where a hundred or a thousand 'may be engaged in the same shop, and still their interests would be entirely individualized.'[23]

This would be a true 'government by consent' where the necessary functions of society could be accomplished by voluntary associations. Then, if some individual, like a Henry David Thoreau, did not wish to join the fire protection company, he would not be required to do so. Of course, if his house burned down, the fire company was also not under the slightest obligation to assist him. Or, if a person wanted protection (although, in a fully libertarian society, where all had been socialized to respect the rights of others, this should be an unlikely need), he or she might band together with others, pay in labor or subscriptions, and organize to meet their requirements.

Of course, the concept of an anarchist police force is likely to raise some objections. What about rivalries? Even if people in a libertarian society were tolerant, individuals and groups could have disputes, or need defense from invaders. Still, most anarchists assume that people would make arrangements among themselves for such occurrences. Perhaps there could be a generally recognized association for adjudication, or local juries.

Juries might consist of twelve people whose names were drawn by lot from a wheel containing the names of all the citizens of the community. Service would be voluntary, although it could be expected for membership in any of the defense associations. The jury would 'shape' the broad suggestions that would comprise anarchist 'rules' to fit each individual case. Their primary activity, since Proudhon had defined the new regime as one of contracts and not of laws, would be to enforce the obligations that individuals had freely assumed. Conviction of a crime could result in public censure, imprisonment or even death. However, anarchists agree that 'punishment is in itself an objectionable and hateful thing, productive of evil even when it prevents greater evil, and therefore it is not wise to resort to it for the redress of trivial wrongs.'[24]

Other forms of non-state governance are also possible. The Oneida

Colony, although centered on the authority figure of John Humphrey Noyes, contributed a remarkable practice called Mutual Criticism. Members of the community were expected to submit themselves to occasional evaluation by a standing committee on criticism. If they were reluctant, such an evaluation could be suggested, or even required. The members of this committee rotated, so that someone might be a critic at one time, and the object of criticism later. The panel analyzed the character and actions of a person while he or she would sit silently. Social virtues were thereby praised and reinforced, while arrogance was deflated by sharply honest words. It was, in effect, an anarchist form of government, supposedly combining the virtues of all other regimes with none of their defects. Noyes predicted that its use in families (children and parents criticizing each other), schools (students 'grading' teachers) or the general community would be strong medicine for a healthy society.[25]

American anarchists further mentioned the possibility of threatening an anti-social individual or group with boycott. This would replace physical coercion with a more subtle form of social control. It would be a reasonable substitute for government. Public opinion is pervasive in democratic societies, where the individual is sensitive about his or her image before other citizens and cultivates their favor.

The boycott technique could take both positive and negative forms. It could be used to discipline or punish some persons or groups, or to gain a larger objective. For example, race prejudice could be attacked by this method: 'The Negroes of the South have the white people of that section in their power, and they can exercise that power without the commission of a single overt act.' If they refused to associate with prejudiced whites – contributing their labor, consuming white products, showing respect or tolerance for them – though racial 'antipathies' might persist, the power of the whites could be broken or at least controlled.[26]

The policy of boycott had been used successfully by Josiah Warren in his City of Modern Times on Long Island, in the 1850s. As one of his friends summarized this policy:[27]

> When we wish to rid ourselves of unpleasant persons, we simply let them alone. We buy nothing of them, sell them nothing, exchange no words with them – in short, by establishing a complete system of noninterference with them, we show them unmistakably that they are not wanted here, and they usually go away of their own accord.

But someone had to be aggressively offensive before the citizens of Modern Times were provoked. The village had some fame (and, among the respectable, infamy) for the political, social and sexual diversity of

its inhabitants. Nor were they all libertarians. Henry Edger, one of the few American disciples of a highly authoritarian Comtean Positivism, lived at Modern Times and openly agitated for followers. He had a perfect right to believe whatever he wished, just as his neighbors had the perfect right to believe the opposite.

Still, one is somewhat uncomfortable with the rude justice of the boycott and similar forms of 'government.' George Orwell, in his writings on the Spanish Civil War, was respectful of anarchist ideals, but suspected that a totalitarianism of public opinion could result. He worried that the beliefs of the majority would be imposed upon everyone. Much earlier, Tucker had admitted that boycotters were no better than other human beings: they could 'sometimes be cruel, sometimes malicious, sometimes short-sighted, sometimes silly.'[28] There is undeniably a fervent element of moral crusade in such writers as Godwin, Proudhon and Kropotkin. This could threaten spontaneity and diversity.

The American anarchists have been aware of this hazard. Tucker had repudiated idealism because he feared the 'invasive' possibilities of ideals. People should be free to be themselves. Warren had called fashion and habit the greatest obstacles to such liberation: 'Fashion – more tyrannical than tyranny itself! . . . A power which controls all other controllable powers.'[29] The anarchists, conscious of this danger, struggled for a society that respected peaceable 'nonconformists.'

They were convinced that such a tolerant society was possible. They ridiculed the existing repression found in laws, courts and jails for denying this democratic hope. The continued existence of the state implied that:[30]

> education goes for nothing; example goes for nothing; public opinion goes for nothing; social ostracism goes for nothing; increase of material welfare goes for nothing; decrease of temptation goes for nothing; health goes for nothing; approximate equality of conditions goes for nothing. . . . The Christian doctrine that hell is the only safeguard to religious morality [becomes the doctrine] that a hell on earth is the only safeguard of natural morality.

Today, the internationalization of capital and conflicts between competing interests have promoted the emergence of prototypes for super states. Such organizations as the Common Market and the United Nations are attempts to create regional and international umpires for various problems. Anarchists condemn these institutions, dominated by the wealthy and privileged elites of the world, as congresses of thieves. If they succeed in organizing the world, the majority of humanity will gain little. If they fail, society may be destroyed in a nuclear war. The

latter is especially ominous. While states often justify their existence, and the necessity for international police, by the dangers posed by other states, it is the state itself that is the greatest threat to humanity. Let us suppose that the US government was not present to block a Russian invasion. Assuming that this actually happened, there would be no state apparatus to seize; there would be a hostile population, 'passive resistance' and guerrilla warfare. 'No occupying force can long keep down a native population determined to resist. . . . Surely the anticipation of this sea of troubles and the enormous costs and losses that would inevitably follow would deter any theoretical invader.'[31]

We would be foolish to ignore such arguments. The modern state is everywhere, and we must judge the pieties about its necessity and sanctity. Is it, or can it be, a 'servant of the people'? The anarchists reply that its own history condemns it.

Notes

1 Kathleen Gough, 'The Decline of the State,' *Our Generation*, 2 (Fall 1962), 22–31; 'The State' (articles by Morton Fried, Frederick M. Watkins, and – on stateless societies – Aidan Southall), in *The International Encyclopedia of the Social Sciences* (New York: Macmillan and The Free Press, 1968), XV, 143–69 (including bibliographies).

   Let me stress the subtitle of my essay, 'Some Basic Notes.' This is only one possible rendition of some anarchist themes.

2 The major theoreticians of anarcho-communism, syndicalism and Marxism have tended to agree on the foundations of the state: Frederick Engels, *The Origin of the Family, Private Property and the State* (1884) – recent editions with introductions by Eleanor Burke (New York: International, 1972) and Evelyn Reed (New York: Pathfinder, 1972); *The Political Philosophy of Bakunin*, ed. G. P. Maximoff (New York: The Free Press, 1953); Peter Kropotkin, 'The State; Its Historic Role' (London: Freedom Press, 1969 [1896]). Some of Marx's comments were elaborated (or transformed) by Karl Wittfogel in *Oriental Despotism* (New Haven: Yale University Press, 1957).

3 Bakunin, quoted in *Fifth Estate* (Detroit), 11 (August 1976), 1; Daniel DeLeon, 'Haywoodism and Industrialism' (1913), in *Self-Governing Socialism*, ed. Branko Horvat and others (White Plains, New York: International Arts and Sciences Press, 1975), 98.

4 This literature includes issues of *Kapitalistate* (1973–present); David Gold, Clarence Y. H. Lo, and Erik Olin Wright, 'Recent Developments in Marxist Theories of the Capitalist State' (a summary and critique, in two parts), *Monthly Review*, 27, nos. 5, 6 (October and November 1975); David Harvey, 'The Marxian

Theory of the State,' *Antipode*, 8:2 (May 1976), 80–9; and Fred Block, 'The Ruling Class Does Not Rule: Notes on the Marxist Theory of the State,' *Socialist Revolution*, no. 33 (May–June 1977), 6–28.

5 David McLellan, 'The State,' in *The Thought of Karl Marx* (texts and commentary) (New York: Harper and Row, 1971), 179–95.

6 B. R. Tucker, *Liberty*, 7 (March 7, 1891), 1. He further remarked that 'when people begin to hate their governments, they will begin to love one another' (*Liberty*, 9 (September 24, 1892], 1). The only comprehensive anarchist study of nationalism is Rudolf Rocker's *Nationalism and Culture* (Los Angeles: Rocker Publications Committee, 1937). By and large, early anarchists such as Tucker and Goldman seldom wrote elaborate tomes on their major concepts. Proudhon wrote disjointed treatises, but Kropotkin was quite unusual, in the nineteenth century, as a systematic anarchist thinker.

7 See Ernst Cassirer, *The Myth of the State* (New Haven: Yale University Press, 1946).

8 This is discussed in Murray Rothbard's introduction to *The Politics of Obedience*, by Étienne de la Boétie (New York: Free Life, 1975 [1550s]). The edition includes a blurb by Stanley Milgram, the author of *Obedience to Authority* (New York: Harper and Row, 1974), that la Boétie has uncovered 'the psychological foundations' of subservience. A libertarian thesis on the role of psychology is also presented in Alex Comfort's *Authority and Delinquency in the Modern State* (London: Routledge & Kegan Paul, 1950).

9 Fritz Pappenheim, 'Politics and Alienation,' in *The Alienation of Modern Man* (New York: Monthly Review, 1968 [1959]), 45–60; M. Bakunin, in *The Fifth Estate*, 12 (June 1977).

10 F. Engels, *The Origin of the Family, Private Property and the State* (New York: International, 1972), 232.

11 August Bebel, 'The Withering Away of the State,' in *The Society of the Future* (Moscow: Progress Publishers, 1971), 84–7.

12 Most of these questions are polemically addressed in *Anarchism and Anarcho-Syndicalism*, by Marx, Engels, and Lenin (New York: International, 1972), 153.

13 P. J. Proudhon, quoted in J. Hapden Jackson, *Proudhon, Marx and European Socialism* (New York: Macmillan, 1957), 182. Tucker commented that 'anarchy is equal liberty; democracy is reciprocal tyranny' (*Liberty*, 5 (November 5, 1887), 1).

14 Karl Marx, 'American Split,' in *Documents of the First International*, 5 vols (London: Lawrence and Wishart, n.d.), V, 323–32.

15 Karl Korsch, 'The Crisis of Marxism' (1931), *New German Critique*, 1 (Fall 1974), 10.

16 Lenin, quoted in Paul Mattick, 'The Inevitability of Communism' (New York: Polemic Publishers, 1935), 20. See also Emma Goldman, *My Disillusionment in Russia* (New York: Apollo, 1970); Errico Malatesta, 'Anarchy' (London: Freedom Press, n.d.)–

including his comment that, 'should it survive, [the state] would continually tend to reconstruct, under one form or another, a privileged and oppressing class' (p. 22); Marie-Louise Berneri, *Neither East nor West* (London: Freedom Press, 1952); 'Towards Workers' Control' (London: Freedom pamphlet, n.d.).

17 Unidentified; quoted in *Communalism: From Its Origins to the Twentieth Century*, by Kenneth Rexroth (New York: Seabury, 1974), x. Many of Lenin's central writings on government have been conveniently collected in *On the Soviet State Apparatus* (Moscow: Progress Publishers, 1975).

18 From *The Knouto-Germanic Empire*, in *Quotations from the Anarchists*, ed. Paul Berman (New York: Praeger, 1972), 73. See, in addition, Daniel Guerin, *Anarchism* (New York: Monthly Review, 1970), April Carter, 'Anarchism and the State,' in *The Political Theory of Anarchism* (New York: Harper and Row, 1971), 28–59, and Colin Ward, 'Anarchy and the State,' in *Anarchism in Action* (New York: Harper and Row, 1974), 17–27.

19 Tucker, *Liberty*, 1 (October 1, 1881), 3. He once confessed that it was easier for him to demonstrate why he was not anything else than to tell why he was an anarchist: 'Archism once denied, only Anarchism can be affirmed. It is a matter of logic.' ('Why I am an Anarchist,' *Twentieth Century Magazine*, 4 (May 29, 1890), 5–6).

20 Tucker, *Liberty*, 3 (June 3, 1885), 4.

21 Peter Kropotkin, *Paroles d'un Révolté* (Paris: Marpon, Flammarion, 1885), 117; S. P. Andrews, *The Science of Society*, no. 2 (New York: T. L. Nichols, 1854), 179–81.

22 Josiah Warren, *Equitable Commerce* (New York, 1852), 69.

23 S. P. Andrews, *Science of Society*, no. 2, 49. While this implies craft labor, not factory jobs, he was not merely an archaic spokesman for a simpler agrarian and petty capitalist period. None of the major anarchists repudiated modern technology. Instead, they hoped to use technology to free humanity. Godwin, in the 1790s, had eloquently expressed the possibility that machines could liberate people for a fuller life. He made the fantastic prediction that the members of a properly functioning society would work a half-hour every day! Warren and Andrews more modestly estimated that two hours of daily labor might provide all necessities. Kropotkin was also confident that mechanization could free men and women from innumerable tedious and degrading tasks.

24 Tucker, *Liberty*, 11 (February 8, 1896), 5. Kropotkin was fearful that these defense associations would be the seed for recreating the state, but he offered no realistic alternative for the defense of anarchism. His criticisms are scattered throughout *Kropotkin's Revolutionary Pamphlets*, edited by Roger Baldwin (New York: Dover, 1970 [1927]).

25 John Humphrey Noyes, *Mutual Criticism* (New York: Syracuse University Press, 1975 [1876]); William Hinds, *American Communities* (New York: Corinth, 1961 [1878]), 135; Maren Lock-

wood Carden, *Oneida* (Baltimore: Johns Hopkins University Press, 1969).

26 Clarence Lee Swartz, 'The Solution of the "Negro Problem",' *Liberty*, 15 (December 1906), 47.

27 Quoted in John B. Ellis, *Free Love and Its Votaries* (New York: US Publishing Co., 1890), 398. This book's information on Modern Times is more reliable than its interpretations.

28 Tucker, *Liberty*, 14 (April 1903), 4.

29 Warren, *Equitable Commerce*, 117.

30 Tucker, *Instead of a Book, by a Man Too Busy to Write One* (New York: B. R. Tucker, 1893), 57-58.

31 Murray N. Rothbard, *For a New Liberty* (New York: Macmillan, 1973), 250-1. The reader is also directed to several other general studies that are frequently cited by radical individualists: Franz Oppenheimer, *The State*, with an introduction by C. Hamilton (New York: Free Life, 1975 [1st Eng. ed. 1914]); Albert J. Nock, *Our Enemy, the State*, with an introduction by Walter Grinder (New York: Free Life, 1973 [1935]); R. N. Nozick, *Anarchy, State and Utopia* (New York: Basic Books, 1974); and Peter Manicas, *The Death of the State* (New York: Putnam, 1974).

5 Towards a decentralist commonwealth*

Gar Alperovitz

Where to begin a dialogue on long-term program? Historically, a major radical starting point has been socialism – conceived as social ownership of the means of production primarily through nationalization. Although the *ideal* of socialism involves the more encompassing values of justice, equality, co-operation, democracy, and freedom, in practice it has often resulted in a dreary, authoritarian political economy.

Alternatives to centralization

A number of traditions have attempted to confront difficulties inherent in the centralizing tendencies of state socialism; consideration of some of their alternatives suggests an initial approach to defining elements of a positive program. It is helpful to acknowledge, frankly and at the outset, that some traditional conservatives (as opposed to rightist demagogues) have long been correct to argue that centralization of both economic and political power leaves the citizen virtually defenseless, without any institutional way to control major issues which affect his life. They have objected to state socialism on the grounds that it destroys individual initiative, responsibility and freedom, and have urged that privately held property (particularly that of the farmer or small capitalist entrepreneur) at least offers a man some independent ground to stand on in the fight against what they term 'statism.' Finally, most have held that the competitive market can work to make capitalists responsible to the needs of the community.

Some conservatives have also stressed the concept of 'limits,' especially limits to state power, and like some new radicals have emphasized the importance of voluntary participation and individual personal responsibility. Karl Hess, Murray Rothbard and Leonard Liggio, among

---

* This is excerpted from the original which appeared in *Our Generation*, vol. 9, 1973.

others of the Libertarian Right, have recently begun to reassert these themes against old socialists, liberals, and more modern 'statist' conservatives like William Buckley Jr. The conservative sociologist, Robert A. Nisbet, argues as well that voluntary associations should serve as intermediate units of community and power between the individual and the state.

Few traditional conservatives or members of the Libertarian Right, however, have recognized the socialist argument that private property (and the competitive market) as sources of independence, power, and responsibility have led historically to other horrendous problems, including exploitation, inequality, ruthless competition, individual alienation, the destruction of community, expansionism, imperialism, war etc.

A second alternative – also an attempt to organize economic power away from the centralized state – is represented by the Yugoslav argument for workers' self-management. Whereas private property (in principle if not in practice) implies decentralization of economic power to individuals, workers' self-management involves decentralization to the social and organizational unit of those who work in a firm. This alternative may even be thought of as a way to achieve the conservative anti-statist purpose but also to establish different, socially defined priorities over economic resources.

The Yugoslav model of decentralization raises a series of difficult problems. Though the Yugoslavs proclaim themselves socialists and urge that the overall industrial system must benefit the entire society, the various workers' groups which actually have direct control of industrial resources are each inevitably only one part of society. And as many now see, there is no obvious reason why such partial groups will not develop special interests ('workers' capitalism') which run counter to the interests of the broader community.

Indeed, problems very much akin to those of a system based on private property in production have begun to appear in Yugoslavia. Over-reliance on the market has not prevented inequality between communities, and has led to commercialism and exploitation. Both unemployment and inflation also plague the Yugoslav economy. An ethic of individual gain and profit has often taken precedence over the ideal of co-operation. Worker participation in many instances is more theory than practice. Meanwhile, as competitive tendencies emerge between various worker-controlled industries, side by side there have grown up anomalies produced by the need for some central co-ordination. The banks now control many nationwide investment decisions, severely reducing local economic power; the Yugoslav Communist Party takes a direct and often arbitrary hand in both national and local decisions. In general, it has been extremely difficult for social

85

units to develop a sense of reciprocal individual responsibility as the basis for an equitable community of mutual obligation.

The Yugoslav model recalls the historic themes of both guild socialism and syndicalism. It is also closely related to the 'participatory economy' alternative recently offered by Jaroslav Vanek, and the model of workers' participation proposed by Robert A. Dahl. All alternatives of this kind, unfortunately, suffer from a major contradiction: it is difficult to see how a political economy based primarily on the organization of groups by function could ever achieve a just society, since the various structural alternatives seem inherently to tend towards the self-aggrandizement of each functional group – as against the rest of the community.

The point may perhaps be most easily understood by imagining workers' control or ownership of the General Motors Corporation in the United States of America – an idea close to Dahl's alternative. It should be obvious that: (1) there is no reason to expect white male auto workers easily to admit more blacks, Puerto Ricans, or women into 'their' industry when unemployment prevails; (2) no internal dynamic is likely to lead workers automatically or willingly to pay out 'their' wages or surpluses to reduce pollution 'their' factory chimney might pour onto the community as a whole; (3) above all, the logic of the system militates against going out of 'their' business when it becomes clear that the automobile-highway mode of transportation (rather than, say, mass transit) is destructive of the community as a whole though perhaps profitable for 'their' industry.

Dahl, for one, is aware of some of these shortcomings; he hopes through interest group representation that somehow an 'optimum combination' of worker and general community interest might be worked out. Clearly, were a socialist framework substituted for the capitalist market such problems might in part be alleviated. The Yugoslav experience (where both the commune and the nation have extensive powers), however, teaches that socialism does not automatically resolve either the market's difficulties or the root contradiction inherent in a context which structurally opposes the interests as a whole.

Some basic distinctions must be confronted. First, while management by the people who work in a firm should be affirmed, the matter of emphasis is of cardinal importance: 'workers' control' should be conceived in the broader context of, and subordinate to, the entire community. In order to break down divisions which pose one group against another and to achieve equity, accordingly, the social unit at the heart of any proposed new system should, so far as possible, be inclusive of all the people – minorities, the elderly, women, youth – not just the 'workers' who have paid 'jobs,' and who at any one time number only

some 40 per cent of the population and 60 per cent of the adult citizenry.

A second, perhaps more difficult, point is that the only social unit inclusive of all the people is one based on geographic contiguity. This, in the context of national geography, is the general socialist argument; the requirement of decentralization simply reduces its scale. In a territorially-defined local community, a variety of functional groups must coexist, side by side. Day-to-day communication is possible (indeed, individuals are often members of more than one group); and long-term relationships can be developed. Conflicts must inevitably be mediated directly by people who have to live with the decisions they make. There are, of course, many issues which cannot be dealt with locally, but at least a social unit based on common location proceeds from the assumption of comprehensiveness, and this implies a decision-making context in which the question 'How will a given policy affect all the community?' is more easily posed.

When small, territorially defined communities control capital or land socially (as, for instance, in the Israeli kibbutz or the Chinese commune), unlike either capitalism or state socialism, there is no built-in contradiction between the interests of owners or beneficiaries of industry against the community as a whole. The problem of 'externalities,' moreover, is in part internalized by the structure itself. Since the community as a whole controls productive wealth, it, for instance, is in a position to decide rationally whether to pay the costs of eliminating the pollution its own industry causes for its own people. The entire community may decide how to divide work equitably among all its citizens.

Although small-scale ownership of capital might resolve some problems, it raises others. The likelihood that if workers owned General Motors they might attempt to exploit their position, or oppose changes in the nation's overall transportation system, illuminates a problem which a society based on co-operative communities would also face. As long as the social and economic security of any economic unit is not guaranteed, it is likely to function to protect (and out of insecurity, extend) its own special interests even when they run counter to the broader interests of the society. The only long-run answer to the basic expansionist tendency of all market systems is to establish some stable larger structural framework to sustain the smaller constituent elements of the political economy.

A pluralist commonwealth?

To review and affirm both the socialist vision and the decentralist ideal is to suggest that a basic problem of positive alternative programs is to

define community economic institutions which are egalitarian and equitable in the socialist sense of owning and controlling productive resources for the benefit of all, but which can prevent centralization of power, and finally which over time can permit new social relations capable of sustaining an ethic of individual responsibility and group co-operation which a larger vision must ultimately involve.

The sketch of a long-term vision might begin with the neighborhood in the city and the county in the countryside (and pose as a research problem which industries from shoe repair to steel refining can usefully be decentralized) and what scale (say between 30,000 and 100,000) is appropriate for communities. Its longer thrust however is more complicated. In place of the streamlined socialist planned state which depends upon the assumption of power at the top, I would substitute an organic diversified vision: a vision of thousands of small communities, each organized co-operatively, each working out its own priorities and methods, each generating broader economic criteria and placing political demands on the larger system out of this experience. The locality should be conceived as a basis for, not an alternative to, a larger framework of regional and national co-ordinating institutions.

In its local form, such a vision is obviously greatly supportive of the ideal of community proposed by Percival and Paul Goodman in their book *Communitas*. More specifically, a community which owned substantial industry co-operatively and used part of its surplus for its own social services would have important advantages: it could experiment, without waiting for bureaucratic decrees, with new schools, new training approaches, new self-initiated investments (including, perhaps, some small private firms). It could test various worker-management schemes. It would be free for a range of independent social decisions based upon independent control of some community economic resources. It could grapple directly with efforts to humanize technology. It could, through co-ordination and planning, reorganize the use of time, and also locate jobs, homes, schools so as to maximize community interaction and end the isolated prison aspects of all these presently segregated units of life experience.

Communities could work out in a thousand diverse localities a variety of new ways to reintegrate a community – to define productive roles for the elderly, for example, or to redefine the role of women in community. They could face squarely the problem of the 'tyranny of the majority' (and the concomitant issues of minority rights and individual privacy), and experiment with new ways to guarantee individual and minority initiative. The anarchist demand for freedom could be faced in the context of a co-operative structure. The issue of legitimate leadership functions might be confronted rather than wished away; and various alternatives, including rotation, recall, apprenticing,

etc., might be tested. Communities might even begin
selves as communities – communes, if you like – in
co-operative, humane sense of that term.

In their larger functions communities obviously h
together, for both technological and economic reasons.
nology, in fact, permits great decentralization – and new n
can produce even greater decentralization if that is a consc   ~ject-
tive. In cases where this is not possible or intolerably uneconomical
(perhaps, for example, some forms of heavy industry, energy production, transportation) larger confederations of communities in a region
or in the integrated unit of the nation state would be appropriate – as
they would be for other forms of co-ordination as well.

The themes of the proposed alternative thus are indicated by the
concepts of co-operative community and the Commonwealth of
Regions. The program might best be termed a 'Pluralist Commonwealth'
– 'Pluralist' to emphasize decentralization and diversity; 'Commonwealth' to focus on the principle that wealth should co-operatively
benefit all.

Levels of community

There is no doubt that co-operative development proceeds best in communities sufficiently small that social needs are self-evident. Voluntarism
and self-help can achieve what centralized propaganda cannot – namely,
engender group involvement, co-operative enthusiasm, spontaneity.
This is a primary reason to emphasize small-scale local structures at the
outset – even if it may entail short-term disadvantages. The hope is that
thereafter, with the benefit of a real basis in some co-operative experience, it may be possible to transend historical starting points in the
longer development of a larger framework.

A key question is how to prevent local centralization of power:
individuals as well as small groups must obviously retain some power
as against the local collectivity as a whole. (And the organization of
individuals and small groups is power – power to prevent bureaucratic
domination, even in small settings.) One answer is self-conscious individual responsibility – and therefore another requirement in the achievement of local practices and relationships which build the experience of
responsibility at the same time as they constrain bureaucracy. This will
require a further breakdown into smaller subgroupings organized both
by function and neighborhood geography within communities. (A 'city'
might be understood as a confederation of smaller communities.)

Another answer might be to distribute 'vouchers' to individuals so
they could freely choose different forms of public services like education

.nedicine. Such a financial mechanism would permit substantial eedom of operation for a variety of semi-competitive, non-profit service institutions.

The need for a larger-scale framework becomes obvious when problems of market behavior are considered more closely. What if every community actually owned and controlled substantial industry? Even if each used a share of surpluses for social purposes as democratically decided; even if each began to evolve the idea of planned economic and social development; even if its people began to develop social experiences and a new ethic of co-operation – there would still be competition in the larger unit of the region or nation. Community industry would vie with community industry, neighborhood versus neighborhood, county versus county, city versus city. If communities were simply to float in the rough sea of an unrestricted market, the model would likely end in 'community capitalism,' trade wars, expansionism, and the self-aggrandizing exploitation of one community by another. As in modern capitalism, there also would likely be both unemployment and inflation, ruthless competition and oligopoly, etc. (And within communities one result would be a tendency to exploit wage employees, as some kibbutzim exploit Arabs.)

Such problems can never be fully resolved unless a context of assured stability is established. Above all, the conditions of insecurity in which local expansionism and exploitation arise as defensive strategies, even when the best intentions prevail, must be eliminated. A larger structure capable of stabilizing the economic setting is necessary, and, if it is to rationalize the economic environment facing each community, it will have to control substantially much wholesale marketing, longer-term capital financing, and taxation.

Other issues which cannot be resolved by one community in isolation point up further functions of a larger framework and a larger decision-making body. These include: managing the ecology of a river system, deciding the location of new cities, establishing transportation between population centers, committing capital in large societal investments and balancing foreign trade.

Since the socialist argument for a large unit appears to be correct in all these instances, the issue becomes: How large? And how might it be established without generating a new dynamic towards centralized power? A governing, continental-scale 'state' would be far too large for any hope of democratic management by localities – and totally unnecessary for technical efficiency save, perhaps, in continental transportation and some forms of power exploitation. (But co-operation between areas is feasible, as present international air transport or American tie-ins with Canadian energy sources illustrate.)

Accordingly, once again, as William Appleman Williams and Robert

Lafont have suggested, regional units organized on the principle of 'commonwealth' become significant elements in a solution. This is the least developed area of theory; however, some intermediate unit larger than a 'community' but smaller than a nation of 300 million people appears to be required. The unit must be capable of taking over directly (and decentralizing!) capital and productive functions now controlled by, say, the 500 largest economic corporations – without escalating to the scale of the entire social system.

We should begin to conceive of a system in which the USA, by the end of the century, might be broken into eight or ten confederated regions of 20 to 30 million people, each region made up of confederated communities. Each region might perhaps approximate the scale of the four Scandinavian countries taken together (New England, Appalachia, Tidelands, Deep South, Mid-West, Plains and Mountain States, Southwest, West, Coast).

Part of the answer might also involve regional units of different sizes for different purposes. The metropolitan area as a unit, for example, might control certain heavy industries or specialized public services such as intra-urban transportation. Some state units might control power development and, building on the state park tradition, could also appropriately manage expanding recreational industries like skiing. A grouping of regions like New England and Appalachia might control electric power production and distribution; the Pacific Coast and the Mountain States might unite for a variety of functions, particularly for rational ecological planning and watershed control. In such instances, organization across regions is more rational. Black Americans and other minorities may for political reasons also wish to establish racially organized associations across the nation. The point of regional organization as a guideline is not to exclude collaboration but rather to attempt to solve some problems of co-operation and power by building up units of rational scale which are still manageable by the localities implicit in a decentralist vision.

Planning power and process

In general, the difficult broader principle in a three-level vision of co-operative community, economic region, and confederated nation is to anchor units in new social structures which preserve sufficient independence of decision and power (without which neither freedom nor responsibility is possible), but which are not so powerful as to produce unrestrained competition and deny the possibility of a substantial measure of rational planning. The rule should be to leave as many functions as possible to localities, elevating only what is absolutely

ıl to the higher unit.

identify socialism with streamlined, computerized planning, as
o, is a fatal error. 'Planning' would more likely be an 'iterative'
phenomenon, involving, first, information, priorities and criteria
generated at local levels; next, an integration at a higher order 'planning
stage'; then the implications calculated; a return to smaller units for
reconsideration; and finally back up again.

One must recognize that decentralized, democratic planning inevitably involves inefficiencies and considerably more time. However, if
successful, the gains in released energies, to say nothing of the quality
of life, are likely to more than compensate what is lost.

But this returns us to the question of whether the basic social units
in which day-to-day life occur are, in fact, likely to sustain new, more
humane experiences of community. It should again be clear why it
is important to place priority on local social structures and processes
which have a potential for developing and prefiguring a new ethic of
co-operation, even if this may mean local communities initially function
to an extent competitively as market operators. Staging is critical:
could social relationships within communities be strengthened so as to
alter values and modify external relations over time? Could a co-
operative development process permit the subsequent establishment
of the necessary co-ordinating structures between communities and,
in combination with national political efforts, the larger framework
for the overall economy?

There are no easy answers to such questions and very little guidance
available from foreign experience or past history. Chinese and Israeli
developments suggest that communities may be able to sustain and
deepen the quality of internal social relations at the same time external
relations involve both the limited use of market competition and a larger
framework. Marxist theoreticians as different as Charles Bettelheim and
Paul Sweezy agree, too, that the use both of a limited competitive
market and of planning seem inevitable at certain stages of development
under all forms of socialism. Competition can then be viewed not as a
method of exploitation but as a tool of rational administration. One
challenge, it accordingly appears, is to be able to recognize the latter
and eliminate the former, and (if the social system is to overcome its
origins in capitalism) to attempt shrewd trade-offs between competition
and co-operation at different stages of development, as a new experiential
basis emerges, as mutual needs develop, as larger national political
possibilities open up, and as a new vision is created.

In such a long process of development, as Martin Buber urged, the
permissive environment which may be attainable if localities are not
totally subservient to central agencies is more important, initially, than
the apparent top-down rationality of centralized planning systems. The

conservative, the Yugoslav, the Israeli, the Chinese, and the anarchist all seem right also to argue that a degree of local autonomy and a degree of competition must be assured if freedom and spontaneous innovation are to continue over time.

There are, I think, two answers to the dilemma of equality. First, and this is crucial, America is so far advanced technologically that with different organization, it ultimately would not be a huge burden to pull lagging areas of the nation up. The society is not a Yugoslavia fighting to climb the steep hill of capital accumulation. Even now, at the top of the system, young people are falling away from the false affluence of consumerism. Were the waste of unemployment, militarism, and unnecessary consumption ended, the resources available would be enormous. Poor communities could be aided without intolerable cost. It would also be possible to allocate huge resources to other nations.

Second, politics would not die were the nation organized as a many-level pluralist commonwealth. (Indeed, what we are talking about might best be defined not as an achieved, static goal, but as a stage-by-stage process of increasing mastery of rational and irrational limitations on man's potential.) Especially as a new vision and ethic develops, it is possible to imagine a considerably reinvigorated politics which could concentrate on helping under-developed communities – perhaps progressively narrowing the range of inequality by setting (and gradually lowering) maximum income ceilings, by setting (and gradually raising) minimum income floors, and by regularly introducing a greater share of such free goods as education, medical care, housing, and basic food stuffs.

But a progressive process of this kind is not the same as total equality, and the distinction should make it clear that a fundamental point is at issue. The only alternative to the process of politics is a central decision-making authority which forces its program upon all communities. You simply cannot have it both ways. A basic problem of both democracy and equality is when and what is to be centralized and what is not – and at which stages of development very specific trade-offs between conflicting values are made. There is an obvious trade-off at one level of theory between equality and decentralization; place absolute priority on the former and you must have enormous power at the centre to end variations between localities. On the other hand, if diversity and democracy are priorities, they bring with them a substantial degree of inequality between areas.

Other considerations make it appear that the nature of the trade-offs is even more complex. Although centralization in theory can establish equality between areas, historically, simply to function, most hierarchical systems have required highly stratified, unequal patterns of individual incentives. (The resulting inequality of state-socialist systems

in practice is often ignored by their proponents and apologists.) Motivation is potentially quite different, however, in small units (like the kibbutz), in which almost the only historic examples of substantial equality between individuals are known. But at the outset, semi-autonomous small unit development inevitably means inequality between areas. Therefore, while centralization seems the short cut to equality, it is likely in practice to be a dead end. And while diversity and democracy seem to be antagonistic to equality, this appears to be the only way to build up different motivational patterns out of which an ethic of universal equality might eventually develop.

For this reason, too – and because voluntary, individual choice is critical to the development of a new ethic – a 'second tier' to the economy might also be appropriate. Paul and Percival Goodman (and Arthur Waskow) have suggested that individuals be free to largely opt out of the overall economy, if they so choose, and that they be guaranteed a minimum subsistence income much less than the basic economy's norm. They could then choose freely whether or not to accept the more stringent disciplines (and greater material benefits) of the larger system.

Over the long haul the trade-offs between centralization and decentralization are likely to diminish as increasingly productive technology makes it easier to satisfy more needs – and as rational ecological judgments reduce the pressure for economic growth. If individual and community motivation for exorbitant living standards can be reduced, there will also be less need for the hierarchical and centralized controls that ever-expanding production seems to require. Finally, as true (and voluntary) agreement with the principles of a new vision of equality develops, centralized decision-making to achieve it can, in fact, become more a matter of rational co-ordination and administration than of bureaucratic compulsion. In the final analysis, therefore, the tension between the socialist vision and decentralist alternatives may perhaps best be understood not as an ultimate contradiction but as a transitional problem of societies moving towards the post-industrial era.

Hannah Arendt has urged that we give renewed attention to the history of the 'council' movement – the spontaneous eruption in history of local, people's governing bodies. The contemporary trend towards community control is, in fact, best understood as part of a tradition which includes Jefferson's idea of 'ward republics,' and extends through the Paris Commune, the soviets, the Mexican *ejida*, the Algerian autogestion system, etc.

Though not the result of national upheaval, some of the new American institutions, moreover, emphasize explicitly (as did not all the previous institutions) the socialist concept of direct (local) common ownership of property. That community-owned efforts are at this stage

only fragmentary and partial is obvious; their importance may be more as educative vehicles which teach basic concepts related to the vision of a pluralist commonwealth than as ultimate structures. The question is whether the social and economic forms that are suggested can be extended (and combined with the development of regional and national alternatives) in the longer struggle to build new political power.

Gar Alperovitz, co-director of the Exploratory Project for Economic Alternatives, is a political economist, historian and social theorist. His works include *Atomic Diplomacy* (1965); *Cold War Essays* (1970); *Strategy and Program* (1972); and numerous articles.

6 Anarchism and formal organizations- some notes on the sociological study of organizations from an anarchist perspective*

Howard J. Ehrlich

A prefatory note

The study of human social organization is central to both academic sociology and anarchist theory. American sociology, however, is explicitly a capitalist enterprise; and it has never recognized anarchism or anarchist theory. Critical analyses of sociology conducted by its Marxist critics have also ignored anarchist principles, but at the same time these critiques have also ignored the sociology of organizations.

Why bother to develop a formal critique? What political purposes are served by it? Let me answer in two ways. First, we should examine what the consequences of the sociology of organization can be. To begin with, it presents a view of human organizations that is less than what organizations could be. In the process, sociologists legitimate what is and, I think, contribute to people's alienation and cynicism about the character of organization. It suppresses people's thinking about alternatives, and it promotes individualistic solutions and escape.

It is important to understand that sociology and the other social sciences are socially recognized as legitimate - in fact, preferred - modes of social inquiry. Quite obviously my claims based on my being a sociological theorist will arouse far more positive response in most circles than my claims to being an anarchist theorist. Anarchism is a political ideology and is therefore to be distrusted. Sociology, however, is a scientific discipline and warrants your trust.

In actual practice, social scientists regularly introduce ideological statements under the guise of presenting an objective analysis. Since most of the time this happens without scientists knowing they have done so, it is understandable that most people without formal analytic training are also misled. And so political assertions clothed as scientific

---

* This article was written for the anthology and is published here for the first time. It is also available as a separate pamphlet published by Research Group One.

claims come to be accepted, while naked political claims confront an often embarrassed or indignant audience.

Second, the social sciences do differ from other sciences. Social science is reflexive. That is to say, people can and do read social science materials; and they can and do act upon what they read. The social sciences do not just discover laws or organize knowledge, they also create it.

1

Those familiar with the state of the social sciences would not be surprised to learn that there is no singular definition of 'organizations' or any consensual scheme for their classification. Just the same, social scientists know what an organization is, and a mass of data on their structure and operation has been accumulated. The arrangement of these data is, of course, dependent on the formal or implicit theory of the scientist. There is, however, a paradigm for organizational sociology that is consensual. For example, almost all organizational theorists accept 'control' as a core concept in their theory. They see organizational authority as legitimate, non-coercive, and fundamentally rational. They view leadership and hierarchy as inescapable, if not actually desirable. There are more such paradigmatic statements, to be sure, and we will discuss them as we go along.

The character of this paradigm is essentially authoritarian. Theorists do range across a narrow spectrum. On the right are those who explicitly advocate maximizing control as the means of increasing organizational effectiveness (Price, 1968); and just a step over the center are those who see bureaucracy as the superior mode of organization and the best designed to protect the rights of individuals (Perrow, 1972).

American sociologists of organization are also capitalists. That is, they accept the idea of profit and the accumulation of capital, of the private ownership of organizations, and of mass production and mass consumption. Certainly, statements about the political economy almost never directly enter organizational theories. Nevertheless, as I shall try to show, these theories are built upon, and in turn buttress, the ideology of capitalism.

2

It would be almost totally unprecedented for an anarchist analysis to omit 'the state', however defined. Similarly, it is almost totally unprecedented for an organizational theorist to include 'the state'. Theodore

Caplow's *Principles of Organization* presents one of those rare statements by an academic sociologist (Caplow, 1964, p. 23):

> In modern society, almost all official organizations turn out, on close inspection, to be ultimately authorized by the state, which licenses marriages, charters corporations, and registers voluntary associations. There appear to be two reasons for this phenomenon. First, property cannot be securely held without the sanction of the state. Since official organizations of any consequence have collective property, it is evident why they require authorization. Second, any organization that wields substantial power must occasionally resort to violence. In modern society, in which the state's monopoly of violence is nearly unquestioned, the state must usually provide the means of coercion for private organizations, although there are exceptions, such as criminal syndicates.
>
> The phenomenon of authorization is often overlooked. It may seem implausible that the memorandum establishing a new janitor crew in a branch factory of a manufacturing corporation is authorized ultimately by the state, but the state *does* confer the corporate charter from which the company's board of directors derives its right to appoint the executives who are entitled to do such things as hiring a new janitor crew.

Despite that solid beginning, the state never again appears in his 'principles of organization.'

3

There is no concrete theory of anarchist organization, nor is there an anarchist sociology. What there is, rather, are numerous stipulations of how organizations ought to be structured. Anarchists have indicated a clear preference for small organizations where social relationships may be personalized and spontaneity in behavior maximized.

The preference for small size should not be mistaken for a rigid organizational principle. It is, rather, an expression of beliefs that (1) the size of an organization should not exceed the comprehension of the persons who make it up, and (2) the size should not exceed the point at which social relationships become impersonalized. Since that critical size will vary as people gain experience in anarchist collectives, it is premature to talk about the optimum size of anarchist organizations. For now, I think the simple preference for smallness is sound.

The fulcrum of anarchist organizational thought is the principle of the diffusion of power. Derived from the fundamental belief in human

equality, this principle has been expressed in a variety of ways when applied to social organizations. Primary has been a model of equal participation in decision-making, that is collective decision-making.

More radical, I think, is the conception that organizations be designed as impermanent, that is actually be abolished at intervals. This idea of organizational impermanence is exploratory. It originates from many considerations: (1) the idea that an organization be socially useful and that its members disband when it is no longer of utility; (2) the idea that organizations are often formed to solve particular problems and that they are no longer necessary when the problems have been resolved; (3) the idea that the rigidification of behavior in an organization may be inescapable; and (4) the idea that over time people tend to identify organizational interests with their personal needs. In short, the principle of a temporary organization represents an attempt to prevent or to avoid the pathologies of organizations as we know them today. As we proceed in this essay, other anarchist principles should become more apparent.

4

Caplow provides us with a model sociological view of an organization: 'An organization is a social system that has an unequivocal collective identity, an exact roster of members, a program of activity, and procedures for replacing members' (Caplow, 1964, p. 1). Contrast this with Drabek and Haas: 'Organizations, then, are *relatively permanent and relatively complex interaction systems*' (1974, p. 41; italics in original). Now there are many formal, theoretical reasons why Caplow's definition is sound and Drabek and Haas's one is not. But that is not our immediate concern. What is of concern is that Drabek and Haas would exclude from consideration virtually all organizational forms that an anarchist would take to be central to community life.

5

There are some anarchists who would object even to Caplow's model sociological definition. For them, the very character of organizations would be different in an anarchist society. Anarchist organizations would be the assembly of people who came together in time and place for specific activities. What we call an organization, they would call 'freespace.' There would be no membership roster and certainly no formal procedures for the replacement of members. Basically, the free-spacers would argue, anyone could 'join.' The space would be open to

all of those who sincerely accepted the agenda of those already engaged in the group's activities. Problems of the usurpation of the space would presumably be minimal in a freespace society.

The freespace idea is not fully developed. It ignores conflict and it skirts reductionism (i.e. reducing social relations to matters of individual psychology). Nevertheless, it is a radical organizational model, and some present-day anarchists are attempting to work in freespace.

6

The 'effectiveness' of an organization has been defined 'as the degree of goal achievement' (Price, 1968; Etzioni, 1964). An organization's goals are presumably what the organization through its policy-makers is trying to do. To study effectiveness, sociologists will generally examine the written goals of organizations as well as interview or observe those in leadership positions. All of this is very straightforward, and certainly sounds reasonable.

Price in his inventory of research on organizational effectiveness provides us with a reasonable illustration. 'For example, a prison which has a custodial goal, and which has a low escape rate among its inmates, would be considered an effective organization' (p. 3). And another: 'The successful strike indicates low degrees of morale, conformity, and effectiveness' (p. 143, slightly removed from context). Now you may want to argue that you are opposed to prisons and certainly to custodial goals. As an anarchist you certainly would take that position, but the logical correctness of Price's illustration is unimpeached. Similarly, you may view a worker's strike as representing the high morale and co-operative effort of an effective union. But the definition is written from the perspective of the bosses and not from that of the workers.

As a supposedly neutral sociologist, Price could have said that judgments of organizational effectiveness depend on one's social position. (Having said that, he could have even written the same book by adding the qualification that he was only writing from a management perspective.) He didn't do this – not that it really would have made him neutral – and in not qualifying his inventory, he leaves us with an elitist and distorted view of organizational behavior.

The anarchist conceptualization of organizational effectiveness requires additional considerations: Who set the goals and what are their social consequences? And so an organization would be defined as effective to the degree to which all of its participants were involved in formulating its goals, to the degree to which its goals did not contribute to human discomfort, and to the degree that it achieved those goals.

Organizations work because management has power. Its power is stable because it is accepted by everyone as legitimate (moral, right, correct, true, all of the above). Although sociologists seldom state it openly, they assume that persons who own or manage an organization have the right to dispose of their property as they choose. Those who control the organization contract with workers for their labor. The major conditions of that contract are dictated by the owners in the context of the scarcity of jobs and some regulation by the state. Unions are scarcely 100 years old; and minimum wage, fair employment practices, and health and safety regulations all represent fairly modern innovations in which the liberal state has restricted the nature of the contract.

The intervention of the state has added to the legitimacy of the capitalist's power. And this is partly because the state is presumed to be an entity independent of those who control the workplace. Organizational authority is exercised in the workplace through the legitimacy of ownership and under the protection of government.

Today, the character of that authority – and sociologists love to recite their Weberian catechism – is 'rational–legal.' As Drabek and Haas put it, 'It is legal in the sense that it stems from a set of written rules and rational in that compliance is thought to achieve valued ends' (1974, p. 13).

In the modern organization, where authority is presumptively rational but certainly legal, people know how to behave. The defining characteristic of rational–legal authority is that proper behavior is circumscribed by written rules (Drabek and Haas, 1974, p. 15):

> Through these rules, specific jobs or tasks are identified for individuals, groups of individuals, and the entire collectivity. The general purposes, goals, missions, or products of the organization, and sub-units within, are specified. And there is a division of labor . . . . All of these individuals, each involved in diverse activities, must be co-ordinated and controlled in some way.

Co-ordination and control are the recurrent themes of all organizational theory. Certainly no anarchist would object to a call for co-ordination. What about control? Control, in this context, refers to the control of the decision-making processes – who decides what to do?

For the anarchist, there is no simple solution. What I will call the *minimalist* solution is the position that control can never be held by an elite. That is, it would be unacceptable for some set of people to be able always, or almost always, to control the outcome of decisions.

Now the organizational theorist might reply that the essence of

legal-rational authority is that the power to control decisions resides in positions and roles, not people. What that means to the social scientist is something like this: people are recruited to positions because they have satisfied some qualifying criteria and they can remain only as long as they perform their roles competently. Of course the anarchist response to that should be 'Bullshit!' It is unlikely that organizations ever worked that way, and it probably represents nothing less than the social scientist's shaping of reality for the convenience of a neat theoretical package.

But the appeal to a 'role theory' could be countered on its own. That is, a proper anarchist response is that it makes no difference to have power invested in positions. And there are three quite different reasons why this is so.

First, in so far as we are talking about a work organization within a capitalist society, the decisions controlled by persons in positions of authority must be constrained by the objective of maximizing profit. This is, after all, *the* criterion of effectiveness in a capitalist organization. Thus all decisions must rationally be biased against the workers.

Elitist decision-making in a work organization within a state socialist society must also be constrained by objectives that do not necessarily correspond with those of the workers in a given organization. To be sure, the likelihood of correspondence is greater under socialism and, in some states, worker involvement in determining objectives is greater. Nevertheless, state interests are generally non-negotiable and, to that degree, will also be biased against the workers. (In the classic Marxist-Leninist formulation, only when the dictatorship of the proletariat is established will the interests of the state be identical with those of the workers. Needless to say, no anarchist expects that to happen; nor for that matter do many sociologists. But that of course is another can of theoretical worms.)

There is a second objection to the idea of power and authority being appropriate to certain positions within an organization. In modern capitalist and socialist societies, work is organized into occupational careers. A career is typically defined as some progression of jobs in the same domain, with the implication that each new job or position entails increases in responsibility and usually authority as well as increases in wages or other compensation. Now most workers are tracked. They don't have careers, or they have careers that are highly limited in the span of increased income or responsibility. In fact, the conception of careers is popularly reserved for professionals and managers.

Few persons ever get to occupy positions of power. Partly this is a consequence of the differential life chances associated with class position, sex, and ethnicity in modern society; and partly it is a consequence of the limited number of positions of power in society.

(Neither of these consequences is invariant, even in a capitalist society.) While social scientists are divided in their attitudes about the necessities of class, they do seem to be in accord that positions of power are scarce and that this is the way things ought to be.

So it is that a small set of the total population holds careers that permit them to move across positions of power. So acceptable is the idea of such a career that colleges and organizations provide some people with the option to train in administration, that is, to acquire certain resources of power and knowledge of their use. Careerists in power inevitably acquire further resources of organizational knowledge as well as administrative skills that only come with actual role performance. Thus access to organizational power resources typically has a cumulative effect.

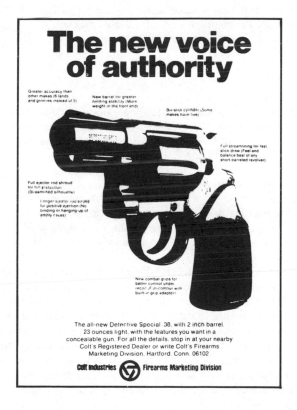

That people can make a career of managing the lives of others is patently unacceptable within an anarchist framework. However, still

within the framework of a minimalist solution, the anarchist could accept the idea of the scarcity of positions of power. There would be an obvious set of qualifications to that acceptance, namely that this scarcity is neither desirable nor inevitable, nor would it be allowed to persist. In keeping with those qualifications, the minimalist program would require that no one be permitted to make a career of positions of power. Put positively, people would rotate through such positions, and tenure would be highly limited. The consequence of this program would diffuse organizational and administrative knowledge.

There is, finally, a third objection to allocating power to positions that are held in limited number. Freedom is not just a matter of social structure; it is also a habit. The concentration of power makes followers of us all. We not only do not have the opportunities to learn how to act autonomously; we are constantly rehearsing our repertory of compliance, passivity and subordination. Having removed the constraints of oppressive institutions doesn't automatically free people. That comes only with a practice now denied to most people.

8

There is a basic premise in organizational sociology that the centralization of decision-making is a requisite of good organizations. This premise sustains the intellectual's distrust of the intentions and capabilities of most people (Price, 1968, p. 81):

> Strategic decisions must be concentrated at a single place if the organization is to attain a high degree of effectiveness. This concentration may involve either a single individual, or a group of individuals . . . what is imperative is that the making of strategic decisions be concentrated at a single place in the organization.

In his inventory of research, Price distinguishes two types of decisions. There are the long-term decisions, mainly concerned with goals and policy-making. These are the *strategic* decisions. *Tactical* decisions are those that are mainly administrative, and these are the routine, day-to-day operational decisions. With regard to both types, Price concludes that centralization – the concentration of decision-making power – is the key to effectiveness. Organizations that have a greater concentration of power in *both* strategic and tactical decision-making, he concludes, will be more effective than those that have a lower concentration of power.

Within the confines of his capitalist criterion of effectiveness, it is likely that Price's conclusions are true as empirical generalizations.

Without accepting that criterion, we could pose the question of whether the rotation of persons through positions of power in highly centralized organizations would modify organizational effectiveness. And the answer is that there is normal turnover in managerial positions without long-term consequences. Such rotation does not have any inescapably negative impact on organizational effectiveness.

A final note: Price's conclusions do not necessarily imply that the most effective organizations are those directed by a small group of individuals. But in the context of his monograph, and in the absence of a disclaimer, I think that is the inference most people would derive. Within the context of this society it may, in fact, be a valid inference. If so, its validity must be regarded by the anarchist as an index of the failure of present-day organizational forms.

9

Since Max Weber wrote the first, now classical, sociological defense of bureaucracy as the form of organization most suited to capitalism, there have been few serious challenges to the belief in the necessity of bureaucratic forms. And the rationalizations for it seem never to end (Perrow, 1972, p. 58):

> Critics, then, of our organizational society, whether they are the hippies of the New Left emphasizing spontaneity and freedom, the new radical right demanding their own form of radical decentralization, or the liberals in between speaking of the inability of organizations to be responsive to community values, had best turn to the key issue of who controls the varied forms of power generated by organizations rather than flail away at the windmills of bureaucracy. If we want our material civilization to continue as it is, we will have to have large-scale bureaucratic enterprises in the economic, social, and governmental areas. This is the most efficient way to get the routine work of a society done.

There are four essential components of a bureaucratic organization that concern us here: (1) there is a hierarchy of positions; (2) there is a specialized division of labor; (3) salaries and other rewards are distributed according to rank in the hierarchy; and (4) there are formal rules and procedures regulating organizational behavior.

It is my belief that bureaucracies are defended more because of the societal effects that social scientists *do not talk about* than because of their supposed efficiency as an organizational form. These four components may be necessary for a bureaucracy, but they are also necessary

to maintain class stratification, to promote ideas of social mobility and competition, to preclude self-management and foster separatism and isolation. Bureaucratic forms – worst of all – deny people opportunities for growth and self-development; and they perpetuate a political-economic standard of self-assessment – 'if you're so smart, how come you're not rich?'

10

Bureaucratic forms in state socialist societies have the same social consequences; that is, they are also supportive of the political economy. While collective goals, co-operation and comradeship are emphasized, hierarchy and specialization persist. In some state socialist settings, there has been a serious attempt to minimize income differences and involve workers in larger organizational decisions. And one should not overlook the guarantees of employment, housing and health care – guarantees that certainly make the life circumstances of people more secure. Just the same, the secure worker in the socialist organization is no more autonomous, no more independent, and no more free than workers in capitalist organizations.

Subordination to authority, indoctrination in the ideological justifications for hierarchy and differences in knowledge and access to information, and the lack of freedom to make basic decisions about one's life – all of these can foster in both the capitalist and socialist worker their dependence on others and a lack of self-respect.

11

We learn to identify authority and power early. The nuclear family with its age- and sex-based division of labor and power is the initial training ground. The school with its demands for regimentation, for discipline, and for the acceptance of the teacher as authority becomes the second level of indoctrination. Autonomy – being in charge of one's self – is not in the teacher syllabus of most public schools.

Matriculating to the workplace, most young people have already adapted to authoritarian institutions. While people are well socialized to follow orders, they are seldom engaged in the learning of modes of autonomous behavior. More likely, they have learned neither to trust nor to like themselves. Psychologically, the two go together; authoritarian acceptance and self-rejection are reciprocating characteristics of

personality. Sociologically, they are necessary conditions for conforming behavior.

Everyday life in most work organizations is stultifying. Rarely is there an opportunity to conceptualize anything better. So one does what one has to do. And by going about one's work, people reaffirm their negative self-conceptions and revalidate the organizational form as something positive.

12

In an extraordinary collection of political sociological essays directed at a defense of liberalism, Barrington Moore attacks the Left, anarchists and neo-Marxists for wanting people to share in decisions. 'A very precious part of human freedom is that *not* to make decisions' (Moore, 1972, p. 69). Mr Moore, contemplating his future oppression in political forums presumably in contrast to his present freedom as a Harvard professor, neglects one critical point. There is at least one universal act which is 'forbidden' in anarchy as it is in all humane forms of social organization: people are not free to give up their freedom.

Moore himself recognizes that some decisions are routinized and need not be reviewed constantly, such as whether to drive on the left- or right-hand side of the road (1972, p. 69):

All that matters is that there should be *some* decision. In others [areas of life] the problem is simply to get the right decision according to some easily agreed-upon criterion. In such areas it is possible to formulate standards of competence about ways to make the decision, and, with considerably greater difficulty, find ways to enforce them. In still other areas of life it may be impossible to persuade people to accept clear criteria that distinguish between good and bad decisions.

Unlike most social scientists who seldom examine their own politics, Moore is quite self-consciously and explicitly antagonistic to anarchism (see particularly pp. 72-6). Even in the brief passage above one can discern his elitist orientation in his concern with persuasion and enforcement. It is clear that Moore casts out these observations to indicate the absurdity of total participation. But on that point, I suspect, most anarchists would agree. For the problem remains for Moore's unrealized liberal democratic state just as it does for anarchy: Is there an optimum level of participation? And that problem, I maintain, will be solved through social practice – and long years of wrong decisions.

13

Even an optimum level of participation would not in and of itself mean that: (1) the right decision will be made; (2) the decision will be less arbitrary than one made by a single person; (3) that no one will necessarily suffer as a result.

By itself, no system of decision-making can guarantee social justice. It is a tenet of anarchist theory that social justice is more likely to be obtained through optimizing the participation of the members of an organization or community.

14

Anarchy is not without leadership. It is without followership. Anarchists do not deny that a person may be *an* authority about some technical or practical or intellectual matter. Anarchists do deny that a person may be *in* authority. An authority may extend leadership in the matter in which s/he is authoritative. But such leadership can never be coercive.

Leadership under anarchism has two other characteristics that leadership in authoritarian organizations does not have. First, it is exercised within an egalitarian framework; that is, it is based not on the presumption that the leader is a superior person but on the presumption that the leader knows more about the subject for which s/he is providing leadership. Second, leadership is exercised within an educative framework. Anarchist leaders attempt to influence outcomes through education, not through issuing directives.

15

Sociologists have never been able to fathom 'voluntary associations.' As someone who reviewed the literature and proposed a new classificatory scheme a number of years ago, I think – in retrospect – that social scientists have been intellectually fascinated but confused by the subject. 'Voluntary associations' in the sociologist's special language are those everyday groupings such as garden clubs and civic associations, tenant's unions and softball teams, self-help groups and that ever-present display of animal clubs like the Lions, Elks, Eagles, etc. Organizational theorists typically treat these voluntary associations as something different from the other organizations they study. Why is that? I think it is because it doesn't correspond with a strictly capitalist model of work or an organizational theorist's model of control.

Drabek and Haas ask with no embarrassment, 'Since member partici-

pation isn't based on wage and salary payment, how is it that participation exists at all?' (1974, p. 61). How can they explain such puzzling behavior? *Boredom.* Membership helps 'avoid boredom.' There are, the authors mention, 'activities' and 'symbolic rewards . . . promoting participation' (p. 62), but the authors leave the impression that they view the whole thing with disbelief. Voluntary association membership, they imply, is transitory – a phenomenon stemming from the fickleness of bored people and the absence of a 'high degree of boundary control.' What that means is that people 'may enter and exit with relative ease' (p. 62).

Now I know of no evidence indicating that membership in voluntary associations is any more or less transitory than residence or place of employment, and the authors cite no evidence. I also know of no evidence that would permit a sociologist to assert what the average life-span of such associations is or was in a given time or place. But should associations live for ever? Should any organization be permanent? Or is longevity a built-in value premise of organizational theorists?

We do know, for example, in the United States alone between 30,000 and 40,000 formal business organizations fail each year, if we take bankruptcy as a criterion. And thousands more simply close down for a variety of other reasons. Organizational theorists seem to be rather unconcerned about these. This is, presumably, the natural outcome of a market economy. And what sociologists study are the survivors of organizational competition. Thus, permanence appears to be an issue only with regard to voluntary associations.

Voluntary associations are viewed also as relatively more ineffective than formal organizations: 'The nature of most voluntary organizations means that it is more difficult to mobilize them for unusual and sustained action' (Drabek and Haas, 1974, p. 62). Why is that? Because 'the notion of command and control by top management is unusual in these organizations' (p. 62).

In case the premises underlying the Drabek-Haas analysis are not clear, let me state them directly. First, the primary incentive for organizational participation is money. Second, in addition, effective participation requires some form of entrance exam and some obstacles to leaving that are built into the organizational structure. Finally, effective organizations have a central command and control unit that can require sustained action on the part of its membership.

Another general critique of voluntary associations, and one that appears in most texts, is that they become more formal over time. That is, they become larger, develop a division of labor, a hierarchy, a paid staff, routine procedures and so on. This ostensibly simple, noncontroversial generalization, in fact, masks a complex of ideological presuppositions.

109

To begin with, the statement is probably neither entirely true nor entirely false. Some associations have grown and become formalized, and some have not. Why make a point about those that have? I think that there is a good reason why sociologists do so. If voluntary associations become formal organizations, and if this is construed as a natural tendency, then they no longer constitute an intellectual problem. That is, they either die or become formalized. Now this may not be good theory or rigorous science, but it is a way of writing off a social phenomenon that does not easily fit the political economics of organizational thought.

Organizations that expand and move to paid positions are surely by conventional criteria a 'success.' On the other hand, the anarchist critic would argue that becoming larger, expanding specialization of the membership, and even hiring a paid staff may well be erroneous decisions; and that these are indicators of failure. For the anarchist organizer, one criterion of success might be that the membership help other people organize their own voluntary associations. For example, instead of becoming larger, the membership would limit itself but assist others in building their own autonomous associations.

16

People who work 'together' in large formal organizations sometimes have difficulty in recognizing their co-workers in other contexts. They are frequently surprised at discovering that people they have worked with for years have 'hidden' interests and talents; that they are real people. The regulation of behavior in the workplace is designed to suppress genuine personal relations. For the manager, this ostensibly increases people's work time and productivity. It also decreases the likelihood of worker solidarity.

People have to learn how not to be sociable, starting with the extraordinary efforts of many parents in teaching children to avoid strangers. At the adult level, privacy becomes the symbolic reward for achievement. At higher levels of achievement, it may mean one's own toilet in one's own lavatory in one's own office; eventually a stove, refrigerator, bar and bed – and the top executive need never have an accidentally non-private moment in her or his corporate life.

There may be a fine line between privacy and isolation. But the sociologist of organizations is not the one to sketch it in. For most workers there is no privacy, only isolation. For most sociologists there is little isolation, only the rewards of privacy. Drabek and Haas (1974, p. 16):

Persons may work in the same organization, indeed on the same substage for a period of years and remain strangers to one another if they so choose. But as inhuman and undesirable as this may seem at first, think of the freedom it provides. You may not wish to become acquainted with everyone. Thus, not only do such arrangements afford greater efficiency, they greatly extend the limits of personal privacy.

If there is any singular flaw in that statement, it is this: people in formal organizations are seldom free to choose *not* to remain strangers.

17

The discipline of a workforce has its roots in personal self-denial. Play is subversive to formal organizations.

Organizational sociologists don't like to talk about it. It has defied social theorists, and its occurrences are not predictable. There is no room for play in the theories of formal organization. Drabek and Haas actually mention the issue, devoting slightly less than a page to it – which is more than is presented by most of their colleagues. Their concern is business-like and very sociologistic: 'Spontaneity of interaction is largely curtailed within any organization' (Drabek and Haas, 1974, p. 100).

As a revolutionary tactic, the anarchist advocates the introduction of play into all formal organizations. As a component of anarchist theory, the relation of work and play is an unresolved equation. As the meaning of work becomes transformed in the process of building anarchist organizations, so the relation of work and play will be changed. These initial theoretical principles would probably be contained in an anarchist theory. Work becomes play to the extent that:

– it is not a matter of survival, or otherwise coercive;
– it is not producing commodities primarily to be exchanged for something else;
– the conditions and process of work are controllable by the worker;
– it is intrinsically satisfying.

(the beginning)

Works cited

Caplow, T. (1964), *Principles of Organization* New York: Harcourt, Brace & World.

Drabek, T. E. and Haas, J. E. (1974), *Understanding Complex Organizations* Dubuque, Ia: Brown.

Etzioni, A. (1964), *Modern Organizations* Englewood Cliffs, N.J.: Prentice-Hall.

Moore, Jr., B.. (1964) (1972), *Reflections on the Causes of Human Misery* Boston: Beacon Press.

Perrow, C. (1972), *Complex Organizations* Glenview, Ill.: Scott, Foresman.

Price, J. L. (1968), *Organizational Effectiveness* Homewood, Ill.: Richard D. Irwin.

Acknowledgements

My thanks to the Group for Anarchist Studies – GAS – regulars. Carol Ehrlich, Glenda Morris, Bob Palmer and Dave Westby all provided helpful criticisms.

Part Three

Criticisms of the left: old and new

57 VARIETIES

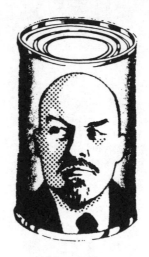

**All unfit for
human consumption**

Introduction

Why the New Left was not enough

In the 1960s, a decade in which it seemed that revolution was imminent in many Western nations, a major new political movement was born. It became known as the New Left; and in the dozen or so years of its existence, it had an enormous impact upon the lives and political development of perhaps hundred of thousands of people.

The New Left struggled to define a radical politics that fit the conditions of the present. In doing so, its adherents consciously rejected the organizational forms of the Marxist–Leninist Old Left, as well as many (though by no means all) of the Old Left's strategies and long-term goals. In their search for a new political analysis, many people on the New Left reinvented anarchy. Sometimes this was a conscious process, often not; but the parallels between much of New Left and anarchist theory and practice are striking.

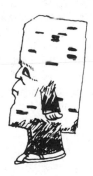

1 From the start, the New Left had a much broader political perspective than the Old Left did: there was a strong concern with defining

and fighting against all oppressions, not just those directly related to capitalism. Perhaps the basic issue was finding a means to end authority relations and to create the conditions for individual freedom and dignity. It was not cadre from the Old Left who spoke of 'participatory democracy' or who found it important to avow, 'I am a human being. Do not fold, spindle, or mutilate.'

2 The New Left also defined its constituency much more broadly than the Old Left did. Revolution would come through the efforts of all sectors of society; it was not the exclusive property of a narrowly defined vanguard.

3 Recognition of the oppressive nature of contemporary culture, especially in culturally approved forms of the family and sexuality, led to a search for the liberation of self.

4 The New Left concern with organization and structure often took anarchist forms. There was a strong tendency towards developing local and decentralized groups that were anti-hierarchical and operated by consensus. And there was no room for a disciplined cadre following the directives of a centralized bureaucracy which took *its* orders from a set of received texts.

Although the New Left had certain things in common with anarchism, its anarchist tendencies were rudimentary and not systematically developed. Participation in New Left organizations did start some people on the path toward anarchism, but by itself it was not enough.

What were the deficiences of the New Left? As we look back nearly a decade later, we can see that the organizations of the sixties were overly locked into time and place. They were typically blatantly sexist – of course, so were most Old Left groups; but the New Left, with its emphasis on personal liberation and the integrity of the individual, seemed especially hypocritical. Many women left what they called 'the male Left' and set up independent organizations (many of them based on anarchist principles).

Paradoxically, although the New Left attempted to reach a much broader constituency than the Old Left did, they were increasingly limited by their own membership. The New Left was predominantly middle-class, campus-based, young, white, and – as time went on – male. The limitations of this group for making a revolution became increasingly evident.

Finally, one could argue that, if the New Left had become self-consciously anarchist, it would have had a theoretical basis for broadening its perspective beyond the immediate concerns of many of its members; it would not have been vulnerable to the inroads of the Old Left (the result of which was to drive all too many people away from radical politics altogether); and it might – just might – have been able to survive the massive police repression that intimidated many of its

members into silence and non-participation.

Perhaps the prototypical New Left organization was Students for a Democratic Society (SDS). Many people date the birth of the North American New Left from the Port Huron Statement of 1962, and mark the beginning of its lingering death from the June 1969 national convention in which SDS tore itself apart into various Old Left sects and Weatherman. The first paper in this section – by the Radical Decentralist Project – illustrates some of the best idealism and spirit of SDS. Ironically, it was written in May 1969, shortly before the self-destruction of the organization. The paper comes from the anarchist wing of SDS, and is strikingly similar in spirit and content to Murray Bookchin's 'Listen, Marxist!' Both documents were written for circulation at the June convention, in an effort to show the organization that it was going in the wrong (i.e. Old Left) direction – a direction that must be reversed immediately. The Radical Decentralist Project urged SDS to realize that conditions were ripe for a different kind of revolution – based on equality and freedom, and one that can transform every area of life. 'We fight on the most advanced terrain in history – a terrain that opens the prospect of a post-scarcity society, a libertarian society, not a substitution of one system of hierarchy by another.' But SDS, at the most critical juncture in its history, did not follow the anarchist path.

Three years later, the California Situationist group Point-Blank! published their critique of the now-'harmless' New Left. They announced that it was a mistake to say the 1969 SDS convention was the beginning of the end: the end of the New Left was in its very beginning, its nearsighted refusal to see that it was merely a product of the American spectacle. As part of the spectacle (i.e. as part of the culture created by capitalism for sale to all of us in our role as passive spectators/consumers), the New Left was a safety valve for capitalism.

The analysis presented in 'The Storms of Youth' has a kind of value. It reminds us that oppression exists inside each of us, in the culture we have internalized, and not only in external conditions such as war, racism and pollution. Thus, a genuine revolution must transform all areas of life. However, to say that the New Left's battles against the Vietnam war, racism and pollution were 'reforms' carefully planned by capitalism can lead only to cynicism and despair, and ultimately to the passivity which Point-Blank! so eloquently attacks.

Why Marxism is not enough

'Once again the dead are walking in our midst – ironically draped in the name of Marx, the man who tried to bury the dead of the nineteenth century.' So said Murray Bookchin in 'Listen, Marxist!' – a stirring

polemic written in a desperate attempt to change the direction of SDS in 1969. To Bookchin, Marxism is an appropriate revolutionary strategy for societies afflicted with harsh poverty, with conditions of great scarcity – such as Europe in the nineteenth century or Third World countries today. But Marxism is inappropriate for Western societies today, because the material conditions of post-scarcity societies make it possible to have revolutions based on the primacy of the individual, on self-management, freedom and human dignity. In short, conditions are ripe for anarchist revolutions. Marxism is not enough.

There are, of course, broad similarities between Marxism and social anarchism. Both are totally opposed to capitalism; and both work to create socialist societies that will provide freedom and equality for their members. Beyond these general goals, however, the two philosophies are in sharp disagreement.

The articles by Benello and Wieck both point out that one fundamental difference lies in conceptions of power. For Marxists, human history is inherently progressive, so that in the far distant future, after communism is fully realized, power in all its forms (including state power) will cease to exist. Anarchists see two problems with this. They have no faith that history will automatically move in this direction, so they work to dissolve power in the present; and they understand that – as Benello phrases it – 'freedom, to be understood, must be lived.' People begin to end authoritarian relationships by constructing egalitarian ones; they construct different relationships by behaving differently.

Anarchists place strong emphasis on the psychosocial origins of inequality, while most Marxists are indifferent to this. Not all Marxists are economic reductionists, of course, but they do see economic factors as primary. Anarchists, on the other hand, are well aware (in Wieck's words) that 'the secret of human liberation' is not to be found in 'something so specific as the politics of property.' Anarchists have at once a more hopeful and a more complex view of humanity's ability to act in a multiplicity of ways to free itself. It is not part of anarchism's strategy, as Benello says, 'to rely on history to do its job for it.'

The differences between anarchism and Marxism are based upon more than abstract philosophical speculation. Anarchists look at the living products of Marxist theory – the nation-states of China, the USSR, Cuba, Eastern Europe, North Korea and all the rest of them – and see that open dissent is not permitted; that revolts in the direction of greater freedom are systematically smashed (Hungary, Czechoslovakia, Poland . . .); that, since the death of Mao Tse-tung, China has apparently moved in the direction of greater bureaucratization and tighter control from the top; that attempts at self-liberation and artistic expression are actively discouraged; and that dissenters are usually not even permitted to leave. Granted, the material conditions for people living in all these

countries have greatly improved since their pre-socialist days – but they are, in many ways which anarchists consider important, not free.

There is a lesson in all these melancholy details: a state socialist society can erode extremes of wealth and poverty; it can end material want; it can provide all the conditions necessary for people to live in health and physical comfort; it can end foreign domination. All these things are not to be taken lightly. Anarchists want them too. But no government can set anyone free. To be free, people must liberate themselves. And anarchists want this too. Indeed, they insist upon it.

7   Toward a post-scarcity society:
the American perspective and the SDS*

Radical Decentralist Project, Resolution No. 1

The twentieth century is the heir of human history – the legatee of man's age-old effort to free himself from drudgery and material insecurity. For the first time in the long succession of centuries, this century has elevated mankind to an entirely new level of technological achievement and to an entirely new vision of the human experience.

Technologically, we can now achieve man's historical goal – a post-scarcity society. But socially and culturally, we are mired in the economic relations, institutions, attitudes and values of a barbarous past, of a social heritage created by material scarcity. Despite the potentiality of complete human freedom, we live in the day-to-day reality of material insecurity and a subtle, ever-oppressive system of coercion. We live, above all, in a society of fear, be it of war, repression, or dehumanization. For decades we have lived under the cloud of a thermonuclear war, streaked by the fires of local conflicts in half the continents of the world. We have tried to find our identities in a society that has become ever more centralized and mobilized, dominated by swollen civil, military and industrial bureaucracies. We have tried to adapt to an environment that is becoming increasingly befouled with noxious wastes. We have seen our cities and their governments grow beyond all human comprehension, reducing our very sovereignty as individuals to ant-like proportions – the manipulated, dehumanized victims of immense administrative engines and political machines. While the spokesmen for this diseased social 'order' piously mouth encomiums to the virtues of 'democracy,' 'freedom' and 'equality,' tens of millions of people are denied their humanity because of racism and are reduced to conditions of virtual enslavement.

Viewed from a purely personal standpoint, we are processed with the same cold indifference through elementary schools, high schools and academic factories that our parents encounter in their places of work. Worse, we are expected to march along the road from adolescence

---

* Excerpt from a mimeographed leaflet, Chicago, May 1969.

to adulthood, the conscripted, uniformed creatures of a murder machine guided by electronic brains and military morons. As adults, we can expect to be treated with less dignity and identity than cattle: squeezed into underground freight cars, rushed to the spiritual slaughterhouses called 'offices' and 'factories,' and reduced to insensibility by monotonous, often purposeless, work. We will be asked to work to live and live to work – the mere automata of a system that creates superfluous, if not absurd, needs; that will steep us in debts, anxieties and insecurities; and that, finally, will deliver us to the margins of society, to the human scrapheap called the aged and chronically ill – desiccated beings, deprived of all vitality and humanity.

The process of social breakdown

The debasement of social life – all the more terrifying because its irrational, coercive, day-to-day realities stand in such blatant contradiction to its liberatory potentialities – has no precedent in human history. Never before has man done so little with so much; indeed, never before has man used his resources for such vicious, even catastrophic ends. The tension between 'what-*could*-be' and 'what-*is*' reaches its most excruciating proportions in the United States, which occupies the position not only of the most technologically advanced country in the world but also of the 'policeman of the world,' the foremost imperialist power in the world. The United States affords the terrifying spectacle of a country overladen with automobiles and hydrogen bombs; of ranch houses and ghettoes, of immense material superfluity and brutalizing poverty. Its profession of 'democratic' virtue is belied daily by racism, the repression of black and white militants, police terrorism, Vietnam, and the prospect of Vietnams to come.

Is it surprising, then, that a basic, far-reaching disrespect and a profound disloyalty is developing toward the values, the forms, the aspirations and, above all, the institutions of American society? On a scale unprecedented in American history, millions of people, especially among the young, are shedding their commitment to the society in which they live. They no longer believe in its claims. They no longer respect its symbols. They no longer accept its goals, and, most significantly, they refuse almost intuitively to live by its institutional and social codes.

This growing refusal runs very deep. It extends from an opposition to the Vietnam War into a hatred of political manipulation in all its forms. Starting from a rejection of racial discrimination, it brings into question the very existence of hierarchical power as such. In its detestation of middle-class values and life-styles, it rapidly evolves into a

rejection of the commodity system; from an irritation with environmental pollution, it passes into a rejection of the American city and modern urbanism. In short, it tends to transcend every particularistic critique of the society and evolve into a generalized opposition to the bourgeois order on an ever-broadening scale.

What we are witnessing is the breakdown of a century and a half of embourgeoisement and an erosion of all bourgeois institutions *at a point in history when the boldest concepts of utopia are realizable.* And there is nothing that the present bourgeois order can substitute for the erosion of its traditional institutions but bureaucratic manipulation and state capitalism. This process is unfolding most dramatically in the United States. That revolution is envisionable in the United States is due precisely to the fact that the process of de-mythification, of de-bourgeoisement, of de-institutionalization began earlier and is occurring more decisively here than anywhere else in the world. Whether this process will culminate in revolution or in a disastrous form of fascism will depend in great part on the ability of revolutionaries to extend social consciousness and defend the spontaneity of the revolutionary development from authoritarian ideologies, both from the 'Left' and the Right.

The role of SDS

SDS and the youth revolt

As historic processes bring us increasingly closer to the threshold of a *classless* society, we are faced with the decomposition of the culture and institutions that emerge from class society. The elemental demands of the youth revolt for uninhibited sexuality, community, and mutual aid, spontaneity, indeed for communism, and its rejection of the commodity relationship, the work ethic, the patriarchal family, the degradation of women, the existence of hierarchy, and the use of coercion – all of these demands do not emerge accidentally. They prefigure culturally the possibilities opened by the development of a post-scarcity technology, however intuitive and inchoate these demands may seem. And it is precisely from the fact that these demands are intuitive and inchoate that we know we are dealing, here, with elemental social forces – forces that emerge not from books and formulas, but from the very social development itself.

If SDS chapters are to play any role in this youth revolt, if they are to contribute to its extension and consciousness, there should be a reconsideration by every chapter of its structure, aims and internal relations. It is patently absurd to believe that a chapter structured

along bureaucratic lines and dominated by an elite of 'politics' can have any relevance to the youth culture that is percolating in this country. Either the chapter will develop the revolutionary post-scarcity forms of relations within themselves – the relations of brothers and sisters, not merely of ideological 'associates' or 'comrades' – or they will isolate themselves completely. Either they will place a new emphasis on life-style or they will ossify along bureaucratic lines.

There is no formula for achieving these internal changes. The atmosphere and structure of a chapter is ultimately determined by its goals. If the chapter is occupied entirely with the conventional political issues of the Old Left, it will become an Old Left organization: elitist, bureaucratic, and centralized in structure, held together primarily by conventional programmatic issues. If, on the other hand, political issues are organically combined with life-style issues, the internal relations within the chapter will change accordingly.

SDS is above all a youth movement, and particularly a youth movement on college campuses. If the measure of its achievement is the influence it exercises on youth and students, it has failed miserably. For all the talk of a 'student–worker alliance,' we have not even won over a substantial number of students, much less youth generally. In withdrawing into a hardening sectarian shell, we will be well on the way toward losing whatever influence we have exercised in the past on campuses.

To avoid this deadening stagnation, we believe that chapters should try to deal with campus issues in *all* their forms, to carry on a struggle *whose essential goal is to convert the campus into a liberated space for students and the community*. Together with the issues of racism and concrete expressions of American imperialism, our chapters should also deal with the authoritarian nature and structure of the university, the idiocy of grading, bourgeois ideology masquerading as education, the right of students to form their own classes (with teachers merely as consultants), the determination of campus policy by student assemblies – and ultimately to transcend the university, converting it into a liberated space, a community center in the fashion of the Sorbonne and particularly of Censier in the French revolt of May–June 1968.

SDS chapters should also become an organic part of the youth revolt both on campus and off. The ties established between students and street people in Berkeley over the People's Park issue are, in many ways, a model of the kind of development chapters could follow in breaking out of the sectarian shell that has enveloped them. Similar possibilities undoubtedly exist throughout the country, and off-campus youth involve not only street people but also high school and vocational school youth, ghetto youth, and young workers. Few if any of these young people will be drawn to SDS because it has the 'correct transi-

123

tional program on imperialism:' they will be drawn to SDS only if it expresses their drive for life and articulates their detestation of deadening middle-class and proletarian values.

SDS and the community

SDS should follow the paths of least resistance in its struggle against an archaic society that is decomposing unevenly but still retains a tremendous inner strength at its core. By 'paths of least resistance' we do not mean that we should compromise our principles, modes of struggle or goals, but simply that we should devote our main efforts to those sectors of the population that are most susceptible to radicalization. If these are minority groups or workers or sectors of the middle classes, the energies of the chapters should be distributed to those sectors. To preconceive issues in advance of a struggle, to straitjacket reality by formulas borrowed from the past, would be a grave error. The revolt of our time cuts across virtually all class lines.

It goes without saying that there can be no successful social revolution in the United States without the full and active participation of the industrial proletariat. The May–June events in France in 1968 provided almost a paradigm of how the revolutionary process can develop today in an advanced industrial country. If we do not try to learn from these events, we will learn nothing. The French students approached the workers at the factory gates without pretensions about their position as students. They did not pretend they were workers – and the French workers acknowledged them for what they were: students. The alliance between workers and students was possible precisely because both recognized each other as distinct but oppressed strata – oppressed in different ways by the same social enemy.

SDS and the Third World

The best way we can help the Third World is by changing the First World. To declare that the main priority of SDS is to create an anti-imperialist 'front' is to guarantee that imperialism will have no problem from SDS in shaping public opinion in the United States along imperialist lines. If imperialism is presented in abstract terms, its concrete manifestations – which can have a profound effect upon the social development in the United States – will float in a limbo. To the vast majority of the American people, the word 'imperialism' is an abstraction unless its *concrete* manifestations are clearly and decisively fought. The casualty figures in the Vietnam War have meanings; conscription has

meaning; a youth overshadowed by the prospect of military service has meaning; the bombing of villages and the killing and maiming of people has meaning; the repressive way of life in military units has meaning; even the wholesale destruction of Vietnamese forests by defoliants and fire has meaning. As revolutionary internationalists, it is our responsibility to explain and fight imperialism in *all* its manifestations – its sinister day-to-day exploitation of the Third World as well as the military barbarities it inflicts on the Third World. But these features of imperialism must be presented *concretely* to the American people, with a clear emphasis on how it also victimizes them. Only in this concrete way will it be possible to mobilize the American people against the social system at home that produces these barbarities abroad.

The struggle going on in the Third World is a struggle within the domain of unavoidable scarcity. China, Vietnam and Cuba are struggling not only to retain their independence, but also to industrialize. They are confronted by tasks that were overcome years ago in the United States and Western Europe – hence the organizational and political forms they adopt. To attempt to emulate these forms in the United States, to borrow the hierarchical, centralized political organizations adopted in varying degrees by the ruling elements of China, Cuba and North Vietnam, would literally amount to a turning back of the historical clock. We must take our point of departure from the sweeping material opportunities provided by technological developments in the United States and Western Europe. The First World has problems and possibilities that differ qualitatively from those of the Third World and from those of the past. We fight on the most advanced terrain in history – a terrain that opens the prospect of a post-scarcity society, a libertarian society – not a substitution of one system of hierarchy by another.

Conclusions

The revolution we seek is centered around the elimination of man's domination by man. Domination is not a problem of social structure alone; it is also a human condition. The poison of domination is fed to us almost at birth – in the family milieu, in the games we play, in schools and universities, in the army, in jobs, in the market place, in periodicals, books and the mass media, in religion, in organizations of all kinds, *ad nauseam*. Rarely are we conscious of the extent to which domination flows into us from our entire sensory apparatus and reveals itself in the way we think, talk and even walk. Unless we begin to remake ourselves, unless we begin to alter our life-styles and values, domination will mold all our concepts of social change, our estimates of what constitutes 'effectiveness' and 'efficiency.' Life-style is related as

intimately to revolution as revolution is to life-style. This is not a tautology; it is an interplay, a dialectical relationship which must be resolved. A 'revolutionary' movement that fails to take account of this relationship – indeed, that fosters the spirit and reality of domination by its structure, theories, strategies and tactics – is destined to achieve only one kind of 'success:' counter-revolution.

In seeking to function within the youth revolt of our time, we seek also to rid ourselves of all the elements that so often betray the revolutionary to the very society he is fighting. We seek to make our own movement the liberated space that we strive to achieve in society as a whole. The revolution that ushers us into a post-scarcity society must be a *complete* revolution or it will be no revolution at all. It must eliminate not only the exploitation of man by man but also the domination of man by man, the splits between man and nature, town and country, work and play, mind and physical activity, theory and practice, reason and sensuousness, survival and life. If we do not overcome and transcend these splits, if we do not decentralize our cities into ecologically balanced communities, if we do not produce for human needs instead of profit, if we do not restore the balance of nature and find our place in it, if we do not replace hierarchy, the patriarchal family and the state by genuine, open, human relations, social life itself will be annihilated.

Our movement should attempt to reflect in its own structure and human relations the kind of society it is trying to build. It should decentralize so that it will not dominate the future society but rather will dissolve into it. It should leave the power with the people in the only sense that is meaningful: it should dissolve power so that every individual will have control over his everyday life. It should decentralize for tactical as well as strategic reasons: each chapter should be free to evaluate local issues without 'directives' from above, for it alone has the closeness of contact with an immediate situation that allows for a proper determination of priorities. Either we will understand that we are living in a period of *general* breakdown, a dissolution of bourgeois society as a *whole*, with a multitude of issues that cut across virtually time-honored social strata, or we will remain blind to events, their victims rather than catalysts of consciousness and revolutionary change.

May 1969

8   The storms of youth*

Point - Blank!

Nothing has preoccupied American capitalism so much in the last ten years as its youth. Faced with the apparent refusal of a younger generation to participate in its structures, capitalism has expended much effort in analyzing the sources of this revolt; sociologists, psychologists, and other ideologues have been called into service to explain the reasons for youth discontent. Initially, their forecasts were optimistic; the alienation of youth was treated as another symptom of the eternal 'rebellion of the generations' which would supposedly end once youth acceded to the 'responsibilities' of adulthood. As the crisis developed, however, the ideologists proclaimed the 'generation gap' to be a permanent *division*, attributable either to a mysterious, socially manifested Oedipal conflict or as a result of 'permissive upbringing' – the operatives of American society feared that no solution was possible and that a real threat had been posed. But suddenly all these grim predictions have disappeared; the bourgeoisie and their analysts have breathed a sigh of relief – they now talk of the youth vote instead of the youth revolt. This new situation has not been the result of some social *coup* in which capitalism has only now retrieved its errant children – the 'youth revolt' has collapsed of its own dynamic.

The suddenness with which this crisis has dissipated casts suspicion on its origin; curiously, the 'enemy' once singled out by capitalism, the New Left, now appears as harmless. The Yippies, who in their heyday scorned all political parties and the electoral process in general, have become campaign workers for McGovern; the Black Panthers, who once openly armed themselves against the police, field slates of anti-poverty workers and distribute bags of groceries at 'survival conferences.' All of these changes have not been merely tactical; the New Left is not simply regrouping its forces for a fresh assault – it is, in fact, in a state of *decomposition*, and a post-mortem is already underway among those

* Reprinted from the journal *Point-Blank!* no. 1, October 1972, Berkeley, California.

127

ideologists who pretend to speak for what is left of the Movement. In their examinations, they have attempted to locate an exact time at which the New Left began its decline. Some have chosen the SDS convention in 1969 as a convenient date, attributing the adoption of a 'Marxist-Leninist' platform there as a sign that the Movement had betrayed its initial vision; others have derided the New Left's 'sexism' or the 'terrorism' of certain factions as being the cause of its downfall. But the real cause of the death of the New Left will always escape these morticians.

The decline of the Movement stands in direct relation to its *development*; the New Left was a product of the American spectacle and as such was defined as much by capitalism as by itself. The history of the New Left bears witness to the ability of modern capitalism to package rebellion as a *commodity*, as a socially necessary safety valve for the rejuvenation of the system. Purely *spectacular* revolt has taken its place in capitalism's show; it is presented as an image to be consumed or contemplated so that people will forget *how* to rebel. Despite the radical impulses which generated its appearance, the New Left remained on this spectacular terrain throughout its existence.

The New Left began at a time when American capitalism seemed secure from any kind of serious challenge; through a combination of overt repression and ideological control, it had succeeded in unifying itself on a basis rarely attained in the past. But this unification was more apparent than real, and the sterile uniformity of life in bourgeois society was to engender the first stirrings of youth revolt, expressed in the bohemian 'beat movement' of the fifties. This revolt was initially confined to a cultural rejection of bourgeois values, but it eventually merged with the more profound social movement which had begun among those who were systematically excluded from participation in the system, notably the blacks. Although the early civil rights movement was generally reformist in that it only sought to correct certain defects within bourgeois society by demanding that blacks be treated as equals, it did open up serious contradictions in the American system. It tapped a source of radical discontent not only among the so-called 'outcasts' of society but among all those powerless over the use of their lives. Students joined the Southern blacks in attempting a total rejection of the roles allotted them in society; in their naive enthusiasm, the early Freedom Riders recognized the truth of many aspects of the American system, however much they may have seen themselves as a mere auxiliary of the black movement. When this nascent revolt spread to the universities, it was initially centered around the issue of civil rights, but its implications went far beyond any particular issue: the American university had long

since ceased to be the training ground of the elite – it had become a *mass* institution, designed to fill the needs of an expanding modern economy which required millions of educated specialists and functionaries. The call for 'free speech' that issued from the revolt of Berkeley students in 1964 rapidly developed into a critique of the 'multiversity's' role in maintaining society – unlike much of what followed, the FSM's analysis of student life focussed on the immediate conditions of alienation confronted daily by everyone in bourgeois society.

But while these positive tendencies could have provided a basis for a radical critique of American capitalism as a whole, the Movement in 1964 contained the seeds of the destruction of its own radicalism. Any critique of the university became lost in the ideology of student power and academic reform: this movement chose its name well – they were little more than Students for a Democratic Society. The guilt impulses that motivated many of the activists in the civil rights movement gradually dominated and defined the later trends in the New Left. The sacrificial militantism and the spirit of renunciation present in the beginning were to form the basis of later Movement ideology. The New Left did not assume a definitive form until the mid-sixties, however. The end of the civil rights movement provoked an adolescent existential crisis within the Movement – with the rise of Black Power, the white movement was temporarily deprived of a Cause, and correspondingly, an effective base to *organize*. As the black movement began to develop its own recuperators, the white students, who had always regarded the struggle of the blacks as an external force, were increasingly relegated to a marginal position. When they were ousted from SNCC, the militants of the white New Left took refuge in proclaiming their support for the new black activist hierarchy. Having been leaders themselves, the white movement maintained that the blacks *deserved* the manipulators who sought to impose the ideologies of 'black power' and separatism upon them: Stokely Carmichael and H. Rap Brown succeeded Martin Luther King and Bob Moses in their esteem. The New Left was at a complete loss to understand the spontaneous and radical violence of Watts, Newark, and Detroit – these revolts did not fit into the reformist schemes of Movement organizers.

The escalation of the Vietnam War resolved the crisis of the early New Left and at the same time accentuated its tendencies towards sacrifice and hierarchy. In Vietnam, the Movement found another cause to serve: organizing anti-war demonstrations succeeded the registration of black voters, and the Freedom Riders became peace marchers. Vietnam provided the New Left with an issue ('ending the war') which could easily be endorsed by large numbers of people, and it became the central focus of action and discussion, in university 'teach-ins' as well as in petitions and marches. The anti-war movement was a new moral

crusade in which the New Left could present itself as the 'conscience of America;' its reformism was made explicit in its call for a 'redress of grievances.' Henceforth, the direction that the Movement was to take had been determined – everything that it accomplished was to be carried out on the system's terms.

The positive content of the New Left was rapidly lost in its subsequent development. Although it had arrived at a partial critique of some aspects of society, it was never able to extend these insights into a coherent explanation of bourgeois domination as a whole – the New Left's opposition to capitalism was always *fragmentary*. Arising from a visceral response to the admitted 'excesses' of American society (Vietnam, racism, pollution), the Movement consumed the image of oppression presented by *capitalism*. The revolt of the New Left remained a spectacular revolt precisely because it was engendered by the stimuli of the spectacle. The Movement was an authentic product of a society where critical attention is everywhere diverted from looking at *oneself* – it was inherently *reactionary*. The traces of the subjective revolt against the conditions of bourgeois society became lost as the Movement developed according to the objective 'demands' presented by capitalism. The New Left admitted this dependence on capitalism for its survival; its leaders boasted that 'the system is our best organizer.' As a result, the New Left was only 'revolutionary' in a sense defined by bourgeois society; in identifying with capitalism's 'enemies' (NLF, China, Cuba), it only sought to replace one form of domination with another. The naive 'anti-imperialist' ideology put forth by the Movement was restricted to support of the Stalinist bureaucracies of the Third World. While profoundly disillusioned with American society, the Left accepted the counter-revolutionary Leninist 'vanguard party' as an organizational paradigm.

Internally, the Movement developed its own hierarchy of cadre and 'base,' and a manipulative practice supposedly 'serving the interests of the people.' This process of Bolshevization was only one extension of earlier attempts at community organizing; in both cases, the Movement conceived of itself as the representative of various abstract constituencies on whose behalf the militants would carry out the struggle. Whenever the possibilities for organizing one set of constituents had been exhausted, the New Leftists would attempt to find another group to manipulate – whether it was voter registration, building the anti-war movement, or 'going to the workers,' the basic motive was the same. If any struggle arose which threatened to go beyond partial issues, the Movement leadership, in almost every instance, would attempt to divert it into the channels of conventional 'protest.' Radical acts like the seizure of land at People's Park became lost in the issues of 'police brutality;' disruptions carried on by left-wing elements (Motherfuckers,

Yippies) were subsumed in the Movement as a whole – despite their pretensions to an authentic radicalism, these 'leftists' were nothing more than a quasi-anarchist sideshow to the New Left in general. The spontaneous violence that accompanied many street actions was easily recuperated by the Movement; riots were viewed as an acceptable complement to the New Left's *spectacle* of protest. All marches became carefully orchestrated performances, produced as much for the TV cameras as for the participants. The Movement consciously evoked a theatrical atmosphere in its panoply of slogans and banners; its leaders were aware of their role as *performers* and played this part in the courtroom as well as on the podium.

The New Left's histrionics, however, were only part of a larger show staged by capitalism. The Movement, which emerged as a revolt against a spectacular *image* of oppression, was in turn presented as an *image* of revolt by capitalism. For a time neither could do without the other and both were conscious of this symbiotic relationship – their ideologies were mutually contingent. The New Left served as a convenient 'threat' to bourgeois society, which attempted to use the specter of a 'generation of freaks' as a means of unifying the 'silent majority.' But while denouncing a revolt which it had itself packaged, capitalism incorporated many of the Movement's demands into its own structure, reforming itself with the Movement's unwitting assistance. This reform was in no way a result of some mysterious 'co-optation' of the New Left – although it proclaimed itself to be a 'revolutionary' alternative, the Movement's practice demonstrated that the transition from the reform of the early sixties to a 'revolutionary' posture was purely a change in semantics. The 'contradictions' within the system which the New Left saw as definitive could easily be resolved by capitalism; blacks and other minorities could be allowed to participate in society, the war could be phased out, the problems of the environment could be alleviated – all without altering the basic structures of modern capitalism. Once the Movement had revealed the 'faults' of the system, it was rendered irrelevant – the spectacle proved far better able to implement reform than the New Left, which began to fade as soon as it was deprived of an effective basis for its activity.

Since it drew its initiative from capitalism's actions, the New Left could only sustain itself as long as the system appeared openly repressive – its zenith was reached during the spring of 1970, with the invasion of Cambodia, raids on Black Panthers, the shootings at Kent State, etc. But by this time, the decline of the Movement had already set in; a once physically unified New Left had degenerated into sectarian disputes between different bureaucratic factions, and with the advent of

terrorism it was to leave the scene in a display of ideological and tactical pyrotechnics. The rise of groups such as Weatherman, however, cannot be considered as an aberrancy attributable to the 'excesses' of a decomposing New Left – rather, the *truth* of the Movement was revealed in these tendencies. These organizations represent the ultimate consequence of the weaknesses inherent in the early New Left; the Weathermen and their ilk took their New Leftism *seriously*.

The Weathermen were Movement veterans who had been through the civil rights and student movements. The initial motivations of guilt and sacrifice that brought them into the New Left was taken to their logical conclusion in Weatherman, whose history demonstrates not only the futility of terrorism but that of the New Left in general. Rather than simply acting on *behalf* of the blacks, the Vietnamese, etc. the Weathermen actually attempted to *become* part of the Third World themselves – they desired to join themselves physically to the 'anti-imperialist' forces of the world. The new 'Americong' terrorists intended to act as a 'fifth column' for the exterior 'proletariat' in the underdeveloped countries, and as such they attempted to translate the latent guerrilla fantasies of the New Left in general into reality.

The triumph of guilt in Weatherman was accompanied by a triumph of ritual. Its actions had a dual aspect – while ostensibly 'fighting imperialism,' Weatherman was more importantly negating the 'bourgeois' attributes of its background, as shown in a Weatherman statement, 'We began to feel the Vietnamese in ourselves.' With its avowed goal of 'smashing' its 'honky' origins. Weatherman could present itself as the most *moral* group of militants. For Weatherman, every aspect of the struggle became a quasi-spiritual test, an act of faith in which the militant purified himself and his ideology. This ritual cleansing could only be accomplished in the cathartic act of violence, where the individual 'put his body on the line' for the cause. The violence of Weatherman, exhibited in such acts as the 'Days of Rage' in Chicago, was designed not only to 'bring the war home' but to establish a line of demarcation for the Movement as a whole. Those who did not come to Chicago would be 'punking out'; if Weatherman was prepared to die for the Vietnamese, anything less would be 'counter-revolutionary.'

Weatherman's extremism lies only in that it played the role demanded of it by capitalism to an *extreme*. Weatherman took its mythic status literally, to the point of consuming the image of itself presented by the bourgeois media. It revelled in its own notoriety, progressively enhancing its mystique of violence and bravado as if to suit the public's taste for titillation. Weatherman was the most spectacular faction of the New Left in that myth became its only rationale; politics became secondary – from violent Maoists, they became satanic harbingers of apocalypse. By the time Weatherman convened the Flint 'War Council,'

its 'solidarity' embraced Ho Chi Minh and Charlie Manson – its actions became black rites of exorcism in which the Weatherman would expiate the sins of their 'privileged' past. This masochism led inevitably to self-destruction; while the Black Panthers only talked of revolutionary suicide, Weatherman was prepared to put it into practice.

The decline of Weatherman was a prelude to the decline of the Movement as a whole; ideologically, Weatherman had been the heir to all the New Left's mystifications. It accepted the *false* divisions promoted by the spectacle between young and old, 'hip' and 'straight,' and proclaimed youth as the only revolutionary force in American society. The later Weatherman carried these divisions one step further; the Third World became the true agent of revolution – all those who reaped the 'privileges' of the 'mother country' were by definition 'honkies,' and 'white-skin privilege' became the sole criterion for Weatherman's conception of the 'bourgeoisie.' This ideology was to be Weatherman's undoing: once it had been deprived of its ephemeral base, Weatherman turned in on itself, exerting an internal terror against its own members, who were accused of 'bourgeois' or 'racist' traits. A Stalinism of everyday life was practiced in Weatherman collectives – these communes, which were supposed to produce the 'new men and women of the revolution,' only succeeded in creating a pitiful breed of obedient android. The truth of militantism was revealed in the burnt-out shells of these activists: the 'revolution' of the New Left disappeared as rapidly as it had developed.

The revolt of youth cannot be discussed solely in terms of the New Left, however – it was not a purely 'political' phenomenon. The personal transformation which was attempted on a political level by groups like Weatherman was mirrored culturally by the proliferation of Bohemian life-styles among the young. In a sense, this 'counter-culture' was more radical than the New Left ever was, because from the beginning it attempted to define itself in opposition to politics and sought to create an alternative to a society based on power. The appeal to the counter-culture lay in its apparent rejection of the attributes of bourgeois society; those who dropped out did so with the intention of creating something out of their lives. Yet, like the New Left, the counter-culture did not pose an authentic opposition to capitalism – far from signalling a radical transformation of all values, it remained *subservient* to the existing values, being merely a hip parody of the dominant spectacle. In its rituals and its 'alternate' institutions, the counter-culture reproduced the hierarchy and the commodity relations of bourgeois society. Its festivals and rock concerts were nothing more than mass displays of *passivity*; its businesses were only modern rivals to conventional firms.

133

In the end, the counter-culture was easily absorbed as another cultural fragment within the spectacle. The Youth Culture only challenged the *form* of modern society; the trappings which it developed to distinguish itself from the rest of society were largely superficial differences in music, clothing, chemicals, etc. The experiments in new social relations that were attempted in the communes resulted in most cases in a simple reproduction of the family unit. The 'isolation' of the counter-culture from the rest of society was always a myth – since it conceived of revolt in *cultural* instead of social terms, its 'rejection' of bourgeois society was easily recuperated. The counter-culture soon became another market for capitalism, which developed new commodities to pander to the tastes of youth. The successful integration of the new culture within the ruling order has disproved all the hopes of the bourgeois ideologists (Marcuse, etc) who entertained various illusions about a 'radical' life-style. The decomposition of the counter-culture – reflected in the growth of mysticism and religion, the sordid misery of the 'drug scene,' and the 'riots' at rock concerts – revealed it to be simply one alienation among many in spectacular society.

Despite the decay of the 'radical' political and cultural movements of the past decade, many of their characteristics and illusions linger on. The collapse of the New Left has engendered various *partial* critiques of its practice, all designed to save the Movement from itself. Women's liberation criticized the hierarchy and manipulation prevalent in New Left sects and attempted to analyze the inter-personal relationships of the Movement, but in the process evolved into merely another separatist movement with a fundamentally reformist ideology. The male New Left redeemed itself through 'men's groups,' where the participants would flagellate themselves for their 'male chauvinism.' Other groups have attempted to overcome the New Left by fusing both political and cultural tendencies; their criticisms of the Movement (especially Anti-Mass) deride its forms of protest (mass movements, etc.) and pose the ideal of the collective or 'affinity group' as constituting the nucleus of the future revolutionary society, which will somehow emerge with the proliferation of these collectives. But far from presenting a radical alternative, this idealization of the collective erects a banality – a particular *living arrangement* – as the major focus of the revolutionary process; in place of the New Left, groups like Anti-Mass can only offer communalized misery. Further to the left are the assorted anarchist denunciations of the Movement; while occasionally perceptive, the anarchists have also been unable to see any way beyond the New Left other than to resurrect the faded anarcho-syndicalist ideology of the IWW or to embrace the modernist confusionism of Bookchin. None of these reformist critiques have ever aimed at the *supersession* of the Movement – all of the New Left's saviors are incapable of seeing that it is already *dead*.

In the wake of the New Left's demise, it has become fashionable to discuss the general mood of 'apoliticism' among youth – the sociologists have attributed this to a sudden upsurge of 'introspection,' while the last remnants of the Movement decry it as 'apethetic.' The fact that many have become disillusioned with the manipulative practice of the Left, however, does not mean that American capitalism has achieved any kind of final victory. While the relics of the New Left are reduced to applauding prison rebellions from the sidelines, the real discontent which resulted in the revolt of American youth *remains*. The New Left was a *false* start in the process of genuine revolution; if the rise and fall of the Movement has shown that a true opposition to capitalism cannot be *partial* or limited in scope, the commodity spectacle, which invades the whole life, can only be answered by *total revolt*.

A desire to change *everything* in this world is what separates us from the feeble reformers of the Left. It is the subjective experience of alienation, and not any external force or issue, which forms the basis of a truly revolutionary opposition to capitalism. The refusal of the constraints imposed by the spectacle does not stem from a need to right any particular wrong, but from a recognition of the absolute *impoverishment* of life in bourgeois society. Any practical rejection of sacrifice and hierarchy must necessarily be made over the ruins of the New Left. Our critique of the New Left is a critique of all spectacular revolt and constitutes the premise for the formation of an authentic revolutionary movement in the United States. While the death of the Movement has revealed the true nature of false opposition, it is still necessary to show how its errors can be avoided, since any movement which proclaims itself to be 'radical' but speaks in the language of Power only stands in the way of the development of a true radicalism.

In our theory and practice, we present ourselves as a group which has opposed the reactionary New Left. An identical opposition has been implicit in the general contempt for the Movement which exists among its former constituents. The alternative to the New Left, however, does not lie in aimless nihilism or in a simple rejection of revolt in favor of passivity. While rejecting *quantitative* change, we do not mean to 'wait' for radical activity to occur: the development of a revolutionary situation in the US requires a practice equal to our theoretical critique. The society that the New Left set out to change is still in power, but capitalism has not succeeded in destroying all opposition to it – the spectacle continues to produce the forces of its possible negation, and from now on, no one can have any illusions as to the meaning of real change – revolution begins when people speak *for themselves* and seize control over everything affecting their lives. If anything, the 'youth revolt' has shown that no one is really young in this society; there are only varying degrees of *age*. The destruction of the *old* world

and the reaffirmation of youth begins when people challenge everything *openly*; instead of allowing itself to be defined by capitalism's rules, the revolutionary movement must define *itself* as the complete negation of existing society through the positive construction of a qualitatively new social order.

The individual, *lost* in the alienation of society and the counter-alienation of the New Left, must form the starting point for real socialism. Throughout its brief existence, the Movement offered nothing more than a vision of sacrifice on behalf of an external cause – its fate proved once again that revolution is not a duty – it is *pleasurable* or it is nothing. Revolt always begins with the individual, whenever he refuses to submit to the mindless routine to which he is subjected daily, and he must take himself and his desires seriously if this revolt is to be extended. Individual subjectivity is the means and the end towards the development of collective revolutionary activity. The 'individualism' that capitalism prides itself on having achieved is merely the alienated subjection of the individual; *self*-management implies the creation of a collectivity where individuals find the possibility for their self-realization in the freedom of others, where they affirm themselves as subjects in a world which they have made their own.

The group, Point-Blank!, was started by Chris Shutes, David Jacobs and Chris Winks in 1971 in Santa Cruz, California. They mainly published leaflets and pamphlets. *Point-Blank!* was to be their theoretical journal, but it was issued only once before the group dissolved.

On the Correct Handling of Nuclear Fallout Upon the People

A MESSAGE
FROM THE NATIONAL STEERING COMMITTEE OF THE U.S. CHINA PEOPLES FRIENDSHIP ASSOCIATION

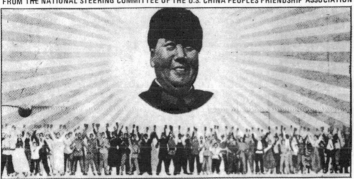

U.S. Getting Radiation From China A-Blast

WASHINGTON — (AP) — Light radiation from a Chinese atomic test is sprinkling parts of the eastern United States, leading health officials in one state to warn residents to wash garden vegetables carefully before eating them.

Pennsylvania officials were first to report detection of the fallout from a Sept. 26 blast at Lop Nor in western China. Other areas reporting some radiation include New Jersey, southern Connecticut, Long Island, Delaware and South Carolina.

The Energy Research and Development Administration (ERDA) in Washington said that "the fallout is of low level and presents no cause of concern." However, a spokesman added that data on radiation levels is still being collected.

Thomas M. Gerusky, head of the Pennsylvania bureau of radiological health, issued a warning that garden vegetables should be washed carefully before being eaten. He said radioactivity had been found in samples of milk.

Detroit Free Press, Oct. 5, 1976

A great and wise man once said that, if handled properly, contradictions among the people can be resolved beneficially so that what was once a bad thing can become a good thing.

There are many contradictions existing between the peoples of the U.S. and China today, but for us the principal contradiction from which all others emanate is not between the people but between the social systems under which they labor; the principal contradiction is between *Capitalism* and *Socialism*.

It is our position that this contradiction has thus far been a bad thing; this much, we think, is self-evident. But it is also our conviction that, armed with the correct political line and a revolutionary will, the working people of America, emulating their brothers and sisters in the People's Republic, can smash the yoke of Capitalism and, in resolving the principal contradiction, transform a bad thing into a good thing.

The Imperialist media recognize this possibility and it terrifies them to think that it might happen. And so they do everything within their power to confuse and divide the workers. The recent furor over "nuclear fallout" from Chinese weapons testing is only the latest and most obvious attempt to divert workers' attention from the real enemy, *Capitalism*, and onto the imagined enemy of Chinese Socialism.

Of course newspapers like the one cited above make no mention of the fact that in the state of Nevada 250 square miles of land have been rendered unliveable for 24,000 years by U.S. nuclear testing. Nor do they note that the fallout introduced into the earth's atmosphere by U.S. testing far exceeds all the fallout that China can possibly produce for many years to come. Nor, finally, do they point out that the U.S. is the only nation in history to use atomic weapons directly against human beings in time of war, not once, but twice.

Still, it is undeniably true that China has nuclear weapons, that she has and will test them in the atmosphere, and that, inevitably, there is going to be fallout from them.

But there is one crucial distinction which, try as they may, the media cannot overlook: the fallout from Chinese atom bombs is *Socialist* fallout.

Capitalism, assuredly, means production, but more importantly, it means production *for profit*. If production is not profitable it does not take place.

Socialism also means production, but it is not production for profit; it is production for *people*.

In China then, production of nuclear weapons is not for profit, it is for people. *The American people have nothing to fear from Socialist fallout, it is only Capitalist fallout which is dangerous because it is not produced for the benefit of the laboring masses.*

We feel it is of the utmost importance to grasp this crucial difference between Capitalist and Socialist nuclear fallout if American working people and oppressed minorities are not to fall into the bourgeois trap of equating the forces of Socialist liberation with those of the Imperialist oppressors.

a paid political advertisement, paid for by the USCPFA

THE FIFTH ESTATE

9 The negativity of anarchism*

David Thoreau Wieck

[*Author's note* In the essay from which these selections are taken, I have sought to express the meaning of 'the anarchist ideas' that have (I believe) been the foundation and inspiration for anarchism as a social and intellectual movement. In terming anarchism an idea (rather than an ideology), I mean to convey specifically that it is non-doctrinal; that it has always been 'understood' rather than defined; that it gives shared meaning to deep-felt longings; that it indicates an ideal aim for which a social movement of everyday human beings, who in practice will often enough contradict their ideals, is called forth; that it expresses an 'ought' that is an anticipation of its object of striving; that it serves as object of faith, as ground of solidarity and mutual aid; that it has been enriched but not transformed essentially by supporting speculations and reasoned argument; and that it has remained continuously and intensely in touch with its originating ideals.

Anarchism is not merely anti-statist. It is, more broadly, an idea or theory of freedom, and the anarchist conception of freedom has not always been clearly articulated. The importance of the anarchist conception becomes manifest, I argue in the essay, once we recognize that anarchism is anti-political in the sense of opposing *all political relationships*, that is all power-structured relationships. We shall have in mind a panoply of 'political' relationships, among them masters and slaves, governors and governed, propertied and propertyless, employers and employees, male and female, teachers and students, old and young (and young and old), dominant and subjugated races, party leaders and party members, bureaucrats and clients, labor leaders and rank and file, commanders and troops, priests and their flocks (and on some views: God and human beings), imperial nations and subject-peoples, liberators and those whom they propose to liberate.]

---

* Excerpted from a longer article which appeared in *Interrogations: International Review of Anarchist Research*, December 1975.

Anarchism can be understood as the *generic* social and political idea that expresses negation of *all* power, sovereignty, domination, and hierarchical division, and a will to their dissolution; *and* expresses rejection of all the dichotomizing concepts that on the grounds of nature, reason, history, God divide people into those dominant and those justly subordinated. Anarchism is therefore more than anti-statism. But government (the state), because it claims ultimate sovereignty and the right to outlaw or legitimate particular sovereignties, and because it serves the interests, predominantly, of those who possess particular spheres of power, stands at the centre of the web of social domination; it is, appropriately, the central focus of anarchist critique. Anarchism is anti-political, therefore, in a comprehensive sense for which electoral and parliamentary abstentionism is a fitting symbol.

Anarchism then is the social and political philosophy that proposes the eradicating of all divisions between (political) haves and have-nots, the dissolving rather than the redistributing of power; and the abolishing of identities of ruler and subject, leader and led, learned and ignorant, superior and inferior, master and servant, human and inhuman. If the anarchist ideal were realized, all persons in their unique individuality would be related to each other in multiple non-stratified societies of voluntary (freely chosen) association.

Today, individuality signifies, almost invariably, membership in an élite class or caste, opposite a mass, and depends on (is given definition by) that membership; such individuality is not authentic because not properly individual. What is presently thought of as socialization is a stabilized, preferably frictionless politics to which the subordinate assent. The aim of anarchism is universal and genuine individuality and complete socialization, their antithesis overcome by, precisely, the elimination of constraining and distorting contexts of power. Then all persons would be political equals, not in the sense of equality of power (for anarchism negates social power) or necessarily of goods but in the sense that no one, no group, and no institution would rule, control, decide for or dominate another. There would be society, but no polity.

Individuality (uniqueness) and the socialization of human existence, so reconceived, can be identified as basic values of anarchism, values in turn describable as social freedom. Justice will no longer be defined in terms of distribution, or of rights that presuppose sovereignty, certainly not by lawfulness. If slavery be taken as metaphor for domination, applicable literally or nearly so to many of its forms, justice and injustice of institutions can be defined in terms of 'slavery': so that an institution is unjust if and in so far as persons implicated in it are the 'slaves' of others. However benign and altruistically intentioned, 'slaveries' violate human beings systematically and essentially, and this cannot be made good. The 'master' of course thinks otherwise, and otherwise say his ideologies.

Plainly, to strive for the total abolition of 'slaveries' is not the only possible mode of response to their recognition: if it were, there would be no liberalisms or Marxisms and anarchists would be everywhere. If convinced that abolition is impossible, one may choose to mitigate, reform or exchange systems of power; without devaluing freedom, one might not hope for more than marginal and sporadic realization of it. Except for incidental remarks, I shall avoid discussion of practicality and the philosophical problems concerning judgment of it, problems that are particularly difficult because the generalization of anarchist attitudes toward institutions might have significant results, in keeping with anarchist values, even if the ideal aim were never approximated. I limit myself to trying to exhibit the meaning of the anarchist Idea, a project prior to, even though not fully distinguishable from, judgments of practicality, and necessary (I believe) because the degree to which an anarchist perspective restructures perception and anticipation of human being, of society, and of history, is rarely appreciated sufficiently.

Sometimes the characteristics of anarchism discussed here are expressed, by anarchists and others, as *anti-authoritarianism*. This is an unhappy mode of expression, first because anti-authoritarianism is professed by numerous and diverse political groups; second because there are forms of authority that do not entail power over persons; third because authority is that to which power pretends and which its ideology claims for it; and for other reasons. Authority that is specifically and voluntarily delegated is not power-over-persons, although it may be converted to such power. Recognition of the authority of technical competence is not submission to power, unless the technically competent are permitted to determine ends as well as means, or to determine means in a fashion that determines ends. The authority of each in his or her own sphere of activity is a way of enunciating the freedom of each. Analysis of authority, to distinguish the genuine from the spurious, has been lacking in anarchist literature; the problem is met squarely by Giovanni Baldelli's *Social Anarchism* (New York: Atherton Press, 1971), from which I have learned much.

Anarchism and Marxism

Persons familiar with 'early Marx' might suggest that I have just described uncorrupted Marxism. The matter is worth pursuit both for its own sake – since I believe Marxism and anarchism to represent truly basic alternatives – and in order to bring out other important dimensions of the anarchist Idea, especially its temporality.

Marx might be called a philosophical anarchist in the sense of the phrase that signifies affirmation of anarchy as an ideal without present

relevance. The conflict between Marx and the anarchists in the First International makes it clear that Marx did not in organizational practice or revolutionary program share the anarchists' negativity toward power. He demanded control by the central organization over the sections; he insisted on programmatic unity, in effect the enforcement of agreement to truths of a leadership-élite; he destroyed the International rather than permit it to be an association of solidarity in diversity; he emphatically rejected the anarchist thesis that the abolition of the state was a present concern. Anarchist criticism of Marxism, in addition to unjustly identifying Marx with later dialectical materialism, sometimes overstresses the historical personage Karl Marx, but, besides foreshadowing the political and ideological practice of future socialism, including the Leninist monoliths, his behavior reflects his conception of power and freedom.

The ideals sometimes (not so very frequently) affirmed in Marxism may not be significantly opposed to those of anarchism; but for all the time between the present and, in Marxism, the eventual realization of the ideal there is systematic variance. For Marx as for Marxism, no-power, to the extent acknowledged, is beyond history, while for anarchists it is within history, within the present, immanent as potentiality in the present.

Anarchism provides a critique of the politics of liberation itself – a critique that only a few Marxists have attempted. Basic to Marxism is the view that economic power is the key to a liberation of which the power of a party, the power of government, and the power of a specific class are (or are to be) instruments. Basic to anarchism is the opposing view that the abolition of dominion and tyranny depends upon their negation, in thought and when possible action, in every form and at every step, from now on, progressively, by every individual and group, in movements of liberation as well as elsewhere, no matter the state of consciousness of entire social classes. Thus, anarchists see in Marxism an illusion of liberation and the creation of new structures of power that forever defer it and that nullify spontaneous liberations briefly tolerated. Correlatively, in the anarchist view the choices and actions of individuals are important for those persons, for their milieu, and for all of us; in the view of Marxists, collectivities and their actions alone have significance, are alone objectively real (this has turned out to be the operational meaning of Marx's famous Feuerbach thesis on the individual).

Congruently with theory, the strategies of Marxist movements have been strategies for conquest and use of power, strategies of affirmation of politics. In every country ruled by Marxists the basic politics, i.e. the basic structures of state, have been perpetuated, or if in collapse reinstituted and revivified, a fact that lends support to the claim that anarchism is the only social philosophy that asserts an alternative to the politics of power.

141

In the light of the preceding, certain familiar Marxist polemics against anarchism can be subjected to inversion. Rather than anarchism, it may be Marxism, with its vision of post-historical transcendence, that is apocalyptic and utopian. Anarchism rather than Marxism may be capable of sustaining a conception of genuine social dialectic, for Marx's theory of superstructure and the primacy of impersonal economic forces inhibits, if it does not entirely rule out, an apprehension of continuous interplay among the many arenas of politics and liberation. It may be anarchism that implies the more complete view of *anthropos* because it does not by abstraction obscure and ignore the psychology and the now so important sociology of power. And it may be not anarchism but Marxism, with its econocentrism, its controlling dialectic of technology and property, that is simplistic and naive.

In the section that follows, part of the meaning of the above theses will be developed.

The new relevance of anarchism

Recent revival of interest in anarchism, and the tendency of some North American and Western European Marxists to revise Marxism in libertarian directions, allow explanation in terms of the present discussion.

First, anarchism is the natural generic expression for the many particular movements of liberation, including a number that have emerged in force only recently. As such a generic idea, anarchism *implies* these liberations, and most lines of argument against particular power-and-dominance relations tend conversely to generalize to the anarchist position. Not merely awareness of twentieth-century extensions of state-power, therefore, has given anarchism contemporary 'relevance' both for radical youth and for various intellectuals and social philosophers.

Anarchism does more than unify the many themes of liberation. For those who suspect that power rather than wealth may be the root of oppression, and that power may be the more comprehensive concept, anarchism offers a framework of explanation. Marxists have generally derived racism from the interest of the wealthy classes in dividing the mass of the people against one another; one does not have to deny this interpretation all validity to see that the psychology of social or ethnic domination, for the sake of domination, may be a deeper theme. It has been difficult, in view of the imperialist actions of the Russian state, to attribute imperialism and wars to economic and profit considerations primarily. In many other spheres, the sphere of 'liberation', included, we see power sought after from motives deeper than a theory centered

upon economics accounts for; while a theory centering upon power is capable of explaining also the seemingly irrational intensity of acquisitive behavior.

Third, it is becoming increasingly apparent that to speak about a 'ruling class' in the present era is totally inadequate. Nationally and internationally, the economics of capitalist distribution retains its disproportionality of wealth and poverty but now power is corporate and bureaucratic. Even that statement falls short, and phrases like 'military-industrial complex' seem ineluctably apt. Individuals and groups face elaborate structures of power, national and transnational and their self-sense, even at relatively high levels of privilege, is likely to be one of powerlessness, helplessness, insecurity. The 'class' that rules is not exactly a class of persons but more like an institutional complex whose administrative and managerial technicians work, one may say with only slight exaggeration, to job-description. Even if we define this personnel, together with the major beneficiary individuals and families, as 'the ruling class,' it remains none the less, in the USA as in the USSR, an impersonal power with replaceable figureheads. The 'power' demands of the American sixties expressed a sense of contemporary society's, not America's alone, central problematic: the abstraction of power from persons in the form of 'bureaucratic society,' 'managerial society,' etc. Anarchism becomes more plainly relevant when power itself, not this group or that class of person, reveals itself as the truth of the nation-state and of international capitalism and nationalistic socialism, and when power rather than wealth is the prime image of success, the one model presented for emulation.

Fourth, from many sources have come reasons to believe that any theory that finds the secret of human liberation in something so specific as the politics of property neglects the interdependence of the many liberations. Each species of dominance and power reinforces other species, directly in ways that can be mapped sociologically, indirectly by requiring and engendering habits of rule and/or submission. Children who have undergone hierarchically structured families and schools will be most fortunate if enabled by countervailing experiences to affirm themselves thereafter in non-power-structured situations, or to relate freely and responsibly as persons with persons, or to resist power rationally rather than by brief rebellion. Solidarity among professedly antagonistic groups against challenge from below – the solidarity of union officials and corporate managers, to name a familiar type – is in striking contrast to the normal and self-defeating non-solidarity, most often mutual hostility, of oppressed groups from different categories. As we proceed more deeply into a world of institutional management of human existence, and in that evolution might be approaching, if we have not already passed, a point of no return, questions of liberation

increasingly reveal themselves as a single issue of manifold human liberation.

Fifth, the interdependence of the many liberations suggests that human liberation must be a continuous process and that the anarchist method of seeking to transform qualitatively the scene of one's life, of trying to create spheres of freedom even when one cannot affect large social institutions of property and government directly, may be a meaningful and necessary part of a multidimensional process of liberation in which many are active in varied and particular ways. This can be expressed by saying that anarchism proposes the *continuous realization* of freedom in the lives of each and all, both for its intrinsic, immediate values and for its more remote effects, the latter unpredictable because they depend on the unpredictable behaviors of persons not known and of non-personal historical processes.

Nevertheless, anarchism remains extraordinarily difficult to adopt other than 'philosophically,' i.e., intellectually, for it makes a severe dialectical demand: that persons envision and find ways to overcome a condition of objective and subjective powerlessness and futility, not by seeking power or planning its seizure, or by pleading with power, and so on, which are the ways of politics and the ways also by which people attempt to cope with everyday oppressions, frustrations, and resentments, but by negating power absolutely *and choosing powerlessness*. (Choice of powerlessness does not, however, imply passivity or lack of militancy. Anarchism and T'aoism have much in common – but anarchism is not a way of merely personal salvation.) The demand is severe, given, in the USA, for specific example, a society that is barren of public ideas other than the power-oriented; given a prevailing ethic that allows one to do whatever one wants so long as no one is hurt very directly; given that authentic models of liberty, individuality, and free cooperation are scarce; given a superficial but malignant pessimism about human beings; given a complex of overlapping hierarchies such that all but a few people are relatively superior to others who are institutionally inferior; given a communications technology that provides a year-round circus of politics for the entertainment and mystification of the citizenry; given the rage, hatred, fear, envy that pervade the nation. Neo-Marxisms that retain a basic affirmation of power and a reassuring vision of power-through-history, while seeking to qualify themselves by incorporating libertarian themes, make lesser psychological and ethical demands.

Whether, in a society (and world) in which the reality and ideality of power are ubiquitous, anarchism, in the sense of generic liberation, can have meaning other than to be a way of life for a small number, would seem to depend on the possibility that the transcendence of power, i.e. integral freedom, becomes by many persons concretely imaginable,

concretely thinkable, as the resolution and liquidation of the power-and-powerlessness polarity. Because such a consciousness has never yet been realized on a large social scale, with the partial exception of a certain period in Spain, its potentialities have never been tested. But the choice of powerlessness, the choice, if run one must, to run with the hares and not with the hounds, and, beyond that, the choice to reject such definition of options, is a choice open to each person as a life-choice, and its intrinsic meanings are not invalidated either by choices others make or by verdicts of mindless history.

Anarchist ethics

Anarchist principle

I should like now to begin to present certain implications of an anarchist view of power and liberation.

In theories justificatory of anarchism one encounters a confusing variety of ethical arguments – a variety attributable in part but not entirely to the authors' desire to emphasize either the theme of individuality or the theme of sociality. In anarchist movements and the lives of anarchists, however, one finds something simpler – a consistent emphasis upon *principles* and *action from principle*. Herein I believe lies a key to the ethical meanings of anarchism.

To the bourgeois, anarchist principle signifies fanaticism, to Marxists, an unrealistic and irresponsible unadaptibility to objective circumstance and historical necessity. 'On principle' anarchists abstain from all elections, refuse to form or support political parties or party-like organizations, refuse to appeal to or accept the aid of government to achieve immediate desired ends, refuse to accept positions of power, oppose and seek the downfall of liberal as well as overtly tyrannical states, oppose all wars and resist military service, refuse to be married by state or church, and so on. Anarchists refuse to 'recognize' laws, courts, and police authorities, refuse to defend themselves by accepted legal procedures. Anarchists make a principle of direct (i.e., personal and non-mediated) action, a principle of solidarity, a principle of personal responsibility. In general the word 'compromise' means for anarchists compromise of principles, and has only pejorative connotations. The conclusion would be difficult to avoid, that this 'inflexibility' is somehow intrinsic to anarchism.

Action from principle has in different contexts very different meanings. In the anarchist context these various principles, this attachment to principle, this ethics and politics of strict (but not absolute) principle, all this becomes intelligible and coherent when the various principles are

145

referred to a single principle, *that one should neither exercise nor submit to power over persons,* either by collectivities or persons; with the correlative belief that the downfall of power depends upon action from this principle. By this interpretation, negation of power can be described as the principle-of-principles of anarchist action: in the end, perhaps it is, or should be conceived as, the *only* principle.

(It is important to note that the principles mentioned are nearly all *negative* principles. Plainly they call for the supplement of concrete alternative actions fitted to circumstances, and an anarchist movement that knows nothing but its negative principles is a movement in decay.)

I believe that the central anarchist principle is best understood in interconnection with certain more general ideas: that the individual is the basic social reality; that individual voluntary consent is the ground of cooperation ('giving one's word,' in the traditional anarchist movements, is the bond that unites); that everyone, oneself not excepted, is responsible for their actions; that social freedom depends on the self-discipline of each; and that the assumption of power or submission to power in any sphere of human activity is a negation of the fundamental reality of individuals, a negation intrinsically incapable of offset by other types of considerations.

Power and violence; fraternity and love

In two areas besides the question of property – which will be discussed separately – anarchists have differed sharply about principles. The dispute between anarchists who distrust formal organization, anarchist as well as other, and for whom the term 'organization' is pejorative, and those who hold organization to be essential, would seem chiefly to represent a difference in sociological and psychological judgment, disguised by semantics of 'organization' and 'association,' as to conditions under which the individual is lost and power emerges. No fundamental questions of ethics seem implicated.

The other area, deeply problematic, is that of pacifism, violence, and revolution. The main anarchist tradition has been revolutionary in a sense that endorses violence as a means of resisting and destroying the apparatus of force and violence by which power is maintained. (That the free society should be non-violent is agreed.) Within the framework of anarchist principle, it can be argued reasonably that violence against an oppressor who maintains his position by violence is not itself an act of oppression since one does not seek to (and will not) enslave or bring into subjection that person. The violence-affirming or violence-condoning tendency would seem to be asserting that negation of master/servant ('slave') relationships takes priority over the claims to respect for life

of those who insist on being masters and, by violence, direct or indirect, make that insistence good. Unfortunately, major social oppression defends itself usually by hired or conscript instruments – and, when defeated, by foreign armies. All these persons are oppressors in their instrumental roles, and subject to seduction and corruption by those roles, yet many in their own way are victims.

Here the anarchist who accepts violence is beyond clear guidance of principle. Even in its terrorist phases, however, anarchist violence has almost always been directed expressly and scrupulously against principals or executives of political and economic oppression, so that, by comparison with the anti-civilian terror-warfare of governments, or nationalist guerrilla warfare, or routine police terrorism in countless nations, to say nothing of the savage reprisal taken upon defeated working classes all through history, anarchist terrorism is ridiculously misnamed. Prevalence of an ethics of principle, rather than a utilitarianism that lends itself to self-deception, may be a major ground for this (self-) control; while the centering of principle in power negation rules out the taking of hostages or other instrumental treatments of persons that are the usual transition from resistance to militarized warfare. (The breakdown of anarchist principle in the Spanish anarcho-syndicalist movement, especially during the civil war and revolution, is a large and complex topic into which I cannot enter here.)

In twentieth-century anarchism, not merely within the Tolstoyan tradition, pacifism has been an important minoritarian tendency. Whether evolutionary or non-violently revolutionary, pacifist anarchism asserts that violence is even clearer negation of human being than is power, is perhaps even the genus of power, and introduces into anarchism a concept of love much stronger than the 'fraternity' of the main tradition – universal, because unlike fraternity not restricted to solidarity of the oppressed – and tends thereby to transform the concept of the individual and the concept of freedom. Love will then be the ultimate positive concept, opposite to violence. I think that one can say that an anarchist, of whatever specific persuasion, who does not feel (more than *think*) such love and non-violence as ultimate values has not fully experienced the meaning of anarchism, although love and non-violence are not easily lived in the midst of the oppression and suffering of others. In a sense, therefore, the motion of anarchism toward a full ethics of love, although a motion intrinsic to the Idea, remains to be realized, and may be realizable only in transition to anarchist society.

The ethics of freedom

The role of principle in anarchist thought and action, as I understand it,

is to liberate the positive ethical life of human beings. Thus the principle of power negation is rather a constitutive principle of the desired society than a rule for life within the society. Put more concretely: an authentic relationship between persons, as understood by anarchists, presupposes the absence of power of some over others, but 'absence of power' says nothing positive about the content of that relationship, and that content will be the creation of those persons.

If such is the meaning of anarchist principles, it would seem to follow that intercourse in an anarchist society would be conducted under conditions of voluntary agreement (often tacit, of course) and personal responsibility – for this seems to be what one would mean by 'absence of power.' Faith in the possibility of anarchist society, then, would signify faith that, in the absence of structured power, of dominant and subordinate classes, and of habits of deference to authority and exercise of power, human beings can use the gift of speech and other subtle forms of communication to resolve their intercourse into mutually beneficial patterns or into intelligent confrontation and disagreement and if necessary pacific disassociation, without need for commandments of morality.

One would not, however, say of such a society that it is post-ethical – as one might of a Marxist society, after the state has withered at last, in which the economic form of communism would be the sociological realization of the ethical. Of anarchy one might say instead that ethics had resolved itself into new human beings, a metaphor that would signify that faith and trust of persons toward persons, rather than contingent modes of cooperation, would be the vital center. Put otherwise: nothing secures an anarchist society, whether of large extent or of commune-size or consisting of just two persons, except continuous realization of the human potentiality for free agreement and disagreement, always in recognition of the personhood of the other. If anarchism does not remain clear to the last of the institutional thinking that Marxists call materialist, it must finally become incoherent and the individualism (or personalism) that, twinned with the corresponding version of sociality, is the soul of anarchism would be threatened with extinction.

In a society of hierarchies – of discriminations against classes or castes and condemnation of various large numbers of persons to particular kinds of limited existence to others' advantage – coercive institutional machinery is everything and its guarantee and enforcement by state-power is of the social essence. If we think of voluntary action, decision, autonomy, as central to the meaning of being human – as the main philosophical traditions assert – then anarchism can be understood as seeking to dissolve those institutions of power that make life-decisions for us, that offer to substitute themselves for our freedom and relieve

us of burdens of responsibility, and·do so whenever they successfully coerce us to accord our will to their demands. Then, anarchism is expressive of a will to restore, and/or create, personhood and human being; whereas in surrendering to *or exercising* dominion one substitutes for oneself an institutional definition, an institutional being; one ceases to be oneself. It will be plain, I think, given these premises, that by voluntary surrender of freedom, by submission to a protectorate such as the Hobbesian state is claimed to be, one yields far more than the exercise of certain liberties.

Anarchism as negative

It may now be clear why a name (an-archist) negative by etymology is appropriate to the import of anarchism.

This appropriateness can be illustrated with respect to a familiar species of power, that of racial oppression. If the thoroughgoing negation of racial oppression is, as one might reasonably think, a society in which recognition of 'racial' identity has vanished, or in which racial terms, if indeed sense can be made of them when oppression does not define them, have become minor descriptive terms without social consequence, then it would be foolish to ask what the theory of this raceless society would be or how it would deal with racial relations. For the US integrationist movement of the 1950s the slogan 'Freedom Now' *said* all that needed be *said*, just as, more than a century before, 'Abolition,' a saying that of course earned one the title 'fanatic,' a title yet to be repealed, was all that needed be said of chattel slavery.

A second illustration, less obvious because even now barely thinkable, would be a society, usually called androgynous, in which recognition as male and female would make reference to nothing but certain physiological matters and reproductive capacities and would be non-indicative of personality, economic role, or worth. Sexes would not constitute classes (or more exactly castes) and sexual identity would have only the significance that each chose to give to it. What this means requires no elaborate explanation, only a certain imagination, an ability to rid oneself of preconceptions and to conceive of what *seems* incapable of being thought without contradiction. 'What will be the relations between the sexes in such a society?' – the question makes erroneous assumptions.

From every locus of power, it has always been inconceivable, because contrary to the *a priori*s of the sustaining ideology, that its system be abolished. From the standpoint of the priesthood it has always been inconceivable that religion dispense with it, that its flock survive bereft of shepherd.

149

With respect to the anarchist concept of social existence, the questions 'Who will rule?', 'Who will govern?' and – what is less obvious intuitively – 'Who will decide?' become non-relevant questions. No theory of total-society decision-making would be called for. 'Power to the people', 'Let the people decide,' although of idealistic intention, perpetuate the sovereignty of the whole and are not anarchist. In practice such qualified (democratic) sovereignty means that 'representatives' of the people constitute a class of decision-makers over against a mass that makes no decisions except (perhaps) to choose their rulers, a choice inevitably reconstrued as majoritarian. Where the *demos* rules, power and its problems remain; a people represented, as Rousseau said, is enslaved. Anarchy means the dissolution and disappearance of democratic sovereignty (or its pretense) also.

In an anarchist society every person decides and there is no class of deciders. Cooperative actions result from voluntary agreements. This is easier to visualize in a small society lacking complex relations of production and distribution; larger-scale cooperation presumes longer-term agreements, reliance on the good will of others as norm, agreement to standard procedures (non-coercive, non-power-based institutions) to achieve commonly desired ends and to resolve differences and conflicts. (A principle of individual decision and voluntary agreement does not mean that driving on right or left, using metric or nonmetric measures, not to say basic economic practices, are continually in question and one knows not what to expect in a topsy-turvy world.) What must be premissed is that the people involved shall by and large be willing – as the way they live and are, rather than by reflective commitment – to affirm each other's humanity and uniqueness and to pursue their differing interests under conditions of voluntary agreement and responsibility for their actions.

In saying that everyone decides, one does not mean that each can cause the world to be as s/he would wish it: for there can be just one actual world, and if I willed the world effectively then I would will it for, and in lieu of, others. The others, instead, present me with their spontaneity, their choosings, which of course foreclose many practical possibilities for me; in more than compensation for which, one would hope, my possibilities are enriched by living in a world of persons who are themselves choosing rather than living out the consequences of technology, market, and other impersonal forces that have preempted their freedom and mystified their intelligence.

Nor, in saying that everyone decides, does one mean that everyone conceivably affected by a particular decision participates in it. No doubt we have, in our everyday experience, little ground for confidence that the people on whom we depend, economically and otherwise, will reliably do their best; and so we put faith in complex systems of control

over others, and of course over ourselves. But the anarchist thought is that social co-operation can be founded upon the autonomy and responsibility of individuals and groups in their spheres of activity, so that the society is the product of the decisions of all, both individually and jointly by agreement.

But it is obvious that 'no class of deciders,' 'non-collectivity,' even if realizable in a moderately complex world, cannot well be applied to all the familiar kinds of social processes, even if the society were disburdened of many functions, such as the military, that would have no possible place in an anarchy.

Practically, if we are all by our choosings to participate in making our world, it would seem necessary that a principle – a practical rather than an ethical principle – of minimum large-scale change be followed generally, so that communication and intelligence be most effective and so that individual choices, and in consequence agreements, contractual and tacit, be made within a world one somewhat understands. The restless technology of our centuries flourishes in a world where institutions of power impose its innovations, provide its workforce, and manipulate its consumers, and where dominant classes are eager to magnify their power and wealth through technological supremacy. Anarchy would not provide these conditions, nor could anarchist decision-making be expected to cope with continuous major technological revolution. Ceaseless and rapid demographic expansion that forces constant dissolution and reformation of life-complexes (neighborhoods, towns, cities, regions) creates a turmoil that free people cannot deal with any more intelligently than can the present institutions. Many technological patterns already existing may also make demands for decision-making that cannot well be met except on a basis of collective institutions that create bureaucratic and other forms of power. That is, anarchist society would not be readily compatible, if compatible at all, with certain practical goals or ways of life or with certain societal rhythms.

In the era of unchallenged technological ideology, to which Marxism contributed its share, such concessions would have been regarded as determining conclusively the reactionary nature of anarchism. In the era of ideologies of progress, they would similarly have stamped anarchism as impossible of realization just because it does not extrapolate what was then thought of as progress, and as undesirable because unsuited to spiralling future progress. Today it may be easier to agree that incompatibility with certain practical goals is not necessarily a defect or limitation. The kinds of things that cannot be done well in an anarchist society may be just those that release the blind and uncontrolled historical processes that determine much of our existence in a manner that renders our will ineffectual and that even determines our will.

Perhaps the major thrust of serious social thinking for two centuries

has been toward solution of the problem of determination by history, by the past, by yesterday: how shall we be free today to solve today's problems? Virtually all of this thinking, however, has posed the question as one of achieving control. By sheer force, and sometimes also by social sciences, statist societies seek to master these historical processes, and have given very little evidence of ability to do so. (Besides which, the values and interests in terms of which the attempt is made are plainly those of the controlling groups or institutions.) This ambition of control is a way of human pride.

In anarchist society human beings would, presumably, seek to free themselves from processes of institutional momentum by consciously choosing rhythms of change, and technologies, harmonious with viable rhythms of life-choice, in order to avoid a need, for survival, to create institutions of power. That we should cease to court disaster, that we should simplify and make possible the solution of primary life-problems in the mode of freedom, should not, especially in view of the number and magnitude of disasters our species produces for itself, be an unreasonable negative principle, particularly because there appear to be no reasons why a comparatively stable and comparatively simplified society need be reduced to spinning-wheel technology or to changelessness. We might, if such a society were realized, become able at last to apply an authentic spirit of experimentation to the practical problems of life.

Anarchism as social philosophy

The chief thing that I have wanted to show is that anarchism represents a fundamental ideal of human existence: that it represents something other than mere absence of government, something other than the freedom to do anything one wants, something different than a freedom limited by what will harm others. It represents instead the aim of social union, on a ground of unique individuality, where no class or caste divisions exist between people and where integral individuality and integral society, non-antithetical, have become two aspects of the same life. The deepest meaning of this anarchist freedom, if I see rightly the implications of what I have written, is that certain significant barriers to the realization of potentialities of human beings will have been broken. Integral individuality and integral society are ancient as well as modern values, and every system of ethics and social philosophy could be said to have endeavored to accommodate them to each other. I suggested that anarchism is a social idea of importance, and not merely a peculiar kind of member in the series 'tyranny, monarchy, oligarchy, democracy . . . anarchy,' because it claims to identify, in *power*, the missing clue. It presents both a conception of general and ultimate

social/personal harmony, which may well turn out to be an ideal beyond reach, and a conception of social/personal harmony in any circumscribed realm, any relatively closed human 'system,' as small as the sphere of one's immediate life-circle, where the negation of ideologically justified, socially divisive patterns of domination are (by hypothesis) a necessary condition for social/personal harmony. As a practical goal, the 'free society' can hardly recommend itself for its probability, whatever exactly probability means in such matters; but the idea reflects itself, sometimes as a secular philosophy of love, into the daily life of persons who derive from it their values.

If we are to discuss anarchism as a 'social philosophy,' we will want it to be more than a set of 'feelings' at the core of an 'idea,' and something more than an abstract resolution of power-and-powerlessness. During the course of this article I have set down a number of propositions, beyond the initial propositions of the first sections, that I would like to recapitulate here:

- that the individual is the fundamental social (but not necessarily metaphysical) reality;
- that voluntary agreement is the foundation of cooperation;
- that everyone is responsible for their actions;
- that general freedom depends on the self-discipline of each;
- that the assumption of power or submission to power in any sphere is negation of the fundamental human reality;
- that a morality of principles that apply the theme of power-negation affirms the free development of individuality as the condition of realizing our sense of humanity;
- that faith and trust toward persons is the vital ethical center of anarchy;
- that anarchism represents and demands a transcendence of power/powerlessness that can be described as integral freedom;
- that the alternative to the sovereignty of collectivities is 'every person decides';
- that power is the root evil of human being;
- that integral freedom is immanent in human life and history as an always realizable potentiality;
- that freedom is the reversal of the substitution of institutional definition, institutional being, institutional will, for oneself;
- that the breakdown of sovereignties prepares the way for liberation from the determinism of history;
- that 'individual' and 'society' are a dynamic tension that find their ground of union in freedom;
- that the 'program' of action is the continuous realization of freedom in the lives of each and all;
- that individuals are the loci of social change as well as the founda-

tion of free society;

– that in the continuous realization of freedom values are won continuously.

About these propositions I wish to claim that they indicate a non-
simplistic view of society and human being that provides a mode of
social analysis, an image of the ethical potentiality of man, and a
proposal of method for realizing that potentiality.

If one is to consider anarchism as a 'philosophy,' one will of course
ask about the nature of metaphysical and epistemological commitments
and their foundation. This question threatens to reintroduce the fragmentation into 'schools' that I have sought to overcome, for on these
questions anarchists differ sharply and I have chosen to view anarchism
in a way that avoids such commitments. I should like now, however, to
give a positive sense to this avoidance, and I offer the following
thoughts, intended to be no more than suggestive; their elaboration will
have to wait another occasion.

We are a puzzle to ourselves, I believe, because we do not fully
experience our own humanity, and this in turn is because we cannot
fully experience the humanity of others so long as we exist in the many
interlocking relations of masterhood and servitude. We yield to those
structures of power in order to live in a human world that pre-exists
each of us and demands that we discipline ourselves to culture organized
around insignia, languages, persons, institutions, mythologies, and
philosophies of power. We move dialectically to a plane of consciousness of our common humanity, instantiated uniquely in each person, as
we move dialectically to a plane of social existence in which we wield
no power over others and do not allow ourselves to be determined in
our being by the power that they wield. Only then do we realize the
meaning of subjectivity in another or, authentically, in ourselves. By
that move, we bring love to reality, for such recognition of subjectivity
is what I understand by love.

Put otherwise: certain truths must be brought to be, must be made
living, before their meaning can be apprehended more than negatively.
(Thus anarchism, in this respect like Marxism, transposes the philosophical questions into questions of actualization and realization.) What
I see in anarchism is the indication that human beings will become
adequately self-conscious, and therefore free toward the future, and
dichotomies of thought and action will dissolve, only when human
beings free themselves from one another and, in certain significant
senses from themselves.

Thus anarchism can be seen as proceeding from the hypothesis that
there is a negative task to be accomplished before we can genuinely
experience ourselves as human beings and grasp our relationships to
one another. Throughout, therefore, anarchism is, ideationally, essen-

tially negative. Whereas with respect to particular social problems this would be a gross defect, anarchism is concerned with a far more fundamental kind of question, and from its vision of the potentialities residing in our actual human situation, its thoroughgoing negativity would seem to follow and to be the foundation of creation.

David Wieck was born in 1921. He was imprisoned for thirty-four months for refusal of military service during World War II. He was a member of the editorial groups of *Why?* and *Resistance* in New York City, 1946–54; and a contributor to *Liberation* during the 1960s. He has been a professor of philosophy at Rensselaer Polytechnic Institute since 1960.

10 Anarchism and Marxism: a confrontation of traditions*

C. George Benello

The division of labor is the central feature of modern industrial society because it is equally evident within major institutions of industrial society, but more clearly so within those organizations, corporations and state-owned firms that are the main manifestations of production and technological advance.

For Marxism, the division of labor arises out of the interplay between man and nature.[1] Originally society is perceived as communal. But at the point that a surplus is created, it is appropriated by those who maintain a commanding position within society. Out of this emerges the class structure of all subsequent societies, manifested in its purest and most heightened form, since they are shorn of the traditional relations of mutual obligation and shared values, in capitalism. The division of labor is thus responsible both for the specialization of work into narrow job categories, and for the separation of the worker from control over the means of production. The result of this is alienation, both from control over the processes of production, and from the products as well. The only solution to this, for Marxism, is to abolish the division of labor and reintegrate man both with the tools of his labor and the fruits of his labor. Here Marx took a resolutely utopian stand, refusing to admit that the division of labor was essential to either technological advance or industrial productivity. This stand was congruent with Marx's view, expressed in his early writings,[2] that not only class divisions, but the divisions of town and country should be abolished, and it represents a basic principle of utopian thought, which has always sought to reintegrate man in such a way that all members of the society could share holistically in the major areas of social life.

The anarchist tradition, although it is far less unified on many points than Marxism, shares with it the belief that the division of labor must be abolished in order to create a liberatory society. If anything, it is

* Excerpted from a longer article that appeared in *Our Generation*, vol. 10, 1974.

clearer in its stress that, not only must the division of labor be abolished, but the division between work and community life, and between manual and intellectual work, must also be abolished. The Chinese have espoused this goal, but it is worth remembering that Mao Tse-tung had once been an anarchist himself. Anarchism parts company with Marxism most clearly in perceiving the necessity of building integrated social forms as the precondition of a successful revolution, conceived of as a fundamental social transformation of the society. For while anarchism shared with Marxism its utopian view of the goal – an egalitarian and libertarian society in which self-determination extended into the forms of daily life, dispensing with all forms of coercion and authoritarian power – on the question of strategy anarchism parts company with Marxist thought.

Marx conceived of class struggle as the basic social fact, seeing divisions of class as the result of a process of social evolution involving the creation of a productive surplus. Because Marx defined class in terms of the relations of production, Marxism has tended to restrict its class and analysis to the capitalist model, wherein class is defined in terms of ownership of the means of production. Anarchism, however, has focused on the question of human organization in a much more general way, seeking to understand the psychosocial mechanisms out of which domination and power relationships derive. It sees class as based on the control of the means of production as a particular case of a more general form of class division. Hence anarchist thought is more easily able to comprehend within the realm of its theory the existence of 'New Classes' based on Communist Party elites; the monopolization of the means of production and of capital are only one form of power. The authoritarian state, which in addition to controlling capital possesses a monopoly on its other instrumentalities as well – its bureaucracies, its means of violence, its ideological control – has far more powerful means at its disposal. To call fascist dictatorships or the USSR 'state capitalist' is to fit the more general conditions of state domination and imperialism, which anarchism has always pointed to as *sui generis*, on the Procrustean bed of a more limited theory. It is domination as such which must be understood, and on its own terms, not as manifested exclusively through capital and its control.

Marxism, however, reifies class conflict as a historical universal: 'The history of all past societies has consisted in the development of class antagonisms . . . . One fact is common to all past ages, viz., the exploitation of part of society by the other.'[3] This formulation fails in two ways. It fails to account for the continued existence throughout history of bureaucratic forms which combine domination with a capacity to subdue antagonism by a system of rewards and status, and by a rationalization of domination through the use of rules which mystify and conceal it. Second, it fails to recognize the extent to which

primitive societies vary widely in their manifestation of a whole pattern of traits which tend toward the formation of a coherent gestalt or system. Some societies are egalitarian, co-operative, pacifistic, and relatively permissive; at the other end of the spectrum one finds societies riddled by social divisions and hierarchy which are property-oriented, competitive and aggressive. Both forms seem to be equally stable and enduring.

It is true that recent Marxism has taken cognizance of bureaucracy as a phenomenon occurring within socialism as well as capitalism.[4] Also, it has combined its class analysis with a psychoanalytic theory of authoritarianism[5] which explains the power orientation in terms very similar to those used by contemporary anarchists such as Comfort and Goodman. But it can nevertheless be argued that the focus on the psychosocial origins of domination and hence of class has never been resolved with the macro-analysis of class found in early Marxist thought and in Marx himself. For one may argue that you cannot have it both ways: either class is perceived as a product of a historical dialectic, which of itself leads progressively to higher stages of human development, into the stage in which class itself is transcended in the classless society; or class is to be understood as the particular product of a fundamental and continuing psychosocial dynamic which occurs under given conditions throughout human history, the overcoming of which constitutes the central radical project.

The strategic implications of this difference in perspective are profound: in the case of the Marxist view of the process of historical development, capitalism must be accepted as a necessary stage, since only through the ultimate clarification of class divisions through the dominance of the economic forms over all others can the internal contradictions of class itself be made to give way. This constitutes a reliance on historical forces which in its modern form is expressed by a reliance on technological advance to create the conditions for the abolition of class. Involved in this debate, in somewhat complex ways, is the question of the role of scarcity in leading to a state of liberation. For Marxism, it is the evolution of the technology of production, out of which a surplus is created, that creates both classes and class society, and at the same time the continuing dynamic whereby class itself can be transcended.

The reading of human history as inherently progressive, following the Darwinian ideas of evolution, is in fact the major basis for distinguishing Marxism from anarchist thought, which has in the main refused to grant that history is revelatory of any geist or inherent dynamism which can be relied on to create the good society.

Refusing to rely on history to do its job for it, it seeks where possible to build the future into the present by creating the nuclei of the good

society within the existing situation. As a consequence, anarchists have tended to rely more on pre-industrial and pre-capitalist social forms out of which to build the libertarian values required by a good society.

Engels saw factory structure, which imbued the workers with authoritarianism and hierarchy, as the necessary basis capable of giving discipline to a workers' movement; the anarchists, in quite opposite fashion, saw the necessity of building a movement on those who were least imbued with such forms of consciousness. The anarchist focus on the psychosocial aspects of the problems of organization is central; for anarchism, theory must confront this central fact of authoritarian organization, whether economically exploitative or political, whether class-determined or bureaucratic, and build an alternative to it. It is the central problem.

Such an approach has strategic significance today, within the context of the debate on whether Marxian categories have been superseded or are still relevant. Marxist methodology still dictates the search for the 'objective contradictions' within the capitalist system which will lead to the possibility of class division and struggle. But with the continuing extension of the areas of bureaucratized organization characteristic of the modern welfare–warfare state, the major contradiction has less and less to do with relation to the means of production, and more and more to do with the contradiction between the democratic myth system and the official ideology of freedom on the one hand, and the highly oppressive and authoritarian living and work environment on the other. Whether as urban resident, welfare recipient, hospital patient, white-collar worker – and whether it is within the public or private sector matters little – or blue-collar worker, today's citizen confronts at every turn large and authoritarian bureaucracies which process him like an IBM card. The central contradiction is precisely the one the anarchists point to: on the one hand technology has vastly increased the scope of human power, leading to the possibility of human liberation from historic forms of bondage, from disease, and from starvation. It has extended the area of human freedom through communication, transportation and travel, and through the variety of artifacts and products. But it has done this through the construction of a system which is oppressive, bureaucratic, and irrational. The priorities are statist and grandiose: production as such, measured in terms of GNP, the fielding of huge armies and weapons production, huge and dehumanizing industrial complexes. For the anarchist, the contradiction is that of the power orientation, magnified and abetted through technology, coming into conflict with the full play of human purposes. It is a contradiction which both divides man from man, creating the fundamental division of the dominator and the dominated in many complex forms, and, more basically, creates the division within man himself, thus

rendering him both power-crazed and powerless at one and the same time.

The psychology of power

The understanding of the psychology of power is a critical element in the anarchist understanding of the exercise of power within organizations. In such organizations the organizational dynamics and psychological dynamics come together. And if it is true that people accept the system because they are bedazzled by its size, its capacity to manifest forms of abstract power related to their personal aspirations through the mythology of success wherein they see themselves climbing up the various status hierarchies so as to move closer and closer to positions of power, then it is this orientation which constitutes a central problem. The enemy is not a class, even though such a class exists, and through its monopoly of privilege constitutes a central problem. The enemy, basically, is within, represented by the internalization of the authoritarian gestalt. More than theories of alienation, this explains what holds people fast to the system, and validates the anarchist understanding that fundamental changes in the behavior patterns – and beyond that in the forms of consciousness – are necessary in order to move toward liberation. The strategic task then becomes one of building the kind of movement which can provide concrete settings for self-determination and liberation from the authoritarian perspective – exactly what the Spanish anarchists were about.

Applied to contemporary society, characterized by the extension of bureaucratic control, the strategy dictates working with those where the authoritarianism of the work situation is contrasted most clearly with the democratic mythology which still obtains. Certain groups, through their upbringing and conditions of work, have relatively high expectations and the experience of at least intellectual freedom, and it is these groups which have revolted most explicitly, both in socialist societies as well as in the capitalist countries. Thus one finds preeminently students, who have in many cases come from relatively permissive conditions of home life, and who are marginal to the central productive institutions of the society, who have rebelled most explicitly against the oppressiveness and false values of contemporary society. This revolt has also existed among public schoolteachers and social service workers, and here one may generalize. For unlike the Spanish situation with its pre-industrial forms, contemporary industrial society exacerbates the division between the official cultural values and the authoritarian forms of organization. Hence those groups which maintain a professional allegiance to the official cultural values, through educational levels and

the goals of their profession, and yet experience the facts of authoritarian bureaucracy are likely to be the ones to rebel most directly against this contradiction.

The problem with the anarchist perspective in applying its understanding of the psychology of power has been both historical and objective. Historically, it has failed as often as not to develop strategies adequate to its insights. On the one hand, while espousing theoretically the principle of self-determination and escape from authoritarianism, it has tended, as Bakunin did, to see the revolutionary project as requiring a form of vanguardism involving a leadership by the enlightened, thus resulting of necessity in the creation of a centralist elite. In doing this it has fallen into the trap of Leninism. For Lenin, the supreme strategist of Marxism, saw that the objective contradictions of capitalism were insufficient to lead to revolution. Hence the need to create a revolutionary vanguard for whom the seizing of power was the objective to which all else was subordinate: morality, humanity, every value was seen as not only subordinate to the revolutionary objective, but in fact as only definable in terms of that objective. On the other hand, anarchism has tended, as Bookchin suggests, to reject the problem entailed by creating liberatory organization, and has lapsed instead into cultural and individualist forms which seek liberation outside of the social and political arena.

The organizational problem

Objectively, the understanding of the nature of the power system and the psychology of power requires a far broader form of social transformation and indeed a total social reconstruction, rather than a simple mobilizing of the oppressed with the objective of seizing power. Liberatory organization must be created which can both express the psychology of free and voluntary association free of authoritarianism, and at the same time confront the power system so as to challenge it. Only in this way can the revolutionary project result in social transformation. However if this ideal has failed as often as not to be realized in practice, it provides a significant critique of the historical failures of Marxism to transform society. At its worst, Marxism has led to the replacement of early capitalist forms, as in Russia, with a bureaucratic collectivism even more coercive and extensive. In the parliamentary democracies, this strategy has been replaced, as in France and Italy, by the renunciation of revolutionary methods, and the acceptance of access to power through parliamentary means. Here and elsewhere (in Latin America, for instance) the communist parties have tended to become upholders of what in their own terms would be bourgeois parliamentarianism,

against the various movement espousing guerrilla warfare or extra-parliamentary opposition. Some of these movements are also communist, and many of them Marxist, but the division in strategy can be seen as a product of the failure of capitalist societies to develop the revolutionary conditions which have been predicted as part of the historical development of capitalism. Too much can indeed be made of this, inasmuch as, in those countries where wars of national liberation took a communist form, communism was able to develop out of the socialist states exemplifying varying stages of socialism on the way to communism – as in Yugoslavia, China or Cuba.

At the same time, such states have been forced to confront the problem of bureaucratic centralism and the emergence of a class system based on the party or the military, and one may argue that this is consonant – certainly from the anarchist perspective – with a flaw in the Marxian analysis of social organization. Hence the Marxist strategy which centers on the metaphor of the revolution terminating in the taking over of state power is consistent with the social analysis which sees the dictatorship of the proletariat as leading to the classless society. And its failure, from the anarchist perspective, does not derive from any incompleteness of the revolutionary project, but rather from an inherent flaw in the revolutionary project itself, which does not pause to analyze the broader organizational question which underlies not simply economic classes but bureaucracy and state power as well. Seen in this perspective, the revolutionary strategy has on the one hand provided a powerful metaphor which, admittedly using the force of nationalism more than an already developed class consciousness, still enables a revolutionary government dedicated to communism to get into power. And here, contrary to the more simplistic versions of elitist theory, it has shown a significant willingness to decentralize in a number of instances, although maintaining overall ideological and political control.

But on the other hand, the impetus moving toward genuine liberation has been constrained and restricted by the desire to maintain centralized control. Hence Yugoslavia has continued to balance precariously between the forces moving toward greater self-determination, represented characteristically by students and intellectuals, and the forces of government repression in the interests of maintaining centralist control. (cf. the Yugoslav left-wing periodical *Praxis* for a detailing of this dilemma.) China has maintained a strong centralized ideological control while decentralizing the social forms of the society. However, it has struggled with the inevitable bureaucratization of the party structure; and by the insistence on imposing an ideology which elevates the leadership and the state to an almost god-like status, it has failed to realize the libertarian ideal. For the libertarian ideal of anarchism is

unique in locating freedom in the area where the individual and the social meet: in the affinity groups of the Spanish anarchists, in the community associations of the Chilean workers' movement, in short, in face-to-face associations wherein praxis is based on direct experience rather than on the acceptance of a propagated ideology from above. Freedom, to be understood, must be lived, for it is only through this experience that authoritarianism can be conquered.

This approach has been given a broad historical dimension in the recent work of Lewis Mumford,[6] where he has traced through history the periodic arising of mass totalitarian social forms, and the conditions under which this occurs. Mumford diverges critically from Marxism by seeing these forms as originating in certain social, not technological, conditions, and as at all times exemplifying a certain inherent dynamic and pattern wherein the psychology of power is both expressed and reinforced by mass organization, which Mumford terms the 'megamachine.' He does see it as being powerfully reinforced by industrial and technological development, which allowed for the replacement by machines of human parts in the megamachine. But he sees it as above all a social and organizational form, as apparent in preindustrial societies at various times and places as in industrial societies. Its major manifestations are the military, mass organization, the state bureaucracy, and mass industrial organization. While this essay will not deal with the full ramifications of this analysis, its importance lies in two places where it diverges most fundamentally from Marxism. First, it refuses to see the megamachine as in any way progressive or historically determined, but sees it rather as the product of certain historical conditions reinforcing a human tendency which is at all times pernicious. While it is brought forth as a result of a number of historical conditions which are not so much economic as religious and nationalistic, its result is always to enslave and limit the area of human freedom. Second, it sees the historical conditions as themselves only partially explanatory, and sees the logic of domination itself, which is an essentially psychosocial dialectic between objective conditions and subjective response, as the further necessary category of explanation.

For Mumford then, it is the appeal of the mythology of power, seen as both power over nature but also as power over other human beings, which causes not simply class divisions to arise, but also the whole system of rationalized domination concealed by myths of the divine right of kings, the appeal to national destiny, as well as to technological advance which is expressed by hierarchy, rule from the top, extensive specialization, the rationalization of power through bureaucratic regulation, and the division between the dominators and the dominated, seen in the military and state hierarchies as well as in the industrial system. For in this view, just as the basis for values rests in man, not history, so

163

the basis for evil, seen in the power orientation, also rests in man, not history. Hence just as progress must be seen as a result of willed and conscious human achievement, so the megamachine is also neither progressive nor historically determined, but a product of willed and conscious human action, determined by the quest for power.

Such a view, it can be argued, explains how imperialism, a product of the inherent expansiveness of the megamachine, can equally take nationalistic as well as economic forms, and affirms that religious, nationalistic and ideological conflicts must be analyzed on their own terms, not as the superstructural manifestations of essentially economic causes. Moreover, it is consonant with the tradition of anarchist analysis which sees the state, of whatever ideological persuasion, as inherently warlike and coercive, if not of its neighbors, then at least of its own inhabitants. (As Randolph Bourne put it, 'War is the health of the state.') At perhaps its deepest level, seen in the writing of Landauer, anarchism has seen the superabundance of power so consistently made manifest in the state as essentially a product of a certain relationship between people – that of power divorced from and exceeding function. Which is to say that, where the social and institutional structure of a society manifests a proliferation of organizational forms which are primarily oriented and structured to the achieving of power, then the state itself, as the organizational level which comprehends all other organizational levels, will reflect this orientation of becoming the supreme exemplar of power. And given the inherent expansiveness of power, this will inevitably result in various forms of imperialism and the manifestations of military and economic domination.

Human nature

This brings us to the third and final subject of this chapter, the question of human nature. For anarchism this question is primary, since in locating both values and the origins of social evil in man rather than history, it is then faced with the problem of explaining how evil can arise not as a product of the historical process, but directly out of human nature. Here, it must be admitted, anarchist theory is weak, as we shall see, since it tends to posit the natural goodness of man when liberated from the constraints of an unjust society. To the extent that it sees society as the cause of evil, it is left with an asymmetrical and non-dialectical condition in which good comes from man but evil comes from society. This avoids the dialectics of how man creates the social order, and in the process creates himself. For, as the Marxists amply remind us, human nature is a mere abstraction outside of its manifestations in society, and hence if society manifests both human evil as well as good, both must

be sought for in the dialectic whereby man creates himself through constructing the social order.

In its theory of human nature, Marxism exhibits two trends of thought, both in the early Marx, and in its later Freudo-Marxist manifestations. Marx rejected the 'homo duplex' view that has characterized much sociological and psychological thought. This view states that there is an implicit antagonism between man and society, expressed on one level in the biological antagonism which Freud saw between the demands of instinct and the demands of socialization and becoming civilized. At another level it can be seen as the area of human freedom and transcendence in which man remains only partially determined by his culture and can in turn act back and transform it. Marx, on the contrary, believed that 'The individual is the social being . . . . Individual human life and species-life are not different things.'[7] This is consonant with the view that man is historically determined, and that all thought is historically determined – except, apparently, Marxist thought which states that proposition.

It is worth-while pointing out here that contemporary Marxists have sought to grapple with this problem, of how to reconcile a historical determinism with the idea, emphasized in existentialist thought (certainly to an extreme degree in the early writings of Sartre) that man is free. Leszek Kolakowski speaks of man as the center of moral judgment, and attacks a history-centered basis for values.[8] And Sartre, coming to Marxism from existentialism, argues for the addition of an existentialist view of man to Marxist thought: 'It is precisely the expulsion of man, his exclusion from Marxist Knowledge, which resulted in the renascence of Existentialist thought outside the historical totalization of Knowledge.'[9] Kolakowski simply asserts that there is no contradiction between individual freedom and historical and social determinism. But stating this unfortunately does not make the problem go away, since it bypasses a central area of dispute between Marxists on the one hand and anarchists, existentialists and humanists on the other.

In the first place, the ease with which Leninism flowed out of Marxism, and Stalinism out of Leninism was precisely a product of the historically determined view of man wherein all that mattered was species-man, not individual man. Given the man-centered type of radicalism of the anarchists, shared by others in the libertarian tradition, possibly the Russian Revolution might not have come at all; but certainly Leninism and Stalinism – all we find most reprehensible that claims to be within the Marxist tradition – would not have come out of it. Yet we must not forget Bakunin, nor on the other hand the man-centered analysis of Marx himself, which speaks of alienation. What is in question is a profound dilemma of social thought which is reflected on many levels of social and strategic analysis. For on the one hand

man seeks to grasp the pattern of events, the true laws of history, in order to understand the nature of that which oppresses him. This gives rise to the macro-social and macro-historical attitude which observes how history and social forces have their own laws, shaping human beings to purposes beyond their ken. At the same time, in opposition to the view of man as determined by society and by history, there is the stubborn affirmation of the libertarian view which holds precious the area of freedom that man does have, and refuses to allow history to be either the substitute for human action directed toward human liberation, or the bearer of a geist which man has but to follow to be free. Thus anarchism refuses the Marxist distinction beween subjectivity and objectivity, where objectivity alone is considered real (the objectively correct approach) and accords an equally prominent place to the understanding of motives as to the understanding of objective structure.

This is not to say that the experience of Stalinism, and the growth of existentialism in Europe, has not forced changes in Marxist thought, and new confrontations with this dilemma. In addition to Kolakowski, one may go back to Lukács, who took the Marxian concepts of reification and objectification and saw that man as a social being inevitably objectifies through the need to construct a social reality. This can lead to a false form of objectification, to wit the reification of the objects and institutions which he has created, resulting in social productions which are set off against man.[10] This grasp of the inherent dilemma involved in the process of social construction constitutes a profound understanding of how the rationalized structures of bureaucracy can come about, and represents an essential complement and completion to the Marxian analysis of alienation. For in generalizing from the Marxian analysis of alienation as flowing from the processes of production to a broader view in which alienation is seen as a continuing possibility within the broader process of social construction and objectification, Lukács paves the way for an understanding of organizational totalitarianism in all its forms, not simply its productive aspects.

This essay unfortunately does not permit of a full treatment of the anarchist and Freudo-Marxist views of man. To generalize all too briefly, anarchism in its more simplistic forms has tended to see man as naturally good, corrupted by society, and in doing so it has failed to grasp the dilemma of social construction that Lukács expressed. Existentialism, in its one-sided emphasis on the absoluteness of human freedom, has also failed to come to terms with the social side of homo duplex. But the more sophisticated forms of anarchist thought, that of Goodman and Comfort, among others, has allied itself with the Left Freudianism of Wilhelm Reich, and has seen personal liberation in the psychoanalytic sense of a heightened self-awareness and self-understanding as the necessary concomitant of social liberation. To the extent that, as

Lukács claimed, Marxist thought has as its primary characteristic the urge to develop a dialectic conception of the totality,[11] Marxism can be seen as moving toward a more complete and coherent view of social reality through the addition of insights from depth psychology having to do with the nature of personal liberation.

However, Freud and Marx are uneasy bedfellows, despite their convergence on the problem of false consciousness and the similarity between objectification and reification on the one hand and the Freudian views of projection and introjection on the other. The Freudian Left, even more than Freud, has focused on the problem of repression as the major way in which bourgeois society impinges on the individual. Consequently, they have seen de-repression, either in explicitly sexual terms, as with Reich, or in more generalized libidinal terms (as with Marcuse), as the path toward liberation. But here it can be argued that Marx, with his view of liberation as achieved through the 'sensuous human activity' of work, was closer to the truth. This may sound suspiciously like the Marxist moralism that one finds pervasively in the revolutionary societies of Cuba and China, but the response to this is persuasive: erotic de-repression, even if it is expressed more broadly than in sexual terms, is in fact encouraged in contemporary capitalist societies, even though admittedly in distorted form. What is discouraged is not the various privatized forms that the search for the expression of the pleasure principle can take, but rather the opportunity to engage in the productive transformation of the society through control of the reified structures which are the real causes of repression. Such a control would require an integration of affectivity and libido with rationality: the long and difficult job of building a society fit for man, on a scale where social purpose could find full play.

What remains to be done

It can be argued that no school of thought has come up with a comprehensive critique of bureaucratic collectivism sufficient to establish a viable alternative. Such a critique requires above all that technology and scientific rationality be questioned, in order to be able to disentangle what is progressive from what is regressive in its social manifestations. Some image of a society which is both technological and humanized must be put forward which can demonstrate ways in which technology can be managed without leading to the dehumanization of work in both factories and in bureaucracies. Moreover, a theory of community must be developed, seen as a comprehensive and coherent unit wherein the basic activities of work and life can be reintegrated in maximum autonomy and freedom from dependence on statist institutions.

167

Marxism has almost totally failed in its effort to develop a full critique of contemporary industrial society, having for the most part accepted the unholy triumvirate of science, technology and industry as *per se* progressive. Only anarchists such as Goodman and Bookchin, and at an earlier time Kropotkin, have sought to develop such a critique, despite accusations of utopianism. At present libertarian thought is to be found in various places: among anthropologists such as Jules Henry and Stanley Diamond, who seek to enlighten the present by reference to the communal and co-operative forms of primitive society; among thinkers such as Freire and Ivan Illich, who seek to de-school society, and raise individual consciousness; within the ecology and commune movements, where people seek to restore a more balanced and non-exploitative relationship to nature. In various ways these movements and thinkers are seeking new definitions of the social wherein the human demand for scope and freedom to develop can find its place. The focus here is on the social project itself, and the approach is conditioned by the view that, if the oppressions of class and bureaucratic organization are to be avoided, new social forms are necessary. This leads to the view that for strategies to be devised, the understanding of everyday life, as that point where the social meets the individual, must be expanded.

Thus Lefebvre suggests that in the understanding of everyday life one can find the point of imbalance which can lead to change. A contemporary Marxist thinker, Lefebvre has sought to analyze the concrete conditions of contemporary existence both through the categories of everyday life and through the phenomenon of urbanism in order to be able to come up with a more extensive understanding of the psycho-social conditions of contemporary existence. Here we find a coming together of contemporary Marxist and anarchist thought. Bookchin has also studied the conditions of urban life, for both perceive the city as the area where the contradictions of the contemporary society are exemplified in their clearest form. Lefebvre's formulation of the way social structure has its impact on the individual is couched as a dualism which still seems, however, to be socially determined. In his words:[12]

> Everyday life emerges as the sociological point of feed-back; this crucial yet much disparaged point has a dual character: it is the *residuum* (of all possible specific and specialized activities outside of social experience) and the *product* of society in general; it is the point of delicate balance and that where imbalance threatens. A revolution takes place when and only when, in such a society, people can no longer lead their everyday lives; so long as they can live their ordinary lives relations are constantly reestablished.

Here the contemporary Marxist and the anarchist have a common ground. In the words of Theodore Roszak, perhaps the most articulate spokesman for the counterculture:[13]

> The fundamental question of radical politics has always been, why do the people obey unjust authority? Sometimes the answer is as obvious as the threat of starvation or a bayonet held at the throat. But not always . . . . There are far subtler, more effective forms of power. Those who reside in the mainstream of the technocratic society obey because they are trapped in a diminished reality which not only closes out their vision of 'realistic' alternatives, but persuades them that discontent about anything other than superficial inconvenience is inadmissible, a sign of unfortunate maladjustment or failure of reason.

For Roszak, 'the great trick is to discover what it is that holds people fast to the status quo and then to undo the knots – perhaps even on a person-to-person basis.'[14]

Thus strategically, the development of an overall social critique must be rooted in the categories of everyday life. For it is here that the comprehensiveness of the critique as an intellectual construct confronts the experience and consciousness of people as a lived experience, comprising more than simply rational understanding.

To expand on Lefebvre, everyday life is where the society interacts in its concrete totality with the individual, while at the same time the individual responds with a consciousness which is in varying degrees both mystified and critical. An abstract social critique must in the end be evaluated by its capacity to shed light on how the social order is reflected in individual consciousness. To do this, such a critique must be capable of enlightening human possibility and human desire as well as concrete actuality. It must understand both the warping of human consciousness and needs, and also the ways in which the desire for realization and liberation remains. From the libertarian perspective, the desire for freedom is never totally crushed by false consciousness, and the actual experiencing of freedom can bring it to life again. For unless one accepts the notion of man as totally socially determined through socialization and conditioning, one must see self-liberation as the only definitive and lasting form of liberation. As Eugene Debs once said, if somebody can lead people into socialism, somebody else can lead them out again.

C. George Benello's background includes college teaching, serving as a supporting editor of *Our Generation*, and being a founding member of the Federation for Economic Democracy.

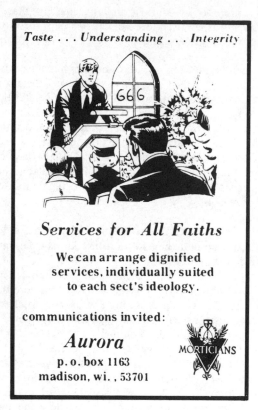
Notes

1 Karl Marx and Frederick Engels, *The German Ideology, Parts I and II*, (New York: International Publishers, 1947). Cf. section on Feuerbach.
2 ibid.
3 Karl Marx and Frederick Engels, *The Communist Manifesto* (Chicago: Henry Regnery, 1954), 53.
4 Georg Lukács, 'Reification and the Consciousness of the Proletariat,' in *History and Class Consciousness* by Georg Lukács (Cambridge Mass.: MIT Press, 1971).
5 Wilhelm Reich, *The Mass Psychology of Fascism* (New York: Farrar, Strauss & Giroux, 1970), and Erich Fromm, *Escape from Freedom* (New York: Rinehart, 1941). Both books are studies of the authoritarian personality.
6 Lewis Mumford, *The Myth of the Machine* (New York: Harcourt,

Brace, Jovanovich, 1970). Cf. especially vol. 1, chs 9 *et seq*.

7 Karl Marx, *Early Writings*, ed. T. B. Bottomore (New York, 1964).

8 Leszek Kolakowski, 'Responsibility and History,' in *Existentialism Versus Marxism*, ed. George Novack (New York: Dell, 1966).

9 J. P. Sartre, 'Marxism and Existentialism' in Novak, op. cit., 203.

10 Lukács, 'Reification and the Consciousness of the Proletariat,' in *History and Class Consciousness*, op. cit.

11 Lukács, 'What is Orthodox Marxism?' in *History and Class Consciousness*, op. cit.

12 Henry Lefebvre, *Everyday Life in the Modern World* (New York: Harper Torchbooks, 1981).

13 Theodore Roszak, *Where the Wasteland Ends* (New York: Anchor Books, 1971), 397.

14 ibid., 398.

11   Why the black flag?

The black flag is the symbol of Anarchy. It evokes reactions ranging
from horror to delight among those who recognize it. Find out what it
means and prepare to see it at more and more public gatherings. . . .
Anarchists are against all government because they believe that the free
and informed will of the individual is the ultimate strength of groups
and of society itself. Anarchists believe in individual responsibility and
initiative and in the whole-hearted co-operation of groups composed of
free individuals. Government is the opposite of this ideal, relying as it
does on brute force and deliberate fraud to expedite control of the
many by the few. Whether this cruel and fraudulent process is validated
by such mythical concepts as the divine right of kings, democratic
elections, or a people's revolutionary government makes little difference to anarchists. We reject the whole concept of government itself
and postulate a radical reliance on the problem-solving capacity of free
human beings.

Why is our flag black? Black is a shade of negation. The black flag is
the negation of all flags. It is a negation of nationhood which puts the
human race against itself and denies the unity of all humankind. Black
is a mood of anger and outrage at all the hideous crimes against humanity perpetrated in the name of allegiance to one state or another. It is
anger and outrage at the insult to human intelligence implied in the pre-
tenses, hypocrisies, and cheap chicaneries of governments. . . . Black is
also a color of mourning; the black flag which cancels out the nation
also mourns its victims – the countless millions murdered in wars,
external and internal, to the greater glory and stability of some bloody
state. It mourns for those whose labor is robbed (taxed) to pay for the
slaughter and oppression of other human beings. It mourns not only the
death of the body but the crippling of the spirit under authoritarian
and hierarchic systems; it mourns the millions of brain cells blacked out
with never a chance to light up the world. It is a color of inconsolable
grief. . . .

But black is also beautiful. It is a color of determination, of resolve,

172

of strength, a color by which all others are clarified and defined. Black is the mysterious surrounding of germination, of fertility, the breeding ground of new life which always evolves, renews, refreshes, and reproduces itself in darkness. The seed hidden in the earth, the strange journey of the sperm, the secret growth of the embryo in the womb – all these the blackness surrounds and protects. . . .

So black is negation, is anger, is outrage, is mourning, is beauty, is hope, is the fostering and sheltering of new forms of human life and relationship on and with this earth. The black flag means all these things. We are proud to carry it, sorry we have to, and look forward to the day when such a symbol will no longer be necessary.

Part Four

The liberation of self

Introduction

Anarchists have always stressed the dual importance of liberating themselves as well as transforming society. For anarchists an essential part of the revolution takes place in everyday life.

We lead such compartmentalized lives that politics is usually defined as having little to do with other aspects of our daily life. In fact, politics is integral to our lives. At its most fundamental level, politics is a system of power relationships, and the institutionalized practices and beliefs that maintain those relationships. In an inegalitarian and alienating society, people will unconsciously act in ways that accept hierarchy and alienation from others and from themselves.

Because anarchism provides an analysis of politics at this most basic level, it can help us to understand our alienation and to end it. Liberation of self involves not only comprehending and transforming our feelings, thoughts and actions, but also learning about and transforming our relationship to our bodies. ·

We can talk about our bodies on two levels. On the surface, our comments may be taken as an analog to the idea of mastery over any *critical* aspect of daily life. Becoming even brilliantly skillful at, say, ballet or frisbee is not critical. It may be exhilarating, gratifying, relaxing, and so on, but such skill and knowledge does not provide any basis to empower people in any societally significant manner. These are not critical in the way in which the mastery of nutritious cooking or electronics may be. Of course, one might turn to haute cuisine or the building of elaborate quadrophonic amplifiers, but these skills do contain the basis for altering a segment of one's power relationships.

On its deepest level learning about one's body can be political, can provide a basis for liberation. We all live in a body and yet we do not have much understanding of how it works, how to care for it, or even its potential. Because of this we find it difficult to make intelligent decisions about our physical selves.

There are billion dollar industries based on the premise that we must make ourselves attractive to other people by using cosmetics, fashionable

clothing, and prepackaged exercise. This emphasis on conforming to market-place ideals has destructive results. Few can live up to the ideals projected in popular culture because they are fictional creations. As long as people are concerned solely about the appearance of their bodies they cannot feel comfortable in them and learn to use them well. This emphasis on appearance rather than on the process of using the body also encourages self-rejection and self-alienation. People who are self-rejecting and alienated cannot be effective political people because they cannot see the objective conditions of their lives and they feel unable to act.

Another aspect of our alienation from our bodies is the militantly heterosexual culture we live in where the only good sexual relationships are defined as heterosexual couple relationships. Women are usually seen as sex objects designed to fulfill men's biological needs. Even the so-called sexual revolution has not defined sex in terms other than genital sex. Instead it eliminated the double standard. Now women are supposedly free to treat men as sex objects and to be more aggressive in sexual encounters. If women wish to remain celibate they are told that they are uptight and repressed. Many feminists sought out lesbian relationships thinking that these would be more satisfying. But just having a woman lover without understanding the political implications did not change anything. The old pattern of relationships often remained so that it was difficult to tell the difference between gay and straight relationships. What was needed was the re-definition of sexual relationships so that sex could become an integrated part of our lives.

This alienation from our bodies also leads to having little knowledge of health care or the confidence to treat ourselves when it is appropriate. Women who joined gynecological self-help groups found that coming to know about their bodies in a supportive group setting helped them to understand that they could learn enough about their bodies and medicine to make intelligent decisions about health care. It also led many of them to understand how this society oppresses women. Put into a larger political framework, many women learned that they could control one aspect of their lives. They also began to grasp the limits of this control when they came up against the medical establishment. So they found they had to provide alternative health care for themselves.

Another area of alienation involves movement. Everyone learns how to walk and develops certain standard ways of moving, usually without giving too much thought to the process. We are taught that exercise is good for us. Physical education is part of most school curricula but the emphasis is on learning competitive sports or calisthenics by imitating someone else, not on really exploring different ways of moving or learning about the structure of the body through movement. As a result, most people believe that they are clumsy, that exercise is painful and

uninteresting, and that someday they should 'get into shape.' When they do seek out exercises that will supposedly get them into shape, they face the same experiences they had in school. So people often become discouraged and give up trying to use their bodies in new ways.

The idea that there is a connection between the mind and body is not new. Recently, however, there has been a revival of interest in movement disciplines including yoga, T'ai Chi Ch'uan, Aikido, bio-energetics, etc. which attempt to make people aware of these connections. Too often they are coupled with mysticism or commercialism or they simply lack any political context, so that they become private therapy or conspicuous displays of skill. It is possible to use techniques from all movement skills to teach people to break old habits by making conscious decisions about how they want to use their bodies in ordinary life.

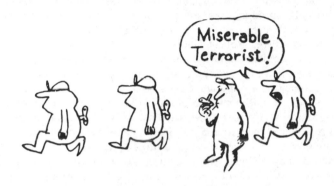

The understanding of how life can be different can come through many experiences. Kingsley Widmer discusses how some of his experiences in school, factory, and prison led him to an anarchist identity. Widmer's strategy for change is to build a community of refusal which challenges the authority of institutions. He points out that this community of refusal already exists in the form of folklore and practice in beating the system – natural anarchism. It remains for us to build on this.

The next three readings are best understood in the context of situationism. The Situationist International (SI) began in Paris in 1957 and had only about seventy members through its fifteen-year life. But it had a great influence on Left ideas and practices. Situationists believed that both capitalism and state socialism were enemies of the working class because they directed every detail of the lives of their citizens. To seize control of their lives, people had to totally *reinvent* everyday life.

In 1966 radical students took over the student government at

Strasbourg University and with the support (and obvious influence) of the SI printed thousands of copies of the pamphlet 'On the Poverty of Student Life.' This pamphlet was one of the major documents that helped touch off the near-revolution in France in May 1968. It was a critique of the university which had become a mass institution designed, they said, not to educate people but to fill the needs of an expanding industrial economy. It joined the students' political struggle to that of the workers, calling for both to change the total structure of their lives.

There are three concepts that are central to Situationist philosophy – capital, commodity, and spectacle. Capitalism is not merely an economic system that controls our economic resources; it is also the system of social relations of people mediated by things. That is to say, capitalism has turned all social relations into commodity relations. A commodity is something that is produced primarily to be exchanged rather than for use by the producer. The producer is only interested in what can be gotten for the product, not the product itself. Thus students get an education so they can get a job, and the better the job the more the education is worth. Robert Cooperstein discusses how children have become commodities under capitalism. These commodity relations produce people who treat each other as objects; who are alienated, isolated, competitive – and unfree.

The spectacle is the culture produced by the commodity economy for consumption by its passive citizens. It is a spectacle because we watch it rather than participate in it. We cannot leave because there is nowhere else to go. Even the opposition to the spectacle is absorbed and recreated as the image of opposition. The only way out is to totally change everyday life. To do this we must create situations that disrupt the ordinary, that jolt people out of their customary ways of thinking and acting. Only this can destroy the manufactured spectacle and the commodity economy.

Jay Amrod and Lev Chernyi focus on the aspect of capital that Wilhelm Reich called 'character.' Character 'is the totality of all internalized or habitual incapacities and limitation of actions within the individual. It is . . . a coherent structure of incapacities and limitations which, as an organized whole, serves its function within the framework of a capitalist society.' Character is a structural phenomenon which exists in such diverse forms as chronic muscular tensions, guilt, dogmatism, racism, mysticism and sexism. But just as this character structure limits free human activity in the service of capital, ideology is the limitation and deformation of thought which justifies self-repression. These two, character structure and fixed ideology, support each other. Only an understanding of both will lead to 'transparent communication and coherent organization.'

This insistence that anarchists evaluate and change their everyday

life can be wearing at times. Activists have often faced a gradual burning out of their personal capacity for sustained effort. David Porter looks at a century of anarchist activity and analyzes some of the factors that give people the motivation to continue the struggle. A revolutionary vision must give people a continually revived sense that alternatives are possible. This, along with the continuing pain of oppression, creates the strongest initial and continuing commitment to revolutionary change.

To maintain their vision of a better society activists must create new structures and life-styles that give a sense of renewal. Only a movement that is already living the revolution will be able to teach people to liberate themselves.

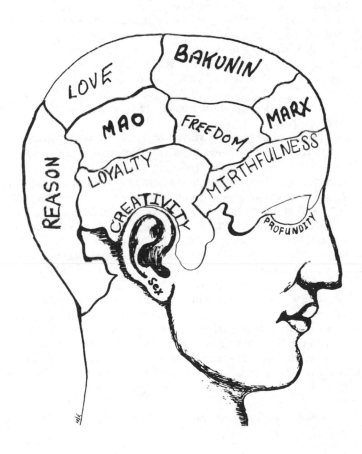

12 Three times around the track: how American workouts helped me become an anarchist*

Kingsley Widmer

When I was in junior high in a midwestern public school system, the genially mean moron who was the gym coach maintained his authority by a graded set of punishing workouts: 'Run once around the track' for any deficiency in obedience or enthusiasm, called 'poor sports spirit;' 'Run twice around the track' for any questioning or criticism of his orders, called 'wise-guy back talk;' 'Run three times around the track' for sardonically smiling, or otherwise looking rebellious, while being punished for crimes one or two, called 'showing your Al Capone character.'

That was a long generation ago, and I've done a good bit of bad-character jogging since. But perhaps that early formulation of the rules of American institutions stayed with me because it was so simple and clear. That has not always been true of the corrective workouts in other of our society's organizations, in the infantry platoons, factory shops, business offices, field crews, prison cellblocks, university departments, political groups, and other coercive orderings I've run through. I don't recall this episode just to attack my particular education. In rather different times and public schools, my sons have found essentially the same pattern of workouts, even the graded trips around the track, though the rhetoric of subordination shows some changes. Nor do I seek to mock especially the common American authoritarian type epitomized in the gym teacher. That one, I am told, later became a highly successful administrator in the educational bureaucracies. I don't see him as really a vicious sort, because 'three times around the track!' quite exhausted his imagination for institutional control. The same cannot be said for the more subtle coercions and denigrations worked out by some of our ostensibly more 'liberal' authorities, in and out of the schools. But 'three times around the track' remains an appropriate metaphor for what encouraged me to become a 'philosophical,' and

* This article was originally published in *Social Policy*, vol. 2, no. 3, 1971.

on certain more or less prudent occasions, an activist, anarchist.

Though starting with an anecdote from adolescence, I want to put the emphasis not on personality development, such as why I spoke out or smiled at the inconvenient moments and got extra laps around the track, but on our institutional order, which makes people unjustly run hard. Of course, I could instead fashionably sketch a psychological profile. No doubt it would be the fairly commonplace rebellious pattern: a first-born child, ambivalent relations to the father, consequent transferred hostilities to authority figures, and a guilty questing for a different identity. Equally standard but pertinent might be a marginal sense of social place, self-definition through anti-roles, and a dependence on 'obsessional defenses' (the self-defensive phrases with which the psychiatrically oriented like to describe the style usual to intellectual radicals). To thus elaborate the personality accounting of an anarchist wouldn't necessarily be wrong; it just wouldn't be enough. For there is a real world outside, a workout social order that often demands radical responses, drastic refusals that are humane and reasonable. So let us just assume the usual rebellious psyche – to elaborate on it would only be to avoid the public issues – and ask what it may find in our contemporary institutions. Suffering people, and most of what I can understand as authentic political issues, exist there, in shop and classroom and street and cell, not just in my, or your, warped head and wizened heart.

Finding the anesthetizing road

Take the usual work. Say 'social order' to me, and I most often associate it with 'unpleasant jobs.' That may be a lower-class trait. Or it could come from certain adolescent traumas linked to working. Perhaps they are the same thing. Anyway, I did some variety of menial and hard jobs over a period of more than half a dozen years, and I'm not satisfied to turn my times as a dock-walloper and seaman and sausage packer and scaffold-jack into mere romantic initiation on the way to something else. Many people never get elsewhere, and there are weariness and pain and rage in me still when memory brings back some of those labors. But could I be an exception – a sensitive kid who went to work too soon in field and factory? I doubt it, not only because when anyone goes to impersonal and exploited work he goes too soon but also because whether one were early or late, tough or tender, those were often arbitrarily harsh and dehumanized jobs. And they still are. To understand working, and the people who do it, requires awareness of bitter pains and resentments.

What else could come from stoop-hoeing carrots in a hot sun for a few cents an hour, with the sweat-caked peat burning on my skin and

the constant scatological threats of the field boss burning in my brain? Bitterness, indeed, comes from unloading by hand boxcars of bagged cement, 800 pounds to a dolly, choking on limestone dust and a steep ramp. A better job, I thought, was running a big steam-filler in a canning factory. It paid more – mandatory overtime, usually twelve-hour shifts. But I soon learned why such rich, machine-happy work was so available; with the required speed, and the 120-degree heat, no one lasted long. In spite of trained Protestant stoicism, I, too, collapsed. It was a nice company, though, for when I got well they rehired me to tend the newest semi-automatic filler – much easier, and less pay. But I was irresponsible. After hours of watching thousands of shiny cans wind through the conveyer, I would be so hypnotized that I didn't always punch the reject lever in time to flip out the defective ones, and so cream-style corn sprayed everything. Appropriately? Fired, I took off down the anesthetizing road, and then there was. . . .

However, I realize that literate people no longer care for this style of reportage – bathetic old proletarian novel stuff. It happens, of course, to be true, not only of my history but, with perhaps a little less variety and overt rebellion, of the work lives of millions of Americans, not to mention most of the rest of the human world. The rasping sense of arbitrary, monotonous, body-and-mind-dulling labor, without autonomy or reasonable reward – the injustice of it an essential part of the pain – remains a basic and harsh noise in my perception of our social reality. And it has made me a bit deaf when I read political moralists, and economists and sociologists, on our Gross National Product affluence and our technologically marvelous social order. Neither wealth nor automation has, in fact, eliminated a lot of our painful and unjust labor. The assembly lines still go on, with their nagging pressures – my recalled image is a grim over and over and over again, of nothing – and the damned hierarchy of supervision. Just about everybody rightly hates the line, and its destructive sense of being overcontrolled by machines as well as people. That's three times three around the track. . . .

The trauma of my labors

When it comes to the work most people do, we're still a long way from those fantasies of bureaucratic technology with nonhuman machines tending other machines in pure, mad productivity. Scientific techniques, and their liberal–bureaucratic rationalizations, contain no necessary imperatives for humaneness and individual autonomy. Superior machines promise no product of ordinary justice. My rounds of work convinced me, for example, that for a society to recognize the burdens of labor fairly would mean that no business man would receive higher

rewards than the field hand hacking with a short hoe; that no exalted professional would merit as much money and honor as those mucking out our coal and crap. No artist in the culture centers or entertainer in the media towers should receive more than those in home and shop and street. I know on my nerves, having been both, that the garbage man deserves to be better paid and comforted than the college professor. Such perfectly sensible conclusions, I later learned, made me an anarchist.

So be it. Freedom and justice must be testable on the independence and vitality – and yes, the eroticism – of the body, not just in realms of abstract manipulation. We must judge a society by the equity and solace and merit it allows for doing our unpleasant and boring labors. A society that does not redeem the Edenic curse will be rotten even in its most polished fruits.

But let me carry the issue of dehumanized laboring beyond the essential moral revulsion. No longer so young, and an academic drop-out – a decent man scorns the impersonalizing identification with 'professional' aggrandizements – I went back to laboring, this time at the somewhat skilled trade of airframe 'template-maker' (which is a sort of metal version of a ladies' dress pattern) in various plants and job-shops in three Western states. After some months of making templates in one of the largest, and reputedly most 'progressive,' plants, my boredom reached such excruciation that some gesture toward critical change became imperative. From the better writings on the subject as well as from my co-workers, I know that much of my reaction was unexceptional. Many a factory hand, not just a *poète maudit* with a power drill, finds his routine painful, his conditions of work arbitrary, and his sense of life emptied.

My resentments took form neither in chauvinistic rage nor in bleary degeneration but in an oddly naïve learning. I combined my responses to the tooling shop with things I had read on industrial organization and came up with a list of moderate, rational requests for humanization of the work. When I then consulted a noted academic specialist on how I might initiate these improvements, he exhibited acute embarrassment. He did provide two pieces of wisdom on how I might improve my factory life: I should go back to school to 'major in Industrial Relations,' thus both getting out of the shop and 'getting ahead' – the traditional American ideal of 'opportunity' substituting for justice and meaning – and I should immediately become involved in my spare time in politics, in liberal-Democratic chores in a Republican suburb. That's what usually passes for 'realism.'

Next, the union. With some difficulty, I finally presented my critical points to someone at a middling level in that hierarchy. My suggestions included flexible 'breaks' (to fit the job instead of a rigid plantwide

schedule), co-operative decisions on work assignments, and a procedure for electing foremen. All such proposals were indignantly rejected. Individual and flexible rules lacked exploitable drama as bargaining issues. By a logic that still eludes me, the union held that work assignments and promotions were purely corporate prerogatives. Though too dumb to say it, the union official's attitude also suggested that arbitrary work required arbitrary authority, including his own, rather than any independence and co-operation on the part of those doing the work.

Even raising such questions was suspect: 'Just what *are* your politics?' I remembered that I had better have none. Some years earlier I had put some related questions to an official of a different union (a Teamster's local) and obtained my answers from two persuasive gentlemen who wanted me to make contact with the hard realities of the problems, and so repeatedly put my head against a brick wall, before getting me fired. In addition to my cowardice, I felt some reluctance in pushing the argument with the machinists' union because of my experiences in a non-union tooling shop, from which I was fired solely for talking too much.

So I started arguing my way up the aircraft company hierarchy, finally reaching one of the biggest incompetents, the Plant Superintendent. That was a scene of comic pathos in a cubicle high above the assembly line, with the factory Major General trying to get rid of a loquacious third-rate toolmaker inexplicably arguing about perfectly standard shop procedures. He came on with phony geniality, then irritated belligerence, and finally collapsed into self-made-boss intimacy, lamenting that he'd never understood those 'industrial psych' courses the company had made him take in night school back in his foreman days. With a paternal hand on my shoulder, he asked, 'What can I really do for you? Put you in for a promotion?' No! I wanted to be able to smoke my pipe at reasonable intervals and to work out with the other template men the divvying up of the jobs (it might even be more efficient) rather than be trapped by plant schedules and engineering numbers and supervisory caprice. In sum, *we* wanted to be a bit more our own bosses and better our work lives.

Wasn't that reasonable? He agreed, but wearily assured me that such changes would require getting rid of all those 'goddamn personnel people,' redoing the company and union contractual procedures, and not only reorganizing the whole plant but the prime contractor, which happened to be the US Government. System, indeed! From such experiences I think I learned that those in our institutions supposedly running things don't really, except by their acquiescence, their unwillingness to refuse. I had also discovered, though I didn't then know the name or history of it, traditional anarchism's demand for 'worker's control.' No doubt I was temperamentally disposed to workplace democracy as well as radical egalitarianism before I discovered that it was a dehum-

anized system run by over-rewarded people of most dubious competence. Still, it came as a bit of a shock repeatedly to find those at the top essentially agreeing that the whole system was locked up and that the alternatives were to exploit it or get out.

For me to become an 'industrial relations' decorator or climb the shop (or union) hierarchy would only reinforce what was wrong. In the long run, the productive order must be radically transformed (a social revolution of far more import than any merely political one), not just aggrandizingly taken over by others. In the short run, our institutional order must be resisted if we are to retain our humanity. I made trouble, subverted things. A good deal, though not enough, of such screwing the system does go on, providing what decency there is in most jobs. Personal intransigence, though unpopular in pseudogenial American manners, seems essential. Our great unwritten contemporary work in social thought may be 'Humanizing Technological Organization,' by the descendants of Ned Lud. Freedom and equality and community must start where people are at, not in some schizophrenic abstractions. Changing our 'workout' realities, rather than choosing among the competing rhetorics of political power, provides the authentically radical issues in our society.

Prisons and other coercive places

If this be true of our ordinary *custodial* places, such as schools and factories, how much more it must be of our 'total institutions,' the determining skeleton of Leviathan. Such places also show how basically obtuse our order is to equality and freedom and change from below. A reasonably perceptive man forced to spend several years as a private in the US Army infantry can only snigger at many American claims to decency, much less liberty and democracy and justice. Although I'm not going to describe here the My Lai's of World War II that I witnessed, I drew some of the obvious deductions that another generation is drawing from the American Indochina War. Thus, though a decorated infantry combat veteran who was not subject to further military service, I refused, as a point of moral revulsion and anti-authoritarian principle, to complete re-registration when conscription was reinstituted in 1948. I got some of the attention my outraged innocence demanded and was locked into the issue, literally, with a much-publicized conviction for felonious violation of the Selective Service Act. It's a story of characteristic American righteousness, certainly theirs and, I must admit, mine. While I lectured the court on the illegitimacy and criminality of the US Army and conscription – with rhetorical appeals to my middle-European grandfather who came to America in flight from Continental militarism

(but ignoring my British grandfather who came to ride with Col. Teddy Roosevelt) – the prosecutor lengthily demanded that I be given five years for 'conspiracy to treason,' and the judge lectured me, cold war style, on what might happen to me in Russia. But in order to demonstrate American liberality toward a purely technical and principled violation, he sentenced me to only eight months in prison – just another totally arbitrary run around the custodial track. (The judge, too, complained about my sardonically smiling.)

The official American character, if one really comes up against it, is not very tolerant. Yet few of my friends who have not experienced time in our total institutions – as soldiers, convicts, mental patients, police victims – think badly of our national character. Thus I am rather less than half-facetious when I now and again argue that the minimum educational certification for any position of prestige and authority and power in America should be a prison sentence, say, two to five. Nothing less would be sufficiently edifying with respect to our institutional realities.

And perhaps given the innocence of a midwestern, small-town character, such as mine, nothing less than a convictable act of defiance could create a radicalization that went beyond the abstract–sentimental prejudices of usual leftism. Not that federal prison was so mean; indeed, it was physically better than the county jails and army stockades I've studied from the inside. Yet that endless, grim track – the futility and tedium, the unlimited repression of all total institutions – pushes everyone into doing 'hard time.' With a determinate sentence, I could insist, regardless of 'the hole,' on what I would only do – head convict librarian. Since I also focussed little of the usual chauvinist hostility to political prisoners – psychotic criminals and their custodians overcompensate with patriotism – I could come under the protection of the tough extortionist who was an inmate leader. Yet since I was there for having defied an unjust government, esthetic consistency demanded critical action.

But this couldn't take the usual ameliorist ways. For example, the 'joint' was in effect racially segregated; but since the ghetto sections were not the worst, the blacks fearfully rejected any efforts to reduce them to 'equal' conditions – a bigotry with a pragmatic future. And when I objected that the educational system only rarely surfaced as a 'rehabilitation' ritual, I ended up with the additional job of convict-head of the prison school. As with most official educational roles, the main effect was probably moral solace. That discouraged me from very vigorous complaints about the psychiatric and religious services for fear that I might be assigned unnecessary additional lessons in humility. There's nothing like a closed, total system for checking out the usual social and political theorists, for learning better than the usual educa-

tional and elitist theories of change, and for arriving at the conclusion that abolition is somewhat more practical than reform.

If there is a learning-change process in prison, it has to be by way of 'the brilliant psychopaths.' While 'outside' institutions make every effort to remove these deviant and dissident personalities, because they are often superior in intelligence and competence to those in power as well as troublesome, total custodial places cannot be so 'scientific' (i.e. conservative). Any radical theory of change must, in effect, include a table of organization with a major section on 'How To Employ The Madmen.' If it doesn't, it's the usual nonsense, so out with it.

A psychopathic young con, bright autodidact and compulsive captive, got bum-rapped with a bad work assignment. As in most institutions in our society, prison job placements and promotions come about through sycophancy (and other corruption), custodial needs (avoiding trouble), and psychosomatic identifications (unconsciously), not through competence and need and desire. More rational standards would not only lessen power but both destroy the illicit order that pays off with what pleasures there are to be had and threaten the whole system. While advantage and avoiding trouble block revision, the basic warping – the trade-off of power for denied gratifications – must be fundamentally disrupted. To be *rationally* appropriate, efforts at change must be *extreme* in style, breaking not only advantage and identification but overall order. Contrary to the smug pieties of most of our social and political thought, nothing less will work. True politics, then, is the art of troublemaking.

I encouraged my psychopathic friend, after he confided his breakout plans to me, to first refuse to work, which I 'unreasonably' backed up by also refusing. Raising the ante included getting other dissidents to 'act out,' refusing to go to the mess hall as the start of a hunger strike, and making demands about everything. These direct actions depended less on the moral suasion claimed for civil disobedience than on the breakdown of the actual illicit structure of gratification (underground use of the dispensary and bakery), on disproportionate work (trouble for the hacks), on dramatic enlargement (distant cons started choosing up sides), and on the psychic explosiveness. Thus are rebellions made.

As I was staring hungrily at the sky, for a last gulp before they dragged me off to windowless solitary, the chief hack sauntered in and announced, 'You dumb bastard! You can't win. No con ever does!' True enough. But he had just fearfully made some sensible changes in job assignments and privileges; and I soon went back to eating, working, and ineffective liberalism. (My friend later went over the wall anyway and, with proper gesture, stole the warden's personal car.) In the art of drawing the line – something one can learn only by overreaching sometimes – I had been lucky, partly, I believe, because that joint had

some tradition of resistance by political prisoners, and my action was therefore recognized as ideological rather than just selfish or sick. This suggests a crucial function for radicals – political esthetics. They must create not only awareness but scenarios for refusal and revolt.

Perhaps, in prison, I was again guility of excessive moderation – we anarchists often are – of not pushing further and fomenting more extreme disorder. After all, total institutions must be totally negated. Yet that finally may be more possible by way of continuing refusal rather than spastic riot, by selective rebellion rather than chiliastic revolution. Most violence is irrelevant, since the wrong people usually get it in the neck. Just changing those in power doesn't much change the institutional order. What I was later to learn to call 'radical de-mythification' and 'anarcho-syndicalist direct action' suggests more continuity, humaneness, and effectiveness than mere revolutionism. They can in practical use undercut the custodial 'workouts.'

Toward a community of refusal

This brief highlighting of some radical libertarian motifs – awareness of arbitrary institutional coercions, the methods of 'worker's control' and 'direct action,' the crucialness of egalitarianism and refusal, and the basic aim of social–institutional liberation – hardly gives a complete syllabus for anarchism. Nor do my three brief anecdotes of the custodial similarities of school, factory, and prison cover all our problems. Granted, we sometimes need to recognize institutional differences as well as the basic school–factory–prison template of society. (To my intellectual discomfort, since I would like to advocate small, communal forms, I must admit that I usually ended up opting to be in large and inefficient bureaucracies – big, muddled factories rather than disciplined job shops, rule-ridden federal prisons rather than brutality-ridden county jails, confusedly massive and mediocre state colleges rather than pretentious and ruthless prestige schools. We must take personal freedom where we can find it, without confusing its present location with a better order.)

Nor have I intended to reject all authority, though most that I know of is illegitimate even when not contemptible. We can acknowledge real authority – the ability to know, to say, to exemplify, and to do – and even grant it appropriate circumstances without giving to any authority continuing force and privilege. If we must have 'leaders,' such as institu-tional figureheads and celebrities and culture heroes, a lottery of random drawings would probably give us a better selection than we currently have and rightly devalue most claims to prerogative and power. In my skeptical anarchism, I want Oedipus and Laius in topsy-turvy order so

they no longer rage when they meet each other and their guilts. To dissolve the ancient curse of authority means to turn it into a daily comedy. And to lessen our curses of American power and control, 'de-authorization' must continue specifically as well as broadly, reaching from school-factory-prison to our cultural sanctities and the megalomania of the state.

Though refusing does not provide a total social politics, it may provide the crucial tests. Institutions that cannot bear considerable refusal, always evident in their running us around an arbitrary track, deserve on that basis alone to go under. Since we should never reduce humans to equations with their institutions, better them than us. Negative? Real destruction belongs not to anarchists, but to those who never claim it, the 'positive' saviors and orderings that advance the great historical crimes. Better the little negations that help move us toward a communal order of more voluntary and human proportions, which we so desperately need.

Here, of course, I must diverge from a leftism with a declared or implied model in political revolutionism. Such subordination to mass external methods of power and institutional manipulation – in the controlling name of *le peuple*, or the proletariat, or a party, or a resentful minority, or 'modernization' and other historical processes – must reject actual social and cultural revolution. Instead of depowering our institutions it heightens their arbitrary and punitive workouts. It also gives itself away in often agreeing with reaction in condemning liberating refusals as romantic and utopian and deviationist and 'unrealistic.' Political revolutionism is not nearly radical enough.

What would be, would be a community of refusal, a libertarian praxis in which ideological radicalism – the vision of an institutionally transformed society – and personal radicalism – from intransigent behavior to Joachimite life-styles – would go together. For 'deconversion' from our institutional faiths may require 'unreasonable' social politics of traumatic breaks in consciousness and radical disruptions of submission. We may be learning from our current social-cultural radicals that a politics of refusal and style and fancy and polymorphous difference can be more pertinent than the usual organizing of the bureaucracies of reform and the barricades of revolutionism. The truly radical criticism, the dissident way, the resistant method, the selective troublemaking, all the other ways of refusal must be put against and inside our institutional orderings. Furthering rebellious life-styles constitutes radical change now. So does institutional subversion, such as that considerable folklore and practice of 'beating the bureaucracy' and 'fighting the system.' They already exist in an expansive state – natural anarchism. Otherwise, our institutions would be quite unbearable, since patently not designed for passionate human freedom and fullness. Far more than

political postures, the manifold ways of refusal may redeem the curse of labor by transforming its justice, decorrupt authority by removing its legitimacy, and humanize power by making it limited and communal and personal. Such libertarianism is also of this time and place, at one with the often wonderful anarchy of the social and cultural revolutions around us, the rebellions that provide contemporary community.

The favorite myth of those who would master others is that denial is bad – bad manners, bad policy, bad psychology. Do they most fear its truth, its effectiveness, or its pleasure? By a fraudulent calculus they conclude that an order of human attritions and arbitrary workouts comes out less destructive than a liberating human negation. But the simple truth, discoverable here and now, is that a richer human life often comes from a joyous *no*, three times over, to running the track.

Kingsley Widmer is a professor of comparative literature at San Diego State College. His collected writings on anarchism, *The End of Culture: Essays on Sensibility in Contemporary Society*, were published by San Diego State University Press in 1975. He is now completing a book on the intellectual history of anarchism.

13   Revolutionary letter no. 1

Diane di Prima

I have just realized that the stakes are myself
I have no other
ransom money, nothing to break or barter but my life
my spirit measured out, in bits, spread over
the roulette table, I recoup what I can
nothing else to shove under the nose of the maitre de jeu
nothing to thrust out the window, no white flag
this flesh all I have to offer, to make the play with
this immediate head, what it comes up with, my move
as we slither over this board, stepping always
(we hope) between the lines

Diane di Prima is an anarchist who can trace her background to her
grandfather who was an anarchist from southern Italy. She has been
active in the peace movement and in the anti-nuclear campaign in
California. Several books of her poems have been published, including
Revolutionary Letters (1970) and *Selected Poems* (1975).

14 On the poverty of student life

(Once upon a time the universities were respected)*

Modern capitalism and its spectacle allot everyone a specific role in a general passivity

The student is no exception to the rule. He has a provisional part to play, a rehearsal for his final role as an element in market society as conservative as the rest.

Being a student is a form of initiation, an initiation that echoes the rites of more primitive societies with bizarre precision. It goes on outside history cut off from social reality. The student leads a double life, poised between his present status and his future role. The two are absolutely separate, and the journey from one to the other is a mechanical event 'in the future.' Meanwhile, he basks in a schizophrenic consciousness, withdrawing into his initiation group to hide from that future. Protected from history, the present is a mystic trance. . . .

Nowadays, the teenager shuffles off the moral prejudices and the authority of the family to become part of the market even before he is adolescent; at fifteen he has all the delights of being directly exploited. In contrast the student covets his protracted infancy as an irresponsible and docile paradise. Adolescence and its crises may bring occasional brushes with his family, but in essence he is not troublesome: he agrees to be treated as a baby by the institutions that provide his education. There is no 'student problem.' Student passivity is only the most obvious symptom of a general state of affairs, for each sector of social life has been subdued by a similar imperialism. . . .

* Excerpts from a pamphlet written by Situationist students at Strasbourg University in 1966. We are using a translation published in New York City in 1969 by the 'eyemakers.' We have made some editorial changes based mainly on a 1970 translation and pamphlet publication by an unidentified group in Berkeley.

The student persists in the belief that he is lucky to be there. But he arrived too late: the bygone excellence of bourgeois culture has vanished. A mechanically produced specialist is now the goal of the 'educational system.'

A modern economic system demands mass production of students who are not educated and who have been rendered incapable of thinking. Hence, the decline of the universities and the automatic nullity of the student once he enters its portals. . . .

There was once a vision – if an ideological one – of a liberal bourgeois university. But as its social base disappeared, the vision became a banality. In the age of free trade capitalism when the 'liberal' state left it its marginal freedoms, the university *could* still think of itself as an independent power.

Of course, it was a pure and narrow product of that society's needs – particularly the need to give the privileged minority an adequate general culture before they rejoined the ruling class (not that going up to university was straying very far from class confines). . . .

The real poverty of his everyday life finds its immediate, fantastic compensation in the opium of cultural commodities

In the cultural spectacle he is allotted his habitual role of the dutiful disciple. Although he is close to the production point, access to the Sanctuary of Thought is forbidden, and he is obliged to discover 'modern culture' as an *admiring spectator*. Art is dead but the student is necrophiliac. He peeks at the corpse in cine-clubs and theaters, buys its fishfingers from the cultural supermarket. Consuming unreservedly, he is in his element; he is living proof of all the platitudes of American market research: a conspicuous consumer, complete with induced irrational preference for Brand X (Camus, for example) and irrational prejudice against Brand Y (Sartre, perhaps). Impervious to real passions, he seeks titillation in the battles between his anemic gods, the stars of a vacuous heaven: Althusser, Garaudy, Barthes, Lefebvre, Lévi-Strauss, Halliday, De Chardin, Brassens . . . and between their rival theologies, designed like all theologies to mask the real problems by creating false ones: humanism, existentialism, scientism, structuralism, cyberneticism, new criticism, dialectics-of-naturism, metaphilosophism . . . .

We must add in all fairness that there do exist students of tolerable intellectual level, who without difficulty dominate the controls designed to check the mediocre capacity demanded from the others. They do so for the simple reason that they have understood the system, and so

despise it and know themselves to be its enemies. They are in the system for what they can get out of it – particularly grants . . . .

At the same time, since the student is a product of modern society just like Godard or Coca Cola, his extreme alienation can only be fought through the struggle against this whole society. It is clear that the university can in no circumstance become the battlefield; the student, in so far as he defines himself as such, manufactures a pseudo-value which must become an obstacle to any clear consciousness of the reality of his dispossession.

The best criticism of student life is the behavior of the rest of youth, who have already started to revolt. Their rebellion has become one of the *signs* of a fresh struggle against modern society.

It is not enough for thought to seek its realization in practice: practice must seek its theory.

After years of slumber and permanent counter-revolution, there are signs of a new period of struggle, with youth as the new carriers of revolutionary infection. But the society of the spectacle paints its own picture of itself and its enemies, imposes its own ideological categories on the world and its history. Fear is the very last response. For everything that happens is reassuringly part of the natural order of things. Real historical changes, which show that this society can be *superseded*, are reduced to the status of novelties, processed for mere consumption.

The revolt of youth against an imposed and 'given' way of life is the first sign of a total subversion. It is the prelude to a period of revolt – the revolt of those who can no longer *live* in our society. . . .

The revolt is contained by over-exposure: we are given it to contemplate so that we shall forget to participate

In the spectacle, a revolution becomes a social aberration – in other words a social safety valve – which has its part to play in the smooth working of the system. It reassures because it remains a marginal phenomenon, in the apartheid of the temporary problems of a healthy pluralism (compare and contrast 'the woman question' and the 'problem of racialism'). In reality, if there is a problem of youth in modern capitalism it is part of the total crisis of that society. It is just that youth feels the crisis most acutely.

Youth and its mock freedoms are the purest products of modern society. Their modernity consists in the choice they are offered and are already making: total integration to neo-capitalism, or the most radical

refusal. What is surprising is not that youth is in revolt but that its elders are so soporific. But the reason is history, not biology - the previous generation lived through the defeats and were sold the lies of the long, shameful disintegration of the revolutionary movement.

In itself youth is a publicity myth, and as part of the new 'social dynamism' it is the potential ally of the capitalist mode of production. The illusory primacy of youth began with the economic recovery after World War II. Capital was able to strike a new bargain with labor: in return for the mass production of a new class of manipulable consumers, the worker was offered a *role* which gave him full membership in the spectacular society. This at least was the ideal social model, though as usual it bore little relation to socioeconomic reality (which lagged behind the consumer ideology).

The revolt of youth was the first burst of anger at the persistent realities of the new world - the boredom of everyday existence, the *dead* life which is still the essential product of modern capitalism, in spite of all its modernizations. A small section of youth is able to refuse that society and its products, but without any idea that this society can be superseded - they opt for a nihilist present.

Yet the destruction of capitalism is once again a real issue, an event in history, a process that has already begun. Dissident youth must achieve the coherence of a critical theory and the practical organization of that coherence.

At the most primitive level, the 'delinquents' (*blousons noirs*) of the world use violence to express their rejection of society and its sterile options. But their refusal is an abstract one: it gives them no chance of actually escaping the contradictions of the system. They are its products - negative, spontaneous, but none the less exploitable.

All the experiments of the new social order produce them: they are the first side-effects of the new urbanism; of the disintegration of all values; of the extension of an increasingly boring consumer leisure; of the growing control of every aspect of everyday life by the psycho-humanist police force and of the economic survival of a family unit which has lost all significance.

The 'young thug' despises work but accepts the goods. He wants what the spectacle offers him - but *now*, with no down payment. This is the essential contradiction of the delinquent's existence. He may try for a real freedom in the use of his time, in an individual assertiveness, even in the construction of a kind of community. But the contradiction remains, and kills. (On the fringe of society, where poverty reigns, the gang develops its own hierarchy, which can fulfill itself only in a war with other gangs, isolating each group and each individual within the group.)

In the end the contradiction proves unbearable. Either the lure of

the product world proves too strong, and the hooligan decides to do his honest day's work (to this end a whole sector of production is devoted specifically for his co-optation: clothes, records, guitars, scooters, transistors, purple hearts beckon him to the land of the consumer), or else he is forced to attack the laws of the market itself – either in the primary sense, by stealing, or by a move towards a conscious revolutionary critique of commodity society. For the delinquent, only two futures are possible: revolutionary consciousness, or blind obedience on the shop floor. . . .

The banality of everyday life is not incidental, but the central mechanism and product of modern capitalism

. . . The proletariat is the motor of capitalist society, and thus its mortal enemy: everything is designed for its suppression (parties, trade union bureaucracies, the police, the colonization of all aspects of everyday life) because it is the only really menacing force. . . .

Idle reader, your cry of 'What about Berkeley?' escapes us not. True. American society *needs* its students; and by revolting against their studies they have automatically called the society in question. From the start they have seen their revolt against the university hierarchy as a revolt against *the whole hierarchical system*, the dictatorship of the economy and the state. Their refusal to become an integrated part of the commodity economy, to put their specialized studies to their obvious and inevitable use, is a revolutionary gesture. It puts in doubt that whole system of production which alienates activity and its products from their creators.

For all its confusion and hesitancy, the American student movement has discovered one truth of the new refusal: that a coherent revolutionary alternative can and must be found *within* the 'affluent society.' The movement is still fixated on two relatively accidental aspects of the American crisis – the blacks and Vietnam – and the mini-groups of the New Left suffer from the fact. There is an authentic whiff of democracy in their chaotic organization, but what they lack is a genuine subversive content. Without it they continually fall into dangerous contradictions. They may be hostile to the traditional politics of the old parties; but the hostility is futile, and will be co-opted, so long as it is based on ignorance of the political system and naive illusions about the world situation. *Abstract* opposition to their own society produces facile sympathy with its apparent enemies – the so-called socialist bureaucracies of China and Cuba.

Many American students can in the same breath condemn the state

and praise the 'Cultural Revolution' – that pseudo-revolt directed by the most elephantine bureaucracy of modern times.

At the same time, these organizations, with their blend of libertarian, political and religious tendencies, are always liable to the obsession with 'group dynamics' which leads to the closed world of the sect. The mass consumption of drugs is the expression of a real poverty and a protest against it; but it remains a false search for 'freedom' within a world dedicated to repression, a religious critique of a world that has no need for religion, least of all a new one.

The beatniks – that right wing of the youth revolt – are the main purveyors of an ideological 'refusal' combined with an acceptance of the most fantastic superstitions (Zen, spiritualism, 'New Church' mysticism, and the stale porridge of Ghandi-ism and humanism). Worse still, in their search for a revolutionary program the American students fall into the same bad faith as the Provos, and proclaim themselves 'the most exploited class in our society.' They must understand one thing: there are no 'special' student interests in revolution. . . .

The tradition of dead generations still weighs like a nightmare on the minds of the living

Opposition to the world offered from within – and in its own terms – by supposedly revolutionary organizations can only be spurious. Such opposition, depending on the worst mystifications and calling on more or less reified ideologies, helps consolidate the social order. Trade unions and political parties created by the working class as tools of its emancipation are now no more than the 'checks and balances' of the system. Their leaders have made those organizations their private property; their stepping stone to a role within the ruling class. The party program or the trade union statute may contain vestiges of revolutionary phraseology, but their practice is everywhere reformist – and doubly so now that official capitalist ideology mouths the same reformist slogans.

Where the unions have seized power – in countries more backward than Russia in 1917 – the Stalinist model of counter-revolutionary totalitarianism has been faithfully reproduced. Elsewhere, they have become a static complement to the self-regulation of managerial capitalism. The official organizations have become the best guarantee of repression – without this 'opposition' the humanist–democratic facade of the system would collapse and its essential violence would be laid bare. In the struggle with the militant proletariat, these organizations are the unfailing defenders of the bureaucratic counter-revolution, and the docile creatures of its foreign policy. They are the bearers of the most blatant falsehood in the world of lies, working diligently for the perennial and universal dictatorship of the state and the economy.

As the Situationists put it,

a universally dominant social system tending toward totalitarian self-regulation, is apparently being resisted – but only apparently – by false forms of opposition which remained trapped on the battlefield ordained by the system itself. Such illusory resistance can only serve to reinforce what it pretends to attack. Bureaucratic pseudo-socialism is only the most grandiose of these guises of the old world hierarchy and alienated labor.

As for student unionism, it is nothing but the travesty of a travesty, the useless burlesque of a trade unionism itself long totally degenerate.

A first principle of all future revolutionary organizations must be the theoretical and practical denunciation of Stalinism in all its forms. In France at least, where economic backwardness has slowed down the consciousness of crisis, the only possible road is over the ruins of Stalinism. It must become the *delenda est Carthago* of the last revolution of pre-history. Revolution must break with its past, and derive all its poetry from the future. . . .

The revolutionary project must be reinvented, as much as the life it announces. If the project is still essentially *the abolition of class society*, it is because the material conditions upon which revolution was based are still with us. . . .

The fight between the powers-that-be and the new proletariat can be only in terms of the totality. And for this reason the future revolutionary movement must be purged of any tendency to reproduce within itself the alienation produced by the commodity system; it must be the *living* critique of that system; and the negation of it, carrying all the elements essential for its transcendence.

As Lukacs correctly showed, revolutionary organization is this necessary mediation between theory and practice, between man and history, between the mass of workers and the proletariat *constituted as a class* (Lukacs's mistake was to believe that the Bolsheviks fulfilled this role).

If they are to be realized in practice, 'theoretical' tendencies or differences must be translated into organizational problems. It is by its present organization that a new revolutionary movement will stand or fall. The final criterion of its coherence will be the compatibility of its actual form with its essential project – *the international and absolute power of workers' councils* as foreshadowed by the proletarian revolutions of the last hundred years. There can be no compromise with the foundations of existing society – the system of commodity production; ideology in all its guises; the state; and the imposed division of labor from leisure. . . .

Ideology, however 'revolutionary,' always serves the ruling class; false consciousness is the alarm signal revealing the presence of the enemy fifth column. The lie is the essential product of the world of alienation and the most effective killer of revolutions: once an organization that claims the *social truth* adopts the lie as a tactic, its revolutionary career is finished.

All the positive aspects of the workers' councils must be already there in an organization that aims at their realization. All relics of the Leninist theory of organization must be fought and destroyed. The spontaneous creation of soviets by the Russian workers in 1905 was in itself a practical critique of that baneful theory, yet the Bolsheviks continued to claim that working-class spontaneity could not go beyond 'trade union consciousness' and would be unable to grasp the 'totality.' This was no less than a decapitation of the proletariat so that the Party could place itself 'at the head' of the Revolution. . . .

Workers' control is the abolition of all authority; it can abide no limitation, geographical or otherwise: any compromise amounts to surrender. 'Workers' control must be the means and the end of the struggle: it is at once the goal of that struggle and its adequate form' (*International Situationniste 10*).

A *total* critique of the world is the guarantee of the realism and reality of a revolutionary organization. To tolerate the existence of an oppressive social system in one place or another, simply because it is packaged and sold as revolutionary, is to condone universal oppression. To accept alienation as inevitable in any one domain of social life is to resign oneself to reification in all its forms. It is not enough to favor workers' councils in the abstract; in concrete terms they mean the abolition of commodities and therefore of the proletariat.

Despite their superficial disparities all existing societies are governed by the logic of commodities and the commodity is the basis of their dreams of self-regulation

This famous fetishism is still the *essential* obstacle to a total emancipation, to the free construction of social life. In the world of commodities, external and invisible forces direct men's actions; autonomous action directed toward clearly perceived goals is impossible. The strength of economic laws lies in their ability to take on the appearance of natural ones, but it is also their weakness, for their effectiveness thus depends *only* on 'the lack of consciousness of those who help create them.'

The market has one central principle – the loss of self in the aimless and unconscious creation of a world beyond the control of its creators.

The revolutionary core of workers' control is the attack on this principle. Workers' control *is* conscious direction by all of their whole existence. It is not some vision of a workers' control *of the market*, which is merely to choose one's own alienation, to program one's own survival (squaring the capitalist circle). The task of the workers' councils will not be the workers' control of the world that exists, but its continual qualitative transformation. The commodity and its laws (that vast detour in the history of man's production of himself) will be superseded by a new social form.

With workers' control ends one of the fundamental splits in modern society – between a labor that becomes increasingly reified and a 'leisure' consumed in passivity. The death of the commodity naturally means the suppression of *work* and its replacement by a new type of free activity. . . .

Far from being a 'Utopia,' its suppression is the first condition for a break with the market. The everyday division between 'free time' and 'working hours,' those conplementary sectors of alienated life, is an *expression* of the internal contradiction between the use-value and exchange-value of the commodity. It has become the strongest point of the commodity ideology, the one contradiction that intensifies with the rise of the consumer. To destroy it, no strategy short of the abolition of work will do.

It is only beyond the contradiction of use-value and exchange-value that history begins, that men make their activity an object of their will and their consciousness, and see themselves in the world they have created. The democracy of workers' councils is the resolution of all previous contradictions. It makes 'everything which exists apart from individuals impossible.'

What is the revolutionary project? The conscious domination of history by the men who make it. Modern history, like all past history, is the product of social praxis, the unconscious result of human action.

In the epoch of totalitarian control, capitalism has produced its own religion: the spectacle

In the spectacle, ideology becomes flesh of our flesh, is realized here on earth. The world itself walks upside down. And like the 'critique of religion' in Marx's day, a critique of the spectacle is now the essential precondition of any critique. . . .

We must destroy the spectacle itself, the whole apparatus of commodity society, if we are to realize human needs

We must abolish those pseudo-needs and false desires which the system manufactures daily in order to preserve its power.

The liberation of modern history, and the free use of its hoarded acquisitions, can come only from the forces it represses. In the nineteenth century the proletariat was already the inheritor of philosophy; now it inherits modern art and the first conscious critique of everyday life. With the self-destruction of the working class, art and philosophy shall be realized.

To transform the world and to change the structure of life are one and the same thing for the proletariat – they are the passwords to its destruction as a class, its dissolution of the present reign of necessity, and its accession to the realm of liberty. As its maximum program it has the radical critique and free reconstruction of all values and patterns of behavior imposed by an alienated reality. . . .

Already, in the highly industrialized countries, the decomposition of modern society is becoming obvious at a mass level. All previous ideological explanations of the world have collapsed and left the misery and chaos of everyday life without any coherent dissimulation at all. Politics, morality and culture are all in ruins – and have now reached the point of being marketed as such, as their own parody, the spectacle of decadence being the last desperate attempt to stabilize the decadence of the spectacle.

Less and less masks the reduction of the whole of life to the production and consumption of commodities; less and less masks the relationship between the isolation, emptiness and anguish of everyday life and this dictatorship of the commodity; less and less masks the increasing waste of the forces of production, and the richness of lived experience now possible if these forces were only used to fulfill human desires instead of to repress them. . . .

The consumption of hysteria has become a principle of social production, but one where the real banality of the goods keeps breaking the surface, and letting loose a necessary violence – the violence of a man who has been given everything, but finds that every *thing* is phony. . . .

The real revolution begins at home: in the desperation of consumer production, in the continuing struggle of the unofficial working class. As yet this unofficial revolt has an official ideology. The notion that modern capitalism is producing new revolutionary forces, new poverties of a new proletariat, is still suppressed. Instead, there is an *a priori*

fascination with the 'conversion' or 'subversion' of the old union movement. The militants are co-opting themselves (and their intellectual 'advisors' urge on the process).

The *only* real subversion is in a new consciousness and a new alliance – the location of the struggle in the banalities of everyday life, in the supermarket and the coffee house *as well as* on the shop floor. The enemy is centrism, cultural or political. Art and the labor movement are dead! Long live the Situationist International!

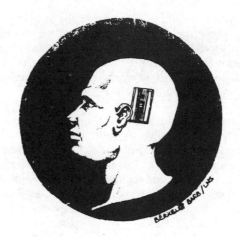

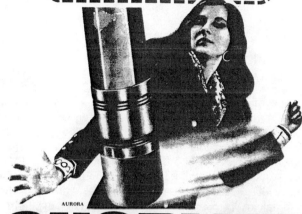

HOW TO ERASE A GOOD PART OF CAPITALISM...

SHOPLIFT

NO IFS, ANDS, OR BUTS!

By learning the proper techniques you can steal a fair portion of the things you need to live, which amounts to not having to work as much at some type of slave job. Private property is a disease which we can begin to combat by realizing that everything in the world of capitalist businesses is social wealth, and therefore is free.

Of course shoplifting has its drawbacks, if the pigs get you it may land you in jail. But the chief drawback is that shoplifting doesn't go far enough in destroying capitalist social relations. Qualitative looting takes things a step further, but hopefully we will see a day when we can pull off the final theft and destroy capitalism altogether. Then such terms as shoplifting and money will be shelved in pre-history.

S.T.E.M.
Skillfull Theft can Eliminate Money!

15   The production and consumption of humans*

Robert Cooperstein

The production of humans differs from almost all other commodity production in that it is still the direct production of use-value. This was obviously true in the past wherever parents in a state of dire material poverty required the production of humans as a means of human capital accumulation, in order to supplement the family income (with respect to industrial child labor, the condition being that the parents could still extract surplus value from the child even after the capitalist had taken his share; on the farm this did not apply, child labor was directly exploitable). Furthermore, children could assure economic security later on in the form of a life-long pension to the parents when they would have become economically obsolete. These motivations for human production are still prevalent in the poor countries, and locally in more developed countries.

In the spectacle, direct material necessities only rarely engender the reproduction of children, which none the less remains an *economic* decision; here the difference being that the use-values attributed to children take on different forms, often in the sense of developing attitudes formerly possessed in an embryonic form in less wealthy epochs. The following is a list of some of the economic reasons for which humans are produced, or why parents seek to *own* children:

1 as a source of consumable entertainment, like TV;
2 as a shared possession, a kid serves to preserve an otherwise unstable, because miserable, relation between the parents, whose survival instinct compels them to stay together 'for the sake of the children' (and of the state as well, which will take any measures necessary to preserve the family: divorce laws, free marriage counseling, family planning centers, etc.);
3 as a trap by means of which one parent can compel the other to form a survival relation in the first place, s/he having recognized the

* Excerpted from the pamphlet, *Some Notes on the Reproduction of Human Capital*, April 1974.

enormous offensive power of this weapon: child as shared possession, as detailed in #2;

4 as a vehicle of conspicuous consumption: the attributes of the child (his cuteness, good looks, spontaneity, vitality, precociousness, etc.) are conferred upon the owners, in the same way that money can confer personal wealth upon qualitatively poor people, as detailed by Marx;

5 as a means by which the parents can use self-sacrifice in order to escape the practical task of rectifying otherwise unbearable conditions – that is, parents can realize their own unfulfilled desires vicariously: unwilling to live for themselves, they decide to 'live for the children' as a compensatory substitute;

6 as a proof of normality: a childless couple will be thought strange (even in the ecological era where 2.1 children will suffice), and the ownership of a nuclear family is still a vital business asset ('business' must be broadly interpreted since all social life is a business);

7 as a means by which one can preserve his property in perpetuity, even after death (this is true whether property is defined as material possession proper, which is to say *having*, or as the ownership of an organized appearance, or *appearing*): to the extent you can pass on to him your material wealth and/or character traits, the child eternalizes your existence. (Producing an heir is the spectacular analog of going to heaven.) (Just as the modern corporations occasionally sacrifice short-run profits in return for their long-run security, so the parent bears a child which is expensive in money terms but priceless in so far as it can confer immortality.);

8 as a proof of virility or fertility: those who are creatively sterile and orgastically impotent can exhibit and consume the child as the *living image* of their potency;

9 as a vehicle upon which one who has had his love, care, and affection rejected everywhere else can practice such: the infant cannot reject love if only he can be made absolutely dependent upon it – this is the pet syndrome (born of loneliness, children are raised as dogs).

Capitalism has always resolved the contradiction between use-value and exchange-value in favor of the latter. Hence even if humans are not directly produced for sale in a visible market, their use-value in itself is that of a depository of exchange-value, a subjective money which can buy social recognition, survival, etc. – all the returns to human reproduction listed above. Moreover, the slavery of old might reappear, albeit in a more rationalized and humanized form, as the reconstitution of the right to bear a child as a *marketable asset*; the economists have already detailed the plans. Prospective parents are to be issued coupons with which they can either bear children or sell their rights to another couple, which for example is infertile or perhaps desires to produce more than

its fair share of 2.1 children per couple. (The social planners find the coupon system by which commodities are rationed in wartime quite suited for turning the 'population problem' into a population market.) Another more imminent device to ration and control the baby market will be in the form of tax disincentives, the elimination or reduction of child exemptions in income taxes. As always, in short, the legal codification of property rights serves to sanctify pre-existing *de facto* relations of production, in this case, of human reproduction. . . .

Sometimes parents will desire to produce children for non-economic reasons. Perhaps the possibility of uninhibited play with them, i.e., they 'like' kids; but even then this borders on the economic when, perchance, this serves as a compensatory substitute for the inability to play with other individuals, which is to say the abandonment of the practical task to radicalize existing social relations. And sometimes, of course, there are bound to be accidents, due to the failure of contraception, or a moral opposition to contraception and/or abortion. In these cases, even though he is not born of economic motivations, the infant will be raised as a commodity anyway.

16 Beyond character and morality: towards transparent communications and coherent organization*

Jay Amrod and Lev Chernyi

1

To create a *revolutionary* organization, it is not sufficient mechanically to link up a number of people with revolutionary pretensions. The creation of such an organization must involve the conscious project of aggressively destroying all barriers to communication, thought, and action both from within and from outside the organization. It involves the conscious elaboration of a theory and practice adequate to its task. And it involves a commitment to change which never questions the need for self-change. You can't change the world if you expect to remain unchanged.

2

The first step in the destruction of all barriers to communication, thought, and action is logically the identification of these barriers. When we examine our situation closely we inevitably find that these obstacles can all be subsumed under the general label of 'capital,' understood as the coherent totality of all the aspects that together make it up. It is only logical that what restrains all our attempts to destroy capitalist society is in the end only capital itself.

3

For our theoretical and practical purposes we will focus our attention on that moment or aspect of capital that Wilhelm Reich called 'character.'

* Excerpted from a paper which was presented in May 1976 to a regional anarchist organizing meeting in Des Moines, Iowa. Published here for the first time.

Character is 'capital' as it appears to us within the individual. It is the totality of all the internalized or habitual incapacities and limitations of action within the individual. It is not an aggregate sum of arbitrary limitations, but a coherent structure of incapacities and limitations which, as an organized whole, serves its function within the framework of capitalist society. Character must never be viewed as a thing in itself, detached from any other social reality. It only exists as one moment of the totality of capital. To act on any other perception of character is to miss the whole point.

4

Recall your childhood. In doing so you will recall the formation of your character structure, the formation of the pattern taken by your defeat at the hands of (and your submission to) the logic of capital as it was presented to you by your family, your peers, your church or temple, the media, and your school. You can see the same process going on every day if you observe the lives of the children around you. They are learning the logic of capital the hard way, just as we all did. Each time a child is born her/his capacity for self-regulation is systematically attacked by the people who are closest to him/her. It usually begins with rigid feeding times, which are not only a convenience to mothers and hospitals, but serve the added function of introducing the child early in the game to the 'reality principle' ('You'll eat on schedule, not when you're hungry'), otherwise known as the logic of character and capital. For most newborn males there is the added trauma of circumcision which serves him notice as to the kind of care to expect from his parents. In quick succession the child is exposed to more and more types of conditioning when s/he is least able to understand and fight it. Often children who cannot yet walk are 'potty-trained.' Any touching of the genitals is quickly rewarded by most conscientious parents, and children are taught to *always* wear clothes ('It's not *nice* for people to see you naked'). Parents impose rigid sleeping schedules on children, who know well enough when they are tired and when they want to get up. And in general, children are allowed to investigate their environment, and exercise their powers only within the limits allowed by their captors – whether their captors be parents, schools, etc.

5

The one basic message that is always received with each conditioning is that the child isn't in control; someone else is. Children react to this in

the only way they can, they adapt themselves to the situation through a trial-and-error process. The first time a child is slapped for what s/he thought was a natural act, there is a look of astonishment and wonder. After being punished more than a few more times for the mysteriously simple act, the child learns to avoid it when in the presence of the seemingly irrational aggressor. The child eventually acquires a deference to figures of authority (arbitrary power) within the family. This is eventually generalized to a 'respect' for and deference to all authority as the child is exposed to ever-wider spheres of perception and action. One thing that needs to be made clear is that few people consciously condition children. The pervasive conditioning that takes place is usually a result of a whole organization of forces working through the parents and others. These forces include those of the economy, the parents of the parents, social mores, etc. Capital must continually reproduce itself or it will cease to exist.

6

We live in a society without natural scarcity. Our natural desires are often temporarily frustrated by the natural world. This usually has no lasting effect on our lives, though, since we eventually learn what we did wrong, or the natural circumstances change such that we are then able to fulfill our wish. Unfortunately, we also live in a society dominated by capital, which is to say that we live in a society dominated by chronic, socially enforced (artificial) scarcities. These scarcities result in chronic frustrations of certain desires. And when important natural desires are chronically frustrated, not just denied but also often punished, we are soon forced to collaborate with this denial. In order to avoid the punishment that we will receive for trying to satisfy this need, we learn to suppress it as soon as it begins to intrude upon our awareness. We use some of the energy that would otherwise have been used to fulfill our desire to suppress it in order to satisfy our secondary desire to avoid punishment. Once this self-repression exists for any prolonged period, it becomes a habit, an unconscious habitual attitude of our character structure. Our awareness of the original situation of chronic frustration is repressed because it is too painful to maintain. We learn that our desire is 'irrational,' 'bad,' 'unhealthy,' etc. We internalize the logic of capital as character traits, and they become 'natural' for us and the original desires become 'irrational' desires. Even when there is no longer a threat of punishment for acting within the logic of the original desire, we continue to suppress it automatically. We have learned to cripple ourselves *and like it*.

7

Throughout the first years of our lives we were forced not just to internalize a few aspects of capital, but to build up a structure of internalizations. As our capacity for coherent natural self-regulation was systematically broken down, a new system of self-regulation took its place, a coherent system, incorporating all the aspects of self-repression. We participated in capital's ongoing project of colonization by colonizing ourselves, by continually working at the construction of a unitary character structure (character armor), a unitary defense against all the drives, feelings, and desires which we learned were dangerous to express. In the place of our original transparent relations to our world, we created a structure of barriers to our self-expression which hides us from ourselves and others.

8

The ramifications of character can be found in all aspects of our behavior because character is a unitary deformation of the entire structure of our existence. It produces a deterioration of our capacity to live freely and fully by destroying the structural basis of free life. Character is not a mental phenomenon. It is a structural phenomenon of our entire existence. It exists as: inhibitions, chronic muscular tensions, guilt, perceptual blocks, creative blocks, psychosomatic or psycho-genetic diseases (in many of the cases of 'illnesses' as diverse as chronic insomnia, arthritis, obsessive–compulsive neuroses, chronic headaches, chronic anxiety, etc.). It exists as: respect for authority, dogmatism, mysticism, sexism, communications blocks, insecurity, racism, fear of freedom, role-playing, belief in 'God,' etc., ad nauseam. In each individual these character traits take on a coherent structure which defines that person's character.

Just as character is a limitation and deformation of the free human activity in general in the service of capital, so ideology is the limitation and deformation of *thought* in the service of *capital*. Ideology is always the acceptance of the logic of capital at some level. It is the form taken by alienation in the realm of thought.

9

With ideologies, I justify my complicity with capital, I justify my self-repression (my submission, my guilt, my sacrifice, my suffering, my boredom, etc. – in other words, my character). On the other hand, my

character structure, by existing as fixed, conditioned behavior, naturally tends to express its existence in thought as fixed ideas which dominate me. Neither character nor ideology could exist without the other. They are both parts of one unitary phenomenon. All ideology is revealed as the impotence of my thought, and all character is revealed as the impotence of my activity.

10

A particularly insidious form of ideology is the pervasive moralism which has always plagued the libertarian revolutionary movement. It destroys possibilities for transparent communication and coherent collective activity. To limit one's behavior according to the proscriptions of a morality (to seek the 'good' or the 'right') is to repress one's own will to satisfaction in favor of some ideal. Since we cannot possibly do anything else but seek our own satisfaction, alienation results, with one part of ourselves subduing the rest – one more instance of character. Wherever morality exists, communication is replaced by manipulation. Instead of speaking to me, a moralist tries to manipulate me by speaking to my internalizations of capital, my character, hoping that his brand of ideology may give me a hold on my thought and behavior. 'The projections of my subjectivity, nurtured by guilt, stick out of my head like so many handles offered to any manipulator, any ideologue, who wants to get a hold of me, and whose *trade skill* is the ability to perceive such handles' (*The Right To be Greedy*). The only really transparent, and thus revolutionary, communication is that which takes place when our selves and our desires are out in the open, when no morals, ideals, or constraints cloud the air. We will be amoralists, or we will be manipulators and manipulated. The only coherent organization is that in which we unite as individuals who are conscious of our desires, unwilling to give an inch to mystification and constraint, and unafraid to act freely in our own interests.

Jay Amrod grew in Saugerties, New York, and writes stories to his friends. Lev Chernyi is an artist who lives in Columbia, Missouri.

17 Revolutionary realization: the motivational energy*

David Porter

Many political activists of the last decade experienced a gradual 'burn-ing out' of their personal capacity for sustained radical effort. To their despair, the struggle for change drained too much energy, too fast, and with no source of replenishment. They wrote off the revolutionary project for a distant future – at best, something others might see. Feelings of deprivation, pain and anger seemed an inadequate basis for sustaining creative political effort.

This generation's experience, however, is not unique. Activists failed to recognize that equally formidable systems in the past caused the same personal torment and defection from radical movements then. Our ahistorical perspective, then, not only increased our sense of isola-tion and despair, but also hid from us those lessons of survival painfully learned by our predecessors.

Of particular importance in the past, as now, was a continually revived sense that alternatives are possible. The truly revolutionary vision is an imagery compelling enough to motivate intense activism *and* to renew activity regularly as time goes on. It is the awareness or 'real-ization,'[1] gradually or suddenly acquired, that social experience *can* be qualitatively satisfying. It is a phenomenological conviction, that is, based on some actual lived experience. The barriers to fulfilled existence *can* be conquered. While the effort to break these is painful, the pain is tolerable when it permits entry into the utopian realm already glimpsed. The vision offers a world where people respect, glorify and delight in each other's uniqueness and mutual interests; yet such a world is attainable only if distorting social lenses are removed. In sociological terms, the vision entails awareness of the arbitrary limits of the roles and institutions of everyday life as well as damaging socialization and the institutional mechanisms that maintain social control. It is the convincing power of this vision, in addition to

* Published here for the first time.

214

the pain of oppression, that creates the strongest initial and continuing commitment to revolutionary change.

Images of consciousness from other experiential realms help explain the significance of revolutionary 'real-ization' in politics as well. (Indeed, they also suggest the strong possibility of common features in the core experience of altered consciousness states in various realms – psychological, aesthetic, religious and political.) Literature on millennial movements, disaster communities or front-line war experience, artistic creativity, encounter groups, meditative and drug experience, nonlinear time consciousness, surrealism, peak emotional experiences, and the sociology of de-reification and de-legitimization all describe common periods of heightened intensity, in which the world is far more real than before. Undeniably, many will panic when thrust into such an experience without choice or social support. Under the right conditions, however, many prefer the intense new reality to the old. At the least, people perceive vast positive capabilities in themselves and others for the first time. Such situations suspend the normal construction of everyday reality and reveal in its place the indefinable flux of living, the basic sources of spontaneous delight, and the common humanity which predate in each individual and each society the veneer of 'civilization.'

Among major political movements for revolutionary change, anarchists (of socialist rather than individualist orientation) have shown a broad and compelling vision for over a century.[2] The anarchist vision, at its strongest, caused militants to demand the finest now, from and for all. In contrast, most other activists eventually reduced their claims or projected their ideals into a distant future.

Revolutionary consciousness comprehends a vision of alternatives and a knowledge of the forces that hold us back; it also includes strategic and tactical awareness of how best and most rapidly to achieve liberation in the immediate present. Such knowledge is generated by practical experience. There are few maps at best, and environmental conditions change often enough to render even these guidelines obsolete in a few years.

Meanwhile, radical progress draws attention and counter-attack from those who benefit from conditions as they are. Anarchists are first priority targets, since theirs is the vision most in contrast with existing 'law and order.' Ridicule also threatens the militant, especially when it comes from groups with the most to gain from social transformation or from those proclaiming themselves 'realistic' progressives. Finally, constant political activity is mentally and physically exhausting itself.

For many revolutionaries (and all the more for anarchists who suffer the greatest repression and who set the most difficult goal to achieve), the original sustaining vision, however intense it is at first, thus gradually burns out. Consciously or not, the militant becomes too exhausted, too

pained, too demoralized or too obsessed with negative conditions to continue. S/he forgets the intensity of conviction and begins to view him/herself as mentally rigid or even insane. Even if s/he understands the causes behind this fatigue, s/he may simply become cynical and retreat, content now and then to throw knowing barbs at those still in the struggle. The persistent pain that accompanied the original revolutionary vision may drive him/her eventually to a 'safe' individualistic enclave at anesthetic distance from others. Among those still struggling, tension between comrades intensifies, and the movement splits into smaller and smaller hostile fragments. How obvious by now are all of these tendencies among so many of the activists for change in the 1960s and 1970s. How clear the exhaustion, pain, demoralization, self-ridicule, cynicism, opportunism and petty factioning among those whose vision seemed so convincingly strong.

Yet such reactions are not new. Leading figures in the historic anarchist movement suffered similar feelings of discouragement. Among these was Michael Bakunin. The statement below was written toward the end of his life, following the collapse of the Paris Commune and other insurrectionary defeats of the same period:[3]

> You are right, the revolutionary tide is receding and we are falling back into evolutionary periods – periods during which barely perceptible revolutions gradually germinate. . . . The time for revolution has passed not only because of the disastrous events of which we have been the victims (and to which we are to some extent responsible), but because, to my intense despair, I have found and find more and more each day, that there is absolutely no revolutionary thought, hope, or passion left among the masses; and when these qualities are missing, even the most heroic efforts must fail and nothing can be accomplished.
>
> I admire the valiant persistence of our Jura and Belgian comrades. . . .
>
> As for myself, my dear friend, I am too old, too sick, and – shall I confess it? – too disillusioned, to participate in this work. I have definitely retired from the struggle and shall pass the rest of my days in intense intellectual activity which I hope will prove useful.

Similarly, for Emma Goldman, the apparent hypnotic appeal of Stalinist and Nazi totalitarianism mocked her own and others' continuing effort:[4]

> No one is interested any longer in human suffering and in incessant butchery. Yes, they kick when it is in Germany or their own countries. But Russia can and does get away with murder. . . . Hitler is beginning to be praised. Sure, nothing succeeds like success. Fact is,

dearest, we are fools. We cling to an ideal no one wants or cares about. I am the greater fool of the two of us. I go on eating out my heart and poisoning every moment of my life in the attempt to rouse people's sensibilities. At least if I could do it with closed eyes. The irony is I see the futility of my efforts and yet I can't let go. Just clear meshugeh [crazy], that's what I am.

Despite such depression, many anarchists *did* persist. They did so mainly, I believe, because somehow, somewhere, they found sources of new energy[5] to maintain their vision, their sense that utopia was indeed achievable. What concerns me here is precisely those experiences that periodically jolt militants into an intense new certainty of the worth of their ideals. These are the periodic re-energizers, the high points of political consciousness, which are essential to the sustained vitality of individual revolutionaries and the movement as a whole. These are the periodic creations of 'liberated space,' where the vision becomes actuality and the temporary actuality in turn revives the long-range vision. As Emma Goldman stated, 'There is much truth in the saying *Der Appetite komt mit dem Essen* [Appetite comes with eating]. When our interests are alive our capacity grows [and] our mentality revives.'[6] In the most liberated moments and spaces, 'common sense' is meaningless, usual categories and identities collapse, people are responsible for themselves separately and in community, work becomes play, adventure replaces security, 'imagination is in power,'[7] social existence is a spontaneous and endless festival. To actualize these dreams, however temporarily, renews the certainty of their worth and restores the drive to make them an ever-increasing part of human existence.

In humanistic psychology, Abraham Maslow is famed for his identification and analysis of peak emotional experiences. Yet Maslow also distinguishes clearly between these periods themselves and the ensuing high plateaus of expanded consciousness.[8] Transferred to the political realm, my discussion focuses on the first of these, with the understanding that the plateaus of 'after-glow' awareness sustain the movement over time.

'Revolutionary re-energizers' may be described by several different dimensions. These include the size of social unit involved, the degree of personal involvement, the predominant emotional attitude (negative vs positive), and the range of social realms of 'new reality' experienced. Within each dimension, in turn, the relative power of such experiences differs. The following discussion concentrates on the first dimension listed, the size of the social unit.

217

The individual level

A natural setting, by itself, *can* expand political consciousness:[9]

> And on many an evening the sunlight would envelop the whole
> prairie in a brilliant display of light and colour which merged the
> land and the burning sky into a spectacle arousing in one the deepest
> and noblest feelings of admiration for the great glory of nature. In
> the early days [of the intentional community] I would watch these
> magnificent natural phenomena from the upper windows of 'The
> Hotel,' my heart filled with delight, with hope and expectancy, at
> the great things we were going to accomplish under such glorious
> skies.

Yet a fascist as well as an anarchist may enjoy a sunset, a mountain
range, a rocky seashore. Metaphors of domination as well as egalitarian
community are inherent in nature. The crucial difference is the political
framework that exists already in the mind of the perceiver. The objectively fiery skies of sunset can invoke dreams of power and destruction
as well as ideals of human creativity and love. Indeed, for the whole
range of experiences indicated below, the significance of the pre-existing
political framework is paramount for the type of inspiration received.

Renewal may come from works of art as well, creations that sometimes recall forgotten dimensions of human existence and the natural
world. In the view of early twentieth-century German anarchist Gustav
Landauer, for example, since the best artistic creation reflects acute
sensitivity to the most universal levels of the human spirit, it is ultimately logical that 'the consequence of poetry is revolution.'[10]

Also at this level, the matching of high moral standards with self-
chosen action in one's own life may restore faith that such behavior is
a general human potential. In the late nineteenth century, prominent
French anarchist Elisée Reclus, for example, wrote:[11]

> For my part, I struggle for that which I know to be the good cause
> because I thus align myself with my sense of justice. It is a question
> of conscience, not a question of hope. Whether we succeed or not, it
> doesn't matter, we will have been at least the interpreters of the
> interior voice.

One-to-one relationships

A trusting and loving relationship, expressing its beauty reciprocally
through words, glances, touch and the power of orgasmic sex, is poten-

tially a vision renewer of great significance. Gustav Landauer, in an early novel, even used this as a key theme in the life of his hero, a formerly active revolutionary socialist. Temporarily disheartened and withdrawn from life's absurdity, he reawakens to political militance through the life-affirming sensuality of an unexpected love affair.[12] Rudolf Rocker, anarchist writer and lecturer in Germany and abroad during the first half of this century, affirmed related values from a longer-range perspective:[13]

> A man who has stood as I have from his earliest youth in the crush and throng of a movement must have a place where he can find inner peace, and another human being who is not only his wife, but his friend and comrade, to whom he can open his heart and trust her with everything.

Less dramatically, a teacher or a speaker also may notice that certain magic of communication, when comprehension grows among those who were previously ignorant, distracted or confused. Such experiences well compensate for the long gaps in between. After two months of lectures in provincial France, for example, Sébastien Faure happily reflected that the questions posed were now, in 1896, far more intelligent and with a larger understanding of libertarian concepts:[14]

> I sensed, ascertained, that the hour is come to communicate to the crowds chilled by discouragement the flame which burns within us. ... This path we travelled fills us with hope and steels us against the critics who reproach us with wanting too much from a single blow and pursuing – without practical men's patience and wise men's deliberation – the complete transformation of society.

On the opposite side of the relationship, to encounter fortitude of 'presence' in someone else revives one's own forgotten dreams:[15]

> [Reflecting on the strength Alexander Berkman showed during his first years of imprisonment], so often since that day when the steam monster at the Baltimore and Ohio station had snatched him away from me, he stood out like a shining meteor on the dark horizon of petty interests, personal worries, and the enervating routine of everyday existence. He was like a white light that purged one's soul, inspiring even awe at his detachment from human frailties.

Errico Malatesta, himself a great influence in the international movement for half a century from the 1870s on, testified about the amazing personal effect of Michael Bakunin:[16]

[He was] the great revolutionary, he who we all look upon as our spiritual father. . . . [His greatest quality was his ability to] communicate faith, the desire for action and sacrifice to all those who had the opportunity of meeting him. He would say that one needed to have *le diable au corps*: and he certainly had it in him and in his spirit.

Small-group level

At this level is a variety of people all contributing unique modes and contents of expression. The greater potential energy involved is like the difference between a solo musician and a well-integrated ensemble. There is a power here, as in festive outings, effective classes or meetings, group projects or communal sharing, which can re-evoke vivid images of the ideal society. After lifetimes fuller than most, for example, both Rocker and Russian anarchist Peter Kropotkin recalled still-inspiring memories of their youthful activism:[17] [18]

The publication of the new periodical [*Germinal*, in 1900] was bound up with difficulties and hardships which cannot be easily described. We started with empty hands. From the material point of view it was perhaps the hardest time in the whole of my life. We were often without the barest necessities. Yet I think of those days with nostalgia. My old heart warms at the memory of those fine young people who worked at my side, and gave so much devotion and love and self-sacrifice to the cause. They were wonderful young people.

The two years that I worked with the Circle of Tchaykovsky, before I was arrested, left a deep impression upon all my subsequent life and thought. During these two years it was life under high pressure, – that exuberance of life when one feels at every moment that full throbbing of all the fibres of the inner self, and when life is really worth living. I was in a family of men and women so closely united by their common object, and so broadly and delicately humane in their mutual relations, that I cannot now recall a single moment of even temporary friction marring the life of our circle. Those who have had any experience of political agitation will appreciate the value of this statement.

Small community

A small community might contain several dozens or several thousand

220

people. In any case, it is simply too large for the intense personal communication of a small group. Nevertheless, a shared new awareness can still be attained. Confident of support and interest, the individual can now express previously contained thoughts and desires throughout the community. Satisfaction of deepest yearnings and imagination now takes priority. To experience this among strangers or with friends who had never been so open before relights that previous vision.

Consider the feelings of French anarchist Emile Pouget during a labor strike in the late nineteenth century:[19]

[The general strike in Paris] gave to the people that consciousness of their own strength which they had lost since the crushing of the Commune [of 1871].... The spirit of solidarity was wonderful!... There rests in their hearts a rich ferment of revolt and, one of these mornings, when the clamor of the General Strike reverberates again there will be a colossal thrust forward.... The most chicken-hearted will awaken with energy! In a period of revolutionary ferment, individuals change rapidly and radically under the influence of the new and super-charged milieu: it takes not much to produce a zealous fellow from the bedrock of prejudice where the unconscious individual sleeps.

Large community

The strength of feelings associated with 'real-ization' within a small community is amplified when whole regions or nations are simultaneously involved. Dynamic protest movements, insurrections and revolutions all validate the universal appeal of the utopian vision. The power of such events for restoring revolutionary energy is unsurpassed.

Rudolf Rocker, for example, describes the passionate interest aroused by Russian events among Jewish workers in London in 1905:[20]

Each time something happened there was a big mass meeting in the East End, which thousands of people attended.

A number of our younger comrades made their way back to Russia, to take part in the events. We were all elated. We were sure that we stood on the threshold of Russian Liberation, of a world-shaking event that would like the French Revolution start a new era.

People may shake their heads wisely today over us and call us dreamers, and say that we had no sense of the reality of history. They fail to see that dreams are also a part of the reality of life, that life without dreams would be unbearable. No change in our way of life would be possible without dreams and dreamers.

For Emma Goldman, her first direct exposure to the constructive revolutionary activity of the Spanish anarchists in 1936 validated her lifetime of effort and especially melted that bitterness she had felt since the authoritarian outcome of the Russian Revolution:[21]

> I cannot possibly go into details about the situation after only three days in Barcelona. I can only say that I feel I have come to my own, to my brave and heroic comrades who are battling on so many fronts and against so many enemies. The most impressive of their achievements so far is the marvelous order that prevails, the work in factories and shops of those I have seen now in the hands of the workers and their organizations. . . . I think it is the first time in history that such stress has been laid on the superior importance of running the machinery of economic and social life as is being done here. And this by the much maligned, chaotic Anarchists, who supposedly have 'no program' and whose philosophy is bent on destruction and ruin. Can you imagine what this means to me to see the attempt made to realize the very ideas I have stressed so passionately since the Russian Revolution. Why . . . it was worth all the travail, all the pain and bitterness of my struggle to have lived to see our comrades at work. I am too overjoyed, too happy to find words to express my exaltation and my admiration for our Spanish comrades.

Some concluding remarks

Guided by revolutionary vision, the present-day movement for social change must criticize and seek eventually to eliminate those conditions of society – in workplace, market, home, school and cultural activity – which repress rational and emotional self-responsibility. At the same time, it must persist *in the present* to maximize that 'liberated space' where people are unrestrained.[22] On the basis of this dual agenda, the Chicago anarchists struggled for the ten-hour work-day in the 1880s. Similarly, Malatesta stated that even the desired social revolution, by opening free realms, would provide merely rough preconditions for the eventual development of anarchist society.

Clearly, progressive liberation of more free space is not an exclusively anarchist strategy. Historically, however, anarchists have been acutely sensitive to ways in which such zones are co-opted for the ultimate ends of existing society. While Pouget praises workers who finally decide to strike, for example, he sees partial (as opposed to general) strikes as mere 'haggling, shabby affairs', nearly always in the long run doomed to defeat.[23] Referring to personal relationships, Emma Goldman likewise states that:[24]

the struggle to maintain my own individuality and freedom was always more important to me than the wildest love affair. You see, I had never trusted love that tends to enslave, fetter and possess. I do not mean to say it was easy to break away when love proved that and nothing else. It was a painful process. It would have been much more so to remain. Always I had to go my way.

Malatesta, in turn, denounces those who seek personal liberation at the expense of others:[25]

There are strong, intelligent, passionate individuals, with strong material or intellectual needs, who finding themselves, by chance, among the oppressed, seek, at all costs, to emancipate themselves and do not resent becoming oppressors. . . . Sometimes, when they are well read, they think of themselves as *supermen*. They are unhampered by scruples; they want 'to live their lives'; they poke fun at the revolution and at every forward-looking aspiration, they want to enjoy life in the present at any cost and at everybody's expense; they would sacrifice the whole of mankind for one hour's 'intensive living'.

In the present-day factory or office, such 'human relations' innovations as respect for different hair-lengths or better lighting conditions or more autonomous work activity can remove certain alienating aspects of the workplace. Yet obviously they do nothing to challenge the premises that govern working conditions. Even the emergence, here and there, of radical forms of workers' control remains still confined by the capitalist political and economic infrastructure, economic competition, linear time consciousness and a consumer orientation.

It is useful here to recall the four dimensions of revolutionary re-energizers. Each dimension provides contexts of greater and lesser potential power. In general it seems that the smaller the potential, the easier it is for a renewing experience to emerge. But as it does, it also risks easier co-optation as an escape valve for the system's survival. Thus, *small*-scale free space, expression of *rage* or *destructive* activity, *passive* enjoyment of *others*' liberation, and *single* realms of freedom are generally easier to achieve, but also are more readily used by the system. By contrast, liberating action on a *large* scale, including *direct constructive* involvement in *several* different realms (cultural, social, political and economic), though most difficult to attain, also holds the greatest guaranteed rewards. Nevertheless, it is also true that *any* liberated areas, however limited, are a challenge to the capitalist order. The challenge lies in their visceral resistance to and struggle against the system and in their offering time and space for potentially less sub-

limated behavior. If those who benefit from such zones are encouraged to understand the *political* nature of this challenge, such achievements *can* provide greater and greater revolutionary momentum. This is especially true if such comprehension exists *before* space is won.

Such zones sustain the energy of militants, in particular, given the political framework they already possess. (Though with the zeal and frustrations of revolutionary struggle, occasional reductionists wrongly proclaim certain single zones as *the* exclusive road to the ultimate goal.) For militants, liberated experiences are reminders; while for the non-activist the initial exposures to freedom, a love relationship, a demo-cratized classroom, a playful workplace or an insurrection may seem quite threatening. Some feel overwhelmed when too many landmarks are destroyed, however oppressive these may be. By contrast, the threat to militants is of another sort. Precisely because energy is re-charged to such a degree, the inconsistencies, collapse or repression of liberated zones is more bitter.[26]

> I have been out of Russia now five months, but my Russian experi-ence will never leave me. The tragedy is too overwhelming to ever get away from me. I wish I could write about just how it impressed me. . . . It is not the events that took place during my two years in Russia which are so difficult to describe; it is much more the effect they have had upon my spirit and the scars they have left upon my soul which I will never, never be able to make known.

Nevertheless, even the present likelihood of only temporary durations of success *can* become part of the movement's wisdom. This is valuable, of course, only if such limits are viewed not as inherent in 'human nature' but rather as the product of social and therefore changeable conditions. Once again, Emma Goldman articulates this point as she seeks to adjust to the fact of the repression of anarchists in Spain by their republican 'allies:'[27]

> Something I have been thinking very deeply about since the May events in Spain. It is whether we Anarchists have not taken the wish for the thought. Whether we have not been too optimistic in our belief that Anarchism had taken root in the masses? The war, the Revolution in Russia and Spain and the utter failure of the masses to stand up against the annihilation in all countries of every vestige of liberty have convinced me that Anarchism even less than any other social idea has not penetrated the minds and hearts of even a sub-stantial minority, let alone the compact mass. . . . In Spain alone has the ground been fertile. But even in Spain the harvest is still small. . . . In our enthusiasm we forgot the natural forces the young, tender

plants will be subjected to, the storm and stress, the drought and winds. . . . We Anarchists imagined our ideas can be realized in one jump, rise from the depths of enslavement and degradation to the very heights of fulfillment, come to full fruition from the hard rocks of the past in Spain. It was our mistake and we are now paying for it in the agony of our bitter disappointment.

. . . I am convinced it will take more than one revolution before our ideas will come to full growth. Until then the steps will be feeble. . . .

Does that mean I have lost faith in Anarchism, or that I think we ought to sit hands folded? Of course not. In point of truth I think now more than ever we must strain every nerve to bring our ideas before the world. . . . However the Spanish revolution will end it has already given us marvelous material to enhance the logic of our ideas.

New wisdom, in such a case, allows the militant and the movement to analyze reasons for failure and propose appropriate correctives for later attempts.

Without denying the significance of rational analysis, anarchists must also sensitize themselves to the range and power of renewing energy sources. Sustained consciousness and activity demands creation of those structures and life-styles within the movement that regularly renew militants with the scope and wonder of the revolutionary vision. Only a movement that is already living the revolution, even if partially, will be capable of assisting non-activists in finding their own liberation. And only when the vast majority of people themselves possess such vision can an enduring anarchist society be established.

Notes

1 The term is used here in the more subtle sense of apprehending 'reality' (see Peter Berger and Thomas Luckmann, *The Social Construction of Reality* (Garden City, New York: Anchor Books, 1967), 66, for one example of such usage). Its more common connotation of accomplishment, as well, is implied in the title of the article and later in the text.

2 Numerous observers have commented on the near-mystical intensity of vision in the strongest anarchist movement historically, that in Spain. See, for example, Gaston Leval, *Collectives in the Spanish Revolution* (Montreal: Black Rose Books, 1976) and Murray Bookchin, *The Spanish Anarchists: The Heroic Years, 1868–1936* (New York: Free Life Editions, 1977) for descriptions by committed anarchist authors themselves.

3 Bakunin letter to Elisée Reclus, February 15, 1875; reproduced in

Sam Dolgoff (ed.), *Bakunin On Anarchy* (New York: Alfred A. Knopf, 1972), 354–5. That Bakunin in the late 1860s and early 1870s had a pre-eminent revolutionary reputation among his contemporaries makes this quotation all the more striking. During this same decade, his inspiration and leadership of the international anarchist movement led to a fundamental clash with Karl Marx in the First International and a subsequent split between the two socialist groups.

4   Emma Goldman letter to Alexander Berkman, January 5, 1935; reproduced in Richard Drinnon and Anna Maria Drinnon (eds), *Nowhere At Home: Letters From Exile of Emma Goldman and Alexander Berkman* (New York: Schocken Books, 1975), 57–8. Emma Goldman emigrated from Russia to the United States in her teens and soon, by the late 1880s, became a devoted and energetic activist in anarchist ranks. Because of her own unmatchable courage and talents as a speaker and writer, she became one of the leading figures in the American anarchist movement. Deported with her close comrade Berkman from the United States, in part because of their anti-conscription propaganda during World War I, she was sent to Russia where she spent the next two years observing directly the realities of Bolshevik ascendence over the revolution. In despair at authoritarian developments, she left Russia (again with Berkman) and remained a permanent exile in Europe, except for short periods in Canada (and the United States again for ninety days in 1934), until her death in 1940.

5   I use the term 'energy' intentionally. *Intellectual* reminders, in the form of rational analysis and ideology, are simply not adequate to restore motivation for sustained activity. Another dimension, affecting deeper levels of the psyche, clearly is needed.

6   Emma Goldman letter to Alexander Berkman, May 15, 1934; reproduced in Drinnon and Drinnon (eds), op. cit., 234.

7   This slogan and the other themes in this sentence which describe the vision of liberated society at its best were articulated most recently on a large scale during the May 1968 upheaval in France. Literature describing and analyzing this period abounds.

8   Abraham H. Maslow, *Toward A Psychology of Being* (Princeton: Van Nostrand, 1962) and *The Farther Reaches of Human Nature* (New York: Viking Press, 1972). In the latter book, Maslow himself specifically acknowledged that the political and economic implication of his 'self-actualization' theory was anarchist society.

9   Joseph J. Cohen, *In Quest of Heaven: The Story of the Sunrise Co-operative Farm Community* (New York: Sunrise History Publishing Committee, 1957), 42. Cohen edited the Yiddish-language anarchist newspaper, *Freie Arbeiter Stimme*, in New York from 1923 to 1932 and was an active figure in the American movement from 1903 until 1946, when he moved abroad.

10 Gustav Landauer, *Ein Weg deutschen Geistes* (Munich, 1916), 15, as quoted in Charles B. Maurer, *Call To Revolution: The Mystical*

Anarchism of Gustav Landauer (Detroit: Wayne State University Press, 1971), 140. Landauer was a leading German anarchist writer, closely involved with progressive literary and artistic circles from the early 1890s to 1919, the date of his murder by right-wing troops suppressing the Bavarian revolution. Unfortunately little known in this country, Landauer heavily influenced, among others, his friend Martin Buber, as acknowledged in the latter's *Paths In Utopia* (Boston: Beacon Press, 1958).

11 Elisée Reclus letter to Victor Buurmans, April 25, 1878; reproduced in Elisée Reclus, *Correspondence*, vol. II (October 1870–July 1889) (Paris: Librairie Schleicher Frères, 1911), 202–03. Reclus was a leading geographer, a friend of Bakunin, and a major French anarchist writer until his death in 1905.

12 The novel, *Der Todesprediger* (*The Preacher of Death*) (1893) is discussed in Maurer, op. cit., 32–3, 74–5.

13 Rudolf Rocker, *The London Years* (London: Robert Anscombe, 1956), 99. (This edition is an abridged English-language translation of the second volume of his autobiography.) Rocker was another pre-eminent figure in the international anarchist movement, best known for his writing, speaking and organizing talents among Jewish workers of London's East End from the turn of the century to World War I and similar efforts among the German working class during the 1920s. Following the Nazi rise to power, Rocker fled to exile, eventually to the United States where he died in 1958.

14 Sébastien Faure, 'Le mouvement en province,' *Le Libertaire*, 31 (June 13–19, 1896). Faure played a major role in the French anarchist movement from the 1890s on, in great part through his steady editorship of *Le Libertaire*, which he founded in 1895. He died in 1942.

15 Emma Goldman, *Living My Life* vol. I, (New York: Dover Publications, 1970 [1931]), 177.

16 Errico Malatesta, in *Pensiero e Volontà* (Rome), July 1, 1926; quoted in Vernon Richards (ed.), *Errico Malatesta: His Life and Ideas* (London: Freedom Press, 1965), 208–09. Malatesta also was the leading figure in the Italian anarchist movement from the 1870s through the 1920s. He died under house arrest during the Mussolini regime in 1932.

17 Rocker, op. cit., 145.

18 Peter Kropotkin, *Memoirs of A Revolutionist* (New York: Dover Publications, 1971 [1899]), 317. After Bakunin's death, the exiled Russian geographer Kropotkin was generally acknowledged to be the most influential anarchist writer until his pro-Allied stand in World War I. Returning to Russia in 1917 after an exile of forty-one years, he died in 1921. His funeral in Petrograd was the occasion of the last open anarchist demonstration permitted by the Bolshevik regime.

19 Emile Pouget, *Père Peinard*, series II, no. 105 (1898). Pouget was active leader of the French anarchist movement during the years of

its greatest influence, from the 1880s to World War I. He died in 1931.

20 Rocker, op. cit., 174.
21 Emma Goldman letter to Stella Ballantine, September 19, 1936 (from the Emma Goldman manuscript collection, New York City Public Library).
22 Malatesta, for one, explicitly proposed such an evolutionary 'education for freedom' strategy (including revolution as an integral part). See his article in *l'Adunata dei Refrattari*, December 26, 1931, and 'The Anarchist Program' which he drafted in 1920, both of which are reproduced in Richards (ed.), op. cit., 179, 195.
23 Pouget, *Père Peinard*, series II, nos. 37 and 38 (1897), and 105 (1898).
24 Emma Goldman letter to Ethel (Mannin?), May 15, 1933 (from the Goldman collection, New York City Public Library).
25 Malatesta in *Volontà*, June 15, 1913, as quoted in Richards (ed.), op. cit., 24–5.
26 Emma Goldman letter to Ellen Kennan, April 9, 1922; reproduced in Drinnon and Drinnon (eds), op. cit., 22–3.
27 Emma Goldman letter to Mollie Steimer and Senia Fleshin, September 1937 (from the Goldman collection, New York City Public Library).

Acknowledgment

Emma Goldman's letters of May 15, 1933, September 19, 1936 and September 1937 are reproduced by permission of Ian Ballantine and the New York Public Library (Emma Goldman Papers, Manuscripts and Archives Division, Astor, Lenox and Tilden Foundations).

David Porter teaches political science at Marlboro College in Vermont. In his graduate research in Algeria, he was strongly influenced by the workers' struggle for genuine self-management in the face of the new post-independence bureaucracy. Other important influences toward anarchism were movement and teaching experiences, student and faculty friends in Montreal and Maryland, and his two children. He is presently preparing an anthology of Emma Goldman's writings on the Spanish revolution.

18 red emma

Peggy Kornegger

'I want freedom, the right to self-expression, everybody's right to
beautiful, radiant things.'   *Emma Goldman*

black and red
you are a flag
flying
black and
red
emma
red emma
you stand out
like
blood
like earth
like black roses
in winter
years of winter
that go on
and on
turning to gray slush
turning to dull brown mud
while you stay
red
emma
red and black
flying
radiant
at the top
of your vision

Peggy Kornegger has been an editor of *The Second Wave* magazine for

two years and was a member of the collective that wrote *Women and Literature: An Annotated Bibliography of Women Writers*. She works part-time as a typist and copy-editor. Currently, she is interested in trying to integrate anarchist lesbian feminism, revolutionary nonviolence, and political spirituality.

Part Five

Anarcha-feminism

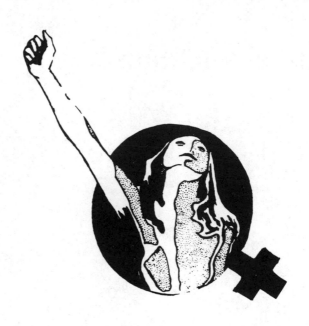

Introduction

People who are familiar with social anarchism and radical feminism are invariably struck by their essential similarity. Both see social and economic inequality as rooted in institutionalized power relationships; both stress the absolute necessity of smashing these power relationships as a precondition for liberation; both work for the realization of personal autonomy and freedom within a context of collective living and working; and both insist on the necessary of total revolution.

Surely, then, one might expect contemporary social anarchist literature to explore the interconnections with radical feminism, and to express a strong commitment to the liberation of women. Even though the bulk of this literature seems to be produced by men (see, for example, the table of contents of this or any other anthology of current anarchist writings), one would expect anarchist men to notice. One would expect their listings of the evils of existing societies to include sexism. But with few exceptions they seem to be completely unaware of the existence of sexist oppression. The state is an unmitigated evil; daily life is a horror; capitalism and state socialism are enemies of freedom; but patriarchy is usually unremarked. (References to Emma Goldman do not begin to make up for the deficit.)

In short, the exploration of the anarcha-feminist connection is being done almost exclusively by women. For the past several years, female anarchists who are feminists have been busy reinventing social anarchism to incorporate the principles and practices of radical feminism.

The articles and manifestoes contained in this section have in common a set of broad themes. First, they affirm the truth of the radical feminist principle, 'the personal is political.' Politics extends far beyond a set of narrowly defined events; it encompasses everything we do in our daily lives, everything that happens to us, and every interpretation we make of these things. All of them have political meanings, because they are integral parts of the culture in which we live. In a society that distinguishes people on the basis of gender, females will have a whole range of experiences that are different from those of males and even

similar experiences will carry different meanings. In a society that makes gender distinctions *and* ties these to superior/inferior status, experiences and the meanings attached to them will serve to keep one group (i.e. women) subordinate to the other. Law, government, education, science, the arts, work, play, living arrangements, language, emotional expression, clothing, sex – our personal experiences with these all have political meanings. Always. There are no exceptions. Of course, many male anarchists have talked about the importance of socialization, the role of education in (de-) forming young children, the sexually repressive character of the traditional family, the way in which authoritarian societies restrict the expression of emotions and abilities, and other examples of the personal as political, but they have seldom extended their analyses to the position of women. It is anarcha-feminists who have done this.

A second theme is the absolute necessity of eroding power as domination, authority and hierarchy. This is central to both anarchist and radical feminist thought. The anarcha-feminist connection is this. Anarchists work to destroy the state, which has the monopoly on 'legitimate' power and authority within a given geographical area. Radical feminists work to end patriarchy – that is, male domination of women through physical force and institutionalized acceptance of masculine authority. To anarcha-feminists, the state and patriarchy are twin aberrations. Thus, to destroy the state is to destroy the major agent of institutionalized patriarchy; to abolish patriarchy is to abolish the state as it now exists. However, anarcha-feminists go a step further than most radical feminists: they caution that the state is by definition always illegitimate. For this reason, feminists should not try to substitute *female* states for the present male states. Some radical feminists argue that a society controlled by women would not have the oppressive features of patriarchal society; anarcha-feminists respond that state control is always evil, because it creates inequities. Anarchism is the only mode of organization that will prevent this from happening.

Because they are anarchists, anarcha-feminists know what radical feminists often have to learn from bitter experience: the development of new forms of organization designed to get rid of hierarchy, authority and power as domination requires structure. Further, the structures must be carefully built and continually nurtured so that the organizations will function smoothly and efficiently, and so that informal elites will not emerge.

A third theme expressed by both radical feminists and anarchists is that each individual must gain control over her life. The fact that this has become a Movement cliché shows how widespread its acceptance now is. Marxists, apolitical dropouts, probably even left-liberals endorse the idea. However, the concept has a particular meaning for radical

feminists and social anarchists: it is an activist orientation (you gain control for yourself, not by sitting back and waiting for it to be handed to you), and autonomy exists within the social context, in a setting of co-operation and mutual aid. In keeping with this perspective, radical feminists and social anarchists have built an impressive number of organizations and networks linking them: media collectives, clinics, printing co-ops, living collectives, alternative schools, anti-profit businesses, and so on.

The organizations built by radical feminists are often developed on anarchist principles – although, as Peggy Kornegger points out in 'Anarchism: The Feminist Connection,' this development is usually intuitive. Now, the intuitive needs to be made conscious, for the linkage between social anarchism and radical feminism will broaden the theory and practice of both.

Perhaps one reason why the similarities stressed in the articles reprinted here are not more obvious to people (including both radical feminists and social anarchists) is that both feminism and anarchism have been almost unknown, too disreputable or alien or frightening to qualify as models of dissent for most residents of England or the United States. Peggy Kornegger said of her 'education' in a small Illinois high school: 'The "his-story" of *man*kind (white) had meant just that; as a woman I was relegated to a vicarious existence. As an anarchist I had no existence at all. A whole chunk of the past (and thus possibilities for the future) had been kept from me.'

In the mid-1970s anarcha-feminists began the attempt to rediscover the rich anarchist tradition and to combine it with contemporary radical feminism to produce models for the present and future. Anarcha-feminists associated with the Chicago mimeographed newsletter, *Siren*, and with the Champaign-Urbana (Illinois) Social Revolutionary Anarchist Federation (SRAF) issued manifestoes declaring 'Who We Are' and calling 'For a General Contestation.'

> From the bedroom to society as a whole, the task of the women's movement *as a liberation movement* is to reject the *totality* of domination and exploitation perpetuated by the male-dominated, capitalist order. ['For a General Contestation']

> We consider Anarcho-Feminism to be the ultimate and necessary radical stance at this time in world history, far more radical than any form of Marxism. ['Who We Are']

Peggy Kornegger ('Anarchism: The Feminist Connection'), Marian Leighton ('Anarcho-Feminism') and Carol Ehrlich ('Socialism, Anarchism, and Feminism') carefully draw the theoretical and organizational

235

connections between feminism and anarchism. Although writings in the area are still sparse (especially in comparison with the literature of socialist feminism), discussion and debate are increasing. With the infusion of anarcha-feminist ideas, perhaps anarchist groups will stop being, as Leighton put it, 'havens of arrogant and isolated men prattling their rhetoric for their own dubious benefit;' and perhaps feminists will see that social anarchist theory makes better sense than does alliance with Marxist socialists, matriarchs, or spirituality-trippers.

After all, anarchists were socialists long before Marxists expropriated the term for their own exclusive and dubious use. Anarcha-feminists don't want to relinquish socialism to authoritarians, and they refuse to hand anarchism over to men who are blind to their own sexism. What do they want? Kornegger answers: 'What we ask is nothing less than total revolution.'

19 Anarchism: the feminist connection *

Peggy Kornegger

Eleven years ago, when I was in a small town Illinois high school, I had never heard of the word 'anarchism' at all. The closest I came to it was knowing that anarchy meant 'chaos.' As for socialism and communism, my history classes somehow conveyed the message that there was no difference between them and fascism, a word that brought to mind Hitler, concentration camps, and all kinds of horrible things which never happened in a free country like ours. I was subtly being taught to swallow the bland pablum of traditional American politics: moderation, compromise, fence-straddling.

I learned the lesson well: it took me years to recognize the bias and distortion which had shaped my entire 'education.' The 'his-story' of *man*kind (white) had meant just that; as a woman I was relegated to a vicarious existence. As an anarchist I had no existence at all. A whole chunk of the past (and thus possibilities for the future) had been kept from me. Only recently did I discover that many of my disconnected political impulses and inclinations shared a common framework – that is, the anarchist or libertarian tradition of thought. It was like suddenly seeing red after years of colorblind grays.

Emma Goldman furnished me with my first definition of anarchism:[1]

> Anarchism, then, really stands for the liberation of the human mind from the dominion of religion; the liberation of the human body from the dominion of property; liberation from the shackles and restraint of government. Anarchism stands for a social order based on the free grouping of individuals for the purpose of producing real social wealth, an order that will guarantee to every human being free access to the earth and full enjoyment of the necessities of life, according to individual desires, tastes, and inclinations.

* Excerpted from a longer article that appeared in *The Second Wave*, vol. 4, no. 1, Spring 1975.

Soon, I started making mental connections between anarchism and radical feminism. It became very important to me to write down some of the perceptions in this area as a way of communicating to others the excitement I felt about anarcha-feminism. It seems crucial that we share our visions with one another in order to break down some of the barriers that misunderstanding and splinterism raise between us. Although I call myself an anarcha-feminist, this definition can easily include socialism, communism, cultural feminism, lesbian separatism, or any of a dozen other political labels. As Su Negrin writes: 'No political umbrella can cover all my needs.'[2] We may have more in common than we think we do. While I am writing here about my own reactions and perceptions, I don't see either my life or thoughts as separate from those of other women. In fact, one of my strongest convictions regarding the women's movement is that we *do* share an incredible commonality of vision.

What does anarchism really mean?

Anarchism has been maligned and misinterpreted for so long that maybe the most important thing to begin with is an explanation of what it is and isn't. Probably the most prevalent stereotype of the anarchist is a malevolent-looking man hiding a lighted bomb beneath a black cape, ready to destroy or assassinate everything and everybody in his path. This image engenders fear and revulsion in most people, regardless of their politics; consequently, anarchism is dismissed as ugly, violent, and extreme. Another misconception is the anarchist as impractical idealist, dealing in useless, utopian abstractions and out of touch with concrete reality. The result: anarchism is once again dismissed, this time as an 'impossible dream.'

Neither of these images is accurate (though there have been both anarchist assassins and idealists – as is the case in many political movements, left and right). What *is* accurate depends, of course, on one's frame of reference. There are different kinds of anarchists, just as there are different kinds of socialists. What I will talk about here is communist-anarchism, which I see as virtually identical to libertarian (i.e. non-authoritarian) socialism. Labels can be terribly confusing, so in hopes of clarifying the term, I'll define anarchism using three major principles (each of which I believe is related to a radical feminist analysis of society – more on that later):

(1) *Belief in the abolition of authority, hierarchy, government.* Anarchists call for the *dissolution* (rather than the seizure) *of power* – of human over human, of state over community. Whereas many socialists call for a working-class government and an eventual 'withering away of the state,' anarchists believe that the means create the ends, that a

strong state becomes self-perpetuating. The only way to achieve anarch-ism (according to anarchist theory) is through the creation of co-operative, anti-authoritarian forms. To separate the process from the goals of revolution is to insure the perpetuation of oppressive structure and style.

(2) *Belief in both individuality and collectivity.* Individuality is not incompatible with communist thought. A distinction must be made though, between 'rugged individualism,' which fosters competition and a disregard for the needs of others, and true individuality, which implies freedom without infringement on others' freedom. Specifically, in terms of social and political organization, this means balancing individual initiative with collective action through the creation of structures which enable decision-making to rest in the hands of all those in a group, community, or factory, not in the hands of 'representatives' or 'leaders.' It means co-ordination and action via a non-hierarchical network (overlapping circles rather than a pyramid) of small groups or communities. Finally, it means that successful revolution involves unmanipulated, autonomous individuals and groups working together to take 'direct, unmediated control of society and of their own lives.'[3]

(3) *Belief in both spontaneity and organization.* Anarchists have long been accused of advocating chaos. Most people in fact believe that anarchism is a synonym for disorder, confusion, violence. This is a total misrepresentation of what anarchism stands for. Anarchists don't deny the necessity of organization; they only claim that it must come from below, not above, from within rather than from without. Externally imposed structure or rigid rules which foster manipulation and passivity are the most dangerous forms a so-called 'revolution' can take. No one can dictate the exact shape of the future. Spontaneous action within the context of a specific situation is necessary if we are going to create a society which responds to the changing needs of changing individuals and groups. Anarchists believe in fluid forms: small-scale participatory democracy in conjunction with large-scale collective co-operation and co-ordination (without loss of individual initiative).

Anarchism and the women's movement

The development of sisterhood is a unique threat, for it is directed against the basic social and psychic model of hierarchy and domin-ation . . .   [*Mary Daly*[4]]

All across the country, independent groups of women began function-ing without the structure, leaders, and other factotums of the male

239

left, creating independently and simultaneously, organizations similar to those of anarchists of many decades and locales. No accident, either.   [*Cathy Levine*[5]]

Anarchist men have been little better than males everywhere in their subjection of women.[6] Thus the absolute necessity of a *feminist* anarchist revolution. Otherwise the very principles on which anarchism is based become utter hypocrisy.

The current women's movement and a radical feminist analysis of society have contributed much to libertarian thought. In fact, it is my contention that feminists have been unconscious anarchists in both theory and practice for years. We now need to become *consciously* aware of the connections between anarchism and feminism and use that framework for our thoughts and actions. We have to be able to see very clearly where we want to go and how to get there. In order to be more effective, in order to create the future we sense is possible, we must realize that what we want is not change but total *transformation*.

The radical feminist perspective is almost pure anarchism. The basic theory postulates the nuclear family as the basis for all authoritarian systems. The lesson the child learns, from father to teacher to boss to God, is to OBEY the great anonymous voice of Authority. To graduate from childhood to adulthood is to become a fully-fledged automaton, incapable of questioning or even thinking clearly. We pass into middle-America, believing everything we are told and numbly accepting the destruction of life all around us.

What feminists are dealing with is a mind-fucking process – the male domineering attitude toward the external world allowing only subject-to-object relationships. Traditional male politics reduces humans to object status and then dominates and manipulates them for abstract 'goals.' Women on the other hand, are trying to develop a consciousness of 'Other' in all areas. We see subject-to-subject relationships as not only desirable but necessary. (Many of us have chosen to work with and love only women for just this reason – those kinds of relationships are so much more possible.) Together we are working to expand our empathy and understanding of other living things and to identify with those entities outside of ourselves, rather than objectifying and manipulating them. At this point, a respect for all life is a prerequisite for our very survival.

Radical feminist theory also criticizes male hierarchical thought patterns – in which rationality dominates sensuality, mind dominates intuition, and persistent splits and polarities (active/passive, child/adult, sane/insane, work/play, spontaneity/organization) alienate us from the mind-body experience as a whole and the continuum of human experience. Women are attempting to get rid of these splits, to live in har-

mony with the universe as whole, integrated humans dedicated to the collective healing of our individual wounds and schisms.

In actual practice within the women's movement, feminists have had both success and failure in abolishing hierarchy and domination. I believe that women frequently speak and act as 'intuitive' anarchists; that is we *approach*, or *verge on*, a complete denial of all patriarchal thought and organization. That approach, however, is blocked by the powerful and insidious forms which patriarchy takes – in our minds and in our relationships with one another. Living within and being conditioned by an authoritarian society often prevents us from making that all-important connection between feminism and anarchism. When we say we are fighting the patriarchy, it isn't always clear to all of us that that means fighting *all* hierarchy, *all* leadership, *all* government, and the very idea of authority itself. Our impulses toward collective work and small leaderless groups have been anarchistic, but in most cases we haven't *called* them by that name. And that is important, because an understanding of feminism *as* anarchism could springboard women out of reformism and stop-gap measures into a revolutionary confrontation with the basic nature of authoritarian politics.

If we want to 'bring down the patriarchy,' we need to talk about anarchism, to know exactly what it means, and to use that framework to transform ourselves and the structure of our daily lives. Feminism doesn't mean female corporate power or a woman President; it means *no* corporate power and *no* Presidents. The Equal Rights Amendment will not transform society; it only gives women the 'right' to plug into a hierarchical economy. Challenging sexism means challenging *all* hierarchy – economic, political, and personal. And that means an anarcha-feminist revolution.

Specifically, when have feminists been anarchistic, and when have we stopped short? As the second wave of feminism spread across the country in the late 1960s, the forms which women's groups took frequently reflected an unspoken libertarian consciousness. In rebellion against the competitive power games, impersonal hierarchy, and mass organization tactics of male politics, women broke off into small, leaderless, consciousness-raising (C-R) groups, which dealt with personal issues in our daily lives. Face-to-face, we attempted to get at the root cause of our oppression by sharing our hitherto unvalued perceptions and experiences. We learned from each other that politics is not 'out there' but in our minds and bodies and between individuals. Personal relationships could and did oppress us as a political class. Our misery and self-hatred were a direct result of male domination – in home, street, job, and political organization.

So, in many unconnected areas of the US, C-R groups developed as a spontaneous, direct (re)action to patriarchal forms. The emphasis on

the small group as a basic organizational unit, on the personal and political, on anti-authoritarianism, and on spontaneous direct action was essentially anarchistic. The structure of women's groups bore a striking resemblance to that of anarchist affinity groups within anarcho-syndicalist unions in Spain, France, and many other countries. Yet, we had not called ourselves anarchists and consciously organized around anarchist principles. At the time, we did not even have an underground network of communication and idea-and-skill sharing. Before the women's movement was more than a handful of isolated groups groping in the dark toward answers, anarchism as an unspecified idea existed in our minds.

I believe that this puts women in the unique position of being the bearers of a subsurface anarchist consciousness which, if articulated and concretized, can take us further than any previous group toward the achievement of total revolution. Women's intuitive anarchism, if sharpened and clarified, is an incredible leap foward (or beyond) in the struggle for human liberation. Radical feminist theory hails feminism as the ultimate revolution. This is true if, and only if, we recognize and claim our anarchist roots. At the point where we fail to see the feminist connection to anarchism, we stop short of revolution and become trapped in 'ye olde male political rut.' It is time to stop groping in the darkness and see what we have done and are doing in the context of where we want to ultimately be.

C-R groups were a good beginning, but they often got so bogged down in talking about personal problems that they failed to make the jump to direct action and political confrontation. Groups that did organize around a specific issue or project sometimes found that the 'tyranny of structurelessness' could be as destructive as the 'tyranny of tyranny.'[7] The failure to blend organization with spontaneity frequently caused the emergence of those with more skills or personal charisma as leaders. The resentment and frustration felt by those who found themselves following sparked in-fighting, guilt-tripping, and power struggles. Too often this ended in either total ineffectiveness or a backlash adherence to 'what we need is more structure' (in the old male up/down sense of the word).

Once again, I think that what was missing was a verbalized anarchist analysis. Organization does not have to stifle spontaneity or follow hierarchical patterns. The women's groups or projects which have been the most successful are those which experimented with various fluid structures: the rotation of tasks and chairpersons, sharing of all skills, equal access to information and resources, non-monopolized decision-making, and time slots for discussion of group dynamics. This latter structural element is important because it involves a continued effort on the part of group members to watch for 'creeping power politics.'

If women are verbally committing themselves to collective work, this requires a real struggle to unlearn passivity (to eliminate 'followers') and to share special skills or knowledge (to avoid 'leaders'). This doesn't mean that we cannot be inspired by one another's words and lives; strong actions by strong individuals can be contagious and thus important. But we must be careful not to slip into old behavior patterns.

On the positive side, the emerging structure of the women's movement in the last few years has generally followed an anarchistic pattern of small project-oriented groups continually weaving an underground network of communication and collective action around specific issues. Partial success at leader/'star' avoidance and the diffusion of small action projects (Rape Crisis Centers, Women's Health Collectives) across the country have made it extremely difficult for the women's movement to be pinned down to one person or group. Feminism is a many-headed monster which cannot be destroyed by singular decapitation. We spread and grow in ways that are incomprehensible to a hierarchical mentality.

This is not, however, to underestimate the immense power of the Enemy. The most treacherous form this power can take is co-optation, which feeds on any short-sighted unanarchistic view of feminism as mere 'social change.' To think of sexism as an evil which can be eradicated by female participation in the way things are is to insure the continuation of domination and oppression. 'Feminist' capitalism is a contradiction in terms. When we establish women's credit unions, restaurants, bookstores, etc., we must be clear that we are doing so for our own survival, for the purpose of creating a counter-system whose processes contradict and challenge competition, profit-making, and all forms of economic oppression. We must be committed to 'living on the boundaries,'[8] to anti-capitalist, non-consumption values. What we want is neither integration nor a *coup d'etat* which would 'transfer power from one set of boys to another set of boys.'[9] What we ask is nothing less than total revolution, revolution whose forms invest a future untainted by inequity, domination, or disrespect for individual variation – in short, feminist–anarchist revolution. I believe that women have known all along how to move in the direction of human liberation; we only need to shake off lingering male political forms and dictums and focus on our own anarchistic female analysis.

Where do we go from here? making utopia real

'Ah, your vision is romantic bullshit, soppy religiosity, flimsy idealism.' 'You're into poetry because you can't deliver concrete details.' So says the little voice in the back of my (your?) head.

243

But the front of my head knows that if you were here next to me,
we could talk. And that in our talk would come (concrete, detailed)
descriptions of how such and such might happen, how this or that
would be resolved. What my vision really lacks is concrete, detailed
human bodies. Then it wouldn't be a flimsy vision, it would be a
fleshy reality.   [*Su Negrin*[10]]

Instead of getting discouraged and isolated now, we should be in our
small groups – discussing, planning, creating, and making trouble . . .
we should always be actively engaging in and creating feminist
activity, because we all thrive on it; in the absence of [it] , women
take tranquilizers, go insane, and commit suicide.   [*Cathy Levine*[11]]

Those of us who lived through the excitement of sit-ins, marches,
student strikes, demonstrations, and *revolution now* in the sixties may
find ourselves disillusioned and downright cynical about anything
happening in the seventies. Giving up or in ('open' marriage? hip
capitalism? the Guru Maharaji?) seems easier than facing the prospect
of decades of struggle and maybe even ultimate failure. At this point,
we lack an overall framework to see the process of revolution in. Without it, we are doomed to deadended, isolated struggle or the individual
solution. The kind of framework, or coming-together-point, that
anarcha-feminism provides would appear to be a prerequisite for any
sustained effort to reach utopian goals. True revolution is 'neither an
accidental happening nor a coup d'etat artificially engineered from
above.'[12] It takes years of preparation: sharing of ideas and information,
changes in consciousness and behavior, and the creation of political and
economic alternatives to capitalist, hierarchical structures. It takes
spontaneous direct action on the part of autonomous individuals through
collective political confrontation. It is important to 'free your mind'
and your personal life, but it is not sufficient. Liberation is not an
insular experience; it occurs in conjunction with other human beings.
There are no individual 'liberated women.'

So, what I'm talking about is a *long-term process*, a series of actions
in which we unlearn passivity and learn to take control over our own
lives. I am talking about a 'hollowing out' of the present system through
the formation of mental and physical (concrete) alternatives to the
way things are. The romantic image of a small band of armed guerrillas
overthrowing the US Government is obsolete (as is all male politics)
and basically irrelevant to this conception of revolution. We would be
squashed if we tried it. Besides, as the poster says, 'What we want is not
the overthrow of the government, but a situation in which it gets lost in
the shuffle.' Whether armed resistance will be necessary at some point is
open to debate. The anarchist principle of 'means create ends' seems to

imply pacifism, but the power of the state is so great that it is difficult to be absolute about nonviolence.

The actual tactics of preparation are things that we have been involved with for a long time. We need to continue and develop them further. I see them as functioning on three levels: (1) 'educational' (sharing of ideas, experiences); (2) economic/political; and (3) personal/political.

'Education' has a rather condescending ring to it, but I don't mean 'bringing the word to the masses' or guilt-tripping individuals into prescribed ways of being. I'm talking about the many methods we have developed for sharing our lives with one another – from writing (our network of feminist publications), study groups, and women's radio and TV shows to demonstrations, marches, and street theater. The mass media would seem to be a particularly important area for revolutionary communication and influence – just think of how our own lives were *mis*-shaped by radio and TV.[13] Seen in isolation, these things might seem ineffectual, but people *do* change from writing, reading, talking, and listening to each other, as well as from active participation in political movements. Going out into the streets together shatters passivity and creates a spirit of communal effort and life energy which can help sustain *and* transform us. My own transformation from all-American-girl to anarcha-feminist was brought about by a decade of reading, discussion, and involvement with many kinds of people and politics – from the Midwest to the West and East Coasts. My experiences may in some ways be unique, but they are not, I think, extraordinary. In many, many places in this country, people are slowly beginning to question the way they were conditioned to acceptance and passivity. God and government are not the ultimate authorities they once were. This is not to minimize the extent of the power of church and state, but rather to emphasize that seemingly inconsequential changes in thought and behavior, when solidified in collective action, constitute a real challenge to the patriarchy.

Economic/political tactics fall into the realm of direct action and 'purposeful illegality' (Daniel Guerin's term). Anarcho-syndicalism specifies three major modes of direct action: sabotage, strike, and boycott. Sabotage means 'obstructing by every possible method, the regular process of production.'[14] More and more frequently, sabotage is practiced by people unconsciously influenced by changing societal values. For example, systematic absenteeism is carried out by both blue- and white-collar workers. Defying employers can be done as subtly as the 'slowdown' or as blatantly as the 'fuck-up.' Doing as little work as possible as slowly as possible is common employee practice, as is messing up the actual work process (often as a union tactic during a strike). Witness habitual misfiling or loss of 'important papers' by

secretaries, or the continual switching of destination placards on trains during the 1967 railroad strike in Italy.

Sabotage tactics can be used to make strikes much more effective. The strike itself is the workers' most important weapon. Any individual strike has the potential of paralyzing the system if it spreads to other industries and becomes a general strike. Total social revolution is then only a step away. Of course, the general strike must have as its ultimate goal workers' self-management (as well as a clear sense of how to achieve and hold on to it), or the revolution will be still-born (as in France, 1968).

The boycott can also be a powerful strike or union strategy (e.g. the boycott of non-union grapes, lettuce, and wines, and of Farah pants). In addition, it can be used to force economic and social changes. Refusal to vote, to pay war taxes, or to participate in capitalist competition and over-consumption are all important actions when coupled with support of alternative, non-profit structures (food co-ops, health and law collectives, recycled clothing and book stores, free schools, etc.). Consumerism is one of the main strongholds of capitalism. To boycott buying itself (especially products geared to obsolescence and those offensively advertised) is a tactic that has the power to change the 'quality of everyday life.' Refusal to vote is often practiced out of despair of passivity rather than as a conscious political statement against a pseudo-democracy where power and money elect a political elite. Non-voting can mean something other than silent consent if we are simultaneously participating in the creation of genuine democratic forms in an alternative network of anarchist affinity groups.

This takes us to the third area – personal/political, which is of course vitally connected to the other two. The anarchist affinity group has long been a revolutionary organizational structure. In anarcho-syndicalist unions, they functioned as training grounds for workers' self-management. They can be temporary groupings of individuals for a specific short-term goal, more 'permanent' work collectives (as an alternative to professionalism and career elitism), or living collectives where individuals learn how to rid themselves of domination or possessiveness in their one-to-one relationships. Potentially, anarchist affinity groups are the base on which we can build a new libertarian, non-hierarchical society. The way we live and work changes the way we think and perceive (and vice versa), and when changes in consciousness become changes in action and behaviour, the revolution has begun.

Making Utopia real involves many levels of struggle. In addition to specific tactics which can be constantly developed and changed, we need political tenacity: the strength and ability to see beyond the present to a joyous, revolutionary future. To get from here to there requires more than a leap of faith. It demands of each of us a day-to-day, long-range commitment to possibility and direct action.

The transformation of the future

> The creation of female culture is as pervasive a process as we can
> imagine, for it is participation in a vision which is continually un-
> folding anew in everything from our talks with friends, to meat
> boycotts, to taking over storefronts for child care centers, to making
> love with a sister. It is revelatory, undefinable, except as a process of
> change. Women's culture is all of us exorcising, naming, creating
> toward the vision of harmony with ourselves, each other, and our
> sister earth. In the last ten years our having come faster and closer
> than ever before in the history of the patriarchy to overturning its
> power . . . is cause for exhilarant hope – wild, contagious, uncon-
> querable, crazy hope! . . . The hope, the winning of life over death,
> despair and meaninglessness is everywhere I look now – like talis-
> women of the faith in womanvision. . . .   [*Laurel*[15]]

I used to think that if the revolution didn't happen tomorrow, we
would all be doomed to a catastrophic (or at least, catatonic) fate. I
don't believe anymore that that is necessarily true. In fact, I don't
even believe in that kind of before-and-after revolution, and I think we
set ourselves up for failure and despair by thinking of it in those terms.
I *do* believe that what we all need, what we absolutely require, in order
to continue struggling (in spite of the oppression of our daily lives) is
hope, that is, a vision of the future so beautiful and so powerful that it
pulls us steadily forward in a bottom-up creation of an inner and outer
world both habitable and self-fulfilling for *all*. (And, by self-fulfilling I
mean not only in terms of survival needs (sufficient food, clothing,
shelter, etc.) but psychological needs as well (e.g., a non-oppressive
environment which fosters total freedom of choice before specific,
concretely possible alternatives).) I believe that that hope exists – that
it is in Laurel's 'womanvison,' in Mary Daly's 'existengial courage'[16]
and in anarcha-feminism. Our different voices describe the same dream,
and 'only the dream can shatter stone that blocks our mouths.'[17] As we
speak, we change, and as we change, we transform ourselves and the
future simultaneously.

It *is* true that there is no solution, individual or otherwise, *in this
society.*[18] But if we can only balance this rather depressing knowledge
with an awareness of the radical metamorphoses we have experienced –
in our consciousness and in our lives – then perhaps we can have the
courage to continue to create what we dream is possible. Obviously, it
is not easy to face daily oppression and still continue to hope. But *it is
our only chance.* If we abandon hope (the ability to see connections, to
dream the present into the future), then we have already lost. Hope is
woman's most powerful revolutionary tool; it is what we give each

other every time we share our lives, our work, and our love. It pulls us forward out of self-hatred, self-blame, and the fatalism which keeps us prisoners in separate cells. If we surrender to depression and despair now, we are accepting the inevitability of authoritarian politics and patriarchal domination ('Despair is the worst betrayal, the coldest seduction: to believe at last that the enemy will prevail.'[19] - Marge Piercy). We must not let our pain and anger fade into hopelessness or short-sighted semi-'solutions.' Nothing we can do is enough, but on the other hand, those 'small changes' we make in our minds, in our lives, in one another's lives, are not totally futile and ineffectual. It takes a long time to make a revolution: it is something that one both prepares for and lives now. The transformation of the future will not be instantaneous, but it can be *total* . . . a continuum of thought and action, individuality and collectivity, spontaneity and organization, stretching from what is to what can be.

Anarchism provides a framework for this transformation. It is a vision, a dream, a possibility which becomes 'real' as we live it. Feminism is the connection that links anarchism to the future. When we finally see that connection clearly, when we hold to that vision, when we refuse to be raped of that *hope*, we will be stepping over the edge of nothingness into a being now just barely imaginable. The womanvision that is anarcha-feminism has been carried inside our women's bodies for centuries. 'It will be an ongoing struggle in each of us, to birth this vision,'[20] but *we must do it*. We must 'ride our anger like elephants into battle':[21]

> We are sleepwalkers troubled by nightmare flashes,
> In locked wards we closet our vision, renouncing. . . .
> Only when we break the mirror and climb into our vision,
> Only when we are the wind together streaming and singing,
> Only in the dream we become with our bones for spears,
>   we are real at last
>   and wake.

Notes

1 Emma Goldman, 'Anarchism: What It Really Stands For,' *Red Emma Speaks* (Vintage Books, 1972), 59.
2 Su Negrin, *Begin at Start* (Times Change Press, 1972), 128.
3 Murray Bookchin, 'On Spontaneity and Organization,' *Liberation*, March 1972, 6.
4 Mary Daly, *Beyond God the Father* (Beacon Press, 1973), 133.
5 Cathy Levine, 'The Tyranny of Tyranny,' *Black Rose* 1, 56.
6 Temma Kaplan of the UCLA history department has done consid-

erable research on women's anarchist groups (esp. 'Mujeres Liberes') in the Spanish Revolution.

7 See Joreen's 'The Tyranny of Structurelessness,' *Second Wave*, vol. 2 no. 1, and Cathy Levine's 'The Tyranny of Tyranny,' op. cit.
8 Daly, op. cit., 55.
9 Robin Morgan, speech at Boston College, Boston, Mass., November, 1973.
10 Negrin, op. cit., 171.
11 Levine, op. cit., 50.
12 Dolgoff ed., *The Anarchist Collectives* (Free Life, 1974), 19.
13 The Cohn-Bendits state that one major mistake in Paris 1968 was the failure to take complete control of the media, especially the radio and TV.
14 Goldman, 'Syndicalism: Its Theory and Practice,' *Red Emma Speaks*, 71.
15 Laurel, 'Toward a Woman Vision,' *Amazon Quarterly*, vol. 1, issue 2, 40.
16 Daly, op. cit., 23.
17 Marge Piercy, 'Provocation of the Dream.'
18 Fran Taylor, 'A Depressing Discourse on Romance, the Individual Solution, and Related Misfortunes,' *Second Wave*, vol. 3., no. 4.
19 Marge Piercy, 'Laying Down the Tower,' *To Be of Use* (Doubleday, 1973), 88.
20 Laurel, op. cit., 40.
21 Piercy, op. cit.

20 For a general contestation!*

Champaign-Urbana SRAF

From the bedroom to society as a whole, the task of the women's movement *as a liberation movement* is to reject the *totality* of domination and exploitation perpetuated by the male-dominated, capitalist order. The strength of the women's movement is its emerging understanding that this rejection must include a radical critique of daily life and a rejection of its negative features (i.e. almost everything). We must reject the reduction of social relations to commodity relations, of creative social relations to passive consumption, of total revolution to participation in our own alienation. We must come to understand what is subversive about love and what is positive in the refusal of constraints. Finally, as proletarians, we must create new forms of organization which shatter the chains of authority that binds us to our past. These new forms of organization (whose preliminary emergences include Kronstadt, 1921; Italy in the early 1920s; Spain, 1936; Hungary, 1956; and France, 1968), inside and outside the workplace, must abolish the production and corollary consumption of useless commodities; must seize, transform, and operate the productive network of society to make it responsive to actual human needs; must transform the lives of their participants so that they are no longer passive 'spectators' but active creators of new life and new values; and, finally, must extend their developing and evolving forms in increasingly wider circles.

---

* Excerpted from a leaflet published by the Champaign-Urbana (Illinois) Social Revolutionary Anarchist Federation, probably 1974.

21 Who we are: the anarcho-feminist manifesto*

We are dedicated to extremism in the cause of liberty.

We consider anarcho-feminism to be the ultimate and necessary radical stance at this time in world history, far more radical than any form of Marxism.

We believe that a women's revolutionary movement must not mimic but destroy all vestiges of the male-dominated power structure, up to and including the apex of that power structure, the state itself – with its whole ancient and dismal apparatus of jails, armies and armed robbery (taxation); with all of its murder; with all of its grotesque and repressive legislative and military attempts, internal and external, to interfere with people's private lives and freely chosen co-operative ventures.

The world obviously cannot survive many more decades of rule by gangs of armed males calling themselves governments. The situation is insane, ridiculous and even suicidal. Whatever its varying forms of justifications, the armed state is what is threatening all of our lives at present. The state, by its inherent nature, is really incapable of reform. True socialism, peace and plenty for all can be achieved only by people themselves, not by 'representatives,' especially 'representatives' ready and able to turn guns on all who do not comply with state directives. As to how we proceed against the pathological state structure, the best word is outgrow rather than overthrow. This process entails, among other things, a tremendous thrust of education and communication among all peoples. The intelligence of womankind has at last been brought to bear on such oppressive male inventions as the church and the legal family; it must now be brought to re-evaluate the ultimate stronghold of male domination, the state.

While we recognize important differences in the rival systems, our analysis of the evils of the state must extend to both its communist

* First published by *Siren, a Journal of Anarcho-Feminism*, Chicago, Illinois, in their first mimeographed issue in 1971. The manifesto was presumably written by the editors.

and capitalist versions.

We intend to put to the test the concept of freedom of expression, which we trust will be incorporated in the ideology of the coming Socialist Sisterhood which is destined to play a determining role in the future of the race, if there really is to be a future.

We are all socialists. We refuse to give up this pre-Marxist term which has been used as a synonym by many anarchist thinkers. Another synonym for anarchism is libertarian socialism, as opposed to statist and authoritarian varieties. Anarchism (for the Greek *anarchos* – without a ruler) is the affirmation of human freedom and dignity expressed in the negative, cautionary term signifying that no person should rule or dominate another person by force or threat of force. Anarchism indicates what people should not do to one another. Socialism, on the other hand, means all the groovy things people can do and build together, once they are able to combine efforts and resources on the basis of common interest, rationality and creativity.

We love our Marxist sisters and all our sisters everywhere, and have no interest in disassociating ourselves from their constructive struggles. However, we reserve the right to criticize their politics when we feel that they are obsolete or irrelevant or inimical to the welfare of woman-kind.

As anarcho-feminists, we aspire to have the courage to question and challenge absolutely everything – including, when it proves necessary, our own assumptions.

22 Anarcho-feminism*

Marian Leighton

There is general agreement among women that we have gone about as far as spontaneity and gut level reactions to our oppression can take us. Many women in many groups are self-consciously attempting to develop a well-thought-out and painstakingly analyzed theory of women's oppression, a theory capable of leading the way in developing strategic priorities in the women's struggle. This article is a preliminary offering to relate several aspects of anarchist theory to organizational preferences shown both historically and contemporarily by the women's movement.

To date, within feminist theory, most work has tended to concentrate upon definition of and analysis of exactly what constitutes women's work, her productive material contributions to society. The principal technique has been the application of and further extensions of Marxist analytical categories, as is to be expected. This is very important work since the bulk of feminist literature has been narrative and descriptive rather than systematically analytical. I think I should make clear at the very beginning that I do not believe the classical Marx/Bakunin or Lenin/Goldman dichotomy applies to the feminist analysis of 'women and work.' The literatures produced thus far by James, Dalla Costa, Mitchell, and Rowbotham are not narrowly dogmatic or opportunistic in the tradition of Marxist/Leninist/Trotskyist sect groups; rather they are exploratory and utilize Marxist analysis in a way that is creatively consistent with the best and intellectually most rigorous of the Marxist approaches. 'To ask feminist questions to receive Marxist answers' is not antithetical, to my way of thinking, to an anarcho-feminist critique of society.

I do feel, however, that in order to develop the most far-reaching and consequently the most transformative feminist theory it is necessary to develop a technique capable of analyzing the psycho-social roots of

* This is the first half of an article entitled 'Anarcho-feminism and Louise Michel,' originally published in *Black Rose: A Journal of Contemporary Anarchism,* no. 1, 1974.

253

the female self-image that serves to reinforce the political and social inequities.

In this country, feminists aware of the anarchist tradition of radicalism early articulated their awareness of certain theoretical and organizational preferences within the women's movement that are clearly anarchist, such as preference for the small group structure, distrust of hierarchically organized groups, distrust of leader figures and leadership positions, and an acceptance of federalized group networks, rather than of centralized organizations. (See Sue Katz in the 'Furies,' an anarchist answer to Rita Mae Brown; Marian Leighton and Cathy Levine, 'Blood of the Flower;' and Arlene Meyer, 'Siren,' for an anarcho-feminist manifesto.)

Is radical feminism inherently anarchist in the above terms? Have revolutionary women's organizations a tradition, perhaps even older than we yet know, that emphasizes voluntaristic creation of groups, mutual aid and co-operation among such groups, a stress upon consciousness-raising at the lowest levels of society as the only true prelude to total revolution, federalized distribution of power among neighborhood groups, and a negative valuation of centralized power-wielding agencies? If such a tradition exists in women's history, from where arise the psycho-social roots for such a concept of one's position in society? How does this relate to positive or creative leadership roles for individual women in the forefront of theoretical articulation? Most importantly, perhaps, how realistic is the anarchist vision of feminists (the oft-repeated criticism of anarchism as beautiful but impossibly utopian)?

In order to provide first steps to answering some of the above questions, I must first make clear what aspects of anarchist theory are particularly applicable to the radical feminist experience and in what areas I feel the anarchist critique offers the most hopeful possibilities in innovative theoretical contributions.

The anarchist tradition

Before setting out to chart a relationship between revolutionary feminism and anarchism, it is imperative that I attempt to state as succinctly as possible just what the chameleon-like term 'anarchism,' as here used, encompasses. Within the socialist movement, anarchism – as old as Marxism – has always existed as an alternate tradition to authoritarian socialism and its accompanying evils, vanguardist manipulation and pseudo-scientific dogmatism. Generally, the anarchist tradition has stressed the need for the total identification of means with ends. In specific structural terms, the anarchist critique of authoritarian socialist

theory has focused upon the incompatibility of vanguard organizations, 'revolutionary' leadership organizations with the projected view of a libertarian socialist theory.

Anarchism has always stressed, more than has any other part of the socialist movement, the importance of the coincidence of the 'personal' and the 'political.' Personal consciousness, as part of social and political analysis, is emphasized equally with revolutionary solidarity and struggle. However, simply because of the consistent emphasis on ethical integrity in each 'revolutionary' individual's life, the popular misconception that anarchists are out to trash all organizational systems as such is certainly not justified.

Some of the most incisive contributions of anarchist analysis, all the way from the First International, but especially since the Bolshevik period, have related to organizational modes. More importantly, many anarchist criticisms of socialist 'movement' groups are identical with those made by feminists who have come out of the male-dominated socialist left. For example, the anarcho-communist Murray Bookchin's characterization of the left seems very relevant to the feminist experience:

> The tragedy of the socialist movement is that, steeped in the past, it uses the methods of domination to try to 'liberate' us from material exploitation. . . . We are beginning to see that the most advanced form of class consciousness is self-consciousness. The tragedy of the socialist movement is that it opposes class consciousness to self-consciousness and denies the emergence of the self as 'individualist' – a self that could yield the most advanced form of collectivity, a collectivity based on self-management.
> [p. 13, 'Anarchos 4,' *On Spontaneity and Organization*]

To state that, because anarchists have criticized certain structural and organizational choices made by authoritarian socialists, they in general trash all forms of organization and arbitrarily opt for personal solutions to liberation, is both unfair and simplistic. However, because anarchists have stressed both psychological struggle and awareness as well as economic/political analysis, a fairer characterization is that made by Sam Dolgoff in his article, 'Anarchism and Modern Society' in *Workers' Opposition Magazine*:

> While the anarchists never underestimate the great importance of the economic factor in social change, they have nevertheless rejected fanatical economic fatalism. One of the most cogent contributions of anarchism to social theory is the proper emphasis on how political institutions, in turn, mold economic life. Equally significant is the

255

importance attached to the will of man, [sic] his aspirations, the moral factor, and above all, the spirit of revolt in the shaping of human history.

This latter emphasis, the 'spirit of revolt,' awakening consciousness or transcendent awareness, accounts in large part for an organic and conceptual link between anarchism and revolutionary feminism.

The anarchist tradition of socialism has been popularly misunderstood as being 'unscientific' socialism. However, historically, this criticism is not terribly justified. Because of the splits between Marx and Bakunin in the First International and disagreement between Goldman, Berkman and Lenin, the differences between anarchists and scientific socialists have usually been overemphasized. Both historically and contemporarily many left-wing anarchists do accept the Marxian technique of class analysis as a basic part of their own radical critique. Anarchists have not in general, it is true, accepted a narrowly determinist function of materialism.

The closeness of the libertarian Marxist and left-wing anarchist traditions is particularly obvious if one looks at the development of mutualism *à la* Proudhon into anarcho-syndicalism and the base of class analysis within the latter tradition. Today these currents come together in the workers' councilist movement. The reason for mentioning this strong relationship is simply to call attention to the similarities in approach and intellectual method of the Marxist socialist and anarcho-communist as a tentative reply to those who feel anarchism is incomprehensible, confused, unsystematic, a far-left fringe movement, as the most dogmatic of Marxist–Leninists have wished us to believe.

However, it is indeed true that the most influential and creative of anarchists can be differentiated further within the socialist movement than by their non-assent to a narrowly economic determinist viewpoint. They have tended to affirm that, without self-consciousness, as a logical concomitant to class-consciousness any revolution will ultimately be a restoration, with new faces in old places. The dichotomy between oppressor and oppressed must not only be comprehended, but transcended, or ultimately it will be perpetuated with a new cast of characters.

Wishing won't stop the vicious circle. Just as the Marxist technique when utilized by a disciplined and committed mind can enable us to form a clear analysis of and concretely based solutions to the economic relationships under capitalism, so, too, there of necessity must be developed a systematic analysis of character and of consciousness and of the ways in which they are projected on to the socio-political environment. The total picture of human life is only comprehended in the interaction of human consciousness and organization of the material world.

Anarcho-feminism

Anarcho-feminism, like socialist feminism, as a movement within the larger women's movement has developed only in recent years. There have always been anarchist women, a few of whom became very well-known and influential, in the male-dominated anarchist movement (analogous to Luxemburg and Zetkin in the male-dominated socialist workers' movement). Unlike this earlier period of 'anarcho-feminism' of Louise Michel, Emma Goldman, Marie Louise Berneri, today the anarchist 'movement,' especially in America, is scarcely worthy of the name.

For the most part, 'anarchist groups' consist of a few irascible men quarrelling with a few others, or of Wobblies nostalgically recalling the labor union strategies of yesteryear, or of neo-capitalist Randists flailing the air with irrelevant and nit-picking abstractions.

Unfortunately, many unfair and inaccurate criticisms of anarchists of earlier periods have become fairly accurate stereotypes for contemporary anarchists, 'undisciplined thinkers,' 'chaotic personalities,' 'extreme egoists,' 'opportunistic individualists.' In respect to this growth of 'in'-group irrelevance, the anarchist movement, such as it is, shares with other male-dominated socialist sectarian groups the distinction of having become havens of arrogant and isolated men prattling their rhetoric for their own dubious benefit. However, this irrelevance is usually even more blatant in the case of anarchist groups which lack even the veneer of pseudo-scientific credibility of their Trotskyist/Leninist/Maoist counterparts in splinterdom.

Even if there were an 'anarchist movement,' anarcho-feminists belong right where they are, which is with other women. Nor should we delude ourselves about consideration of women's issues in the past of the anarchist movement. Feminist priorities were no more positively received by anarchist men than by any others in over-all male socialist circles (an infamous relationship documented often and well in contemporary works by Rowbotham, Mitchell, Morgan. . . .). It is patently untrue that male anarchists usually led lives compatible in practice with the theories, and implications of theories which they originated, Nestor Makhno's rapine practices bearing extreme testimony to this fact.

For current attitudes and responses to feminist issues by anarchist men, the reader is referred to the male/female conflicts in the *Social-Revolutionary Anarchist Federation Bull(etin)* or to editor Fred Woodworth's myopic and paranoid discussion of possible sexist material in the then only regularly-appearing anarchist newspaper, the *Match*. The alienating experiences of anarcho-feminists at meetings of the Wobblies (Industrial Workers of the World) have been recorded in the *Social Revolutionary Anarchist Federation Bull(etin)* as well as in the *Indus-*

trial Worker itself. Significantly enough, the few constructive male anarchists usually prefer to be active in areas other than the 'anarchist movement,' but rather look to other emerging groups as embodying truly anarchist priorities. For example, Murray Bookchin strongly emphasizes the radical ecology, 'counter-culture,' women's and gay movements, while Karl Hess has worked with the draft resistance movement and now with neighborhood-controlled, alternative technology systems.

Since anarcho-feminism's primary commitment is and should be made to the radical feminist movement with only marginal participation in anarchist movement politics, does the term 'anarcho-feminist' possess any functional significance, or is it only a confusing label laden with semantic difficulties? My own feeling is that the refining distinction from radical feminist to anarcho-feminist is largely that of making a step in self-conscious theoretical development. Having perceived that there are 'natural' anarchist tendencies in the women's movement, an anarcho-feminist is one who intellectually identifies with major aspects of the intellectual tradition of anarchist radicalism. If anarchism itself were more well-known as a radical tradition, the term 'anarcho-feminist' would be as self-evident as the term 'Marxist feminist,' i.e., one who has chosen to utilize a particular intellectual analytical method to aid in the development of feminist theory and strategy.

There is no question that Marxism is indispensable in articulating any coherent understanding of economic and material interrelationships. However, many materialist theorists have tended to define 'matter' itself too narrowly, often defining out of existence many crucial areas of human life, such as consciousness, transformation of values except by manipulating the political/economic environment directly, and the relationship of a society's sexual attitudes and its cultural styles. The anarchist tradition has nowhere been so inhospitable to investigation of these areas.

Marian Leighton is a member of the Rounder Records Collective which issues traditional and contemporary folk music of the United States. She was a founding member of Black Rose Anarcho-Feminists in 1971 and, later, of *Black Rose: A Journal of Contemporary Anarchism.* Her freelance writing and research projects include work on women and spirituality, Wilhelm Reich, and radical therapy.

23 Socialism, anarchism, and feminism*

Carol Ehrlich

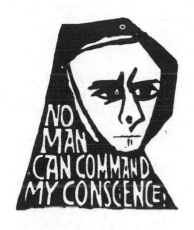

You are a woman in a capitalist society. You get pissed off: about
the job, about the bills, about your husband (or ex), about the kids'
school, the housework, being pretty, not being pretty, being looked
at, not being looked at (and either way, not listened to), etc. If you
think about all these things and how they fit together and what has
to be changed, and then you look around for some words to hold all
these thoughts together in abbreviated form, you'd almost have to
come up with 'socialist feminism.'[1]

From all indications a great many women have 'come up' with socialist
feminism as the solution to the persistent problem of sexism. 'Socialism'

---

* This was originally published as Report no. 26 from Research Group
One, January 1977.

(in its astonishing variety of forms) is popular with a lot of people these days, because it has much to offer: concern for working people, a body of revolutionary theory that people can point to (whether or not they have read it), and some living examples of industrialized countries that are structured differently from the United States and its satellites.

For many feminists, socialism is attractive because it promises to end the economic inequality of working women. Further, for those women who believe that an exclusively feminist analysis is too narrow to encompass all the existing inequalities, socialism promises to broaden it, while guarding against the dilution of its radical perspective.

For good reasons, then, women are considering whether or not 'socialist feminism' makes sense as a political theory. For socialist feminists do seem to be both sensible and radical – at least, most of them evidently feel a strong antipathy to some of the reformist and solipsistic traps into which increasing numbers of women seem to be stumbling.

To many of us more unromantic types, the Amazon Nation, with its armies of strong-limbed matriarchs riding into the sunset, is unreal, but harmless. A more serious matter is the current obsession with the Great Goddess and assorted other objects of worship, witchcraft, magic and psychic phenomena. As a feminist concerned with transforming the structure of society, I find this anything but harmless.

– *Item One.* Over 1,400 women went to Boston in April 1976 to attend a women's spirituality conference dealing in large part with the above matters. Could not the energy invested in chanting, swapping the latest pagan ideas and attending workshops on belly-dancing and menstrual rituals have been put to some better and more feminist use?

– *Item Two.* According to reports in at least one feminist newspaper, a group of witches tried to levitate Susan Saxe out of jail. If they honestly thought this would free Saxe, then they were totally out of touch with the realities of patriarchal oppression. If it was intended to be a light-hearted joke, then why isn't anyone laughing?

Reformism is a far greater danger to women's interests than are bizarre psychic games. I know that 'reformist' is an epithet that may be used in ways that are neither honest nor very useful – principally to demonstrate one's ideological purity, or to say that concrete political work of *any* type is not worth doing because it is potentially co-optable. In response, some feminists have argued persuasively that the right kinds of reforms can build a radical movement.[2]

Just the same, there are reformist strategies that waste the energies of women, that raise expectations of great change, and that are misleading and alienating because they cannot deliver the goods. The best (or worst) example is electoral politics. Some socialists (beguiled by the notion of gradualism) fall for that one. Anarchists know better. You

cannot liberate yourself by non-liberatory means; you cannot elect a new set of politicians (no matter now sisterly) to run the same old corrupt institutions – which in turn run *you*. When NOW's Majority Caucus – the *radical* branch of that organization – asks women to follow them 'out of the mainstream, into the revolution' by means that include electoral politics, they will all drown in the depths of things as they are.

Electoral politics is an obvious, everyday kind of trap. Even a lot of non-radicals have learned to avoid it. A more subtle problem is capitalism in the guise of feminist economic power. Consider, for example, the Feminist Economic Network (FEN). The name might possibly fool you. Ostensibly it was a network of alternative businesses set up to erode capitalism from within by creating economic self-sufficiency for women. That is an appealing idea. Yet FEN's first major project opened in Detroit in April 1976. For an annual membership fee of $100, privileged women could swim in a private pool, drink in a private bar, and get discounts in a cluster of boutiques. FEN paid its female employees $2.50 per hour to work there. Its director, Laura Brown, announced this venture as 'the beginning of the feminist economic revolution.'[3]

When two of the same old games – electoral politics and hip capitalism – are labeled 'revolution,' the word has been turned inside out. It's not surprising that a socialist brand of feminism seems to be a source of revolutionary sanity to many women who don't want to be witches, primitive warriors, senators or small capitalists, but who do want to end sexism while creating a transformed society. Anarchist feminism could provide a meaningful theoretical framework, but all too many feminists either have never heard of it, or else dismiss it as the ladies' auxiliary of male bomb-throwers.

Socialist feminism provides an assortment of political homes. On the one hand, there are the dingy, cramped quarters of Old Left sects such as the Revolutionary Communist Party (formerly the Revolutionary Union), the October League and the International Workers Party. Very few women find these habitable. On the other hand, a fair number of women are moving into the sprawling, eclectic establishments built by newer Left groups such as the New American Movement, or by various autonomous 'women's unions.'

The newer socialist feminists have been running an energetic and reasonably effective campaign to recruit nonaligned women. In contrast, the more rigid Old Left groups have largely rejected the very idea that lesbians, separatists and assorted other scruffy and unsuitable feminists could work with the noble inheritors of Marx, Trotsky (although the Trotskyists are unpredictable), Stalin and Mao. Many reject the idea of an autonomous women's movement that cares at all about women's

issues. To them, it is full of 'bourgeois' (most damning of all Marxist epithets!) women bent on 'doing their own thing,' and it 'divides the working class,' which is a curious assumption that workers are dumber that everyone else. Some have an hysterical antipathy to lesbians: the most notorious groups are the October League and the Revolutionary Communist Party (RCP), but they are not alone. In this policy, as in so many others, the anti-lesbian line follows that of the communist countries. The RCP, for example, released a position paper in the early 1970s (back in its pre-party days, when it was the plain old Revolutionary Union) which announced that homosexuals are 'caught in the mire and much of bourgeois decadence,' and that gay liberation is 'anti-working class and counter revolutionary.' All the Old Left groups are uneasy with the idea that any women outside the 'proletariat' are oppressed at all. The working class, of course, is a marvelously flexible concept. In the current debates on the Left, it ranges from point-of-production workers (period) to an enormous group that takes in every single person who sells her or his labor for wages, or who depends on someone else who does. That's almost all of us. (So, Papa Karl, if 90 per cent of the people of the United States are the vanguard, why haven't we had the revolution yet?)

The newer socialist feminists have been trying in all manner of inventive ways to keep a core of Marxist–Leninist thought, update it, and graft it to contemporary radical feminism. The results are sometimes peculiar. In July 1975, the women of the New American Movement and a number of autonomous groups held the first national conference on socialist feminism. It was not especially heavily advertised in advance, and everyone seemed to be surprised that so many women (over 1,600, with more turned away) wanted to spend the July 4 weekend in Yellow Springs, Ohio.

On reading the speeches given at the conference, as well as extensive commentary written by other women who attended,[4] it is not at all clear what the conference organizers thought they were offering in the name of 'socialist feminism.' The Principles of Unity that were drawn up prior to the conference included two items that have always been associated with radical feminism, and that in fact are typically thought of as *antithetical* to a socialist perspective. The first principle stated: 'We recognize the need for and support the existence of the autonomous women's movement throughout the revolutionary process.' The second read: 'We agree that all oppression, whether based on race, class, sex, or lesbianism, is interrelated and the fights for liberation from oppression must be simultaneous and co-operative.' The third principle merely remarked that 'socialist feminism is a strategy for revolution;' and the fourth and final principle called for holding discussions 'in the spirit of struggle and unity.'

This is, of course, an incredible smorgasbord of tasty principles – a menu designed to appeal to practically everyone. But when 'socialist' feminists serve up the independent women's movement as the main dish, and when they say class oppression is just one of several oppressions, no more important than any other, then (as its Marxist critics say) it is no longer socialism.

However, socialist feminists do not follow out the implications of radical feminism all the way. If they did, they would accept another principle: that non-hierarchical structures are essential to feminist practice. This, of course, is too much for any socialist to take. But what it means is that radical feminism is far more compatible with one type of anarchism than it is with socialism. That type is *social* anarchism (also known as communist anarchism), not the individualist or anarcho-capitalist varieties.

This won't come as news to feminists who are familiar with anarchist principles – but very few feminists are. That's understandable, since anarchism has veered between a bad press and none at all. If feminists were familiar with anarchism, they would not be looking very hard at socialism as a means of fighting sexist oppression. Feminists have got to be skeptical of any social theory that comes with a built-in set of leaders and followers, no matter how 'democratic' this centralized structure is supposed to be. Women of all classes, races and life circumstances have been on the receiving end of domination too long to want to exchange one set of masters for another. We know who has power, and (with a few isolated exceptions) it isn't us.

Several contemporary anarchist feminists have pointed out the connections between social anarchism and radical feminism. Lynne Farrow said, 'feminism practices what anarchism preaches.' Peggy Kornegger believes that 'feminists have been unconscious anarchists in both theory and practice for years.' And Marian Leighton states that 'the refining distinction from radical feminist to anarcho-feminist is largely that of making a step in self-conscious theoretical development.'[5]

We build autonomy
The process of ever growing synthesis
For every living creature.
We spread
Spontaneity and creation
We learn the joys of equality
Of relationships
Without dominance
Among sisters.
We destroy domination
In all its forms.

This chant appeared in the radical feminist newspaper, *It Aint Me Babe*,[6] whose masthead carried the line, 'end all hierarchies.' It was not labeled an anarchist (or anarchist-feminist) newspaper, but the connections are striking. It exemplified much of what women's liberation was about in the early years of the reborn movement. And it is that spirit that will be lost if the socialist feminist hybrid takes root; if goddess worship or the lesbian nation convince women to set up new forms of dominance-submission.

Radical feminism and anarchist feminism

All radical feminists and all social anarchist feminists are concerned with a set of common issues: control over one's own body; alternatives to the nuclear family and to heterosexuality; new methods of child care that will liberate parents *and* children; economic self-determination; ending sex stereotyping in education, in the media and in the workplace; the abolition of repressive laws; an end to male authority, ownership and control over women; providing women with the means to develop skills and positive self-attitudes; an end to oppressive emotional relationships; and what the Situationists have called 'the reinvention of everyday life.'

There are, then, many issues on which radical feminists and anarchist feminists agree. But anarchist feminists are concerned with something more. Because they are anarchists, they work to end all power relationships, all situations in which people can oppress each other. Unlike some radical feminists who are not anarchists, they do not believe that power in the hands of women could possibly lead to a non-coercive society. And unlike most socialist feminists, they do not believe that anything good can come out of a mass movement with a leadership elite. In short, neither a workers' state nor a matriarchy will end the oppression of everyone. The goal, then, is not to 'seize' power, as the socialists are fond of urging, but to abolish power.

Contrary to popular belief, all social anarchists are socialists. That is, they want to take wealth out of the hands of the few and redistribute it among all members of the community. And they believe that people need to co-operate with each other as a community, instead of living as isolated individuals. For anarchists, however, the central issues are always power and social hierarchy. If a state – even a state representing the workers – continues, it will re-establish forms of domination, and some people will no longer be free. People aren't free just because they are surviving, or even if they are economically comfortable. They are free only when they have power over their own lives. Women, even more than most men, have very little power over their own lives. Gaining

such autonomy, and insisting that everyone have it, is the major goal of anarchist feminists:[7]

> Power to no one, and to every one: To each the power over his/her own life, and no others.

On practice

That is the theory. What about the practice? Again, radical feminism and anarchist feminism have much more in common than either does with socialist feminism.[8] Both work to build alternative institutions, and both take the politics of the personal very seriously. Socialist feminists are less inclined to think either is particularly vital to revolutionary practice.

Developing alternative forms of organization means building self-help clinics, instead of fighting to get one radical on a hospital's board of directors; it means women's video groups and newspapers, instead of commercial television and newspapers; living collectives, instead of isolated nuclear families; rape crisis centers; food co-ops; parent-controlled day-care centers; free schools, printing co-ops; alternative radio groups, and so on.

Yet, it does little good to build alternative institutions if their structures mimic the capitalist and hierarchical models with which we are so familiar. Many radical feminists recognized this early: that's why they worked to rearrange the way women perceived the world and themselves (through the consciousness-raising group), and why they worked to rearrange the forms of work relationships and interpersonal interactions (through the small, leaderless groups where tasks are rotated and skills and knowledge shared). They were attempting to do this in a hierarchical society that provides no models except ones of inequality. Surely, a knowledge of anarchist theory and models of organization would have helped. Equipped with this knowledge, radical feminists might have avoided some of the mistakes they made – and might have been better able to overcome some of the difficulties they encountered in trying simultaneously to transform themselves and society.

Take, for example, the still current debate over 'strong women' and the closely related issue of leadership. The radical feminist position can be summarized the following way.

1 Women have been kept down because they are isolated from each other and are paired off with men in relationships of dominance and submission.

2 Men will not liberate women; women must liberate themselves. This

cannot happen if each woman tries to liberate herself alone. Thus, women must work together on a model of mutual aid.

3 'Sisterhood is powerful,' but women cannot be sisters if they recapitulate masculine patterns of dominance and submission.

4 New organizational forms have to be developed. The primary form is the small, leaderless group; the most important behaviors are egalitarianism, mutual support, and the sharing of skills and knowledge.

If many women accepted this, even more did not. Some were opposed from the start; others saw first-hand that it was difficult to put into practice, and regretfully concluded that such beautiful idealism would never work out.

Ideological support for those who rejected the principles put forth by the 'unconscious anarchists' was provided in two documents that quickly circulated through women's liberation newspapers and organizations. The first was Anselma dell'Olio's speech to the second Congress to Unite Women, which was held in May 1970 in New York City. The speech, entitled 'Divisiveness and Self-Destruction in the Women's Movement: A Letter of Resignation,' gave dell'Olio's reasons for leaving the women's movement. The second document was Joreen's 'Tyranny of Structurelessness,' which first appeared in 1972 in *The Second Wave*. Both raised issues of organizational and personal practice that were, and still are, tremendously important to the women's movement.[9]

> I have come to announce my swan-song to the women's movement. . . . I have been destroyed. . . . I learned three and one-half years ago that women had always been divided against one another, were self-destructive and filled with impotent rage. I never dreamed that I would see the day when this rage, masquerading as a pseudo-egalitarian radicalism under the 'pro-woman' banner, would turn into frighteningly vicious anti-intellectual fascism of the Left, and used within the movement to strike down sisters singled out with all the subtlety and justice of a kangaroo court of the Ku Klux Klan. I am referring, of course, to the personal attack, both overt and insidious, to which women in the movement, who have painfully managed any degree of achievement, have been subjected. . . . If you are . . . an achiever you are immediately labeled a thrill-seeking opportunist, a ruthless mercenary, out to get her fame and fortune over the dead bodies of selfless sisters who have buried their abilities and sacrificed their ambitions for the greater glory of Feminism. . . . If you have the misfortune of being outspoken and articulate, you are accused of being power-mad, elitist, racist, and finally the worst epithet of all: a MALE IDENTIFIER.

When Anselma dell'Olio gave this angry farewell to the movement, i

did two things: For some women, it raised the question of how women can end unequal power relationships among themselves without destroying each other. For others it did quite the opposite – it provided easy justification for all the women who had been dominating other women in a most unsisterly way. Anyone who was involved in women's liberation at that time knows that the dell'Olio statement was twisted by some women in exactly that fashion: call yourself assertive, or strong, or talented, and you can re-label a good deal of ugly, insensitive and oppressive behavior. Women who presented themselves as tragic heroines destroyed by their envious or misguided (and, of course, far less talented) 'sisters' could count on a sympathetic response from some other women.

Just the same, women who were involved in the movement at that time know that the kinds of things dell'Olio spoke about *did* happen, and they should not have happened. A knowledge of anarchist theory is not enough, of course, to prevent indiscriminate attacks on women. But in the struggle to learn new ways of relating and working with each other, such knowledge might – just might – have prevented some of these destructive mistakes.

Ironically, these mistakes were motivated by the radical feminist aversion to conventional forms of power, and the inhuman personal relationships that result from one set of persons having power over others. When radical feminists and anarchist feminists speak of abolishing power, they mean to get rid of all institutions, all forms of socialization, all the ways in which people coerce each other – and acquiesce to being coerced.

A major problem arose in defining the nature of coercion in the women's movement. The hostility towards the 'strong' woman arose because she was someone who could at least potentially coerce women who were less articulate, less self-confident, less assertive than she. Coercion is usually far more subtle than physical force or economic sanction. One person can coerce another without taking away her job, or striking her, or throwing her in jail.

Strong women started out with a tremendous advantage. Often they knew more. Certainly they had long since overcome the crippling socialization that stressed passive, timid, docile, conformist behavior – behavior that taught women to smile when they weren't amused, to whisper when they felt like shouting, to lower their eyes when someone stared aggressively at them. Strong women weren't terrified of speaking in public; they weren't afraid to take on 'male' tasks, or to try something new. Or so it seemed.

Put a 'strong' woman in the same small group with a 'weak' one, and she becomes a problem: How does she not dominate? How does she share her hard-earned skills and confidence with her sister? From the other side – how does the 'weak' woman learn to act in her own behalf?

267

How can one even conceive of 'mutual' aid in a one-way situation? Of 'sisterhood' when the 'weak' member does not feel equal to the 'strong' one?

These are complicated questions, with no simple answers. Perhaps the closest we can come is with the anarchist slogan, 'a strong people needs no leaders.' Those of us who have learned to survive by dominating others, as well as those of us who have learned to survive by accepting domination, need to resocialize ourselves into being strong without playing dominance–submission games, into controlling what happens to us without controlling others. This can't be done by electing the right people to office or by following the correct party line; nor can it be done by sitting and reflecting on our sins. We rebuild ourselves and our world through activity, through partial successes, and failure, and more partial successes. And all the while we grow stronger and more self-reliant.

If Anselma dell'Olio criticized the personal practice of radical feminists, Joreen raised some hard questions about organizational structure. 'The Tyranny of Structurelessness'[10] pointed out that there is no such thing as a 'structureless' group, and people who claim there is are fooling themselves. All groups have a structure; the difference is whether or not the structure is explicit. If it is implicit, hidden elites are certain to exist and to control the group – and everyone, both the leaders and the led, will deny or be confused by the control that exists. This is the 'tyranny' of structurelessness. To overcome it, groups need to set up open, explicit structures accountable to the membership.

Any anarchist feminist, I think, would agree with her analysis – up to this point, and no further. For what Joreen also said was that the so-called 'leaderless, structureless group' was incapable of going beyond talk to action. Not only its lack of open structure, but also its small size and its emphasis upon consciousness-raising (talk) were bound to make it ineffective.

Joreen did not say that women's groups should be hierarchically structured. In fact, she called for leadership that would be 'diffuse, flexible, open, and temporary;' for organizations that would build in accountability, diffusion of power among the maximum number of persons, task rotation, skill-sharing, and the spread of information and resources. All good social anarchist principles of organization! But her denigration of consciousness-raising and her preference for large regional and national organizations were strictly part of the old way of doing things, and implicitly accepted the continuation of hierarchical structures.

Large groups are organized so that power and decision-making are delegated to a few – unless, of course, one is speaking of a horizontally co-ordinated network of small collectives, which she did not mention.

How does a group such as NOW, with its 60,000 members in 1975, rotate tasks, share skills, and ensure that all information and resources are available to everyone? It can't, of course. Such groups have a president, and a board of directors, and a national office, and a membership – some of whom are in local chapters, and some of whom are isolated members. Few such groups have very much direct democracy, and few teach their members new ways of working and relating to one another.

The unfortunate effect of 'The Tyranny of Structurelessness' was that it linked together large organization, formal structure, and successful direct action in a way that seemed to make sense to a lot of people. Many women felt that in order to fight societal oppression a large organization was essential, and the larger the better. The image is strength pitted against strength: you do not kill an elephant with an air gun, and you do not bring down the patriarchal state with the small group. For women who accept the argument that greater size is linked to greater effectiveness, the organizational options seem limited to large liberal groups such as NOW or to socialist organizations which are mass organizations.

As with so many things that seem to make sense, the logic is faulty. 'Societal oppression' is a reification, an over-blown, paralyzing, made-up entity that is large mainly in the sense that the same oppressions happen to a lot of us. But oppressions, no matter how pervasive, how predictable, almost always are done to us by some *one* – even if that person is acting as an agent of the state, or as a member of the dominant race, gender or class. The massive police assaults upon our assembled forces are few; even the police officer or the boss or the husband who is carrying out his allotted sexist or authoritarian role interesects with us at a given point in our everyday lives. Institutionalized oppression *does* exist, on a large scale, but it seldom needs to be attacked (indeed, seldom *can* be attacked) by a large group. Guerrilla tactics by a small group – occasionally even by a single individual – will do very nicely in retaliation.

Another unfortunate effect of the 'Tyranny of Structurelessness' mentality (if not directly of the article) was that it fed people's stereotypes of anarchists. (Of course, people don't usually swallow something unless they're hungry.) Social anarchists aren't opposed to structure: they aren't even against leadership, provided that it carries no reward or privilege, and is temporary and specific to a particular task. However, anarchists who want to abolish a *hierarchical* structure are almost always stereotyped as wanting no structure at all. Unfortunately, the picture of a gaggle of disorganized, chaotic anarchist women, drifting without direction, caught on. For example, in 1976 *Quest* reprinted an edited transcription of an interview which Charlotte Bunch and Beverly Fisher had given the Feminist Radio Nework in 1972. In one way, the most

269

interesting thing about the interview was that the *Quest* editors felt the issues were still so timely in 1976.[11] ('We see the same trashing of leaders and glorification of structurelessness that existed five years ago.' - p. 13). But what Bunch had to say at that time was also extremely interesting. According to her, the emphasis on solving problems of structure and leadership was 'a very strong anarchist desire. It was a good desire, but it was an unrealistic one' (p. 4). Anarchists, who are used to being called 'unrealistic,' will note that the unreality of it all apparently lay in the problems that the women's movement was having in organizing itself – problems of hidden leadership; of having 'leaders' imposed by the media; of reaching out to interested but uncommitted women; of overrepresentation of middle-class women with lots of time on their hands; of the amorphousness of the movement; of the scarcity of specific task groups that women could join; of hostility towards women who tried to show leadership or initiative. A heavy indictment! Yet these very real problems were not caused by anarchism, nor will they be cured by doses of vanguardism or reformism. And by labeling these organizational difficulties 'anarchist,' feminists ignore a rich anarchist tradition while at the same time proposing solutions that are – although they apparently don't known it – anarchist. Bunch and Fisher laid out a model of leadership in which everyone participates in making decisions; and leadership is specific to a particular situation and is time-limited. Fisher criticized NOW for 'hierarchical leadership that is not responsible to the vast membership' (p. 9), and Bunch stated, 'leadership is people taking the initiative, carrying things through, having the ideas and imagination to get something started, and exhibiting particular skills in different areas' (p. 8). How do they suggest we prevent the silencing of these women under false notions of egalitarianism? 'The only way women will stop putting down women who are strong is if they are strong themselves' (p. 12). Or, as I said earlier, a strong people needs no leaders. Right on!

Situationism and anarchist feminism

> To transform the world and to change the structure of life are one and the same thing.[12]

> The personal is political.[13]

Anarchists are used to hearing that they lack a theory that would help in building a new society. At best, their detractors say patronizingly, anarchism tells us what *not* to do. Don't permit bureaucracy or hierarchical authority; don't let a vanguard party make decisions; don't tread

on me. Don't tread on anyone. According to this perspective, anarchism is not a theory at all. It is a set of cautionary practices, the voice of libertarian conscience – always idealistic, sometimes a bit truculent, occasionally anachronistic, but a necessary reminder.

There is more than a kernel of truth to this objection. Just the same, there are varieties of anarchist thought that can provide a theoretical framework for analysis of the world and action to change it. For radical feminists who want to take that 'step in self-conscious theoretical development,'[14] perhaps the greatest potential lies in situationism.

The value of situationism for an anarchist–feminist analysis is that it combines a socialist awareness of the primacy of capitalist oppression with an anarchist emphasis upon transforming the whole of public and private life. The point about capitalist oppression is important. All too often anarchists seem to be unaware that this economic system exploits most people. But all too often socialists – especially Marxists – are blind to the fact that people are oppressed in every aspect of life: work, what passes for leisure, culture, personal relationships – all of it. And only anarchists insist that people must transform the conditions of their lives *themselves* – it cannot be done for them. Not by the party, not by the union, not by 'organizers,' not by anyone else.

Two basic situationist concepts are 'commodity' and 'spectacle.' Capitalism has made all of social relations commodity relations: the market rules all. People are not only producers and consumers in the narrow economic sense, but the very structure of their daily lives is based on commodity relations. Society 'is consumed as a *whole* – the ensemble of social relationships and structures is the central product of the commodity economy.'[15] This has inevitably alienated people from their lives, not just from their labor; to consume social relationships makes one a passive spectator in one's life. The *spectacle*, then, is the culture that springs from the commodity economy – the stage is set, the action unfolds, we applaud when we think we are happy, we yawn when we think we are bored, but we cannot leave the show, because there is no world outside the theater for us to go to.

In recent times, however, the societal stage has begun to crumble, and so the possibility exists of constructing another world outside the theater – this time a real world, one in which each of us directly participates as subject, not as object. The situationist phrase for this possibility is 'the reinvention of everyday life.'

How is daily life to be reinvented? By creating situations that disrupt what seems to be the natural order of things – situations that jolt people out of customary ways of thinking and behaving. Only then will they be able to act, to destroy the manufactured spectacle and the commodity economy – that is, capitalism in all its forms. Only then will they be able to create free and unalienated lives.

The congruence of this activist, social anarchist theory with radical feminist theory is striking. The concepts of commodity and spectacle are especially applicable to the lives of women. In fact, many radical feminists have described these in detail, without placing them in the situationist framework.[16] To do so broadens the analysis, by showing women's situation as an organic part of the society as a whole, but at the same time without playing socialist reductionist games. Women's oppression is part of the overall oppression of people by a capitalist economy, but it is not less than the oppression of others. Nor – from a situationist perspective – do you have to be a particular variety of women to be oppressed; you do not have to be part of the proletariat, either literally, as an industrial worker, or metaphorically, as someone who is not independently wealthy. You do not have to wait breathlessly for socialist feminist manifestoes to tell you that you qualify – as a housewife (reproducing the next generation of workers), as a clerical worker, as a student or a middle-level professional employed by the state (and therefore as part of the 'new working class'). You do not have to be part of the Third World, or a lesbian, or elderly, or a welfare recipient. All of these women are objects in the commodity economy; all are passive viewers of the spectacle. Obviously, women in some situations are far worse off than are others. But, at the same time, none are free in every area of their lives.

Women and the commodity economy

Women have a dual relationship to the commodity economy – they are both consumers and consumed. As housewives, they are consumers of household goods purchased with money not their own, because not 'earned' by them. This may give them a certain amount of purchasing power, but very little power over any aspect of their lives. As young, single heterosexuals, women are purchasers of goods designed to make them bring a high price on the marriage market. As anything else – lesbians, or elderly single, or self-sufficient women with 'careers' – women's relationship to the market place as consumers is not so sharply defined. They are expected to buy (and the more affluent they are, the more they are expected to buy), but for some categories of women, buying is not defined primarily to fill out some aspect of a woman's role.

So what else is new? Isn't the idea of woman-as-passive-consumer, manipulated by the media, patronized by slick Madison Avenue men, an overdone movement cliché? Well, yes – and no. A situationist analysis ties consumption of economic goods to consumption of *ideological* goods, and then tells us to create situations (guerrilla actions on

many levels) that will break that pattern of socialized acceptance of the world as it is. No guilt-tripping; no criticizing women who have 'bought' the consumer perspective. For they have indeed *bought* it: it has been sold to them as a way of survival from the earliest moments of life. Buy this: it will make you beautiful and lovable. Buy *this*: it will keep your family in good health. Feel depressed? Treat yourself to an afternoon at the beauty parlor or to a new dress.

Guilt leads to inaction. Only action, to *reinvent* the everyday and make it something else, will change social relations.

The gift[17]

Thinking she was the gift
they began to package it early.
They waxed its smile
they lowered its eyes
they tuned its ears to the telephone
they curled its hair
they straightened its teeth
they taught it to bury its wishbone
they poured honey down its throat
they made it say yes yes and yes
they sat on its thumbs.

That box has my name on it,
said the man. *It's for me.*
And they were not surprised.

While they blew kisses and winked
he took it home. He put it on a table
where his friends could examine it
saying *dance* saying *faster*.
He plunged its tunnel
he burned his name deeper.
Later he put it on a platform
under the Kleig lights
saying *push* saying *harder*
saying *just what I wanted*
you've given me a son.

Women are not only consumers in the commodity economy; they are consumed as commodities. This is what Oles's poem is about, and it is

273

what Tax has labeled 'female schizophrenia.' Tax constructs an inner monologue for the housewife-as-commodity: ' "I am nothing when I am by myself. In myself, I am nothing. I only know that I exist because I am needed by someone who is real, my husband, and by my children." '[18]

When feminists describe socialization into the female sex role, when they point out the traits female children are taught (emotional dependence, childishness, timidity, concern with being beautiful, docility, passivity, and so on), they are talking about the careful production of a commodity – although it isn't usually called that. When they describe the oppressiveness of sexual objectification, or of living in the nuclear family, or of being a Supermother, or of working in the kinds of low-level, under-paid jobs that most women find in the paid labor force, they are also describing woman as commodity. Women are consumed by men who treat them as sex objects; they are consumed by their children (whom they have produced!) when they buy the role of the Supermother; they are consumed by authoritarian husbands who expect them to be submissive servants; and they are consumed by bosses who bring them in and out of the labor force and who extract a maximum of labor for a minimum of pay. They are consumed by medical researchers who try out new and unsafe contraceptives on them. They are consumed by men who buy their bodies on the street. They are consumed by church and state, who expect them to produce the next generation for the glory of god and country; they are consumed by political and social organizations that expect them to 'volunteer' their time and energy. They have little sense of self, because their self-hood has been sold to others.

Women and the spectacle

It is difficult to consume people who put up a fight, who resist the cannibalizing of their bodies, their minds, their daily lives. A few people manage to resist, but most don't resist effectively, because they can't. It is hard to locate our tormentor, because it is so pervasive, so familiar. We have known it all our lives. It is our culture.

Situationists characterize our culture as a *spectacle*. The spectacle treats us all as passive spectators of what we are told are our lives. And the culture-as-spectacle covers everything: we are born into it, socialized by it, go to school in it, work and relax and relate to other people in it. Even when we rebel against it, the rebellion is often defined by the spectacle. Would anyone care to estimate the number of sensitive, alienated adolescent males who a generation ago modeled their behavior on James Dean in 'Rebel Without a Cause?' I'm talking about a *movie*, whose capitalist producers and whose star made a great deal of money

from this Spectacular.

Rebellious acts, then, tend to be acts of *opposition* to the spectacle, but seldom are so different that they *transcend* the spectacle. Women have a set of behaviors that show dissatisfaction by being the opposite of what is expected. At the same time these acts are clichés of rebellion, and thus are almost prescribed safety valves that don't alter the theater of our lives. What is a rebellious woman supposed to do? We can all name the behaviors – they appear in every newspaper, on prime time television, on the best-seller lists, in popular magazines – and, of course, in everyday life. In a setting that values perfectionist housekeeping, she can be a slob; in a subculture that values large families, she can refuse to have children. Other predictable insurgencies? She can defy the sexual double standard for married women by having an affair (or several); she can drink; or use what is termed 'locker room' language; or have a nervous breakdown; or – if she is an adolescent – she can 'act out' (a revealing phrase!) by running away from home and having sex with a lot of men.

Any of these things may make an individual woman's life more tolerable (often, they make it less so); and all of them are guaranteed to make conservatives rant that society is crumbling. But these kinds of scripted insurrections haven't made it crumble yet, and, by themselves they aren't likely to. Anything less than a direct attack upon all the conditions of our lives is not enough.

When women talk about changing destructive sex role socialization of females, they pick one of these possible solutions: (1) girls should be socialized more or less like boys to be independent, competitive, aggressive, and so forth. In short, it is a man's world, so a woman who wants to fit it has to be 'one of the boys', (2) we should glorify the female role, and realize that what we have called weakness is really strength. We should be proud that we are maternal, nurturant, sensitive, emotional, and so on; (3) the only healthy person is an androgynous person: we must eradicate the artificial division of humanity into 'masculine' and 'feminine,' and help both sexes become a mix of the best traits of each.

Within these three models, personal solutions to problems of sexist oppression cover a wide range. Stay single; live communally (with both men and women, or with women only). Don't have children; don't have male children; have any kind of children you want, but get parent and worker-controlled child care. Get a job; get a better job; push for affirmative action. Be an informed consumer; file a lawsuit; learn karate; take assertiveness training. Develop the lesbian within you. Develop your proletarian identity. All of these make sense in particular situations, for particular women. But all of them are partial solutions to much broader problems, and none of them necessarily requires seeing

275

the world in a qualitatively different way.

So. We move from the particular to more general solutions. Destroy capitalism. End patriarchy. Smash heterosexism. All are obviously essential tasks in the building of a new and truly human world. Marxists, other socialists, social anarchists, feminists – all would agree. But what the socialists, and even some feminists, leave out is this: we must smash *all* forms of domination. That's not just a slogan, and it is the hardest task of all. It means that we have to see through the spectacle, destroy the stage sets, know that there are other ways of doing things. It means that we have to do more than react in programmed rebellions – we must act. And our actions will be collectively taken, while each person acts autonomously. Does that seem contradictory? It isn't – but it will be very difficult to do. The individual cannot change anything very much; for that reason, we have to work together. But that work must be without leaders as we known them, and without delegating any control over what we do and what we want to build.

Can the socialists do that? Or the matriarchs? Or the spirituality-trippers? You know the answer to that. Work with them when it makes sense to do so, but give up nothing. Concede nothing to them, or to anyone else:[19]

> The past leads to us if we force it to.
> Otherwise it contains us
> in its asylum with no gates.
> We make history or it
> makes us.

Notes

1 Barbara Ehrenreich, 'What is Socialist Feminism?', *WIN Magazine* (June 3, 1976), 4.
2 The best of these arguments I've encountered are 'Socialist Feminism: A Strategy for the Women's Movement,' by the Hyde Park Chapter, Chicago Women's Liberation Union (1972); and Charlotte Bunch, 'The Reform Tool Kit,' *Quest*, 1:1 (Summer 1974), 37–51.
3 Reports by Polly Anna, Kana Trueblood, C. Corday and S. Tufts, *The Fifth Estate* (May 1976), 13, 16. The 'revolution' failed: FEN and its club shut down.
4 People who are interested in reading reports of the conference will find them in almost every feminist or socialist newspaper that appeared in the month or so after July 4. Speeches by Barbara Ehrenreich, Michelle Russell, and the Berkeley–Oakland Women's Union are reprinted in *Socialist Revolution*, no. 26 (October–December 1975); and the speech by Charlotte Bunch, 'Not For

Lesbians Only,' appears in *Quest*, 2:2 (Fall 1975). A thirty-minute audiotape documentary is available from the Great Atlantic Radio Conspiracy, 2743 Maryland Avenue, Baltimore, Maryland 21218.

5 Lynne Farrow, 'Feminism as Anarchism,' *Aurora*, 4 (1974), 9; Peggy Kornegger, 'Anarchism: The Feminist Connection,' *The Second Wave*, 4:1 (Spring 1975), 31 and Chapter 9 above; Marian Leighton, 'Anarcho-Feminism and Louise Michel,' *Black Rose*, 1 (April 1974), 14.

6 December 1, 1970, p. 11.

7 'Lilith's Manifesto,' from the Women's Majority Union of Seattle, 1969. Reprinted in Robin Morgan (ed.), *Sisterhood is Powerful* (New York: Random House, 1970), 529.

8 The best and most detailed description of the parallels between radical feminism and anarchist feminism is found in Kornegger, op. cit.

9 The speech is currently available from KNOW, Inc.

10 Joreen, 'The Tyranny of Structurelessness,' *The Second Wave*, 2:1 (1972).

11 'What Future for Leadership?,' *Quest*, 2:4 (Spring 1976), 2–13.

12 Strasbourg Situationists, *Once the Universities Were Respected*, (1968), 38 (also Chapter 14 above).

13 Carol Hanisch, 'The Personal is Political,' *Notes from the Second Year* (New York: Radical Feminism, 1970), 76–8.

14 Leighton, op. cit.

15 Point-Blank!, 'The Changing of the Guard,' in *Point-Blank!* (October 1972), 16.

16 For one of the most illuminating of these early analyses, see Meredith Tax, 'Woman and Her Mind: The Story of Everyday Life,' (Boston: Bread and Roses Publications, 1970).

17 Carole Oles, 'The Gift,' in *13th Moon*, II:1 (1974), 39.

18 Tax, op. cit., 13.

19 Marge Piercy, excerpt from 'Contribution to Our Museum,' in *Living in the Open* (New York: Knopf, 1976), 74–5.

277

24 Newspoem

Tuli Kupferberg

Amy to be 1st '75 hurricane

Washington (AP) – The first hurricane of the new hurricane season
that begins June 1 will be named Amy, according to the National
Weather Service.

Other hurricanes will be named Blanche, Doris, Eloise, Fay,
Gladys, Hallie and Ingrid. The 21st and last name on the list is
Winnie. The hurricane season, which officially ends Nov. 30, annually
claims an average of 100 lives and causes $150 million in property
damage in the U.S., the Weather Service said.

New York Post, May 14, 1975

HOLD THE PRESSES!
A SLIGHT CHANGE:
Adolf
Benito
Caesar
Denikin
Esau
Frankenstein
Gerald
Hirohito
Ibn Saud
Jack the Ripper
Kitchener
Lucifer
Moshe
Napoleon
Osman
Pizarro
Quisling
Richard Milhous

Savonarola
Tamerlane
Ulbricht
Van Fleet
Winston
Xerxes
Yamashita
Zaharoff

Part Six

The liberation of labor

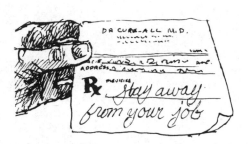

Introduction

In the United States, as well as most other industrialized countries, labor unions have become an integrated mechanism for the maintenance of capitalism. 'The new capitalism,' wrote David Deitch, 'requires a strong centralized trade union movement with which to bargain.' (Deitch, for many years a financial columnist for the *Boston Globe*, was fired soon after he began expounding such ideas in his columns.)

The persistence of union membership reflects the persistence of workplaces that are dangerous, unhealthy and degrading. Declining real wages along with the conditions of the workplace lead many workers to identify the unions as their only defense. And unions do give the appearance of fighting for them. More problematic – at least from an anarchist perspective – most workers do not perceive the validity of alternative forms. As Zerzan so meticulously documents, American trade unions have never challenged the organization of work itself. The 1971–2 strike in Lordstown, Ohio, that Zerzan talks about may have been the first major strike in which American workers demanded some control over the design of their jobs. They were opposed by their union.

Zerzan's documentation of the shared attitudes of union leaders and corporate management is important data. So too are his reports of workers' rejection of contracts negotiated 'in their interest' and their hostility to union leadership. His report is an important backdrop to David DeLeon's 'For Democracy Where We Work.'

DeLeon's essay codifies the standard criticisms of trade unionism. His five-part summary is a cogent statement. He presents an overview of the arguments for workers' self-management and explores the failures of state socialism as a solution to the problems of work. He concludes with the consideration of alternatives from moderate reforms to complete democracy at the workplace.

REVISED FORM F 716

DEATH REGISTRY

SAN FRANCISCO
CONVENTION & VISITORS BUREAU
1390 MARKET STREET, SAN FRANCISCO, CALIFORNIA 94102

CERTIFICATE OF DEATH

STATE OF CALIFORNIA—DEPARTMENT OF HEALTH
OFFICE OF THE STATE REGISTRAR OF VITAL STATISTICS

NAME OF DECEASED

afl-cio

IMMEDIATE CAUSE OF DEATH

A Refusal of workers to be humiliated any longer by union oppression.

DUE TO

B Unions' transparent role as wage labor's last effective police force.

UNDERLYING CAUSE OF DEATH

C The AFL-CIO was the enemy of freedom, creativity, pleasure.

DURATION: from birth

OTHER CONDITIONS

Racism, pollution, bureaucracy, corruption, etc.

DEATH CERTIFICATE

Despite the best efforts of management, government, and leftists, this corpse succumbed to workers' desire to end the disease of Organized Labor. Destroyed with such other relics as authority, representation, private property, duty, mediation, rules, productivity, parties.

DID AN OPERATION PRECEDE DEATH ☒ YES ☐ NO

DATE (several)

KIND OF OPERATION

Unions given progressively greater doses of authority in attempts to discipline members.

DIAGNOSIS FOR OPERATION

(condition: terminal)

ACCIDENT OCCURING DURING HOSPITALIZATION

DATE

VISITING CHIEF M.D.

INTERNE M.D.

HOUSE OFFICER M.D.

PREVIOUS INTERNE M.D.

CORONER NOTIFIED | DATE | TIME A.M. P.M. | BY WHOM | ☐ ACCEPTED ☐ REFUSED | BY WHOM

AUTOPSY DESIRED ☐ YES ☐ NO | PERMISSION FOR AUTOPSY GIVEN BY | RELATIONSHIP | SUPERINTENDENT'S APPROVAL

ANATOMICAL FINDINGS

Subject in advanced state of decomposition.

BODY DELIVERED TO

Unclaimed.

SIGNATURE—AUTOPSY SURGEON

UPSHOT
P. O. BOX 40256
SAN FRANCISCO, CA 94140

25 Organized labor versus 'the revolt against work': the critical contest*

John Zerzan

Serious commentators on the labor upheavals of the Depression years seem to agree that disturbances of all kinds, including the wave of sit-down strikes of 1936 and 1937, were caused by the 'speed-up' above all.[1] Dissatisfaction among production workers with their new CIO union set in early, however, mainly because the unions made no efforts to challenge management's right to establish whatever kind of work methods and working conditions they saw fit. The 1945 *Trends in Collective Bargaining* study noted that 'by around 1940' the labor leader had joined the business leader as an object of 'widespread cynicism' to the American employee.[2] Later in the 1940s C. Wright Mills in his *The New Men of Power: America's Labor Leaders*, described the union's role thusly: 'the integration of union with plant means that the union takes over much of the company's personnel work, becoming the discipline agent of the rank-and-file.'[3]

In the mid-1950s, Daniel Bell realized that unionization had not given workers control over their job lives. Struck by the huge, spontaneous walk-out at River Rouge in July 1949, over the speed of the Ford assembly line, he noted that 'sometimes the constraints of work explode with geyser suddenness.'[4] And as Bell's 'Work and Its Discontents' (1956) bore witness that 'the revolt against work is widespread and takes many forms,'[5] so had Walker and Guest's Harvard Study, *The Man on the Assembly Line* (1953), testified to the resentment and resistance of the men on the line. Similarly, and from a writer with much working-class experience himself, was Harvey Swados' 'The Myth of the Happy Worker,' published in *The Nation* (August 1957).

Workers and the unions continued to be at odds over conditions of work during this period. In auto, for example, the 1955 contract between the United Auto Workers and General Motors did nothing to

* This article was first published in the autumn 1974 issue of *Telos* magazine. It was reprinted in pamphlet form by *Black and Red* (Detroit) and by Solidarity (London).

check the 'speed-up' or facilitate the settlement of local shop grievances. Immediately after Walter Reuther made public the terms of the contract he'd just signed, over 70 per cent of GM workers went on strike. An even larger percentage 'wildcatted' after the signing of the 1958 agreement because the union had again refused to do anything about the work itself. For the same reason, the auto workers walked off their jobs again in 1961, closing every GM and a large number of Ford plants.[6]

Paul Jacobs's *The State of the Unions*, Paul Saltan's *The Disenchanted Unionist* and B. J. Widick's *The Triumphs and Failures of Unionism in the United States* were some of the books written in the early 1960s by pro-union figures, usually former activists, who were disenchanted with what they had only lately and partially discovered to be the role of the unions. A black worker, James Boggs, clarified the process in a sentence: 'Looking backwards, one will find that side by side with the fight to control production, has gone the struggle to control the union, and that the decline has taken place simultaneously on both fronts.'[7] What displeased Boggs, however, was lauded by business. In the same year that his remarks were published, *Fortune*, American capital's most authoritative magazine, featured as a cover story in its May 1963 issue Max Way's 'Labor Unions Are Worth the Price.'

But by the next year, the persistent dissatisfaction of workers was beginning to assume public prominence, and a June 1964 *Fortune* article reflected the growing pressure for union action: 'Assembly-line monotony, a cause reminiscent of Charlie Chaplin's *Modern Times*, is being revived as a big issue in Detroit's 1964 negotiations,'[8] it reported.

In the middle-1960s another phenomenon was dramatically and violently making itself felt. The explosions in the black ghettoes appeared to most to have no connection with the almost underground fight over factory conditions. But many of the participants in the insurrections in Watts, Detroit and other cities were fully employed, according to arrest records.[9] The struggle for dignity in one's work certainly involved the black workers, whose oppression was, as in all other areas, greater than that of non-black workers. Jessie Reese, a Steelworkers' union organizer, described the distrust his fellow blacks felt toward him as an agent of the union: 'To organize that black boy out there today you've got to prove yourself to him, because he don't believe nothing you say.'[10] Authority is resented, not color.[11]

Turning to more direct forms of opposition to an uncontrolled and alien job world, we encounter the intriguing experience of Bill Watson, who spent 1968 in an auto plant near Detroit. Distinctly post-union in practice, he witnessed the systematic, planned efforts of the workers to substitute their own production plans and methods for those of management. He described it as 'a regular phenomenon' brought out by the refusal of management and the UAW to listen to

workers' suggestions as to modifications and improvements in the product. 'The contradictions of planning and producing poor quality, beginning as the stuff of jokes, eventually became a source of anger . . . temporary deals unfolded between inspection and assembly and between assembly and trim, each with planned sabotage . . . the rest was stacks upon stacks of motors awaiting repair . . . it was almost impossible to move . . . the entire six-cylinder assembly and inspection operation was moved away – where new workers were brought in to man it. In the most dramatic way, the necessity of taking the product out of the hands of laborers who insisted on planning the product became overwhelming.'[12]

The extent and co-ordination of the workers' own organization in the plant described by Watson was very advanced indeed, causing him to wonder if it wasn't a glimpse of a new social form altogether, arising from the failure of unionism. Stanley Weir, writing at this time of similar if less highly developed phenomena, found that 'in the thousands of industrial establishments across the nation, workers have developed informal underground unions due to the deterioration or lack of improvement in the quality of their daily job lives.'[13]

Until the 1970s – and very often still – the wages and benefits dimension of a work dispute, that part over which the union would become involved, received almost all the attention. In 1965 Thomas Brooks observed that the 'apathy' of the union member stemmed from precisely this false emphasis: 'grievances on matters apart from wages are either ignored or lost in the limbo of union bureaucracy.'[14] A few years later, Dr David Whitter, industrial consultant to GM, admitted, 'That [more money] isn't all they want; it's all they can get.'[15]

As the 1960s drew to a close, some of the more perceptive business observers were about to discover this distinction and were soon forced by pressure from below to discuss it publicly. While the October 1969 *Fortune* stressed the preferred emphasis on wages as the issue in Richard Armstrong's 'Labor 1970: Angry, Aggressive, Acquisitive' (while admitting that the rank and file was in revolt 'against its own leadership, and in important ways against society itself'), the July 1970 issue carried Judson Gooding's 'Blue-Collar Blues on the Assembly Line: Young auto workers find job disciplines harsh and uninspiring, and they vent their feelings through absenteeism, high turnover, shoddy work, and even sabotage. It's time for a new look at who's down on the line.'

With the 1970s there has at last begun to dawn the realization that on the most fundamental issue, control of the work process, the unions and the workers are very much in opposition to each other. A St Louis Teamster commented that traditional labor practice has as a rule involved 'giving up items involving workers' control over the job in exchange for cash and fringe benefits.'[16] Acknowledging the disciplinary

function of the union, he elaborated on this time-honored bargaining: 'Companies have been willing to give up large amounts of money to the union in return for the union's guarantee of no work stoppages.' Daniel Bell wrote in 1973 that the trade union movement has never challenged the organization of work itself, and summed up the issue thusly: 'The crucial point is that however much an improvement there may have been in wage rates, pension conditions, supervision, and the like, the conditions of work themselves – the control of pacing, the assignments, the design and layout of work – are still outside the control of the worker himself.'[17]

Although the position of the unions is usually ignored, since 1970 there has appeared a veritable deluge of articles and books on the impossibility to ignore rebellion against arbitrary work roles. From the covers of a few national magazines: Barbara Garson's 'The Hell With Work,' *Harper's,* June 1972; *Life* magazine's 'Bored On the Job: Industry Contends with Apathy and Anger on the Assembly Line,' September 1, 1972; and 'Who Wants to Work?' in the March 26, 1973 *Newsweek.* Other articles have brought out the important fact that the disaffection is definitely not confined to industrial workers. To cite just a few: Judson Gooding's 'The Fraying White-Collar' in the December 1970 *Fortune*; Timothy Ingram's 'The Corporate Underground' in *The Nation* of September 13, 1971; Marshall Kilduff's 'Getting Back at a Boss: The New Underground Papers,' in the December 27, 1971 *San Francisco Chronicle*; and Seashore and Barnowe's 'Collar Color Doesn't Count,' in the August 1972 *Psychology Today.*

In 1971 *The Workers*, by Kenneth Lasson, was a representative book, focusing on the growing discontent via portraits of nine blue-collar workers. *The Job Revolution* by Judson Gooding appeared in 1972, a management-oriented discussion of liberalizing work management in order to contain employee pressure. The Report of a Special Task Force to the Secretary of Health, Education, and Welfare on the problem, titled *Work in America*, was published in 1973. Page 19 of the study admits the major facts: 'absenteeism, wildcat strikes, turn-over, and industrial sabotage [have] become an increasingly significant part of the cost of doing business.' The scores of people interviewed by Studs Terkel in his *Working: People Talk About What They Do All Day and How They Feel about What They Do* (1974), reveal a depth to the work revolt that is truly devastating. His book uncovers a nearly unani-mous contempt for work and the fact that active resistance is fast replacing the quiet desperation silently suffered by most. From welders to editors to former executives, those questioned spoke up readily as to their feelings of humiliation and frustration.

If most of the literature of 'the revolt against work' has left the unions out of their discussion, a brief look at some features of specific

worker actions from 1970 through 1973 will help underline the comments made above concerning the necessarily anti-union nature of this revolt.

During March 1970 a wildcat strike of postal employees, in defiance of union orders, public employee anti-strike law and federal injunctions, spread across the country disabling post offices in more than 200 cities and towns.[18] In New York, where the strike began, an effigy of Gus Johnson, president of the letter carriers' union local there, was hung at a tumultous meeting on March 21 where the national union leaders were called 'rats' and 'creeps.'[19] In many locations, the workers decided to not handle business mail, as part of their work action; and only the use of thousands of National Guardsmen ended the strike, major issues of which were the projected layoff of large numbers of workers and methods of work. In July 1971 New York postal workers tried to renew their strike activity in the face of a contract proposal made by the new letter carrier president, Vincent Sombrotto. At the climax of a stormy meeting of 3,300 workers, Sombrotto and a lieutenant were chased from the hall and down 33rd Street, narrowly escaping 200 enraged union members, who accused them of 'selling out' the membership.[20]

Returning to the spring of 1970, 100,000 Teamsters in sixteen cities wildcatted between March and May to overturn a national contract signed March 23 by IBT President Fitzsimmons. The ensuing violence in the Middle West and West Coast was extensive, and in Cleveland involved no less than a third-day blockade of main city thoroughfares and $67 million in damages.[21]

On May 8, 1970, a large group of hard-hat construction workers assaulted peace demonstrators in Wall Street and invaded Pace College and City Hall itself to attack students and others suspected of not supporting the prosecution of the Vietnam War. The riot, in fact, was supported and directed by construction firm executives and union leaders,[22] in all likelihood to channel worker hostility away from themselves. Perhaps alone in its comprehension of the incident was public television (WNET, New York) and its 'Great American Dream Machine' program aired May 13. A segment of that production uncovered the real job grievances that apparently underlay the affair. Intelligent questioning revealed, in a very few minutes, that 'commie punks' were not wholly the cause of their outburst, as an outpouring of gripes about unsafe working conditions, the strain of the work pace, and the fact that they could be fired at any given moment, etc., was recorded. The head of the New York building trades union, Peter Brennan, and his union official colleagues were feted at the White House on May 26 for their patriotism – and for diverting the workers? – and Brennan was later appointed Secretary of Labor.

In July 1970, on a Wednesday afternoon swing shift, a black auto worker at a Detroit Chrysler plant pulled out an M-1 carbine and killed three supervisory personnel before he was subdued by UAW committee-men. It should be added that two others were shot dead in separate auto plant incidents within weeks of the Johnson shooting spree, and that in May 1971 a jury found Johnson innocent because of insanity, after visiting and being shocked by what they considered the maddening conditions of Johnson's place of work.[23]

The sixty-seven-day strike at General Motors by the United Auto Workers in the Fall of 1970 is a classic example of the anti-employee nature of the conventional strike, perfectly illustrative of the ritualized manipulation of the individual which is repeated so often and which changes absolutely nothing about the nature of work.

A *Wall Street Journal* article of October 29, 1970 discussed the reasons why union and management agreed on the necessity of a strike. The UAW saw that a walk-out would serve as 'an escape valve for the frustrations of workers bitter about what they consider intolerable working conditions,' and a long strike would 'wear down the expectations of members.' The *Journal* went on to point out that, 'among those who do understand the need for strikes to ease intra-union pressures are many company bargainers. ... They are aware that union leaders may need such strikes to get contracts ratified and get re-elected.'[24] Or, as William Serrin succinctly put it: 'A strike, by putting the workers on the street, rolls the steam out of them – it reduces their demands and thus brings agreement and ratification; it also solidifies the authority of the union hierarchy.'[25]

Thus, the strike was called. The first order of the negotiating business was the dropping of all job condition demands, which were only raised in the first place as a public relations gesture to the membership. With this understood, the discussions and publicity centered around wages and early retirement benefits exclusively, and the charade played itself out to its preordained end. 'The company granted each demand [UAW president] Woodcock had made, demands he could have had in September.'[26] Hardly surprising, then, that GM loaned the union $23 million per month during the strike.[27] As Serrin conceded, the company and the union are not even adversaries, much less enemies.[28]

In November 1970, the fuel deliverers of New York City, exasperated by their union president's resistance to pleas for action, gave him a public beating. Also in New York, in the following March the Yellow Cab drivers ravaged a Teamsters' Union meeting hall in Manhattan in response to their union officials' refusal to yield the floor to rank-and-file speakers.

In January 1971, the interns at San Francisco General Hospital struck, solely over hospital conditions and patient care. Eschewing any

ties to organized labor, their negotiating practice was to vote publicly on each point at issue, with all interns present.

The General Motors strike of 1970 discussed above in no way dealt with the content of jobs.[29] Knowing that it would face no challenge from the UAW, especially, it was thought, so soon after a strike and its cathartic effects, GM began in 1971 a co-ordinated effort at speeding up the making of cars, under the General Motors Assembly Division, or GMAD. The showplace plant for this re-organization was the Vega works at Lordstown, Ohio, where the workforce was 85 per cent white and the average age twenty-seven. With cars moving down the line almost twice as fast as in pre-GMAD days, workers resorted to various forms of on-the-job resistance to the terrific pace. GM accused them of sabotage and had to shut down the line several times. Some estimates set the number of deliberately disabled cars as high as 500,000 for the period of December 1971 to March 1972, when a strike was finally called following a 97 per cent affirmative vote of Lordstown's Local 1112. But a three-week strike failed to check the speed of the line, the union, as always, having no more desire than management to see workers effectively challenging the control of production. The membership lost all confidence in the union; Gary Bryner, the twenty-nine-year-old president of Local 1112, admitted: 'They're angry with the union; when I go through the plant I get catcalls.'[30]

In the GMAD plant at Norwood, Ohio, a strike like that at Lordstown broke out in April and lasted until September 1971. The 174 days constituted the longest walkout in GM history.[31] The Norwood workers had voted 98 per cent in favor of striking in the previous February, but the UAW had forced the two locals to go out separately, first Lordstown, and later Norwood, thus isolating them and protecting the GMAD program. Actually, the anti-worker efforts of the UAW go even further back, to September of 1971, when the Norwood Local 674 was put in receivership, or taken over, by the central leadership when members had tried to confront GMAD over the termination of their seniority rights.

In the summer of 1973, three wildcat strikes involving Chrysler facilities in Detroit took place in less than a month. Concerning the successful one-day wildcat at the Jefferson assembly plant, UAW vice president Doug Fraser said Chrysler had made a critical mistake in 'appeasing the workers' and the Mack Avenue walkout was effectively suppressed when a crown of 'UAW local union officers and committeemen, armed with baseball bats and clubs, gathered outside of the plant to "urge" the workers to return.'[32]

October 1973 brought the signing of a new three-year contract between Ford and UAW. But with the signing appeared fresh evidence that workers intended to involve themselves in decisions concerning

their work lives: 'Despite the agreement, about 7,700 workers left their jobs at seven Ford plants when the strike deadline was reached, some because they were unhappy with the secrecy surrounding the new agreement.'[33]

With these brief remarks on a very small number of actions by workers, let us try to arrive at some understanding of the overall temper of American wage-earners since the mid 1960s.

Sidney Lens found that the number of strikes during 1968, 1969 and 1971 was extremely high, and that only the years 1937, 1944-6, and 1952-3 showed comparable totals.[34] More interesting is the growing tendency of strikers to reject the labor contracts negotiated for them. In those contracts in which the Federal Mediation and Conciliation Service took a hand (the only ones for which there are statistics), contract rejections rose from 8.7 per cent of the cases in 1964 to 10 per cent in 1965, to 11 per cent in 1966, to an amazing 14.2 per cent in 1967, levelling off since then to about 12 per cent annually.[35] And the ratio of work stoppages occurring during the period when a contract was in effect has changed, which is especially significant when it is remembered that most contracts specifically forbid strikes. Bureau of Labor Statistics figures reveal that, while about one-third of all stoppages in 1968 occurred under existing agreements, 'an alarming number,'[36] almost two-fifths of them in 1972, took place while contracts were in effect.[37] In 1973 Aronowitz provided a good summary: 'The configuration of strikes since 1967 is unprecedented in the history of American workers. The number of strikes as a whole, as well as rank-and-file rejections of proposed union settlements with employers, and wildcat actions has exceeded that in any similar period in the modern era.'[38] And as Sennett and Cobb, writing in 1971 made clear, the period has involved 'the most turbulent rejection of organized union authority among young workers.'[39]

The 1970 GM strike was mentioned as an example of the usefulness of a sham struggle in safely releasing pent-up employee resentment. The nation-wide telephone workers' strike of July 1971 is another example, and the effects of the rising tide of anti-union hostility can also be seen in it. Rejecting a Bell System offer of a 30 per cent wage increase over three years, the Communication Workers' union called a strike, publicly announcing that the only point at issue was that 'we need 31 to 32 per cent,'[40] as union president Joseph Beirne put it. After a six-day walk-out, the 1 per cent was granted, as was a new Bell policy requiring all employees to join the union and remain in good standing as a condition of employment. But while the CWA was granted the standard 'union-shop' status, a rather necessary step for the fulfillment of its role as a discipline agent of the work force, thousands of telephone workers refused to return to their jobs, in some cases staying out for weeks in

defiance of CWA orders.

The calling of the ninety-day wage–price freeze on August 15 was in large part a response to the climate of worker unruliness and independence, typified by the defiant phone workers. Aside from related economic considerations, the freeze and the ensuing controls were adopted because the unions needed government help in restraining the workers. Sham strikes clearly lose their effectiveness if employees refuse to play their assigned roles, remaining, for example, on strike on their own.

George Meany, head of the AFL–CIO, had been calling for a wage–price freeze since 1969,[41] and in the weeks prior to August 15 had held a number of very private meetings with President Nixon.[42] Though he was compelled to publicly decry the freeze as 'completely unfair to the worker' and 'a bonanza to big business,' he did not even call for an excess profits tax; he did come out strongly for a permanent wage–price control board and labor's place on it, however.

It seems clear that business leaders understood the need for government assistance. In September a *Fortune* article proclaimed that 'A system of wage–price review boards is the best hope for breaking the cost-push momentum that individual unions and employers have been powerless to resist.'[43] As workers try to make partial compensation for their lack of autonomy on the job by demanding better wages and benefits, the only approved concessions, they create obvious economic pressure especially in an inflationary period. Arthur M. Louis, in November's *Fortune,* realized that the heat had been on labor officials for some time. Speaking of the 'rebellious rank and file' of longshoremen, miners and steelworkers, he said, 'Long before President Nixon announced his wage–price freeze, many labor leaders were calling for stabilization, if only to get themselves off the hook.'[44]

A *Fortune* editorial of January (1972) predicted that by the fall, a national 'wave of wildcat strikes' might well occur and the labor members of the tripartite control board would resign.[45] In fact, Meany and Woodcock quit the Pay Board much earlier in the year than that, due precisely to the rank and file's refusal to support the plainly anti-labor wage policies of the board. Though Fitzsimmons of the Teamsters stayed on, and the controls continued, through a total of four 'Phases,' until early 1974, the credibility of the controls program was crippled, and its influence waned rapidly. Though the program was brought to a premature end, the Bureau of Labor Statistics gave its ceiling on wage increases much of the credit for the fact that the number of strikes in 1972 was the smallest in five years.[46]

During 'Phase One' of the controls, the ninety-day freeze, David Deitch wrote that 'the new capitalism requires a strong, centralized trade union movement with which to bargain.' He made explicit exactly what kind of 'strength' would be needed: 'The labor bureaucracy must

ultimately silence the rank and file if it wants to join in the tripartite planning, in the same sense that the wildcat strike cannot be tolerated.'[47]

In this area, too, members of the business community have shown an understanding of the critical role of the unions. In May 1970, within hours of the plane crash that claimed UAW chief Walter Reuther, there was publicly expressed corporate desire for a replacement who could continue to effectively contain the workers. 'It's taken a strong man to keep the situation under control,' Virgil Boyd, Chrysler vice chairman, told the *New York Times*. 'I hope that whoever his successor is can exert great internal discipline.'[48] Likewise, *Fortune* bewailed the absence of a strong union in the coalfields, in a 1971 article subtitled, 'The nation's fuel supply, as well as the industry's prosperity, depends on a union that has lost control of its members.'[49]

Despite the overall failure of the wage control program, the government has been helping the unions in several other ways. Since 1970, for example, it has worked to reinforce the conventional strike – again, due to its important safety-valve function. In June 1970, the US Supreme Court ruled that an employer could obtain an injunction to force employees back to work when a labor agreement contains a no-strike pledge and an arbitration clause. 'The 1970 decision astonished many observers of the labor relations scene,'[50] directly reversing a 1962 decision of the Court, which ruled that such walkouts were merely labor disputes and not illegal. Also in 1970, during the four-month General Electric strike, Schenectady, New York, officials 'pleaded with non-union workers to refrain from crossing picket lines on the grounds that such action might endanger the peace.'[51] A photo of the strike scene in *Fortune* was captioned, 'Keeping workers out – workers who were trying to cross picket lines and get to their jobs – became the curious task of Schenectady policemen.'[52]

A Supreme Court decision in 1972 indicated how far state power will go to protect the spectacle of union strikes. Four California Teamsters were ordered reinstated with five years' back pay as 'a unanimous Supreme Court ruled [November 7, 1972] that it is unfair labor practice for an employer to fire a worker solely for taking part in a strike.'[53] Government provides positive as well as negative support to approved walkouts, too. An eighteen-month study by the Wharton School of Finance and Commerce found that welfare benefits, unemployment compensation and food stamps to strikers mean that 'the American taxpayer has assumed a significant share of the cost of prolonged work stoppages.'[54]

But in some areas, unions would rather not even risk official strikes. The United Steelworkers of America – which allows only union officials to vote on contract ratifications, by the way – agreed with the major steel companies in March 1973 that only negotiations and arbitration

would be used to resolve differences. The Steelworkers' contract approved in April 1974 declared that the no-strike policy would be in effect until at least 1980.[55] A few days before, in March, a federal court threw out a suit filed by rank-and-file steelworkers, ruling in sum that the union needn't be democratic in reaching its agreements with management.[56]

David Deitch, quoted above, said that the stability of the system required a centralized union structure. The process of centralization has been a fact and its acceleration has followed the increasing militancy of wage-earners since the middle-1960s. A June 1971 article in the federal *Monthly Labor Review* discussed the big increase in union mergers over the preceding three years.[57] August 1972 saw two such mergers, the union of the United Papermakers and Paperworkers and the International Brotherhood of Pulp, Sulphite, and Paper Mill Workers, and that of the United Brewery Workers with the Teamsters.[58] In a speech made on July 5, 1973, Longshoremen's president Harry Bridges called for the formation of 'one big, national labor movement or federation.'[59]

The significance of this centralization movement is that it places the individual even further from a position of possible influence over the union hierarchy – at a time when he is more and more likely to be obliged to join a union as a condition of employment. The situation is beginning to resemble in some ways the practice in National Socialist Germany, of requiring the membership of all workers in 'one big, national labor movement or federation,' the Labor Front. In the San Francisco Bay area, for example, in 1969, 'A rare – and probably unique – agreement that will require all the employees of a public agency to join a union or pay it the equivalent of union dues was reported in Oakland by the East Bay Regional Park District.'[60] And in the same area this process was upheld in 1973: 'A city can require its employees to pay the equivalent of initiation fees and dues to a union to keep their jobs, arbitrator Robert E. Burns has ruled in a precedent-setting case involving the city of Hayward.'[61] This direction is certainly not limited to public employees, according to the Department of Labor. Their 'What Happens When Everyone Organizes' article implied the inevitability of total unionization.

Though a discussion of the absence of democracy in unions is outside the scope of this essay, it is important to emphasize the lack of control possessed by the rank and file. In 1961 Joel Seidman commented on the subjection of the typical union membership: 'It is hard to read union constitutions without being struck by the many provisions dealing with the obligations and the disciplining of members, as against the relatively small number of sections concerned with members' rights within the organization.'[62] Two excellent offerings on the subject written in the 1970s are *Autocracy and Insurgency in Organized Labor*,

by Burton Hall[63] and 'Apathy and Other Axioms: Expelling the Union Dissenter from History,' by H. W. Benson.[64]

Relatively unthreatened by memberships, the unions have entered into ever-closer relations with government and business. A Times-Post Service story of April 1969 disclosed a three-day meeting between AFL-CIO leadership and top Nixon administration officials, shrouded in secrecy at the exclusive Greenbriar spa. 'Big labor and big government have quietly arranged an intriguing tryst this week in the mountains of West Virginia . . . for a private meeting involving at least half a dozen cabinet members.'[65] Similarly, a surprising *New York Times* article appearing on the last day of 1972 is worth quoting for the institutionalizing of government–labor ties it augurs: 'President Nixon has offered to put a labor union representative at a high level in every federal government department, a well-informed White House official has disclosed. The offer, said to be unparalleled in labor history, was made to union members on the National Productivity Commission, including George Meany, president of the AFL-CLO and Frank E. Fitzsimmons, president of the IBT, at a White House meeting last week . . . labor sources said that they understood the proposal to include an offer to place union men at the assistant secretary level in all relevant government agencies . . . should the President's offer be taken up, it would mark a signal turning point in the traditional relations between labor and government.'[66]

In Oregon, the activities of the Associated Oregon Industries, representing big business and the Oregon AFL-CLO, by the early 1970s reflected a close working relationship between labor and management on practically everything. Joint lobbying efforts, against consumer and environmentalist proposals especially, and other forms of cooperation led to an exchange of even speakers at each other's conventions in the fall of 1971. On September 2, the president of the AOI, Phil Bladine, addressed the AFL-CIO; on September 18, AFL-CIO president Ed Whalen spoke before the AOI.[67] In California, as in many other states, the pattern has been very much the same, with labor and business working together to attack conservationists in 1972 and defeat efforts to reform campaign spending in 1974, for example.[68]

Also revealing is the 'Strange Bedfellows From Labor, Business Own Dominican Resort' article on the front page of the May 15, 1973 *Wall Street Journal* by Jonathan Kwitney. Among the leading stockholders in the 15,000 acre Punta Cana, Dominican Republic resort and plantation are George Meany and Lane Kirkland, president and secretary-treasurer of the AFL-CIO, and Keith Terpe, Seafarers' Union official, as well as leading officers of Seatrain Lines, Inc., which employs members of Terpe's union.

Not seen for what they are, the striking cases of mounting business-

labor-government collusion and co-operation have largely been over-looked. But those in a position to see that the worker is more and more actively intolerant of a daily work life beyond his control, also realize that even closer co-operation is necessary. In early 1971 *Personnel*, the magazine of the American Management Association, said that 'it is perhaps time for a marriage of convenience between the two [unions and management] ,'[69] for the preservation of order. Pointing out, how-ever, that many members 'tend to mistrust the union.'[70]

The reason for this 'mistrust,' as we have seen, is the historical refusal of unions to interfere with management's control of work. The AFL-CIO magazine, *The American Federationist*, admitted labor's lack of interest and involvement in an article in the January 1974 issue entitled 'Work is Here to Stay, Alas.' And the traditional union position on the matter is why, in turn, C. Jackson Grayson, dean of the School of Business Administration at Southern Methodist University and former chairman of the Price Commission, called in early 1974 for union-management collaboration. The January 12 issue of *Business Week* contains his call for a symbolic dedication on July 4, 1976, 'with the actual signing of a document – a Declaration of Interdependence' between labor and business, 'inseparably linked in the productivity quest.'

Productivity – output per hour of work – has of course fallen due to worker dissatisfaction and unrest. A basic indication of the continuing revolt against work are the joint campaigns for higher productivity, such as the widely publicized US Steel-United Steelworkers efforts. A special issue on productivity in *Business Week* for September 9, 1972, highlighted the problem, pointing out also the opposition workers had for union-backed drives of this kind.[71] Closely related to low produc-tivity, it seems, is the employee resistance to working overtime, even during economic recession. The refusal of thousands of Ford workers to overtime prompted a Ford executive in April, 1974 to say, 'We're mystified by the experience in light of the general economic situation.'[72] Also during April, the Labor Department reported that 'the productivity of American workers took its biggest drop on record as output slumped in all sectors of the economy during the first quarter.'[73]

In 1935 the NRA issued the Henderson Report, which counseled that 'unless something is done soon, they [the workers] intend to take things into their own hands.'[74] Something was done; the hierarch-ical, national unions of the CIO finally appeared and stabilized relations. In the 1970s it may be that a limited form of worker participation in management decisions will be required to prevent employees from 'taking things into their own hands.' Irving Bluestone, head of the UAW's GM department, predicted in early 1972 that some form of participation would be necessary, under union-management control, of

297

course.[75] As Arnold Tennenbaum of the Institute of Social Research in Michigan pointed out in the late 1960s, ceding some power to workers can be an excellent means of increasing their subjection, if it succeeds in giving them a sense of involvement.[76]

But it remains doubtful that token participation will assuage the worker's alienation. More likely, it will underline it and make even clearer the true nature of the union–management relationship, which will still obtain. It may be more probable that traditional union institutions, such as the paid, professional stratum of officials and representatives, monopoly of membership guaranteed by management, and the labor contract itself will be increasingly re-examined [77] as workers continue to strive to take their work lives into their own hands.

Notes

1 See Herbert Harris, *American Labor* (New Haven: Yale University Press, 1939), 272; Sidney Fine, *Sitdown* (Ann Arbor: University of Michigan Press, 1969), 55; Mary Vorse, *Labor's New Millions* (New York: Modern Age Books, 1938), 59; Charles Walker, 'Work Methods, Working Conditions and Morale,' in A. Kornhauser, *et al.* (eds), *Industrial Conflicts* (New York: McGraw-Hill, 1954), 345.

2 S. T. Williamson and Herbert Harris, *Trends in Collective Bargaining* (New York: The Twentieth Century Fund, 1945), 210.

3 C. Wright Mills, *The New Men of Power: America's Labor Leaders* (New York: Harcourt, Brace, 1948), 242.

4 Daniel Bell, 'Work and Its Discontents,' *The End of Ideology* (New York: The Free Press, 1960), 240.

5 ibid., 238.

6 Stanley Weir, *USA – The Labor Revolt* (Boston: New England Free Press, 1969), 3.

7 James Boggs, *The American Revolution: Pages From a Negro Worker's Notebook* (New York: Monthly Review Press, 1963), 32.

8 E. K. Faltermayer, 'Is Labor's Push More Bark Than Bite?' *Fortune* (June 1964), 102.

9 J. C. Leggett, *Class, Race, and Labor* (New York: Oxford University Press, 1968), 144.

10 Staughton Lynd (ed.), *Personal Histories of the Early CIO* (Boston: New England Free Press, 1971), 23.

11 Stanley Aronowitz, *False Promises: The Shaping of American Working Class Consciousness* (New York: McGraw-Hill, 1973), 44–6.

12 Bill Watson, 'Counter-Planning on the Shop Floor,' *Radical America* (May-June 1971), 78.

13 Weir, op. cit., 2.

14 Thomas R. Brooks, 'Labor: The Rank-and-File Revolt,' *Contemporary Labor Issues*, Fogel and Kleingartner, eds (Belmont, Calif.:

Wadsworth, 1966), 321.

15 William Serrin, 'The Assembly Line,' *The Atlantic* (October 1971), 73.

16 George Lipsitz, 'Beyond the Fringe Benefits,' *Liberation* (July-August 1973), 33.

17 Daniel Bell, *The Coming of Post-Industrial Society* (New York: Basic Books, 1973), 144.

18 Jeremy Brecher, *Strike!* (San Francisco: Straight Arrow Press, 1972), 271.

19 *Washington Post* (March 27, 1970).

20 *Workers World* (July 30, 1971).

21 *Cleveland Plain Dealer* (May 11, 1970).

22 Fred Cook, 'Hard-Hats: The Rampaging Patriots,' *The Nation* (June 15, 1970), 712–19.

23 William Serrin, *The Company and the Union* (New York: Alfred A. Knopf, 1973), 233–6.

24 Cited by Brecher, op. cit., 279–80.

25 Serrin, op. cit., 4.

26 ibid., 263–4.

27 ibid., 202.

28 ibid., 306.

29 Roy B. Helfgott, *Labor Economics* (New York: Random House, 1974), 506.

30 Aronowitz, op. cit., 43.

31 *Wall Street Journal* (December 9, 1972).

32 Michael Adelman, in *Labor Newsletter* (February 1974), 7–8.

33 *Los Angeles Times* (October 27, 1973).

34 Sidney Lens, *The Labor Wars* (Garden City, NY: Anchor, 1974), 376.

35 Richard Armstrong, 'Labor 1970: Angry, Aggressive, Acquisitive,' *Fortune* (October 1969), 144; William and Margaret Westley, *The Emerging Worker* (Montreal: McGill-Queen's University Press, 1971), 100.

36 Harold W. Davey, *Contemporary Collective Bargaining* (New York: Prentice-Hall, 1972), 153.

37 Norman J. Samuels, assistant commissioner, Wages and Industrial Relations, letter to author, April 19, 1974.

38 Aronowitz, op. cit., 214.

39 Richard Sennett and Jonathan Cobb, *The Hidden Injuries of Class* (New York: Alfred A. Knopf, 1972), 4.

40 Remark by CWA president, Joseph Beirne, *New York Times* (July 18, 1971).

41 Aronowitz, op. cit., 224.

42 See Jack Anderson's 'Merry-Go-Round' column, August 23, 1971, for example.

43 Robert V. Roosa, 'A Strategy for Winding Down Inflation,' *Fortune* (September 1971), 70.

44 Arthur M. Louis, 'Labor Can Make or Break the Stabilization

Program,' *Fortune* (November 1971), 142.

45 Editorial: 'Phasing Out Phase Two,' *Fortune* (January 1972), 63.

46 Bureau of Labor Statistics, *Work Stoppages in 1972: Summary Report* (Washington: Department of Labor, 1974), 1.

47 David Deitch, 'Watershed of the American Economy,' *The Nation* (September 13, 1971), 201.

48 Quoted by Serrin, op. cit., 24.

49 Thomas O'Hanlon, 'Anarchy Threatens the Kingdom of Coal,' *Fortune* (January 1971), 78.

50 Arthur A. Sloane and Fred Witney, *Labor Relations* (New York: Prentice-Hall, 1972), 390.

51 From an anti-union article by John Davenport, 'How to Curb Union Power' (labeled *Opinion*), *Fortune* (July 1971), 52.

52 ibid., 54.

53 *Los Angeles Times* (November 8, 1972).

54 Armand J. Thieblot and Ronald M. Cowin, *Welfare and Strikes – The Use of Public Funds to Support Strikers* (Philadelphia: University of Pennsylvania Press, 1973), 185.

55 *New York Times* (April 13, 1974).

56 *Weekly People* (April 27, 1974).

57 Lucretia M. Dewey, 'Union Merger Pace Quickens,' *Monthly Labor Review* (June 1971), 63–70.

58 *New York Times* (August 3 and 6, 1972).

59 Confirmed by Harry Bridges, letter to author, April 11, 1974.

60 Dick Meister, 'Public Workers Union Win a Rare Agreement,' *San Francisco Chronicle* (April 13, 1969).

61 'Union Fee Ruling on City Workers,' *San Francisco Chronicle* (October 31, 1973).

62 Joel Seidman, 'Political Controls and Member Rights: An Analysis of Union Constitutions,' *Essays on Industrial Relations Research Problems and Prospects* (Ann Arbor: University of Michigan Press, 1961).

63 Burton Hall (ed.), *Autocracy and Insurgency in Organized Labor* (New Brunswick, NJ: Transaction Books, 1972).

64 H. W. Benson, 'Apathy and Other Axioms: Expelling the Union Dissenter From History,' Irving Howe, ed., *The World of the Blue Collar Worker* (New York: Quadrangle Books, 1972), 209–26.

65 *Times-Post Service*, 'Administration's Tryst with Labor,' *San Francisco Chronicle* (April 14, 1969).

66 'Key Jobs Offered to Labor by Nixon,' *New York Times* (December 31, 1972), 1.

67 Phil Stanford, 'Convention Time,' *Oregon Times* (September 1971), 4.

68 See *California AFL-CIO News*, editorial: 'The Convention Caper' (January 14, 1972), for example.

69 Robert J. Marcus, 'The Changing Workforce,' *Personnel* (January-February, 1971), 12.

70 ibid., 10.

71 *Business Week*, 'The Unions Begin to Bend on Work Rules' (September 9, 1972), 106, 108.
72 *New York Times* (April 27, 1974).
73 *New York Times* (April 26, 1974).
74 Quoted from Serrin, op. cit., p. 118.
75 David Jenkins, *Job Power* (Garden City, NY: Doubleday, 1973), 319–20.
76 ibid., 312.
77 The San Francisco Social Services Union, a rather anti-union union of about 200 public welfare workers, has emphatically rejected these institutions since 1968. This, plus its vocal militancy and frequent exposure of 'organized labor's' corruption and collusion, has earned them the hatred of the established unions in San Francisco.

'After quite a bit of work and union experience, I find myself really feeling the force of everyday opposition to authority. It feels good to begin to see how little legitimacy any of the old shit has left. Wage-labor, all unions, and the Left, too, are barriers to be smashed; on with creative destruction.' – *John Zerzan*

26 Revolutionary letter no. 19
(for The Poor People's Campaign)

Diane di Prima

if what you want is jobs
for everyone, you are still the enemy,
you have not thought thru, clearly
what that means

if what you want is housing,
industry
   (G.E. on the Navaho
   reservation)
a car for everyone, garage, refrigerator,
TV, more plumbing, scientific
freeways, you are still
the enemy, you have chosen
to sacrifice the planet for a few years of some
science fiction utopia, if what you want

still is, or can be, schools
where all our kids are pushed into one shape, are taught
it's better to be 'American' than black
or Indian, or Jap, or PR, where Dick
and Jane become and are the dream, do you
look like Dick's father, don't you think your kid
secretly wishes you did

if what you want
is clinics where the AMA
can feed you pills to keep you weak, or sterile
shoot germs into your kids, while Mercke & Co
grows richer

if you want
free psychiatric help for everyone

so that the shrinks
pimps for this decadence, can make
it flower for us, if you want
if you still want a piece
a small piece of suburbia, green lawn
laid down by the square foot
color TV, whose radiant energy
kills brain cells, whose subliminal ads
brainwash your children, have taken over
your dreams

degrees from universities which are nothing
more than slum landlords, festering sinks
of lies, so you too can go forth
and lie to others on some greeny campus

THEN YOU ARE STILL
THE ENEMY, you are selling
yourself short, remember
you can have what you ask for, ask for
everything

27 For democracy where we work: a rationale for social self-management*

David DeLeon

While some of us work in offices, and others in factories, we frequently have common complaints.

First, capitalism has tended to reduce us to simple interchangeable parts that can be readily replaced. It's the same if our jobs are on an assembly line, or in row-after-row of telephone operators or secretaries. Our labor is usually a treadmill of routine that requires speed and mental concentration at an immediate task. For example, if you worked at the auto factory in Lordstown, Ohio, in 1976, the cars went by you at the rate of 101 an hour. Every thirty-three seconds you had to mechanically repeat certain motions. If you were a telephone operator, a keypuncher or a steelworker you might have the same response to such a division of labor:

> You're there just to handle the equipment. You're treated like a piece of equipment.

> You do it automatically, like a monkey or a dog would do something by conditioning. You feel stagnant; everything is over and over and over. . . . This makes the average individual feel sort of like a vegetable.

> That's mechanical; that's not human. . . . We sweat, we have upset stomachs, and we're not about to be placed in the category of a machine.

The images are all non-human: a vegetable, a monkey, a dog, a machine. Already in the 1840s, Emerson observed that industrial

---

* This article was written for this anthology and was published first by us as Research Group One Report No. 28 in June 1977. The original publication contains references to all of the quotations as well as extensive documentation. We have here eliminated all of the footnotes.

304

capitalism had destroyed the independence and satisfactions of craft labor, turning the workers into commodities to be bought, sold and 'used' – into a collection of walking monsters, here 'a good finger, a neck, a stomach, an elbow,' but never a whole person.

Second, our jobs are often in dirty, noisy, unpleasant, and sometimes dangerous places. Capitalism is concerned primarily with profit, not with providing us with an attractive workplace (unless this might increase productivity enough to offset the expense). We are expected to put up with the bad lighting, noise pollution, chemical hazards, radiation, and poor ventilation that produce a host of occupational diseases, from asbestosis, through black lung, brown lung, and the rest of the alphabet. While the Department of Labor reported, in 1975, that the number of job-related health threats had declined (partly because of unemployment!), it still noted 5,300 deaths and 5 million non-fatal injuries.

Government regulations are usually minimal and are generally avoided or subverted by the companies. Federal laws such as the Occupational Safety and Health Act seldom have a dramatic impact since the government does not wish to hinder the profitability of business. Thus, by the mid-1970s, the national government employed only fifty-five industrial hygienists: one for every 1 million workers. The typical factory is still likely to have the following conditions:

> The presses leaked oil. The roof leaked. [Forklifts] drove with faulty brakes. Scraps accumulated in the aisles. The high pressure air-lines screeched through the plant as leaks were left unrepaired. In late '72 when a die setter was killed by a bolster plate blowing loose cutting off his head, the flashpoint was provided that set up an unofficial safety committee. On 7 June 1973 a walkout of the second shift in the press room protested the conditions that removed two fingers from a woman working a bad press.

Third, our jobs deny us many basic rights. While many believe that there is democracy in politics, few would argue that there is democracy where we work. Most factories are like military dictatorships. Those at the bottom are privates, the supervisors are sergeants, and on up through the hierarchy. The organization can dictate everything from our clothing and hair style to how we spend a large portion of our lives, during work. It can compel overtime; it can require us to see a company doctor if we have a medical complaint; it can forbid us free time to engage in political activity; it can suppress freedom of speech, press and assembly; it can use ID cards and armed security police, along with closed-circuit TVs to watch us; it can punish dissenters with 'disciplinary layoffs' (as GM calls them), or it can simply fire us. We are forced, by circum-

stances, to accept much of this, or join the millions of unemployed. Herbert Marcuse once called our society a 'nonterroristic totalitarianism.' In almost every job, we have only the 'right' to quit. Major decisions are made at the top and we are expected to obey, whether we work in an ivory tower or a mine shaft.

Fourth, our jobs are making others wealthy, although we have less than we want. We are living in a society where we are forced to sell ourselves, producing profits for a few, and administering their property and power. Capitalism is a form of institutionalized robbery, depriving us of the full value of our labor, and selling our products back to us for a profit. As one writer has commented: 'laborers can be robbed twice – at the point of production and at the market place.' In a more significant sense, we are really being deprived of the fullness of our lives. Even when capitalists are compelled to make concessions, they have more to give. As one character in *Marat/Sade* remarked: 'even if it seems to you that you never had so much – that is only the slogan of those who still have more than you.'

Most of these complaints are found in this depiction of the world of the assembly line worker:

> Try putting 13 little pins in 13 little holes 60 times an hour, eight hours a day. Spot-weld 67 steel plates an hour, then find yourself one day facing a new assembly-line needing 110 an hour. Fit 100 coils to 100 cars every hour; tighten seven bolts three times a minute. Do your work in noise 'at the safety limit,' in a fine mist of oil, solvent and metal dust. Negotiate for the right to take a piss – or relieve yourself furtively behind a big press so that you don't break the rhythm and lose your bonus. Speed up to gain time to blow your nose or get a bit of grit out of your eye. Bolt your sandwich sitting in a pool of grease because the canteen is 10 minutes away and you've only got 40 for your lunch-break. As you cross the factory threshold, lose the freedom of opinion, the freedom of speech, the right to meet and associate supposedly guaranteed under the constitution. Obey without arguing, suffer punishment without the right of appeal, get the worst jobs if the manager doesn't like your face. . . . Wonder each morning how you're going to hold out until the evening, each Monday how you'll make it to Saturday. Reach home without the strength to do anything but watch TV, telling yourself you'll surely die an idiot.

While I've stressed that life is not much better for the white-collar worker, there are differences between those who work with tools and those who, in effect, administer people. Although neither experiences much dignity or satisfaction, the white-collar worker may be less

oppressed. One student from a blue-collar family made this comparison between the factory worker and the college professor who is compelled to 'produce' scholarship:

> The professor would begin to understand how a factory worker feels if he had to type a single paragraph, not papers, from nine to five, every day of the week. Instead of setting the pace himself, his typewriter carriage would begin to move at nine and continue at a steady rate until five. For permission to go to the bathroom or to use the telephone, the professor would have to ask a supervisor. His salary [would be cut in half], and his vacations reduced to two weeks a year. Finally, if he faced the grim conclusion that his job was a dead end, his situation would then approximate that of an unskilled young worker in a contemporary auto factory.

Still, it must be said that all workers tend to feel little sense of meaning in their work. Few would disagree with the worker who said that 'the things I like best about my job are quitting time, pay day, days off, and vacations.' The nature of capitalism – however reformed and prettified – has not changed since Marx criticized it in the 1840s as 'coerced labor' because it was prompted not by 'the satisfaction of a need; it is merely the means to satisfy needs external to it. Its alien character emerges clearly in the fact that as soon as no physical or other compulsion exists, labor is shunned like the plague.' Or as Marx later summarized the attitude of the worker: '*I work in order to live* and provide for myself the means of living. Working is *not* living.'

Does this mean that all workers are, at all times, seething with resentment against capitalism? No, this essay is not the script for a radical melodrama. Many workers, if they are unhappy or unemployed, believe the official ideology that it is somehow their fault and not that of 'free enterprise.' Others tolerate work because their pay buys them a sense of freedom through being a consumer. It is easy to be narcotized by the vision and partial reality of consumption. Consumerism becomes a kind of spectacle that controls people by convincing them that they have meaning through products: 'come alive, you're in the Pepsi generation,' 'Suzuki [motorcycle] conquers boredom,' and 'take a puff and it's springtime.' Even those who become disillusioned are often caught in 'the golden chains' of installment buying; they now have something to lose if they rebel.

Many observers of the surface of advanced capitalist society see only a rather placid working class. Failing to perceive the fundamental inhumanity of capitalism, such commentators say that all fundamental problems have been solved by the beneficent welfare state and a 'people's capitalism.' Events such as the May–June days in France in

1968 have always startled these pundits, because such events were presumably impossible. For example, in the early 1960s a sociology professor analyzed class consciousness among the Vauxhall auto workers in England. Dr Goldthorpe concluded that the workers had adjusted to the inevitability and necessity of their jobs and were quite apathetic. The workers unexpectedly began to discuss his views. At the same time, Vauxhall issued its yearly report of substantial profits. This discussion, combined with the 'provocation' that the company had made several thousand dollars from each worker, prompted an explosion of anger. As the London *Times* reported:

> Wild rioting has broken out at the Vauxhall car factories in Luton. Thousands of workers streamed out of the shops and gathered in the factory yard. They besieged the management offices, calling for the managers to come out, singing the 'Red Flag' and shouting 'string them up!' Groups attempted to storm the offices and battled the police which had been called to protect them.

This rioting continued for two days, no doubt to the astonishment of poor Dr Goldthorpe! Similar examples of workers being ignited by studies proving their indifference have occurred in such diverse areas as Oslo, Norway and Cologne, Germany.

Yet such open violence is uncommon. While most of us feel a 'diffuse hostility' toward our work, this hostility is seldom so dramatically explicit. Although we have always fought back against monotony, speed-ups, dangerous work conditions and arrogant bosses, we may not go beyond indolence and bad work, just as the slaves often responded to their masters. This level of resistance is easily understandable. Capitalism limits our interest in our jobs. If we produce more, we threaten other workers and ourselves, since the quotas will probably be raised. If we develop a more efficient way to do our work, the time and motion experts may suddenly appear. While we usually adjust to 'doing time' in the industrial prison, our frequent passivity should not be confused with contentment.

Some forms of 'striking back' are more obvious, such as stealing from work, stores and supermarkets ($1 billion a year in the early 1970s), or wildcat strikes, sabotage and other types of spontaneous protest. Sabotage can be one brake to a speed-up in an auto factory. The workers begin to make scratches, cut wires, break instruments, fail to tighten bolts, and similar acts. As cars pile up in the repair lot, management is likely to get the message. Of course, sabotage tends to be individualized and may threaten or irritate other workers since it could bring down more supervision and firings. But it will undoubtedly continue, so long as the circumstances of capitalism continue. Such acts

are important for what they symbolize. Take the case of a black worker who was fired at a Detroit Chrysler plant in 1969. He went home, got a gun, returned to the factory and killed two foremen and a UAW committeeman. The next day, many foremen got anonymous newspaper clippings about this event. The worker's defense was that the brutal conditions of the plant had driven him insane. After the judge and jury visited the factory, he was acquitted!

Most employers are aware of such undercurrents of hostility. Employers are concerned about low productivity, lack of interest, sabotage, absenteeism, and other signs of what was called in the early 1970s 'the revolt against work' or 'the blue-collar blues.' Soon, the Department of Health, Education and Welfare had funded a study on 'work in America,' Senator Edward Kennedy chaired an investigation into 'worker alienation,' and President Nixon declared that 'the need for job satisfaction' was one of the great issues of the day. In 1975, the Hart poll indicated that about 80 per cent of Americans believed that capitalism had reached its peak and was in decline. American capitalism has been able to respond to such challenges with moderate reforms, seeking to convince us that our best interests are served by capitalism. Business has been able to adjust to 'responsible' unionism, and to such techniques as profit-sharing, company pensions, teams of workers, and more flexible hours of work. These are all excellent forms of social control: 'quit and you lose your pension!;' 'We're speeding up the line to increase your profit-sharing;' or, 'buy a share in *your* company!' While most of these changes are cosmetic, merely giving the appearance of 'humanistic management,' most radicals have been insensitive to the power of such devices to minimally meet human needs. Elinor Langer soon realized that the 'busy little world' of small rewards and loyalties can assuage the impersonality of most existing work situations. For business, 'the pattern of co-optation . . . rests on details: hundreds of trivial, but human details.' Business people have generally understood this better than radicals.

Other business experiments have offered some real elements of workers' control. In 'job enlargement,' a petty job is made more complex and thus (presumably) more interesting. In 'job enrichment,' the worker is permitted to make a few decisions, rather than being completely under the thumb of the supervisor. Job redesign involving both of these factors has included a team of workers building individual cars, instead of turning one screw or tying three wires. Elinor Langer noticed other cases in a phone company which had created a mass of minor supervisors and an elaborate system of limited mobility, thus fostering the impression of power and progress. AT T has allowed those who do the sorting and coding of checks and invoices to vary their pace, work with the same clients continuously (thus developing

a sense of 'my' customers) and arrange different hours of work. This resulted in a 27 per cent increase in productivity and a saving of $558,000 a year. General Foods, in the early 1970s, granted a number of rights to the workers in its Topeka, Kansas, factory: they could interview and hire new workers, form teams for particular work projects, and make various decisions. This stimulated 30 per cent higher productivity. Obviously, the workers were more satisfied.

Nevertheless, job redesign will not solve the basic problems of capitalism. While it might alleviate some difficulties, it causes others. Job enlargement usually means doing more work (often in a higher 'skill' classification) without more money; more efficiency will mean fewer jobs; 'team leaders' are, in effect, foremen; and what happens when these novelties are no longer new? After all, the major goal is still profit: 'I participate, you participate, they profit.'

In Europe, pressure from the working class has forced the capitalists to try even more advanced reforms. In Germany, workers have representation on all boards of directors and management committees of major industries. Under this policy of 'co-determination,' labor and business have regular get-togethers to discuss health, safety and production. Such involvement or consultation, of course, does not mean control – it is pseudo-participation. American reformers like Ralph Nader are naturally attracted to such moderation, and have also called for consumer and 'public' members on US corporate boards. Some capitalists will make such changes because they want to decrease worker resentment and to increase productivity, but this will not eliminate the fact that capitalism is based upon the exploitation of labor. It will remain true that, in the class struggle, nice guys finish last. Capitalism has changed, and may still change, but it will always be divided into the owners of the means of production and the rest of us, wage laborers.

What about unions? Won't they protect us? Aren't they for workers' control? No, they are essentially for the control *of* workers. While unions began as self-defense organizations for workers to limit the power of capital, they have become junior partners of business. Even during the 1920s, intelligent capitalists like Gerard P. Swope, the president of General Electric, had praised 'businesslike' unions that insured a stable, orderly work force. Many other liberals and conservatives became convinced of the need for a new form of discipline when 8.2 million workers struck in 1933, and federal troops were used in sixteen states in 1934. Frances Perkins, FDR's Secretary of Labor, reiterated the values of unions to capitalism: 'You don't need to be afraid of unions. . . . They don't want to run the business. You will probably get a lot better production and happiness if you have a good union organization and a contract.' By the 1960s, Clark Kerr agreed that unions were major 'disciplinary instruments,' Daniel Bell lauded

them as part of 'the control system of management,' C. Wright Mills denounced them as 'managers of discontent,' and Paul Jacobs characterized them as 'an integral part of the system of authority.' How do unions keep the workers in line, and facilitate long-term capitalist planning?

1 *The contract.* Companies are pleased by contracts that promise a predictable labor force. Unions are pleased by the prospect of their own organizational stability. Walter Reuther of the UAW once even stressed a five-year contract (which union militants ridiculed as the equivalent of Stalin's five-year plan), and I. W. Abel of the steelworkers urged a three-year contract with a no-strike provision. Of course, the average worker may not share all of this enthusiasm. It is his or her freedom that has been limited.

The content of these long-term contracts may also be unattractive to many workers. 'Responsible unionists' have tended to limit bargaining to industry-wide issues of wages and hours. Workers at a particular factory or office may be more disturbed about work conditions, but the distant bureaucracy negotiates on other issues. While the contract may win certain concessions, it is at the price of the workers' guaranteed passivity. If work conditions deteriorate, if a speed-up eliminates time benefits, if inflation destroys wage gains – the worker is still bound by the contract. The contract is a basic validation of the company's legal authority. It is the legal mortgage or bill of sale of the workers.

Once the leadership has negotiated a contract, the members are seldom given a chance to knowledgeably discuss it, or even, sometimes, to vote on it. The whole process has become so remote and legalistic that most workers are turned off. A recent contract at Lordstown was representative: it was 166 pages long, and written in a language that would require a team of interpreters to tell the average person what was happening. By the end of bargaining, the majority of workers are apathetic, confused or possibly hostile – leaving about 10–14 per cent of contracts rejected. The contract has become a maze of 'proper channels' that baffles the worker.

2 *The right to strike.* Just as the contract is handed down from above, so are strike orders. Most unionized workers have lost the power to strike over local issues. Even the CIO of the 1930s vigorously discouraged sitdowns and direct action. Strikes, under union direction, are supposed to be controlled, quiet, legal actions occurring only at the end of a contract, if at all. Instead of masses of workers outside and inside the plant, there are a few 'official' pickets. Instead of occupying a plant, it is surrendered to the employer. Instead of spontaneous struggle, the strike is planned and announced to the enemy in advance. The workers are virtually expected to be passive spectators during their own strike. The unions say 'go home! We are negotiating for you.' Union

struggles have become so ritualized that 'most official strikes resemble a badminton game more than a boxing match.'

When workers become impudent and act by themselves, the modern union often responds as a strike-breaker. In 1974, a wildcat at one of Chrysler's truck plants was defeated when the union called the police to throw the workers out of the union hall that had been built with their own dues! The sanctity of the contract was everything. In 1976 nearly one-half of the miners of the UMW wildcatted against the contract negotiated by one of the darlings of liberal unionism, Arnold Miller. His response to the rebellious miners was typical of any bureaucrat: if they don't like it, they can quit.

3 *Grievance procedures.* Let us say that a contract has been 'accepted' and the company follows the pattern described in the *UMW Journal*: it begins 'violating the contract on the day it's signed and continues until the day it expires.' If the workers can't officially strike, why don't they protest through the grievance process?

Suppose that a worker is idle and the foreman tells him or her to push a broom across the floor to 'make work.' The worker may reply: 'shove it up your . . .,' but the order will probably have to be obeyed. If the worker wants to refuse, s/he may be required to ask the foreman to *call* the union representative to file a complaint. This, in itself, prevents many from acting. If not, the union rep may be slow in arriving since the number of them has declined over the years. Then, the rep will inform the worker that the order must be obeyed, although a grievance can be filed. If so, the event will be recorded on a piece of paper. Months or years later, you may 'win' your grievance, but it will no longer make any difference. This system is obviously too cumbersome to be effective, and even if the union official is sympathetic s/he is really a kind of cop who compels the worker to continue working while the lawyers or the officials do something – or nothing. In 1974 the St Louis local of the UAW had 18,000 unresolved grievances. Since the union hesitates to endanger its own privileges (even the lowly committeeman often has special pay, no blue-collar work and the right to leave the workplace during the day), it has holstered its most threatening weapons such as the strike, and speaks in soft, legalistic tones. The union is seldom a watchdog for workers' rights. As one militant has said, 'Your dog don't bark no more.'

4 *Dues checkoff.* Well, if workers don't like what's going on, can't they refuse to pay their dues? No, they can't. One of the first goals of many unions was to have all dues automatically deducted from the worker's paycheck *by the company*. The workers then became passive dues payers. 'The union no longer had to come down to the ranks and hustle your dollars.' This tied the union bureaucracy closer to the company and made it more remote from the workers. In the 1880s, the

officers of the American Railway Union 'rode the rails' like paupers; today, AFL leaders have private jets. They are 'tuxedo unionists.' The uncontrolled wealth generated by the dues checkoff, along with the closed shop (which has limited the necessity for organizing), has fostered the corruption documented by the Kefauver and McClellan investigations, and such magnificent salaries as the $100,000 a year received by seventeen officers of the Teamsters in 1975. Unions have become big business. In 1976 they had 170,000 contracts and $3 billion a year in dues and assessments. The money, cars, clothes and status of these 'workers' place them in the same physical context and intellectual perspective as the capitalist – riding the backs of labor. Where was the average worker at one of the 1976 meetings of this elite:

Somehow they didn't look like formidable political foes of reaction as they relaxed in their shorts and colorful sports shirts around the pool of the Americana Hotel in Bal Harbour, a rather swank Florida resort where they had been gathering each winter for more than two decades. And they didn't look like tough leaders of America's workers as they ordered *escargots* and rack of lamb or thick steaks in the dining rooms of Miami Beach, or when they sipped Dry Sack Sherry and talked quietly among themselves at the nightly receptions given for them by supplicants of their good will. With salaries of $50,000 or more, they might not be expected to voice the concerns of the average worker.

Indeed, historically the unions have 'protected' mainly the aristocrats of labor (the better paid occupations), and locked out minorities and the unskilled. Herbert Hill, the national labor director of the NAACP, lamented that the unions were no longer a social movement, but had disintegrated into 'narrow protective service agencies for their dues-payers,' ignoring the masses of unorganized workers – which means especially the black, Puerto Rican and Chicano laborer. Existing unions are more concerned about their bank accounts than about the general interests of the working class. George Meany regretted the money given to the United Farm Workers because they 'make a lot of noise' but 'few contributions to the working of this organization.' Walter Reuther, despite his own limitations, recognized this as 'the banker mentality in the American labor movement.'

5 *Bureaucracy*. If all of this is true, why don't the workers rise up and vote the rascals out of office? This is not impossible, but extremely difficult since most unions are police states. There is little or no local autonomy; there are no legitimate parties or factions within unions; the bureaucracy controls the union press, union patronage, and union treasury; the bureaucracy has few traditions or 'due process' in union

disputes; power is concentrated in the office of the president; dissidents can be broken easily. Frank Marquart, of the auto workers, recalls that when he tried to use the union hall to discuss local issues, the union locked the doors. Jordan Sims claimed that he hadn't seen a contract in ten years, and the union constitution in eighteen – and that the president of the local told him that 'you don't want to read something like this. It'll just mix up your mind and get you into trouble.' Such bureaucrats turn union meetings into puppet shows:

> The tricks of the trade are numerous. They include all-inclusive resolutions that blunt an opposition view; lengthy and technical committee reports which are difficult to follow; stacking convention committees with 'safe' members, advised by experts whose function is to sell predetermined policy; careful choice of speakers from the floor; overloading the guest list as a form of filibuster against too much time for delegates' discussion; postponing controversial resolutions to the last minute, when delegates are increasingly impatient, so that the discussion is either too brief, or else is 'referred to the incoming board'; and finally using the staff's power of patronage to keep things under control.

Sometimes, militants do win, like Arnold Miller of the UMW. Then, because of the imperatives of 'working within the system,' they become rapidly transformed into 'respectable leaders.' Even the election of radicals may change little of the essentially oligarchic structure of trade unionism. Consider the case of the UAW. All three of the Reuthers were once members of the Socialist Party – Walter Reuther had even been a tool-and-die worker in the USSR during the 1930s (and had no basic criticisms of the labor discipline). Emil Mazey, the secretary-treasurer, once belonged to the Proletarian Party and the SPA. Leonard Woodcock (born in England) came out of the sectarian Independent Labour Party and the SPA! Nevertheless, the UAW remains a dictatorship, though, perhaps, a benevolent one. Whatever the case, it suffers from all of the problems that have been mentioned.

This doesn't mean that unions are all alike. It can be argued that, while George Meany represents a kind of narrow 'business as usual unionism,' Walter Reuther was a champion of 'social unionism' – favoring more social planning or engineering. While one type could be said to be more reformist than the other, both are basically procapitalist, although Reuther tended toward state capitalism.

Both kinds of unions have some positive qualities. They do make some quantitative if not qualitative differences in society. Workers may derive certain benefits in wages and hours, along with the power of mass organization. Unions may foster a sense of solidarity – as in the

ritual use of 'brother' and 'sister' at some meetings – and the inclusion (though often minimal) of women, blacks and minorities. Union officials may, like old-time political bosses, perform certain minor favors: notarizing documents, finding jobs, and influencing local judges and politicians. But, in essence, unions have been accepted by much of capitalism because they insure 'social peace,' divide the workers into organizations (each with its own jealous bureaucracy), and allow for long-term planning.

Of course, it is also true that business remains hostile to the organization of non-militant workers, who can be controlled by other means. While unions and capital can work compatibly, business is still reluctant to concede any wage gains, improvements in physical working conditions, 'interference' with management powers, and workers' rights. Many companies still resist union elections or engage in 'surface bargaining' in the hope of defeating the ratification of any contract.

Nevertheless, there are many circumstances where unions can act as buffers or shock absorbers between the workers and the company. Trade unions, after all, accept capitalist legality, private property, the 'harmony of class interests' and strike limitations. Such union officials function as the agents of capital, mediating as middlemen with the workers. If the company is prosperous (for example, if the workers are more exploited), the union – that is, generally, the bureaucracy – also prospers. Unions like the United Steel Workers, the International Ladies Garment Workers, and the United Rubber Workers have preached productivity to their members. The UMW has promoted automation that has eliminated the jobs of thousands of people. Within the values of capitalist competition, these were all reasonable and responsible actions.

It is understandable, then, that many people are skeptical about unions. Only about 32 per cent of American labor is unionized, and the percentage has been dropping in recent years. Why join a union? In 1975, the California Poll and a study by Gallup revealed that, while business ranked lowest in public esteem, labor unions vied for this distinction. In 1965 unions won 60 per cent of NLRB elections; in 1976, 49 per cent. Many blacks consider the unions racist; many women have been excluded or oppressed by union sexism. And American workers are not unique in this pessimism. Over 40 per cent of British labor votes Conservative! Does this prove that they are content, stupid or misled, as many radicals claim? Perhaps – but it may also illustrate that, in many cases, people can see no difference between a Conservative candidate and a Labour one.

Although many of us are unhappy about our jobs, our unions and our politics, there are few alternatives. Radical parties are usually quite as repressive. Radical unions will not succeed at this moment, and

circumstances are not conducive to mass organization. American capitalism has been able to make concessions because of the unique wealth of North American farmlands and mineral resources, and because of its past lack of equal competitors. It has been able to maintain its profits by a high rate of return from foreign investment or by raising prices (ultimately lowering the workers' real gains). But revolutions abroad and competition from such countries as Japan and West Germany limit these options. What remains is to 'rationalize' the work process through automation and a reduction in the number of workers, along with intensified exploitation (making us work harder). American labor, in the future, may be forced to go beyond trade unionism.

Many workers doubt that the major existing alternative, socialism, would be much better, and they are justifiably suspicious of American radical parties. They have heard of the lack of even political democracy in most socialist countries, and many know something about the military battles against the working class in Hungary, East Germany, Poland and Czechoslovakia. They sense that in most socialist systems the working class does not rule. Instead, a single party dominates all, supposedly 'in the interests of the working class.' None of the Marxist–Leninist states – and this includes China – permits the formation of any open opposition, or the printing of opposition literature, or the holding of opposition meetings. The total life of the workers is subject to the will of a few. Now and then, the 'happy proletarians' rebel, as did many Polish workers in 1970 and 1976 when various Communist Party buildings were sacked. Even in China, the struggle for power after the death of Mao Tse-tung was not openly debated. Most socialist countries are a sad parody of socialist ideals.

This is most obvious in the workplace.

First, the division of labor has been maintained with few exceptions. Marx had condemned this fragmentation of life, saying that it 'converts the labourer into a crippled monstrosity' and that 'the subdivision of labor is the assassination of a people.' Yet conventional socialism has not challenged the organization of work. At best, some argue that 'alienation' is less under socialism because the worker may feel that s/he is working for a higher standard of living for all. But this is not enough. As one critic has stated the proper goal of liberation: 'socialism is not a backyard of leisure attached to the industrial prison. It is not transistors for the prisoners. It is the destruction of the industrial prison itself.'

Second, the immediate aims of state socialism and capitalism are the same: efficiency and productivity. If these conflict with happiness, then happiness is sacrificed. Russia, for example, invented Stakhanovite socialism, named after the ox-like worker who always overfulfilled his quota. What laborer is going to applaud the prediction of André Gorz

that 'after the communist revolution we will work more, not less'? Or the special homes, clothing, food and status of the socialist elites? What worker who hears of Soviet productivity will not think 'speed-up'? Consider the description of a Russian factory where the main work area was dominated by a gigantic poster of Lenin ('Lenin is eternally with us'), surrounded by such thrilling banners as 'every day of shock labor is a stride toward communism' and 'discipline is the precondition of success.' Shock labor? Discipline? Or the North Korean newspaper that proudly informed us that 'Fierce Flames of Speed-Up Campaign [are] Raging at Every Construction Site' (onward, comrade serfs!). What all Marxist–Leninist parties call 'the Communist attitude toward work' is apparently marching, rank after rank, toward tomorrow. Yet the denial of democracy today means the defeat of democracy tomorrow. The workers' rights have been subordinated to capital accumulation, just as they are under capitalism, although individual capitalists have been replaced by a collective capitalist, the state. In either case, productivity comes first, people second. While Chinese communism has been a partial exception, with its refusal to repeat the Russian model of rapid industrialization based upon brutal coercion, it may still be bureaucratized in the era following Mao Tse-tung.

Third, the atomized and oppressive work that is generally maintained under socialism is not democratically organized. If it were, it might be abolished. Instead, workers have little voice in what happens in their workplace. They are still subject to appointed managers, their unions are usually powerless, and they cannot strike against 'their' state. Nationalization has failed to replace what Marx called 'the barracks discipline' of industrial civilization. Nationalization is not synonymous with democratization. Rather, power has become more remote. One British coal miner complained that it was 'like working for a ghost' instead of a definite group of capitalists. Another Yorkshire miner added: 'Why is it we must always work under management and never with it?' Michael Polanyi was probably correct when he observed that a worker in a nationalized mine no more felt that he 'owned' the mine than he felt that he owned the Royal Navy.

Nationalization has not solved inequalities of power; it has merely substituted officials for owners. These officials are the realization of Bakunin's fear of a 'red bureaucracy,' what one modern radical has called 'a red bourgeoisie.' Under the direction of this new elite, an enormous and highly centralized bureaucracy rigidly plans everything. The local unit is, in practice, reduced to insignificance. This is bureaucracy, not democracy . . . and Fabians are as guilty of it as Leninists, Trotskyists as much as Stalinists. For all, the workers are still treated like draftees into the industrial army. This is a socialism of five-year plans, growth rates, and dams and factories, but it is not everyday

democracy.

These criticisms have been summarized by one author this way:

> People can no longer satisfy themselves with the system of the
> U.S.S.R. 'Here is a state factory, and the state is the Party, and the
> Party is the masses, thus the factory belongs to the workers. Q.E.D.'
> No, this is no longer tenable. If someone says to me: 'This factory is
> yours, it belongs to the people,' but I blindly obey the orders of the
> directors, I understand nothing of my machine and still less about
> the rest of the factory, if I do not know what becomes of my product
> when it is finished nor why it was produced, if I work quickly, very
> quickly for a bonus, and if, in the meantime, I am bored to death by
> it all week, Sunday and each holiday, if I am, besides, more neglected
> after years of work than at the beginning – in that case this factory
> is not mine, it does not belong to the people.

We must study the alternatives to both traditional capitalism and
socialism. We must draw upon such history as the Paris Commune of
1871, Russia during 1905 and 1917–21, examples of wildcats, the IWW,
the Socialist Labor Party, the sit-ins of the 1930s, Spain during 1936–9,
Hungary in 1956, direct action during the 1960s, Algeria in the early
1960s, France in 1968, Chile in 1972, and Portugal in 1975. Libertarian
theories must be analyzed, such as syndicalism, anarcho-communism,
Oscar Lange's 'market socialism' of the 1930s, the idea of the general
strike, co-operative movements, the 'ultra-Left' critique of Leninism,
and the Council Communism of Karl Korsch, Anton Pannekoek,
Herman Gorter, Paul Mattick, Serge Mallet and André Gorz. Not least,
we must understand existing models in West Germany, Scandinavia,
Israel (*kibbutzim*), Algeria, Yugoslavia and the United States. From
all of this, we may find answers to what Bakunin called the greatest
problem of socialism, 'to integrate individuals into situations which
they can understand and control.'

The largest experiment with such new institutions has been Yugoslav
'self-management.' Since 1950, the 20 million people of Yugoslavia
have been testing many of the ideas of workers' control. This experience
can tell us both what to do, and what not to do. The Yugoslav system
constitutes a direct repudiation of the Soviet argument that regulation
of the workforce was necessary because of the military threat of capitalism and the need for rapid industrialization. After World War II, over
35 per cent of Yugoslavia's industry had been destroyed, 1.7 million
people had been killed, the country was split into five ethnic groups,
and the USSR was condemning the country for its independence. After
a period of conventional centralism, the Yugoslav party rejected the
Russian example and turned to the mottos of 'the factory for the

workers' and 'direction of production through the producers.' For over a quarter of a century, the workers have acquired more and more control within a decentralized socialist economy. This has become a complex system, with both faults and virtues. Local councils of workers generally determine wages, investments, plans and working conditions. The Yugoslav League of Communists is supposed to represent the general interests of the community. Of course, there are many frustrations in a society that is multi-national, that is still industrializing, and that is attempting (not always with success) to achieve a great ideal. Strikes, legally impossible elsewhere, are signs of both freedom and frustration. Elites still exist; the Party does not allow factions; there is unemployment, inflation, and perhaps (by the existence of a free market) a resurgent capitalist mentality. Nevertheless, one should not refuse to study at this living school of socialism.

Not all illustrations of workers' control occur in foreign countries like Yugoslavia. The United States also has some examples of worker-run factories, businesses and co-ops. We could cite the eighteen worker-owned plywood factories of the Northwest, producing 12 per cent of US plywood. Some of these began in the 1930s. Workers elect the 'managers' of the firm, retain considerable control, create special benefits like dental and health care, gas at wholesale, lunches, insurance paid by the company, along with greater concern for safety, 35 per cent higher salaries, and job security in slack times. Other cases include a multi-million-dollar asbestos factory (the Vermont Asbestos Group), the Saratoga Knitting Mills, clothing factories in the Southeast, and various co-ops. In additions to these attempts – often flawed – to achieve workers' control, there are numerous small libertarian associations.

While there are no perfect models of workers' control, these still cause us to reconsider such 'facts of life' as hierarchy, domination and constraining social roles. By comparison, labor unions are social workers for capitalism; radical parties are ideological junkshops, cluttered with overstuffed Victorian social democracy, faded Orthodox icons and cracked china. It is time, perhaps to follow the advice of one of the 'maniacs' in *Marat/Sade*: 'pull yourself up by your own hair, turn yourself inside out and see the whole world with fresh eyes.'

In our radical vision, the very nature of work and the use of technology must be questioned. Our first motto might be: let the machines do the work! Automated trains, printed circuits rather than hand-wiring, prefabricated houses, car factories with only a few workers, and the general application of computers to production are all possible. Machines should be workers, rather than workers machines.

This libertarian society could guarantee, as a simple matter of justice, a minimum of food, shelter, medicine and clothing free to all. Perhaps you say that no one would work. 'Those committed to the present state

of affairs will ask, "How will we eat, how will we get rid of garbage, how will we fly to Italy, if we get rid of wage labor? People only work because of coercion".' This is not self-evident. One study indicated that 80 per cent of the employed would continue to work even if they didn't have to, although many added that they would quickly change jobs if it were possible. Most people feel a sense of wellbeing when something has been accomplished. If they felt self-realization through their jobs, it is improbable that they would abandon them. This would be more likely in a world where jobs were not as trivial, or were more equitably rewarded (to give Fourier's example, garbage collectors should be the highest paid people in any society). None the less, a free society must allow the option of not working, at a socially guaranteed subsistence. As one free spirit proclaimed: 'I don't believe in work; I believe in the no-work ethic. . . . If you have to work for something, it's not worth having' (that is, why work for the future, why not live now?). Our model is not the society of the ascetic revolutionary, but a culture of celebration, festival, pleasure and play.

This libertarian perspective would encompass all of life, from the person's earliest years to old age. Domestic functions, for example, should be communalized, since housework can be as stultifying as factory work. Charlotte Perkins Gilman once suggested collective laundries, dining areas, child-care and cleaning facilities. These could all be organized by their workers, men and women. In the school, the ideal must be 'self-teaching' and the 'self-managed child,' not the student as passive consumer, note-taker and spectator, and the teacher as cop. The school, too is a workplace; it needs student and faculty syndicalism. The same is true of the office, or the factory.

Each libertarian organization can be founded and sustained only by a conscious, well-informed public. Each person would be able to vote where he or she works or is active, on all issues of significant concern. It is vital that people who have direct experience make the decisions, not some remote bureaucracy. Such elections would occur when necessary, since in the era of TV, radio and rapid communication there should be instantaneous democracy. Participation would mean greater experience and thus, in a general way, greater competence. Meetings should discuss all issues, and votes can be taken on local, regional and 'national' questions. Since the individual has the option of refusal, and a socially guaranteed minimum, this 'democracy' does not violate libertarian principles.

By democracy, I do not mean 'state.' The political system as we know it could be abolished as archaic and parasitic. Instead, people might be organized at local units, electing delegates (if representation could not be avoided) with limited mandates which could be immediately revoked. 'Managers' of all sorts would be directly accountable,

and their actions subject to initiative, referendum and recall. Technicians and specialists would still be necessary also, but their status would be transformed. It would not be enough for the workers to decide *what* to do, and then have the technicians tell them *how* to do it. Rather, the technicians would be involved in the original discussions about both the *what* and the *how*.

This might function in the following way. Auto workers could vote for people to speak for their particular shop, for others who would be general representatives for their factory, for industry-wide spokespeople, and for members of a central council of labor that would be necessary for discussion, statistics, and the co-ordination of production. The workers would have direct, continuous control over their representatives. Delegates for general community interests should sit on all of these committees, to speak for those who do not work (including the young and the aged), and to criticize activities that might be racist, sexist, concerned only with local profit, or harmful to the overall community, such as air and water pollution.

Gar Alperovitz has called this system a pluralist commonwealth, combining both diversity and some unity of values. This would not be a state in any usual sense. There would be no geographic capital, but wherever the General Council of Labor was meeting. It would not be a union of states, but a union of unions; it would achieve the goal that Marx stated in the Communist Manifesto: 'a free association of people in which the free development of the individual is the condition of the free development of all,' where organization exists to administer things rather than people.

Doesn't this assume a technologically advanced society? Would it work elsewhere? Well, Yugoslavia and China have two of the most humane forms of existing socialism. They have sought to avoid a centralization that squashes local initiative and experience. Self-management can mean maximum flexibility, experimentation and – perhaps – efficiency. Workers would have greater interest, and therefore greater self-motivation. This could mean higher productivity, along with fewer overpaid, unproductive and interfering managers and supervisory personnel. While it is probably true that state socialism could direct a poor country more rapidly toward a nuclear bomb, a mammoth military, superhighways and an elite with villas in the countryside, this is scarcely the ideal of this author.

That leaves one final question: can we achieve these ideals? Sartre once belittled surrealism's call for total revolution, saying that it 'does not harm anybody precisely because it is total,' and unattainable. We must have both a maximum program (our radical vision) and a minimum program of immediate criticisms and solutions. Within unions, we should waste no energy seeking to have the AFL declare

321

the general strike! Instead, efforts should be made to foster rank-and-file caucuses and to form newsletters in which people could share their experiences. Committees can demand that the company 'open the books' – that is, reveal its true finances and organizational practices. Committees could also discuss grievances, and agitate on issues of speed, scheduling, the right to strike during a contract, hiring, firing and safety and health issues. Libertarians should, whenever possible, use schools, unions and other groups to agitate and inspire. These can be transitional means to move toward radical goals.

Even today, there are small working models of alternative institutions: producers' co-operatives, free schools, co-ops for food and services, tax resistance funds, communes, and community control movements for education, tenant organizing and many other local concerns. These go beyond the rhetoric of democracy to day-to-day reality. While they are small and disorganized, they represent the IWW dream of 'building the new society within the shell of the old.' But such radicals can still learn from Marx's critique of the social limits of such individual projects. While Marx praised the co-ops, in 1866, as a 'beneficent system of the *association of free and equal producers*,' he realized that their political consciousness was limited, and that they often starved because of the lack of capital, were attacked by large businesses, or, if economically successful, were absorbed into capitalist values. Like Marx, modern libertarians must educate themselves and others to understand the problems of the existing order, the potential for a new society, and the difficulties in achieving it.

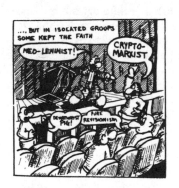

Still, revolutions are not planned. Even 'vanguard' intellectuals and parties are usually stunned by such events as the Paris Commune, the Russian Revolution, the precipitous collapse of the Chinese Nationalists, or the French upheavals in 1968. We can only predict that, just as the

feudal world died in wars and revolutions, so will the capitalist world. But while change may be abrupt, we can prepare for it. Otherwise, when tomorrow brings the equivalent of the Commune or the Soviets, our hopes will once again be suppressed by reaction or become perverted into some new autocracy.

Part Seven

Reinventing anarchist tactics

Introduction

Social anarchists believe that the revolution begins in the present, in every aspect of life. Along with Marxists, they work to end capitalism and create socialism. But unlike Marxists, they leave nothing to the future. As we have seen in the earlier sections of this book, anarchists work to bring down the state (both capitalist and socialist) now; try to destroy all forms of domination now; attempt to behave as autonomous people now; and try to reorganize the nature and structure of work. Right now. This awareness of the indissoluble link between present actions and the shape of the future leads anarchists to place great emphasis on means as well as ends, on employing anarchist tactics to reach anarchist goals. The six articles in this section all explore varying aspects of this crucial problem.

One anarchist tactic is direct action. Contrary to stereotype, it does not mean mindless, random terrorist activity; nor is it the impulsive, anti-intellectual behavior of short-sighted individuals. Rather, as David Wieck states, direct action is 'that action which, in respect to a situation, *realizes the end desired.*' In contrast, indirect action 'realizes *an irrelevant or even contradictory end*, presumably as a means to the "good" end.' This is not an abstract moral issue: people on the anti-authoritarian Left should realize that some frequently used tactics are not only inconsistent with their aims, but may even be harmful. Perhaps the largest category of bad tactics includes those that rely on the government to bring about desired changes. One example is passing laws to abolish inequities. Another is participating in electoral politics.

Everyone can, of course, point to instances in which government or law has acted beneficently. In the United States and other countries, laws designed to end some racist and sexist inequities are on the books; and sometimes they are even enforced. However, inequality will never be ended by the law; it will disappear only when people act as free and responsible individuals, insisting on their own autonomy and respecting that of everyone else. If people can be made to obey a good law, they can be made to obey a bad one as well.

327

If passive reliance on the law is one kind of indirect action (hence, not an anarchist tactic), so is electoral politics. Several years ago, the Anarchos groups suggested that social anarchists might take part in local electoral politics. Judith Malina's article, 'Anarchists and the Pro-Hierarchical Left' strongly rejects voting as a tactic, on the ground that you cannot achieve anarchist ends by hierarchical means. 'The tyranny of the majority is injustice like any other form of tyranny.'

Instead, Malina suggests, anarchists should set up alternative organizations in explicit opposition to the state, to fulfill people's needs better than the state can. These 'action collectives' will be decentralized, non-authoritarian, and controlled by everyone involved. Thus, the construction of alternative institutions is an essential anarchist tactic, because it is directly related to anarchist goals.

Marxists tend to dismiss alternative institutions as ways of dropping out and escaping the struggle with major social institutions, but anarchists disagree. 'Anti-Mass' sums it up very well: 'You make the revolution by actually changing social relations.'

The key, of course, is *actually changing* social relations. Just setting up a clinic, a food co-op, or an alternative paper, or calling a small group made up of you and your friends an 'affinity group' won't do it. In 'The Logic of Alternative Institutions,' Howard J. Ehrlich sets up five criteria for assessing alternative institutions as anarchist organizations: (1) they must offer a genuine service to a politicized constituency; (2) they must develop standards of success and failure, and a means of evaluating their own performance; (3) they must structure themselves on genuine principles of anarchist organization; (4) they must have an ongoing program of internal political education; and (5) they must continue to attack the institutional structures of the larger society (or, as Malina put it, carry out their programs in '*opposition to* the lousy oppressive so-called solutions of the official bodies').

These are high standards, but necessary ones. For without them, the alternative institution as an anarchist tactic becomes corrupted into something that is non-revolutionary. At its very worst, it may actually become counter-revolutionary by taking some of the pressure off capitalist institutional structures.

One of the most striking features of the contemporary political scene is the frequency with which anarchist tactics are chosen by political activists. Doubtless, many would not recognize their actions as anarchist; often these tactics are imperfectly realized – perhaps because imperfectly understood. None the less, the basic forms are there. One recent example is described by Murray Rosenblith, in 'Surrounded by Acres of Clams.' On April 30, 1977, well over 2,000 people occupied a nuclear power plant construction site at Seabrook, New Hampshire, in the north-eastern United States. On the following day, almost 1,500 of

the occupiers refused to vacate the site and were arrested. About 600 eventually spent close to two weeks in prison – refusing release unless guaranteed that all would be released without posting bail.

Were the tactics of the Clamshell Alliance anarchist? In part. In choosing direct action instead of relying on legal measures, they were operating in the anarchist tradition; in their affinity group structure, consensual decision-making, and careful attention to non-authoritarianism, they were acting as anarchists. However, as Rosenblith points out, there were definite problems. People inexperienced in active nonviolence tended to respond passively; and despite all efforts, affinity group representatives at times arrogated too much decision-making power to themselves. Perhaps the key here is political inexperience. Anarchist tactics become sharpened through practice; and practice, as we all know, makes perfect. (Or at least it improves things quite a bit.)

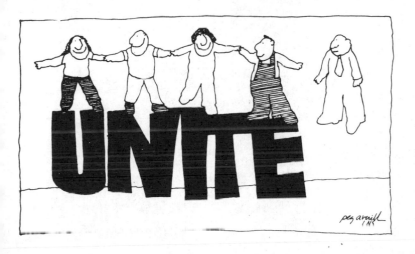

Anarchists tactics can be intellectual as well as organizational: They can involve new ways of understanding the world and of interpreting it. Marxist and feminist intellectuals have, for example, devoted some efforts to developing a revolutionary literary criticism. In 'Notes and Queries of an Anarchist Critic,' HJE makes perhaps the first attempt at an anarchist analysis of literature. For Marxists, feminists and anarchists alike, there are three reasons for doing so: to expose the capitalist political assumptions of the 'accepted' body of criticism; to help readers understand that so-called 'apolitical' literature is in fact profoundly political, in that it reinforces capitalist culture; and to develop

criteria for evaluating radical literature. No doubt, most academics will be enraged. But that, like everything else about their co-optation by the academy, is *their* problem.

28   The habit of direct action*

David Wieck

All action, we can see upon reflection, realizes *some* belief. Indirect action is often criticized on the ground that the means employed are unreliable; a strong point, but perhaps applied too sweepingly, and I think less fundamental than another. I want to distinguish (as direct action) that action which, in respect to a situation, *realizes the end desired*, so far as this lies in one's power or the power of one's group; from action (indirect action) which realizes *an irrelevant or even contradictory end*, presumably as a means to the 'good' end. The most significant – but not the only – distinction lies in the kind of fact thereby created for other persons. It is direct action to present a person with the kind of attitude towards 'race' which one advocates; it is indirect action to rely on legal enforcement because in this is realized the concept that these people must obey the law simply because it is the law, and this may hopelessly obscure the aim.

Persons with no patience often make a bad distinction between 'talk' and 'action.' It can be seen that the important distinction is between talk that is mere moral assertion or propositional argument, and talk (in fact: direct action) which conveys a feeling, an attitude, relevant to the desired end.

To take a homely example. If the butcher weighs one's meat with his thumb on the scale, one may complain about it and tell him he is a bandit who robs the poor, and if he persists and one does nothing else, this is *mere talk*; one may call the Department of Weights and Measures, and this is *indirect action*; or one may, talk failing, insist on weighing one's own meat, bring along a scale to check the butcher's weight, take one's business somewhere else, help open a co-operative store, etc., and these are *direct actions*.

Proceeding with the belief that in every situation, every individual and group has the possibility of *some* direct action on *some* level of generality, we may discover much that has been unrecognized, and the

* Reprinted from *Anarchy*, no. 13, 1962.

importance of much that has been underrated. So politicalized is our thinking, so focused to the motions of governmental institutions, that the effect of direct efforts to modify one's environment are unexplored.

The habit of direct action is, perhaps, identical with the habit of being a free person, prepared to live responsibly in a free society. Saying this, one recognizes that just this moment, just this issue, is not likely to be the occasion when we all come of age. All true. The question is, when will we begin?

FUCK LEGALIZATION

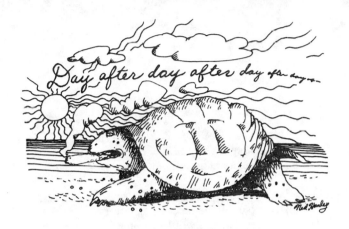

Day after day after day of...

Smoking dope "legally" is no solution to the totality of our oppression. What real difference will it make in our everyday lives if we can "legally" smoke marijuana openly? We smoke it openly right now. Will the loneliness, the anxiety and the boredom of our lives suddenly disappear? Will our bosses be immediately turned to ice? Will police chief Couper choke to death on a roach; and will everything be free? Think about it.

Legalization means: Camel filters, Acapulco Gold, Salem longs..... Singing the praises of the American Tobacco Company:

> "Panama Red, Panama Red,
> Buy till you die and work until you're dead!"

We have had enough of buying and working, enough of pigs and laws. To talk about life today is like talking about rope in the house of a hanged man. So legalizing grass or even acid will not stop us from being outlaws; because we plan to annihilate <u>everything</u> that stands in the way of our desires! We want to abolish the system of wage labor, of profit and of bureaucratic power. We want to decide the nature and conditions of everything we do, collectively and democratically. We want the whole world to be our conscious self-creation, so that our days are full of wonder, learning and pleasure.
For a life without dead time,
and a revolution of untrammeled desire!

AURORA
p. o. box 1163
madison, wi. ; 53701

ABOLISH ALL LAW!

29   Civics I: Nothing Fancy

Dick Lourie

the President is a piece of shit.
I said the President is a piece of shit.
He started out that way if you think back.
There hasn't really been any development.

Second verse: the Vice President is a racist prick.
I ask you only to examine the record objectively.
The so-called cabinet – what a word – cabinet
is a white protestant thing with hands of dirty money.

Your congress eats well (and that's being kind).
Your judges are all thinking about
law law order order and
law and somebody else's real estate.
When I was arraigned the judge
treated me like a distasteful object.

Last verse: you can guess the rest,
             you can guess the rest, and
             you can guess the rest.
Brothers and Sisters, we are all we have.

1969

30 Anarchists and the pro-hierarchical left*

Judith Malina

1 What is voting?

Voting is an agreement by all that the will of the most shall be carried out. When there is unanimous agreement the decision of the people is self-evident.

But when there is no unanimity the vote becomes the tyranny of the many over the reluctant few.

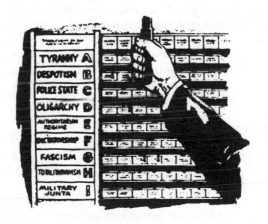

This tyranny is the expression of a principle inherent in the democratic ethic: a tacit understanding that the few will not fight the many

* This was a leaflet distributed in response to an article by the New York City Anarchos Group which suggested that anarcho-communists participate in *local* electoral politics. It was probably written between 1967 and 1971.

because the many would win by virtue of their superior numbers. This form of decision-making originates in the primitive situation where superiority of numbers usually meant victory in battle – all hero stories to the contrary. Therefore, instead of doing battle over each issue, decisions were voted – that is, avowed.* The majority is then considered the victor of the unfought battle.

The myth is that justice consists of a few 'bowing down to the will of the majority;' whereas, the tyranny of the majority is injustice like any other form of tyranny.

2 Action collectives

When the principles of anarchism are understood, it follows that there are increasing numbers of community forums, workers' councils, local committees and other decentralized and non-authoritarian groups which will productively and humanely fulfill the decision-making functions of society.

There are ways of rotating the decision-making functions among all those who are concerned with a particular problem, so that the problem can be solved by all the people concerned. Much heartening experimentation in this direction has already been done in exemplary anarchist experiments of the past – and today in new social structures everywhere.

In the revolutionary process these groupings and these new forms of organization will struggle *against* the existing authoritarian state structures.

3 Smashing the state

In order to overthrow the system effectively so that the new forms will not revert to power structures means to do it without adopting the means of the system.

Yes, the people should take over local control at the community level – but not through the municipal governments which, through party lines, are always closely bound to state and federal governmental structures. Instead, the people should take over control by creating community structures from below. Such structures will not exist parallel to the governmental municipal structures – but will in fact wrest the power from them.

How?

---

* Vote: from the Latin *votum*: vow. 'Votive' and 'devotion' with their implication of servility have the same derivation.

By creating community solutions to local problems that are better – more useful to the people – than the solutions that the municipal government has found.

The municipal government's decisions are always based on laws enacted in the interest of some group's or some individual's profit motive.

Therefore it is inevitable that as soon as community councils activate and begin to carry out *their* solutions, they will come into areas of conflict with the municipal government's decisions. This is inevitable because the municipal government, like any government, is not what the people want.

The local government functions under the law. The people can find a way to function better. A way to carry out their will. And when the people's way confronts the law, and when the will of the people struggles against the law, they will divest the government of its corrupt power – and carry out the will of the people.

The criticism here is not of the forms of local organization that the Anarchos group proposes, but only of the submission to the jurisdiction of the local constitutional government.

It is true that the local municipal councils are frequently in conflict with the larger state and federal bodies, and this does represent an advance from feudal submission to a more populist position.

But it is not true that local radical coalitions can, under the authority of the dreadful power games of the state/federal forces develop their potential as alternatives, precisely because they are affiliated – by the nature of public office – to the larger bodies and always ultimately under their jurisdiction.

The problem is to demonstrate the spurious nature of this jurisdiction. And all jurisdiction is, in fact, invalid.

4 Anarchists and the pro-hierarchical left

The non-hierarchical is a clear goal only among the anarchists. And though the anarchist movement (i.e. those who call themselves – are conscious of themselves as – anarchists), along with the anarchist tendency (among those who do not call themselves anarchists but live and organize their political lives in a more or less libertarian way), is growing daily more strong, more unified and more organized, this anarchist movement is still in the minority.

We must realize that the programs that we envision will necessarily include the participation of the entire spectrum and spectre of the left and probably also the growing radical right – Bookchin's phrase 'these coalitions must be free and non-hierarchical' represents a goal that we

337

do indeed, as anarchists, advocate – but it is not an admissable analysis of the reality of the left in this country, or in most other countries.

It seems outrageously optimistic to imagine that there will be no 'manipulative behavior' no matter how valiantly we struggle against it. These struggles within the left are intrinsic to the development of history, and they must, and will and are already, taking place.

If a radical seat is won on the city councils, as in many European models, and now Berkeley, Ann Arbor and more to come, it will be struggled for in the political arena by all the militants of the left.

It seems apparent that if the anarchists show themselves effective on the city councils, that the Marxists, Marxist–Leninists, socialists, Trotskyists, etc. will seek to share, or even wrest, that representation. But their work is, of course, structured to include political maneuvering within the electoral system and their philosophical basis geared to the older forms of voting and delegated authority, whereas the foundations of anarchism are placed on a rejection of these intrinsically authoritarian forms.

But if the hierarchical left does in fact occupy the municipal councils, and win representation in the local governments, it will be well to see the democrats and republicans move over in their struggle with the voting left; it will help weaken the fabric of the juggernaut and it will help clarify the difference between the anarcho-communist left and the voting left.

The strength of the anarchist movement is sapped by the retreat into old forms: the primary one being . . .

5 The delegation of authority

The delegation of authority is, along with economic pressure and force by arms, the major method of human enslavement in the world today.

The power is wrested from the people and the people bow down.

The people bow down at the ballot box as if to say: 'I agree to obey your laws and follow your decisions, and if I don't, I give you herewith the authority to punish me.'

The delegation of authority is a form of self-demeaning submission like the payment of taxes, or service in armed bodies.

But of course we are all conditioned and educated to regard voting and the delegation of power as a form of noble and humane conduct. Because when voting and the delegation of power become recognizable as forms of submission, then the anarchist principle of human freedom and human possibilities becomes clear also, and then we are ready to make those changes that we anarchists call revolution.

But the anarchist alternatives are *not* clear to the pro-hierarchical

left, and it seems to me that the first task of the revolutionaries is to clarify the nature of authority – and to clarify that fundamentally *all* authority (even tyranny) is delegated by the people – because the power can be taken away from the authority (or the tyrant) and be with the people. (Tolstoy deals with precisely this in 'What is Power?' in which he examines the people's motives that allow a few to have power or authority over so many.)

Now we must begin to make clearer and clearer the processes that lead to this delegation of power and how we all participate in this process. An understanding of this process will hasten revolutionary possibility far more than seeking to infiltrate the electoral party system from below and within.

Action collectives for radical reorganization of local action programs grow and continue.

It is those groups who do *not* join in the electoral battles with their party shit and their lying campaigns and their manipulative corruption –

it is those groups who oppose the old forms with new forms of getting things done –

it is those groups (and precisely *because* of their anarchist forms) that will smash the old forms – because they can get the work done – and the old forms can't.

Anarchism is a higher form of organization. It can't be anything else.

If the anarchists don't prove that the higher forms of organization are attainable and practicable then we weaken our cause and place obstacles to the real changes.

Suggestion for alternative action

– Where there are no local action committees for local alternatives, that anarchist activists help form them;

– where there is community action that is free of state control, that anarchist activists support it;

– where there is opposition to, or ignorance of, the possibilities of local organization, that anarchist activists demonstrate these possibilities;

– that such committees, workers' councils, groups and coalitions – just as Bookchin describes them – form confederations and set up methods for communication and mutual aid;

– that such groups, instead of becoming vulnerable though dissident appendages of the dominant political body, work as opposition forces, especially where it is possible to carry out action programs, action programs that present more functional and more human alternatives, and carry them out in *opposition to* the lousy oppres-

sive so-called solutions of the official bodies.

Thereby the revolutionary possibility is made clear.

As revolutionary groups augment their programs there will eventually be a confrontation on real issues.

Eventually the real nature of government power asserts itself.

At that moment the people can decide between their solution and the governmental solution – and at that moment, if the governmental forces resist the will of the people, then the time is ripe to take the authority away from the authorities so that the people can do things their way.

Judith Malina is a member of The Living Theater Collective.

Do it. Vote.

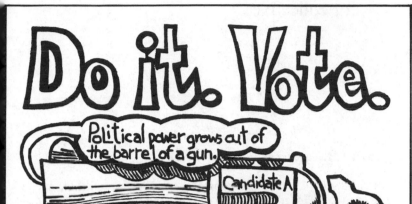

Political power grows out of the barrel of a gun.

Candidate A
Candidate B
VOTER'S SPECIAL

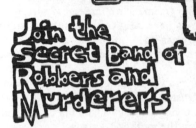

Join the Secret Band of Robbers and Murderers

Terrorism, Stealing & Miscellaneous Bullying— we voters enjoy it! When we vote we sanction government terrorism, tax theft and assorted underworld activities intended to force our will on all. Only 15% of us choose to elect rulers, but since our government has all the guns and goons to use them, the rest of the people who don't support us are forced to pay "protection" money-tax- or suffer. Our morals are made law. We dictate modes of dress, permissable literature and religious customs. We run others' lives! We are a violent terroristic minority.

Our rulers don't have to obey our orders, of course. Try demanding that your "representative" vote as you would. He doesn't have to. Who does he represent? By what authority?

Your card →

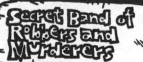

Secret Band of Robbers and Murderers welcomes ___ a fellow voter, to its ranks.
NAT'L CHM. SBRM

31 Anti-mass—methods of organization for collectives*

Primacy of the collective

The small group is the coming together of people who feel the need for collectivity. Its function is often to break out of the mass – specifically from the isolation of daily life and the mass structure of the movement. The problem is that frequently the group cannot create an independent existence and an identity of its own because it continues to define itself negatively, i.e. in opposition. So long as its point of reference lies outside of it, the group's politics tend to be superimposed on it by events and crises.

The small group can be a stage in the development of the collective, if it develops a critique of the frustrations stemming from its external orientation. The formation of a collective begins when people not only have the same politics but agree on the method of struggle.

Why should the collective be the primary form of organization? The collective is an alternative to the existing structure of society. Changing social relations is a *process* rather than a product of revolution. In other words, you make the revolution by actually changing social relations. You must consciously create the contradictions in history.

It is imperative that any people who decide to create a collective know exactly who they are and what they are doing. That is why you must consider your collective as primary. Because, if you don't believe in the legitimacy of this form of organization, you can't have a *practical* analysis of what is happening. Don't kid yourself. The struggle for the creation and survival of collectives at this moment of history is going to

---

* This is excerpted from a pamphlet, *Anti-Mass – Methods of Organiza-tion for Collectives*, published by *the anti-mass* around late 1970 or early 1971, most likely in San Francisco. It was distributed widely through a Vocations for Social Chance reprint; and in 1975 it was typeset by *the black market* and printed with an 'afterword' by Come! Unity Press of New York City.

be very difficult.

The dominant issue will be how collectives can become part of history – how they can become a social force. There is no guarantee and we should promise no easy victories. The uniqueness of developing collectives is their definite break with all hierarchic forms of organization and the reconstructing of a classless society.

The form of a collective is its practice. The collective is opposed to the mass. It contradicts the structure of the mass. The collective is anti-mass.

Size of the collective

Most people cannot discuss intelligently the subject of size. There is an unspoken feeling either that the problem should not exist or that it is beneath us to talk about it. Let's get it out in the open. Size is a question of politics and social relations, not administration. Do you wonder why the subject is shunted aside at large meetings? Because it fundamentally challenges the repressive nature of large organizations. Small groups that function as appendages to larger bodies will never really *feel* like small groups.

The collective should not be bigger than a band – no orchestras or chamber music, please. The basic idea is to reproduce the collective, not expand it. The strength of a collective lies in its social organization, not its numbers. Once you think in terms of recruiting, you might as well join the army. The difference between expansion and reproduction is the difference between adding and multiplying The first bases its strength on numbers and the second on relationships between people.

Why should there be a limit to size? Because we are neither supermen nor slaves. Beyond a certain point, the group becomes a meeting and before you know it you have to raise your hand to speak. The collective is a recognition of the practical limits of conversation. This simple fact is the basis for a new social experience.

Relations of inequality can be seen more clearly within a collective and dealt with more effectively. A small group with a 'leader' is the nucleus of a class society. Small size restricts the area which any single individual can dominate. This is true both internally and in relation to other groups.

Today, the mode of struggle requires a durable and resilient form of organization which will enable us to cope with both the attrition of daily life and the likelihood of repression. Unless we can begin to solve problems at this level collectively, we are certainly not fit to create a new society. Contrary to what people are led to think, i.e. united we stand, united we fall, it will be harder to destroy a multitude

of collectives than the largest organizations with centralized control.

Size is a key to security. But its real importance lies in the fact that the collective reproduces new social relations – the advantage being that the process can begin now.

The limitation on size raises a difficult problem. What do you say to someone who asks, 'Can I join your collective?' This question is ultimately at the root of much hostility (often unconscious) toward the collective form of organization. You can't separate size from the collective because it must be small in order to exist. The collective has a right to exclude individuals because it offers them the alternative of starting a new collective, i.e. sharing the responsibility for organization. This is the basic answer to the question above.

Of course, people will put down the collective as being exclusive. That is not the point. The size of a collective is essentially a limitation on its authority. By contrast, large organizations, while having open membership, are *exclusive* in terms of who shapes the politics and actively participates in the structuring of activities. The choice is between joining the mass or creating the class. The revolutionary project is to do it yourself. Remember. Alexandra Kollontai warned in 1920, 'The essence of bureaucracy is when some third person decides your fate.'

Self-activity

Bad work habits and sloppy behavior undermine any attempt to construct collectivity. Casual, sloppy behavior means that we don't care deeply about what we are doing or who we are doing it with. This may come as a surprise to a lot of people. The fact remains: we talk revolution but act reactionary at elementary levels.

There are two basic things underlying these unfortunate circumstances: (1) people's idea of how something (like revolution) will happen shapes their work habits; (2) their class background gives them a casual view of politics.

A lot of problems which collectives will have can be traced to the work habits acquired in the (mass) movement. People perpetuate the passive roles they have become accustomed to in large meetings. The emphasis on mass participation means that all you have to do is show up. Rarely do people prepare themselves for a meeting, nor do they feel the need to. Often this situation does not become evident precisely because the few people who do work (those who run the meeting) create the illusion of group achievement.

Because people see themselves essentially as objects and not as subjects, political activity is defined as an event outside them and in the

future. No one sees *themselves* making the revolution and, therefore, they don't understand how it will be accomplished.

The short span of attention is one tell-tale symptom of instant politics. The emphasis on responding to crisis seems to contract the span of attention – in fact there is often no time dimension at all. This timelessness is experienced as the syncopation of over-commitment. Many people say they will do things without really thinking out carefully whether they have the time to do them. Having time ultimately means defining what you really want to do. Over-commitment is when you want to do everything but end up doing nothing.

The numerous other symptoms of casual politics – lack of preparation, being late, getting bored at difficult moments, etc. – are all signs of a *political* attitude which is destructive to the collective. The important thing is recognizing the existence of these problems and knowing what causes them. They are not personal problems but historically determined attitudes.

Preparation is another part of the process which creates continuity between meetings and insures that our own thinking does not become a part-time activity. It also combats the tendency to talk off the top of one's head and to pick ideas out of the air. Whenever meetings tend to be abstract and random it means the ideas put foward are not connected by thought (i.e. analysis). There is seldom serious investigation behind what is being said.

What does it mean to prepare for a meeting? It means not coming empty-handed or empty headed. Mao says, 'No investigation, no right to speak.' Assuming a group has decided what it wants to do, the first step is for everyone to investigate. This means taking the time to actually look into the matter, sort out the relevant materials and be able to make them accessible to everyone in the collective. The motive underlying all preparation should be the construction of a coherent analysis.

Self-activity is the reconstruction of the consciousness (wholeness) of one's individual life activity. The collective is what makes the reconstruction possible because it defines individuality not as a private experience but as a social relation. What is important to see is that work is the creating of conscious activity within the structure of the collective.

One of the best ways to discover and correct anti-work attitudes is through self-criticism. This provides an objective framework which allows people the space to be criticized and to be critical. Self-criticism is the opposite of self-consciousness because its aim is not to isolate you but to free repressed abilities. Self-criticism is a method for dealing with piggish behavior and developing consciousness.

32　The logic of alternative institutions*

Howard J. Ehrlich

To be successful, an alternative institution must provide its community with a genuine service. It must do so in an openly politicized context, and one that builds in community control as well as worker self-management. An alternative institution can survive in an un-coopted form only within a politicized constituency.

Second, alternative institutions must develop standards of success and failure, and techniques of assessing their performance. Successes should be publicized everywhere; and failures abandoned and the political struggle begun again. To work to build alternative forms without a clear understanding of what comprises success is self-defeating.

Third, the workers or membership of alternative institutions must operate on principles of collective organization. Decisions must be made collectively, work assignments rotated, and knowledge and skills continually shared. Manifestations of elitist legacies – of sexism, of racism, of egocentrism, of authoritarianism – must all be continually suppressed. As a work group, an alternative institution must be a model.

Fourth, alternative institutions must maintain formal programs of internal education. Experienced members must share their knowledge with the inexperienced. Skills must be taught to the unskilled. And all must study together around the issues of political struggle that unite them.

Finally, a part of the resources and people power of alternative organizations must always be allocated to direct assaults on the institutional structures they are trying to change. Being a model of an alternative structure is important, and it may be personally and collectively gratifying – but it is not enough. An alternative institution must always be a counter-institution.

* Printed here for the first time.

346

33   Surrounded by acres of clams*

Murray Rosenblith

More than a month after the occupation of the Seabrook nuclear power plant construction site, it sometimes is difficult to keep the event in proper perspective. There is a sense that it was a mystical event; something greater than a well planned and executed direct action project. Some have hailed Seabrook as the opening of a new era for social change activism in the US. That it may be, but there is no magic about it. The Seabrook occupation was the result of many hours of hard work by hundreds of people.

Organizing for the mass occupation at Seabrook began last year with the arrest of 180 people after they occupied the site on August 22, 1976. The people of New Hampshire had been fighting the Seabrook nuke to no avail by legal means for many years through the courts, town referenda and lobbying the Public Service Company. The first direct action against the nuke occurred in January 1976, when a Weare, New Hampshire, resident, Ron Rick, climbed a weather tower on the Seabrook site and spent thirty-two hours there in sub-zero degree weather. For most people outside of New Hampshire, publicity of this action brought the Seabrook nuke to their attention for the first time.

Continuing this history of opposition, the Clamshell Alliance began to plan for the mass occupation. The affinity group structure, which had functioned successfully at the early occupation, was central to the organization. The affinity group had been the basic organizational unit of the anarchists during the Spanish Civil War. Operating on the principle that people function best in a situation in which they are familiar with and trust the people immediately around them, the group provides everyone with ongoing feedback into any decision. All participants in the April 30 occupation were members of an affinity group and all groups received nonviolence training before occupying.

Friday night before the occupation was clear and cold. That night

* This article was originally published in *WIN Magazine*, June 16 and 23, 1977.

347

and Saturday morning were a blur of last-minute meetings, training sessions, repacking gear. People were, generally, well supplied. National Guard officers would later comment we were better equipped than they were; looking out over a field of people hoisting 40 and 50-pound packs, I could believe it.

A count finished around 2 am Sunday morning showed that just over 1,200 people were camped out at the five staging areas. Another 500 were expected from Boston early in the morning, and people continued to arrive all through the night.

We did not move out until after 1 pm, Saturday. We woke hours before, ready to roll then, but there were meetings and last minute details to clear up. And, the Clam people reported, there were still people pouring into the Marigold Ballroom, the last-minute staging area south of the site.

Clam organizers had been worried about provocateurs all week, particularly after the Labor Committee, a vehement supporter of nuclear power, became the main source of the violence reports that Meldrim Thomson quoted in the days right before the occupation. However, there was no trouble from provocateurs, and poison ivy, sunburn and blisters became our greatest threats. Most people marched between two and six miles, with heavy packs, to reach the site. Even with good hiking shoes, there were a sizable number of people gingerly limping around the encampment on Saturday night.

Midday Saturday the marchers moved out from Hampton, Newton, the Marigold Ballroom and the North and South Friendly areas bordering the nuke site. A small group boated in through the estuary and landed on the eastern edge of the site.

Miraculously enough, they all converged on the site within minutes of each other. The western march, composed of the Hampton, Marigold and Newton groups numbering over 1,000, had to go through the front gate. The only obstructions were a few sawhorses and a private security guard making a rather tentative request that people not trespass on the site. The main group paused at the gate to allow stragglers to catch up and then swept in.

Just ahead of the march several dozen newspaper and TV photographers struggled to catch a clear picture of the group while walking backwards. The reporters were actually the first trespassers. Some of them would be arrested with everyone else the next day. Only the AP and UPI correspondents, who had some kind of sweetheart deal with the state, were immune. They wandered around the site in funny helmets with flashing lights on top, looking like refugees from a Flash Gordon fan club.

The site itself is not very attractive. It is the former Seabrook town dump (they still haven't found another place to put their garbage),

covered over with a sandy landfill. There are some temporary construction buildings and a five story cement mixer. In all, it looks like a disaster already occurred there.

Clam organizers had not found out until late Friday night that we might be allowed to actually enter the site. The original injunction had covered the entire site, but under the altered injunction only a small, central construction area was fenced off. The change in the injunction indicated that the state might be realigning their tactics. Unfortunately, the organizers had not really worked out a scenario for this possibility.

Once on the site, there was a quick meeting to decide where to camp out. After that we trooped onto the enormous parking lot and pitched camp. The choice of the lot for the campsite would later turn into one of several 'mistakes that didn't have time to become mistakes.'

As the Clam organizers had not worked out an on-site scenario, the inertia of the situation was to do nothing. Many people, particularly those who were veterans of other direct actions, chafed at the inactivity. The occupation was an aggressive action, but somewhere along the way, without a general consultation, some of the more active proposals for confrontation were shelved. Once we got on the site, the energy to do anything seemed to dissipate. Not only did the Clam not have plans for being on the site, but the nonviolence training had emphasized passivity as the proper reaction to any new situation.

Many of the trainers had given the impression during the sessions that nonviolent direct action was more inaction than anything else. Among their examples had been how to nonviolently stop people from breaching the interior fence. Many of us who have been active in the nonviolent movement for a while were surprised at the reappearance of this concept. We didn't get to hold the site long enough to work out these problems, though we did seem to be moving in the right direction. Fortunately, the next two weeks gave many people ample opportunities to explore the possibilities and illustrate the theories of active nonviolence.

After we were on the site there were immediate and constant spokes and DMB (The Decision-Making Body, a smaller group supposedly constituted to make quick, emergency decisions on the march) meetings. The meetings went on into the evening.

For a while the affinity process appeared to have been inverted. Decisions were supposed to come from the affinity groups with the spokes meeting for co-ordination and feedback. But late Saturday afternoon it seemed that spokes were coming back to their affinity groups with 'orders' from above. The discontent among many occupiers was immediate and grew rapidly. People also pointed out that the DMB were supposed to cease functioning once we occupied the site; so why were there DMB meetings?

349

By Saturday night, however, the tide was turning. Spokes carried peoples' anger to their meetings, and there was a growing awareness that the occupation should not continue in a passive vein.

However, there were a significant number of people who felt the occupation's purposes were best served by just sitting tight. The debate began Saturday night. Most of the proposals for action were aimed at Monday morning when workers were to resume construction at the site. The conclusions never came; the State of New Hampshire took the next step.

Police and security activity had followed the site occupation. The fenced-off, injuncted construction area was heavily patrolled by the over 300 state police (Vermont, Maine, Connecticut and Rhode Island had also supplied members of their state forces to patrol the site, and ultimately assist in the arrests) and private guards leading Doberman Pinschers. Police and national guard vehicles were constantly coming and going. And helicopters taking off from a cleared area behind the fence continually buzzed the camp site.

Despite the authorities' good aerial surveillance of the entire area, they still couldn't judge the size of the occupation. On Sunday afternoon, when at least 1,500 people were encamped, the commander of the state National Guard, Adjutant General John Blatsos, flew over the site and estimated there were between 200 and 300 occupiers. The general's statement was a good indicator of how poorly the state was prepared to deal with the large number of occupiers.

Their lack of preparation was ironic, as the Clamshell had never made a secret of anything it was doing or planning. Earlier in the week, Clamshell organizers had informed Colonel Paul Doyon, commander of the New Hampshire State Police, that they expected approximately 1,800 people to occupy the Seabrook site. The media widely reported that this figure was based on a 'mystical formula' – that the Clam was returning with ten times the number of people arrested in the last occupation. In reality, the figure was based on the number of people who had participated in the nonviolence training sessions prior to coming to Seabrook.

It would come out later in testimony in federal court that New Hampshire officials refused to believe the scope of the Seabrook protest until the latest possible moment. They chose to believe unreliable sources and even seemed set on denying what was happening right before their eyes. Colonel Doyon testified that he had expected 400 to 800 people in this occupation. When Clamshell media organizer Cathy Wolff asked him outside the courtroom why he had not believed the figures she had told him before the occupation, he turned away without answering.

As the state was totally unprepared to deal with the over 2,000

people who occupied on Saturday, they decided to play a waiting game, choosing to see if the numbers would evaporate during the night.

Some groups did leave during the night, but by police estimates there were still well over 1,000 people on the site by sunrise, Sunday, May 1, and as the day passed, people continued to arrive.

Governor Thomson, who had been at the site briefly on Saturday, was growing tired of trying to wait the occupiers out. Meldrim Thomson's reputation was a law n' order man and a strategy of appeasement went against his grain. Flown in again by his helicopter, the Governor arrived on the site to consult with Doyon, Attorney General David Souter and other officials on a course of action.

When they were informed of his visit, the Clams decided to send a delegation to seek a meeting. They didn't believe they would change the Governor's mind about nuclear power or anything else, but making the human contact was in keeping with the general spirit of the occupation.

They chose six people, one representing each march route. The meeting was short, terse, but cordial. Thomson immediately informed the Clam representatives, 'You have a right to your opinion, but we cannot permit a violation of the law. We have been patient and tolerant. I doubt that I can persuade you and I doubt you can persuade me; but we all have a place we can go to decide this – to the polls.'

The Clams pointed out that a Seabrook town meeting had voted against the power plant. Thomson retorted that the townspeople had originally approved the plant. This is only half true, as no one in the Public Service Company had told Seabrook residents that the original plans were for a proposed *nuclear* power plant.

Thomson finished with a flourish, 'We cannot as public officials, allow this breaking of the law; it is, after all, Law Day.'

'It's also May Day, Governor,' one of the Clam reps replied.

After once more asking the Clams to leave, Thomson flew off, and Colonel Doyon stepped in. He offered the use of buses, which the police had been stockpiling all morning behind the site, to carry people out to a local destination of their choice. One way or another we would be riding those buses out of the site.

It was about 2.15 pm. Doyon waited until 3 when the Clam representatives returned after a hasty, but spirited spokes meeting. Elizabeth Boardman, a long-time Quaker activist from Acton, Massachusetts, spoke for the Clams, 'We have good news for some of us, we're staying.'

At 3.09, Doyon announced that anyone remaining on the site after thirty minutes would be arrested. The weekend's tactical debates all became moot. The buses rolled onto the site forty minutes later; police emerged and began the arrests. They would continue taking people from the site until 7.30 am, Monday, arresting 1,414 people in all.

351

Arrest was followed by a bus ride to the Portsmouth National Guard armory, where a mass booking facility had been established. We were processed and fingerprinted, then herded into a roped-off holding area.

Louisa Woodman, a bail commissioner for Hampton District court, was there to tell us we could all bail out immediately on personal recognizance (pr). She assured us that this arrangement had been worked out with Clamshell legal representatives. People were tired, anxious, confused and the deal didn't sound right. We had discussed bail solidarity in affinity groups before and there was general agreement that people should not pay any bail and go free unless everyone got out on pr. But this, which sounded like what we wanted, also sounded too easy.

Ms Woodman and the other Hampton court officials didn't understand why people were balking at the deal. They assured people that everyone would be released in this fashion.

New buses, each carrying about twenty people, arrived every five minutes and the holding area quickly became crowded, adding to everyone's confusion and frustration. While some affinity groups, particularly the first ones arrested, were reunited in the holding area, most people were still separated from their groups.

Manny Krasner, a Clam lawyer, finally arrived and tried to explain the pr procedure. He thought it was a good deal and argued earnestly for people to accept. As a show of good faith, Ms Woodman offered to process Medora Hamilton, a third-time occupier from central New Hampshire, so that people could see it was a square deal.

It looked like Krasner was making progress. Some people were still suspicious, but many seemed anxious to get out and regroup. After arrest and release people planned to return to the Hampton camping area to consider the next move. Since a few people held out against consensus, however, most people were reluctant to begin processing.

While the bail debate raged on, Ms Woodman returned to the holding area; she was obviously agitated. She announced that the pr arrangement was scuttled. District court judges had arrived, people would be arraigned and some bail would be required.

What she didn't announce was that Governor Thomson was at the armory. Several people, including me, saw him walk through and heard the arrival and departure of his helicopter. He had obviously been displeased by what he saw, both at the site and here at the armory. People started to realize that the stakes for this game might be higher than we anticipated. Thomson wanted to 'teach us a lesson' and this was one of the first instructions.

With two, and later three, judges sitting, people were arraigned ten at a time. Despite this revolving door justice, the arrestees backed up faster than the court could handle. Some people ended up spending the

night in open trucks and unheated buses outside the armory, waiting for their turn before the law.

In the first arraignment, Manny Krasner asked that people be released on pr, but Assistant Attorney General James Cruse demanded cash bail, claiming the state had evidence showing that people who were released would immediately reoccupy the site. He never proved this, but the judge was satisfied and set $100 bail. Everyone pleaded not guilty, if they pleaded at all, and no one paid bail.

The state would later contend that bail solidarity was part of a Clamshell plot to further hurt the state and damage the criminal justice system. They also tried to prove people were coerced to refuse bail. State officials never understood the discipline of individuals acting in group solidarity. It seemed to them that such a large group of people acting together obviously had to be getting orders from some central authority. When they later attempted to prove this theory and came up against a wall of denials, they wrote that off to further conspiracy. The men from the Attorney General's office admired the Clams' discipline but failed to ever comprehend its actual source.

While Judge Gray assigned $100 bails, Judge Flynn in the next room handed out $200 price tags for people's freedom. It was an excellent lesson in even-handed justice for people participating in their first bust. Bail for second- and third-time occupiers was set at $500. Later, however, when the strain on the state's capacities mounted, New Hampshire residents were urged to take pr. When they refused, some were literally thrown out of the court. They had pr whether they wanted it or not.

General Blatsos says he had not had any plans for holding arrested occupiers in the State's National Guard armories until 6 pm Sunday, May 1. The first armory he opened was in Somersworth. The buses rolled out of Portsmouth for there just after 9 pm. Buses left Portsmouth all night until the armories at Somersworth, Manchester, Concord and Dover were brimming with arrested Clams. Later in the week, the state would move people out of Somersworth and Dover back to the Portsmouth armory to relieve overcrowding in those places.

People arriving at the armories reformed affinity groups or created new ones. The structures differed from place to place, but each group established a process for group decisions. In some armories people stuck with the affinity group and spokes structure; in others they went from affinity groups to mass 'town' meetings. It didn't seem to matter much; it could still take anywhere from fifteen minutes to two days to reach a decision.

The first confrontation and resistance came the first night at Somersworth. Buses of occupiers were arriving every fifteen minutes; by 11 pm there was no room left within the barricades the guard had erected by turning tables on their sides. The guard commander, Captain

Dupee, told us that at least four more buses were due. When we protested the lack of space we were told that we would have to accommodate the newcomers somehow.

We'd just spent two or three nights in the spring chill, and the entire day awaiting arrest, being booked and arraigned, arguing about bail and tactics. We were edgy and pissed off, but we were also still disorganized.

However, when the next bus arrived, people sat down at the door and blocked the new arrivals' entry. They were just as tired and confused as we were, but after a quick explanation they sat down with us. The guardsmen, especially Dupee, did not know how to respond to resistance; they had their orders, but to follow them would have to use force. As the days passed we would realize how important it was for Dupee not to look bad to his superior officers; he would occasionally become absolutely frantic because he could never be sure if a new order would be obeyed. For now, he was just someone who seemed committed to an unreasonable course of action.

We weren't moving, though, and in fifteen minutes another bus would arrive and add twenty more resisters to the confrontation. After a phone call to his superior, Dupee relented and moved the tables out to make more room.

We told him that we would accept two more busloads, not four, and then sit in again. He said he couldn't allow that, but never said how he would stop us. After two more buses arrived, there were approximately 200 people in the armory. We waited for another load and the confrontation. No further buses came to Somersworth, however, so we spread our sleeping bags on the concrete and rested on our apparent victory. That night had revealed the direction the imprisonment would take – resistance, some victories and some defeats.

Each Clam occupier was at the center of decisions; each guardsman was at the mercy of decisions from the top brass. Our 'chains of command' clashed constantly.

Since the guard were so totally unprepared for their role of jailers, they had to improvise in the beginning. Some of their ideas about what they should do were ludicrous, some were merely irritating, some were illegal. For instance, initially, phone calls were censored at Somersworth and throughout the incarceration at other armories.) I got to make a phone call Monday morning, May 2. Chief Warrant Officer Amie Pinard informed me I could not reveal how many people were in Somersworth or what our general conditions were like. I told Pinard what he was doing was illegal; he replied, 'That may be so, but I have my orders.'

I asked him who gave him that order; he said his superior. When I asked who his superior was, he said, 'I can't tell you.' I never heard of anything like that before, but the guard thought their chain of command was some kind of state secret. Pinard's attitude throughout our entire

stay in Somersworth was to treat us like wayward third-graders. It was mildly amusing at first, but by the end of the week it had become a pain in the ass.

As the guard settled into being jailers, their command kept changing the rules, varying the allowed and forbidden from day to day. They changed the times we were allowed to make phone calls at least six times in two weeks. Some of the guardsmen became upset because they realized that their statements might turn out to be false. We were told several times a doctor would come for sick call. When one didn't the guardmen were puzzled; they'd been told to tell us a doctor would come, so why didn't one show up?

Our first meals consisted of coffee and doughnuts. Lunch on Monday was pork and beans. A large number of the occupiers were vegetarians and the Army's standard menu makes little provision for their needs, so one of our first demands was for better and more reasonable food. The guard never did figure out how to feed vegetarians, but at least in Somersworth they allowed support people and friends to bring food in for us. At Manchester the incarcerated Clams had to smuggle cheese and other vegetarian fare past the guards.

Conditions varied widely in the armories. At Somersworth, we were allowed outside only for a half hour in the morning and afternoon, but after Tuesday we had unlimited access to showers. After Thursday we were segregated by sex from 11 pm to 7 am. At Portsmouth they were segregated all the time at first; later it was changed to 9 pm to 9 am. They also only had showers on for an hour during the day.

At the Manchester armory, where almost 700 people were imprisoned, when the guard announced that people would be segregated by sex, the people just laughed. Nothing ever happened. They were allowed outside for recreation all day, until 6 pm. At both the Dover and Portsmouth armories, the guard brought in portable, chemical toilets because the bathroom facilities at both those places couldn't handle hundreds of people.

Most of the resistance inside the armories centered around the moves to segregate men and women and to transfer people away from their affinity groups to other armories.

At first the state authorities had intended to move men and women to separate armories. After encountering resistance to this, they decided just to segregate them within the armories. The most active resistance to segregation occurred at Somersworth where the Clams carried out nonviolent action for over three hours, being dragged apart by guardsmen when they continually crossed into the opposite section of the room.

On Thursday morning, May 5, twenty-one of us left Somersworth for

the first trials in Hampton District Court. We were told to bring our gear but most of us refused, objecting to the idea that we wouldn't be returned to Somersworth and our affinity groups. The state troopers transporting us were hostile and, when we refused to bring our gear, very angry. They were used to having their orders obeyed. But they took us anyway after we refused a second order to pack our stuff.

What happened in court is pretty well known by now. Seventeen of us were found guilty of criminal trespass, sentenced to fifteen days and a $100 fine. We were assigned $500 bail pending appeal.

I had already been tried and given a suspended sentence when the Attorney General of New Hampshire, David Souter, arrived in court to ask for stiffer penalties. The judge obliged him, giving the sixteen people tried after me unsuspended sentences. At the end of the court session, he called me back in and resentenced me, 'unsuspending' my sentence also.

When people went to trial the next week, however, some were found not guilty on technicalities. It was pretty much up to the individual judge's discretion on whether the arrest procedure was in line with the way the law was written. Some judges said it was, some accepted arguments it wasn't. After court, people were being returned to a different armory. Seven people who refused to walk or co-operate with the guard after they were transferred from Somersworth to Manchester ended up being roughly dragged ino the main holding area by the Manchester city police. The guard had refused to do it when the Clams said they would not walk themselves.

When the State attempted to speed up the District Court trials, which stretched into November, they often failed to notify people who were to appear in court until the last minute. This sparked the most dramatic resistance of the second week.

By Tuesday, May 10, there were still over 700 people in the armories, including 300 in Manchester. On Monday night right before 'lights out' (actually lights remained on all night in most of the armories; some were turned off to indicate that it was official bedtime) the guard announced that thirty-three people were going to court at 7.30 the next morning. It was the first time any of the people whose names were read knew their trials had been rescheduled. They held a late-night armory meeting and decided to refuse to go to court in the morning.

Everybody woke up at 6.30 and gathered in the center of the floor. The thirty-three people due for court sat randomly among them. The Clams informed the guard that if they wanted to take these people to court, they would have to come out, find them and drag them away. No one would resist physically, but no one would co-operate either. Whenever the guard announced the people's names, everyone would start to sing and drown out the announcement. This went on until mid-

morning. People were threatened with contempt of court, but no one budged. Finally, the guard announced that the court session had been cancelled.

The day before, Monday, May 9, Judge Hugh Bownes of the Federal District Court in Concord, New Hampshire, had begun hearing a civil rights law suit filed as a class action on behalf of everyone arrested at Seabrook. Nancy Gertner, who had defended Susan Saxe, and John Reinstein were retained by the American Civil Liberties Union to handle the Clams' case. The defendants included Governor Thomson, Attorney General Souter, Blatsos, Doyon and a raft of other state officials.

The suit charged that the state acted irresponsibly and abridged people's rights when it arrested them without having made proper preparations to house them. The Clam hoped the suit would get people released on pr, and it also sought damages for those arrested and held $5000 for the arrest and an additional $5000 for each day an individual was detained. The suit is similar to the May Day legal action in which the courts awarded $10,000 to everyone who was arrested in Washington on May 5, 1971. (Because of the lengthy appeal procedure, people are still waiting to collect.)

The testimony in court revolved around two points: conditions in the armories, and what preparations the state had made when they knew all these people were coming to occupy the Seabrook site and face arrest.

After hearing testimony from occupiers and national guard officials about conditions, the judge seemed inclined to think that while armory conditions had started off bad, they had improved over the two weeks to a reasonable situation.

Assistant Attorney General Tom Rath, who headed the state's defense team, tried to prove that the Clamshell occupiers were purposely clogging the armories and straining the court system. He extensively cross-examined the occupiers about their ability to make bail, the occupiers' internal structure and bail solidarity. The state officials apparently thought the Clam leadership was coercing people into remaining in the armories. The Clam witnesses gave a clear picture of affinity group process, and made it clear that no one was forced to do anything against their will. State officials, and the judge, seemed surprised when people expressed pride in the resistance actions going on in the armories.

The testimony from state officials showed that they had all been informed well ahead of time what to expect from the Clam, but had chosen to put their trust in rather unreliable sources of information, or merely refused to believe the information Clamshell organizers readily told them.

357

When everyone was released from the armories, the part of the suit on conditions was dropped, but the damages section continues. Final depositions will be taken on June 21, but Bownes hasn't set any particular deadline for a decision and legal actions of this kind can be drawn out for years.

When the federal suit had dragged on into the second week, it became obvious that something else would have to be done to get people out of the armories. In the middle of the second week, a team of legal representatives from the Clamshell met with Rockingham County attorney Carlton Eldredge, who was directly responsible for prosecuting the occupiers' cases. The courts were obviously suffering from the case load. Almost two weeks had passed since the arrests and over 600 people still remained in the armories (the normal prison population for the entire state is between 300 and 400). Eldredge and the judges in Hampton district seemed amenable to make a deal to get everyone out and relieve the pressure on the state and the county. And, while the people in the armories had held up for a much longer time than anyone had expected, the strains were showing. People had to return to jobs, schools, commitments. Many were having trouble putting up with the continued incarceration. Spirits were still high, but there was a noticeable drain as more and more people left.

Through an all-night meeting, Eldredge and the Clams hammered out the deal. Finally around 5 am Thursday morning, May 12, they reached what all felt was a workable arraignment. The occupiers would be tried in large groups, and without having any evidence presented either for or against them, they would be found guilty. They would all have an appeal to Superior Court entered for them and they would be released on personal recognizance pending appeal. Most of the appeals would never be heard. In the federal suit, Eldredge had testified that the State was backed up on felony cases in Superior Court and the possibility of getting to these misdemeanor cases, ever, 'was nil.' However, the agreement did stipulate that one of the Seabrook cases would be tried within six months. And people are free to press for their individual appeals.

The agreement also stipulated that as long as a large majority of the people in the armories accepted its terms, the minority was free to pursue their right to an individual trial in district court.

The terms of the agreement were taken to the armories for ratification. Some occupiers felt that the Clam para-legals who presented it to the people came on too strong; that they pressured for its acceptance. At any rate, the people in Somersworth, Dover and Portsmouth accepted the terms with a minimum of debate. However, in both the Concord and Manchester armories, people had a lot of questions about the deal.

As a result of the Manchester and Concord debates, further conditions were included in the agreement guaranteeing that the terms be

applied across the board to all people from the occupation, including second- and third-time occupiers, people in Grafton county jail for contempt, and at Brentwood prison farm (including Gary Donatelli of New York, who had accepted his guilty verdict on May 5). People who had already been found guilty and given $500 bail would have their bails automatically reduced to pr.

The remaining 500-plus detainees were bused to Hampton Court on Friday, May 13. They were allowed to make group statements at their trials, found guilty and released. Despite the abbreviated court procedure, it still took well into the evening to process all the people. The spirit of celebration was marred when, in the last group of people being tried, two women refused to give their real names. The judge cited them for contempt and sent them to jail. Some of the occupiers still hanging around the courthouse tried to sit in front of the police car taking them away. No one was arrested but they were thrown out of the way. Clam legal people tracked the women down, and they were released on Monday morning.

People regrouped at the Smith farm in Kensington for a party; many of us sought a more solitary experience and headed for home or individual retreats.

Some people hailed the pr release as the final victory. But the real triumph is in the solidarity and nonviolent discipline we maintained the entire time, and the thousands of people whose curiosity was aroused by our commitment opposing nukes.

I do not know if the Seabrook occupation was the epochal event some have hailed it to be. It would be gratifying to have been a part of an event which heralds a new era of activism. But I do know, because of what thousands of us have seen and done here, we shall beat the Seabrook nuke – and nukes everywhere.

Murray Rosenblith is a nonviolent, direct-action activist and writer. He has been a cab-driver, waiter, cook, truck-driver, archery instructor and manual laborer. He is currently on the staff of *WIN Magazine*, a radical, pacifist weekly published in the United States.

34   Paris 1968

Anon.

I persist in thinking
That the place of a poet at this moment
Is in the street
You must storm
The ivory towers Raze them to the
Ground
Proclaim
A state of emergency

When I allow myself
To snivel over my misery
If that misery is not also
Your own
Reader
Hit me
There is no more
Absentee poetry.

scrawled on a wall
May 1968

35 Notes and queries of an anarchist critic*

HJE

1

There is little contemporary writing that could be called anarchist literary criticism. Perhaps the reason for this is to be found in the nature of literary criticism. It is, after all, chiefly a classroom exercise. While literary critics exchange their ideas through publications outside the classroom, their publications are read chiefly by those who occupy classrooms.

Literary criticism is not only a classroom exercise; it is also an exercise in class privilege. For the literati, criticism is an end in itself. For the anarchist, it is a prologue. What happens inside a novel (or any literary production) should of course be interesting, but it cannot be the end of a critique; maybe the beginning.

Have I become an apologist for some quaint esthetic?
How is it 7 years ago, when I was first advised of insurrection
My thoughts were all of metre and the New Criticism?
At heart, I tell myself, I am an arsonist.
Yet last evening in the firehouse I was reading aloud
from the selected poems
of Benito Mussolini . . .

That excerpt was from Robert Sward's poem, *Dreams*. The poem ends:

All my poems are burning.
And the cities are burning.

For the anarchist, critical focus should be on the social meaning of the literary work; its origins and its effects. Louis Kampf, in a note about Marxist criticism, writes:

* Printed here for the first time.

Marxist criticism should move in an area marked out by two major questions:

1 From what historical condition does the literary work – both its form and content – emerge? If the form is new or changing, what social transformations does this relate to? In what ways, for example, does practicing the poetry of courtly love and acquiring the skills related to that practice serve to solidify the social position of a certain stratum in feudal society?

2 How does the literary work affect its readers? Does it have any impact on the class structure of a society? Does it serve to justify certain ideologies? Does the act of reading fiction – no matter how realistic the fiction – serve to remove people's minds from the real world? Transforming misery into an art work – even when done by a radical activist – estheticizes that misery; takes it into the realm of beauty, and thereby makes it more acceptable: if it's a work of art, one can live with it. I feel far from certain about this. But I do feel certain that it is such fundamental matters of literary and artistic effect that Marxist criticism must deal with.

As a Marxist critic, Kampf perhaps would give more emphasis than would anarchists to history, and doubtless more emphasis to class. While the anarchist would be less constrained by history and more engaged by all power arrangements (not just class), we are mutually concerned with the radical transformation of the capitalist state.

We need to answer questions dealing with origins and effects in a thorough and historical way not because this will produce better scholarship, but because as Marxists we need to discover what it is we should write and teach and publish in order to advance the struggle for socialism. In short, we need to join theory with practice. So, again, for Marxists, there is no *literary* criticism. There is only the constant attempt to define what it is worth for us to do as social-ist teachers, writers and propagandists. . . .

It will certainly not get done unless we have the courage persis-tently to relate criticism to our political practice. Any criticism which does not concretely relate to practice is, by definition, not Marxist.

It is by definition not anarchist, either.

2

What follows are some questions that anarchist critics might raise about

literary productions.* Their focus is on the underlying themes and formal content of the work. These questions are patently not those that literary critics usually ask. These questions direct us to probe inside a play, a novel, a collection of materials. Our probe is for its unstated premises, its hidden assumptions.

In my own calculus, all art is political. And I raise the question of politics first, artistry second. The calculus is applicable to the literature of both capitalist and socialist states. Literary work is almost always in service to the state. That service is not always obvious to the reader – or even the writer. A major purpose in my formulating these questions is to try to engage people in their own analysis of how literature serves the dominant political interests of the society.

1 What sort of political–economic system is depicted (or implicit) in the work?

2 Are leftist views rejected? Is there an outright contestation of the state? of capitalism?

3 What is the nature of the society portrayed? What aspects of social life are ignored; what is highlighted?

4 What are the work's conflicting forces? What threatens order? (Shor)

5 How does the author cope with the problems of social relationships and social organizations, specifically with power, authority, age, sex, ethnicity, hierarchy? with wealth and property? with crime and deviance? with technology and the ecosphere?

6 Does the author depict egalitarian social relationships? Is there a view of communal life and collective work that is believable? inspiring?

7 Is daily life treated in a realistic manner? What is the ethos of the society?

8 At what points are actions or solutions to problems forced or unreal? (Shor)

9 In terms of characterization, are characters from all social levels equally well sketched? (Shor)

10 What do the characters (or classes of characters) worry about? (Shor)

11 How often, for what reasons, and in what instances does authorial distance from the characters change? Does the author alter her or his detachment, irony or seriousness? (Shor)

12 How does the author cope with the matter of individual auton-

---

* The questions presented here come from a variety of sources. Some are mine, and many come out of the Group for Anarchist Studies of The Baltimore School. I first encountered the idea of preparing a list of questions for critical Left inquiry in an essay by Ira Shor. Shor's questions, as well as those he borrowed, are identified in the text.

omy, and with the relation of individual needs and collective requirements?

13 Are the main problems or solutions in the novel individual or collective? (Shor)

14 Is there any concern with the process of revolutionary change?

15 Is there any indication that social change might improve anything?

16 Is there a view of the 'good' society contained within the work?

17 Which values allow effective action?

a   What values are proposed for the reader's adoption? Which characters are models? (Shor)

b   What is valued most – sacrifice? assent? resistance? How clearly do narratives of disillusionment and defeat indicate that bourgeois values (competition, acquisitiveness, chauvinism) are incompatible with human happiness? (Shor)

c   Does the protagonist defend or defect from the dominant values of society? Are those values in ascendancy or decay? (Shor)

d   What motivates the characters? Who are their significant others?

e   Are characters concerned with the consistency of means and ends?

f   Is anyone caught in a moral dilemma in which social or economic necessity clashes with moral precept? (Shor)

18 Is the work intended for a specific audience, a mass market, an ideological group, a political constituency?

19 If it is intended for a politically sophisticated audience,

a   does its language convey meanings consistent with the content or does it interfere with the ideas the author is trying to develop?

b   is its form appropriate to its political content?

36 Fear and powerlessness*

Love and Anarchy is an appealing movie, often clear in its view of human interaction, but dangerously distorted in its political content. By its sensational use of the word 'anarchy,' it is an obscene comment on the lives and acts of thousands of Italian anarchists. By its use of the word 'love' it is an obscenity to all of us who love enough to fight for a better life.

In the movie, a man chooses to commit an assassination, to be an 'anarchist' true to the simplistic definition he heard at his mother's knee – to kill a powerful ruler and to be killed in return. He is motivated by personal revenge and a gut knowledge of oppression; he acts in spite of being taught that 'it is better to bow down and live than to stand up and die.' It is believable that outrage can move a human spirit to act; this much is beautiful and real. But to succeed, this spirit must be armed, because unarmed, it spells failure and despair. The director betrays Tunin's spirit when she plays on our prejudices toward the 'country bumpkin' who appears to be the perfect dupe in the hands of 'manipulative politicos.'

She goes on to betray the spirit of everyone who loves and everyone who fights by setting them against each other. The battle on the bathroom floor between the women personifying politics/death and love/life is a setup for an anti-political victory. It is a false consciousness. Naturally, everyone wants love and life to win, but to make anarchist politics synonymous with death and reckless suicide is double-think of the first order. An anarchist would perhaps have risked his life, but he or she would not have intended to give it away for nothing. Even the most desperate of the anarchist assassinations came out of the belief that the act would help to destroy the old society and create a new life.

Tunin's act may well be based on a desire for revenge, but it is also

---

* This is excerpted from an eight-page leaflet produced in San Francisco by a small group in late 1974. It was distributed across the United States at showings of Lena Wertmuller's film, *Love and Anarchy*.

apparently based on a desire for suicide. The message is that the two are inextricably linked in Tunin's mind, so much so that when he is deprived of his act, he is still committed to the suicide. This sets us up to conclude that it is really a death wish that motivates political assassination, and not an imperative to defeat tyranny, whatever the cost.

Not only is this political perspective misleading, but love is equally misrepresented as a harness and a betrayal. The ironic, interlocking misuse of 'love' and 'anarchy' is sealed when our hero yells, 'Long live anarchy!' while shooting wildly into a crowd. In the guise of love and anarchy, it is fear and powerlessness that conquers all.

We are revolutionaries who recognize the validity of the anarchist perspective and methods of organization. We also recognize that power-mongers, whatever they may call themselves, have reason to label the anarchists despicable, unrealistic fools. Anarchists are fools because they don't seek power over others or a bureaucrat's position. Anarchists are fools because they know that coercive government (redundant?) is inefficient, and does not protect people from those who prey upon them. Instead, government agencies (FDA, FTC, HEW, etc.) give free rein to and collaborate with those true criminals who would enslave us, who would poison our minds and bodies.

Anarchists are fools because they believe that most 'crimes' result from an interlocking system of laws and economic oppression; they are not a result of a basically evil human nature, needing control by church and state. Anarchists are fools because they believe that if people get together, they can take care of themselves and their communities, that a basic human need is co-operation, not competition. Anarchists are fools because they believe in the elimination of all restraints to life, liberty and the pursuit of happiness. When asked, 'What would you replace it with?' we are the fools who reply, 'With what would you replace a tumor?'

Every day we are treated to glittering spectacles to divert us from the boredom and disintegration of our lives. Death and murder of every description are glutted upon our consciousness by the media. As if to incite the mass of the people to suicidal outbursts or sadistic adventures, everything is depicted in its bloodiest form. People are incited to direct their violent feelings toward one another. Cops shooting people is rampant in the movies and on TV. And the lesson is clear in every sector: fight back, resist, and you will unleash a torrent of annihilating brutality. The authorities made sure to televise the massacre of the SLA. There can be no mistake in the message: be passive, prey on each other, commit suicide, but if you revolt you can expect less than a shoebox of ashes to bear your remembrance.

In spite of, and in response to this cynicism of devastation, we acknowledge that we are fighting *for ourselves*. In a world delirious with destruction, we who have not yet surrendered know that the revolution must be fought on many fronts. We know that one of our mightiest enemies is our own fear and powerlessness. We cannot forget ourselves when we fight the chaos of institutions. We must also fight the chaos and confusion within each of us.

These words are neither the beginning nor the end to our dialogue, to our struggle, to our love.

LOVE AND ANARCHY
MORE TO COME . . . .

37 Letter from the mayor

City of Palo Alto
California
94301

Office of the Mayor

April 16, 1974

For General Distribution

In recent weeks I have been growing increasingly aware of the misery and emptiness of my daily life. I see that I've been spending my working days plowing away at alien tasks, following every dictate but that of my own desires. It seems that I and everyone around me produce an alien world and exhaust ourselves in the process. The only 'reward' for this daily estrangement is the reserve of a certain number of 'leisure' hours and the purchase of a greater or lesser quantity of the same alien activity of ourselves and others – a world of commodities which are diminishing in quality, use, and in their ability to make us feel happy.

Only now am I realizing that with no amount of money I make can I buy back my life.

More and more I find myself retreating from a hostile and indifferent world around me into the isolation of my 'private' and 'family' life. It seems as if I'm struggling to produce an armed camp against the people around me. These are people whom I might be close to and yet somehow I'm unable to be.

In this daily humiliation, I am robbed of all spontaneity and joy. It seems that I and everyone around me exist only to follow commands.

The other day I had a shocking experience. In a conversation I had with one of the office workers, neither of us could remember the last time we did anything that was genuinely voluntary. All I can ever remember doing is useless work, trival errands, eating, sleeping, waiting in lines, consuming worthless entertainment, driving in circles, and following orders. On those few occasions when I'm given a moment to

get in touch with myself or to look back on my life, I'm left with a gnawing and undeniable feeling that somehow I've been burned, that my life has been lost to me – wasted.

As I look around me I see the rise of new religions, mysticisms and pseudo-philosophies which are incessantly thrown at us to distract us from and compensate for our despair. None of these offers any genuine insights or theory of our own practice. They serve the same function (and are as useless) as so many varieties of tranquilizers, alcohol, new cars and drugs. At best they simply make it easy for us to 'live with it.'

Daily we are robbed of real life and then sold back its *representation*. Such 'problems' as the recession, inflation, and the phony energy crisis only bring out and make more dramatic how little control we've had of our lives all along.

Humiliation is nothing other than the experience of being made into an *object*. In the times we are living, conceptions of humanity have become so debased that 'respect' has come to mean little more than the ability to humiliate others. Our society is divided into order givers and order takers. Many people (myself included) are both. My job (as Mayor of Palo Alto) is that of a professional bully. But I've come to realize that giving orders is as alien and unrewarding an experience as following orders. Humiliating others really isn't much fun at all. As a selfless agent of a bureaucracy I am as much removed from my *self* and my desires as anyone else is. It is largely for this reason that I have handed in my resignation from my office as Mayor of Palo Alto – effective immediately. I realize now that I am not an object. I am a *subject* – I have human needs and desires which cannot be satisfied in the world as it now exists. My most personal desires require that it be transformed. In order to become myself I must create a revolution in every aspect of life. This is something I cannot do alone. It requires the conscious and unified action of the overwhelming majority of the world's people – of all of us who are severed from the means of life and who want more in our lives – all of us who want to live in joy and creativity and who are sick of following orders.

Together we must seize direct management of our environment – workplaces, 'public' places, neighborhoods, etc. – and negate their estrangement from us – self-management must be our means and goal. It is only as *free individuals*, bold and guiltless, that we can come together in voluntary association and overthrow all top-heavy institut- tions – the market, the state, etc., and thus create a genuine community of *social individuals*.

The first and most crucial thing we must do is learn to take ourselves and our desires *seriously*. It is time we stopped looking to politicians, capitalists, priests, deities, bureaucrats and pop stars – and start looking

to *ourselves* and to each other. This is the only way we will ever transform our lives. Don't misunderstand me. I am not calling for any kind of stoically internalized 'self-realization.' I am talking about the complete actualization of our most subjective and erotic desires – *in the real world!* We can do this only when together we overthrow every aspect of the commodity system itself and of all the separate powers, materialized reifications, and fragmentation that make our lives unliveable. Where to begin depends largely on the ideas, actions, and desires of other selves (of *your* self). I feel an urgent need for open communication, and I see this as the only way we can begin organizing ourselves to get what we want. Thus I invite you to call me or drop in on me, or to contact my friends at Box 282, Palo Alto, California 94302. Already I can see that *critiques in practice* of the community system are of crucial importance. Shoplifting has its merits – but the inadequacy of such minor forms of theft lies in their limitations. Hopefully shoplifting can be transcended in bold and organized acts of outright pillaging. But the only theft that can get us *permanently* and *totally* what we want is the *total* theft, the biggest crime of all – taking into our own hands the means of production and distribution *everywhere* without any fetishistic illusions about political and legal boundaries; taking back what already belongs to us; taking everything.

Together we can build a world of marvels – a world we create and recreate daily in the image of our desires. This is no mere pipedream. Rather it is more than ever before a genuine and real possibility, and is foreshadowed by the hidden history of the modern world. Never before has human misery been more unnecessary. Never before has the gap between *what is* and *what could be* been greater. Never before has class society – *throughout the world* – had so little excuse for its existence! The kind of social order I foresee and desire is as unlike the so-called 'socialist' and 'communist' countries as it is unlike this one. It has, however, been anticipated throughout modern history. The kind of social movement I am speaking of first emerged in the Paris Commune of 1871 where the primitive proletariat demonstrated its historical capacity to organize all aspects of social life *freely*. Since then, throughout the twentieth century, the phenomenon of *workers' councils* has arisen repeatedly. (Russia 1905 and 1917–21, culminating in Kronstadt 1921; Germany 1919–20; Spain 1936–37; Hungary 1956.) At the highest moments of these councils, everyone formed popular assemblies in workplaces and communities, joined together by means of strictly mandated delegates who carried out decisions *already made* by the assemblies and who could be recalled by their assemblies at any time. These councils organized their own defense and restarted production under their own management. By now, through a system of councils at the local, regional, and global level, using modern telecommunications